ACUTE CORONARY CARE

ACUTE CORONARY CARE

Principles and Practice

edited by

Robert M. Califf
Galen S. Wagner

1985

Martinus Nijhoff Publishing

A member of the Kluwer Academic Publishers Group

BOSTON DORDRECHT LANCASTER

DISTRIBUTORS:

For North America

Kluwer Academic Publishers
190 Old Derby Street
Hingham, MA 02043

For all other countries

Kluwer Academic Publishers Group
Distribution Centre
P.O. Box 322
3300 AH Dordrecht
The Netherlands

Library of Congress Cataloging in Publication Data

Main entry under title:

Acute coronary care:

Includes index.
1. Coronary heart disease. 2. Heart—Muscle—
Diseases. 3. Critical care medicine. I. Califf,
Robert M. II. Wagner, Galen S.
RC685.C6A283 1984   616.1'23   84-10158
ISBN-13: 978-1-4613-3830-7   e-ISBN-13: 978-1-4613-3828-4
DOI: 10.1007/978-1-4613-3828-4

CONTENTS

CONTRIBUTING AUTHORS

A. A. J. Adgey, M.D.
Regional Medical Cardiology Center
Royal Victoria Hospital
Grosvenor Road
Belfast, BT12 6BA Northern Ireland

John T. Baker, M.D.
Durham Cardiovascular Health Center
306 South Gregson Street
Durham, North Carolina 27705, USA

Rudolph M. Ballentine, M.D.
Himalayan International Institute of
  Yoga Science and Philosophy
RD 1, Box 88
Honesdale, Pennsylvania 18431, USA

Lawrence Bergner, M.D.
Project Restart
508 Smith Tower
506 Second Avenue
Seattle, Washington 98104, USA

Wanda Bride, R.N.
Cardiac Intensive Care Unit
7200 Duke North
Duke University Medical Center
Durham, North Carolina 27710, USA

Archer Broughton, M.D.
Baker Medical Research Institute
Alfred Hospital, Commercial Road
Prahran, Victoria 3181, Australia

Bernadine Healy Bulkley, M.D.
Department of Medicine
Johns Hopkins Hospital
600 North Wolfe Street
Baltimore, Maryland 21205, USA

Robert M. Califf, M.D.
Department of Medicine
Box 31123

Duke University Medical Center
Durham, North Carolina 27710, USA

Robert A. Chahine, M.D.
VA Medical Center (111A)
1201 N.W. 16th Street
Miami, Florida 33125, USA

Kanu Chatterjee, M.B.
Department of Cardiology
University of California
1186 Moffitt Hospital
San Francisco, California 94143, USA

Shaun Coughlin, M.D.
Cardiac Unit, Department of Medicine
Massachusetts General Hospital
32 Fruit Street
Boston. Massachusetts 02114, USA

Ralph B. D'Agostino, Ph.D.
Boston University School of Medicine
Boston City Hospital Cardiology Department
818 Harrison Avenue
Boston, Massachusetts 02118, USA

Daniel David, M.D.
Department of Cardiology
Meir General Hospital
44281 Kfar Saba, Israel

Marcus A. De Wood, M.D.
Division of Cardiology
Deaconess Medical Center
West 800 Fifth Avenue
Spokane, Washington 99210, USA

Mickey S. Eisenberg, M.D., Ph.D.
Emergency Medical Service, RC-02
University Hospital
1959 N.E. Pacific Street
Seattle, Washington 98195, USA

Marguerite English, R.N.
Cardiac Catheterization Laboratory

Chippenham Hospital
7101 Jahnke Road
Richmond, Virginia 23225, USA

John T. Fallon, M.D.
Pathology Unit
Massachusetts General Hospital
32 Fruit Street
Boston, Massachusetts 02114, USA

Ginette Ferszt, R.N., M.S.N.
1229 Wharton Street
Philadelphia, Pennsylvania 19147, USA

Harvey Fineberg, M.D., Ph.D.
Institute for Health Research
Harvard School of Public Health
677 Huntington Avenue
Boston, Massachusetts 02115, USA

Walter L. Floyd, M.D.
Department of Medicine
Box 2997
Duke University Medical Center
Durham, North Carolina 27710, USA

William T. Friedewald, M.D.
National Heart, Lung and Blood Institute
National Institutes of Health
Federal Building, Room 212
Bethesda, Maryland 20205, USA

Curt D. Furberg, M.D.
National Heart, Lung and Blood Institute
National Institutes of Health
Federal Building, Room 212
Bethesda, Maryland 20205, USA

Julius M. Gardin, M.D.
Cardiology Section
VA Medical Center
5901 East 7th Street
Long Beach, California 90822, USA

Robert S. Gibson, M.D.
Cardiac Noninvasive Laboratory
Box 468, Medical Center
University of Virginia
Charlottesville, Virginia 22908, USA

Lee Goldman, M.D., M.P.H.
Department of Medicine
Brigham and Women's Hospital
75 Francis Street
Boston, Massachusetts 02115, USA

Sidney Goldstein, M.D.
Division of Cardiovascular Medicine
Henry Ford Hospital
2799 West Grand Boulevard
Detroit, Michigan 48202, USA

Peer Grande, M.D.
Department of Cardiology
Gentofte Hospital
University of Copenhagen
DK-2900 Hellerup, Denmark

Joseph C. Greenfield, Jr., M.D.
Department of Medicine
Box 3246
Duke University Medical Center
Durham, North Carolina 27710, USA

David S. Grierson, M.D.
Department of Medicine
Box 31235
Duke University Medical Center
Durham, North Carolina 27710, USA

Ronald P. Grunwald, M.D.
Department of Cardiothoracic Surgery
Deaconess Medical Center
West 800 Fifth Avenue
Spokane, Washington 99210, USA

Alfred P. Hallstrom, Ph.D.
Biostatistics, F-653
Health Sciences, SC-32
University Hospital
Seattle, Washington 98195, USA

Phillip J. Harris, M.B.
Hallstrom Institute of Cardiology
Royal Prince Alfred Hospital
Missenden Road
Camperdown,
New South Wales 2050, Australia

David G. Harrison, M.D.
University Hospital
Room 406-1
University of Iowa
Iowa City, Iowa 52242, USA

Richard N. W. Hauer, M.D.
Cardiology Department, University Hospital
Utrecht, Catharijnesingel 101
PO Box 16250
3500 CG Utrecht, The Netherlands

Gerald R. Hensley, M.D.
Division of Cardiology
Sacred Heart Hospital
101 West 8th Avenue
Spokane, Washington 99204, USA

Michael L. Hinnen, M.D.
Division of Cardiology
Deaconess Medical Center
West 800 Fifth Avenue
Spokane, Washington 99210, USA

Judith S. Hochman, M.D.
Department of Medicine
College of Physicians and Surgeons
  of Columbia University and
St. Luke's-Roosevelt Hospital Center
Amsterdam Avenue and 114th Street
New York, New York 10025, USA

Raymond E. Ideker, M.D., Ph.D.
Departments of Pathology and Medicine
Box 3140
Duke University Medical Center
Durham, North Carolina 27710, USA

Elieser Kaplinsky, M.D.
Department of Cardiology
Meir General Hospital
44281 Kfar Saba, Israel

Robert Lester, M.D.
The Graduate Cardiology Consultants, Inc.
Suite 505, Pepper Pavilion
Graduate Hospital, 1 Graduate Plaza
Philadelphia, Pennsylvania 19146, USA

K. I. Lie, M.D.
Department of Cardiology and
  Clinical Physiology
University of Amsterdam, Wilhelmina Gasthuis
le Helmersstraat 104
1054 EG Amsterdam, The Netherlands

Melvin L. Marcus, M.D.
Department of Internal Medicine
  and the Cardiovascular Center
University of Iowa
Room E 318-2
Iowa City, Iowa 52242, USA

Randolph P. Martin, M.D.
Ednam Professional Center
2560 B Ivy Road
Charlottesville, Virginia 22901, USA

Kenneth G. Morris, M.D.
Division of Cardiology (111A)
VA Medical Center
508 Fulton Street
Durham, North Carolina 27705, USA

Arthur J. Moss, M.D.
University of Rochester
Medical Center
PO Box 653
Rochester, New York 14642, USA

R. M. Norris, M.D.
Coronary-Care Unit
Green Lane Hospital
Green Lane West
Aukland 3, New Zealand

William P. O'Grady, M.D.
Department of Radiology
University of Iowa
Iowa City, Iowa 52242, USA

Sebastian T. Palmeri, M.D.
National Institutes of Health
Building 10, Room 7B15
Bethesda, Maryland 20205, USA

Harry R. Phillips, M.D.
Department of Medicine
Box 3126
Duke University Medical Center
Durham, North Carolina 27710, USA

Michael W. Pozen, M.D.
(deceased)

David B. Pryor, M.D.
Department of Medicine
Box 3531
Duke University Medical Center
Durham, North Carolina 27710, USA

Eric N. Prystowsky, M.D.
Krannert Institute of Cardiology
Indiana University School of Medicine
1100 West Michigan Street
Indianapolis, Indiana 46223, USA

Martha Radford, M.D.
VA Medical Center
Heart Station
555 Willard Avenue
Newington, CT 06111, USA

Keith A. Reimer, M.D.
Department of Pathology
Box 3712
Duke University Medical Center
Durham, North Carolina 27710, USA

Judith C. Rembert, Ph.D.
Division of Cardiology
VA Medical Center, Room B3003
508 Fulton Street
Durham, North Carolina 27705, USA

William C. Roberts, M.D.
Department of Pathology
National Institutes of Health
Building 10A, Room 3E30
Bethesda, Maryland 20205, USA

Robert A. Rosati, M.D.
Department of Medicine
Box 3337
Duke University Medical Center
Durham, North Carolina 27710, USA

Michael Rotman, M.D.
Austin Diagnostic Clinic
801 West 34th Street
Austin, Texas 78705, USA

Philip A. Routledge, M.D.
Department of Pharmacy and Therapeutics
Welsh National School of Medicine
Heath Park
Cardiff, United Kingdom CF4 4XN

Lewis J. Rubin, M.D.
Pulmonary Section—111F
VA Medical Center
4500 South Lancaster Road
Dallas, Texas 75216, USA

Richard L. Sabina, Ph.D.
Department of Medicine
Box 3491
Duke University Medical Center
Durham, North Carolina 27710, USA

Harry P. Selker, M.D., M.S.P.H.
Assistant Professor of Medicine
Dept. of Medicine, UCLA School of Medicine
Division of General Internal Medicine;
Instructor in Medicine,
Boston University School of Medicine
Boston City Hospital, Department of Cardiology

J. Paul Shields, M.D.
Division of Cardiology
Deaconess Medical Center
West 800 Fifth Avenue
Spokane, Washington 99210, USA

Richard S. Stack, M.D.
Division of Cardiology
VA Medical Center, Room C8001
508 Fulton Street
Durham, North Carolina 27705, USA

Robert K. Stack, M.D.
Department of Medicine
Box 3262
Duke University Medical Center
Durham, North Carolina 27710, USA

W. Wayne Stargel, Pharm. D.
Cardiac Intensive Care Unit
Box 31211
Duke University Medical Center
Durham, North Carolina 27710, USA

Gary L. Stiles, M.D.
Department of Medicine
Box 3444
Duke University Medical Center
Durham, North Carolina 27710, USA

Louis Summaria, Ph.D.
Special Coagulation Research Department
Evanston Hospital, Room G634
2650 Ridge Avenue
Evanston, Illinois 60201, USA

Judith L. Swain, M.D.
Department of Medicine
Box 3828
Duke University Medical Center
Durham, North Carolina 27710, USA

Phyllis Taylor, R.N., E.T.
307 West Mt. Pleasant Avenue
Philadelphia, Pennsylvania 19119, USA

Stephen M. Teague, M.D.
Department of Medicine
The University of Oklahoma Health Sciences
  Center
PO Box 26901
Oklahoma City, Oklahoma 73190, USA

Marc D. Thames, M.D.
Cardiology Section
McGuire VA Medical Center
Richmond, Virginia 23249, USA

Michael Thomas, M.D.
Midhurst Medical Research Institute
Midhurst West Sussex
England GU29 OBL

Frans J. Th. Wackers, M.D.
Director, Cardiovascular Nuclear Imaging
Yale University School of Medicine
Department of Diagnostic Imaging; TE2
333 Cedar Street
New Haven, Connecticut 06510, USA

Galen S. Wagner, M.D.
Department of Medicine
Box 31211
Duke University Medical Center
Durham, North Carolina 27710, USA

Robert A. Warner, M.D.
Cardiology Section
Syracuse VA Medical Center

800 Irving Avenue
Syracuse, New York 13210, USA

S. W. Webb, M.D.
Regional Medical Cardiology Center
Royal Victoria Hospital
Grosvenor Road
Belfast, BT12 6BA Northern Ireland

Richard D. White, M.D.
Box 31211
Duke University Medical Center
Durham, North Carolina 27710, USA

Lewis T. Williams, M.D.
Long 1312
CVRI
University of California
San Francisco, California 94143, USA

R. Sanders Williams, M.D.
Department of Medicine
Box 3945
Duke University Medical Center
Durham, North Carolina 27710, USA

This book is dedicated to Gail McKinnis who is its true editor. Her skills in communication with the various authors and their associates, in changing the words to achieve maximum uniformity and continuity, and her kind way of keeping our noses to the grindstone are manifested on every page.

PREFACE

When a patient develops symptoms suggestive of acute coronary insufficiency, the health care system is presented with a challenging diagnostic and management problem. During the past 20 years, hospitals have been developing coronary care units as the specialized inhospital facilities for such patients. For the past 15 years, many communities have employed paramedical personnel to extend the principles of "coronary care" to the site of the patient who develops the problem. Cardiac rehabilitation programs have also been established to facilitate the return to function of patients who have had acute coronary insufficiency. More recently, aggressive medical and surgical techniques have been developed to either prevent or limit the extent of myocardial necrosis that develops due to acute coronary insufficiency. These developments have dramatically altered the care of these patients during this 20-year period.

It is often difficult to distinguish between "unstable angina pectoris" and "acute myocardial infarction" at the time of the patient's initial presentation to a health care facility. Even those who initially have clear evidence of "an acute myocardial infarction" most likely have some myocardium for which the final outcome has not yet been determined. Conversely, the patient with "unstable angina pectoris" could develop an acute infarct either in the hospital or immediately after hospital discharge.

Since this area has many different facets, a large number of individual chapters have been included. The contributing authors were encouraged to emphasize their own viewpoints in the context of the medical literature. However, we extensively edited the chapters to keep them short, minimize redundancy, and insert cross-references.

Since much has been learned recently about the pathophysiology of acute myocardial ischemia and infarction, this section is emphasized. There are brief sections on prediction and prevention of ischemic events, methods of diagnosing and sizing infarcts, and methods of monitoring the patient with myocardial ischemia. A major focus of the text is on "coronary care." As indicated above, during the past 20 years five distinct phases of coronary care have evolved: (a) prehospital, (b) postadmission, (c) coronary care unit, (d) predischarge, and (e) convalescent.

The section on pathophysiology begins with a chapter by Greenfield and Rembert discussing the factors that determine the transmural distribution of blood flow. Reimer then shows the relationship between coronary blood flow and both reversible and irreversible damage to the myocardium. Swain and Sabina review the biochemistry of both the normal and abnormal myocardium. Fallon describes the steps in the development of the simple atherosclerotic plaque and the changes that occur to produce a thrombogenic state within the diseased coronary vessel. Chahine considers the role of coronary artery spasm and Hueter the role of thrombosis in the development of the acute myocardial ischemic syndromes. It has recently become accepted that thrombosis superimposed upon an occlusive atherosclerotic plaque is the cause of most episodes of acute myocardial infarction. Summaria discusses the basic biochemistry of the thrombolytic agents and Grierson presents the clinical pharmacology of the most currently used thrombolytic agent, streptokinase. Roberts and Gardin discuss terminology based upon ECG characteristics for locating acute myocardial infarcts. A specific form of infarct location is "subendocardial versus transmural." Ideker examines the evidence that the presence or absence of QRS changes is capable of distinguishing "subendocardial" from "transmural" involvement. Hemodynamic monitoring has become common in coronary care units, and Baker presents the physiologic considerations that pertain to the peripheral circulation and to the heart. Thames considers the state of the autonomic nervous system during acute myocardial ischemia and infarction, and indicates the rationale for either sympathetic or parasympathetic predominance.

Computerized data banks have now facilitated our prediction of patients at high risk for the acute ischemic syndromes. Califf documents the changing prognosis of patients with both unstable angina and acute infarction over the past ten years; however, these events are continuing to occur and Harris and Rosati identify the risk factors that predict the occurrence of both nonfatal infarction and death. Prevention can occur at the primary (prevention of atherosclerosis), secondary (prevention of the acute syndromes in patients with underlying coronary artery disease), and tertiary (prevention of the complications of acute myocardial infarction) levels. Ballentine discusses the role of nutrition in primary prevention of atherogenesis. Coughlin and Williams present the evidence for using antithrombotic therapy in high-risk patients to prevent the development of the acute ischemic syndromes. Friedewald and Furberg briefly review the outcomes of the large number of clinical trials of modification of mortality during acute myocardial infarction.

In the section on methods for diagnosing and sizing infarcts, only commonly used techniques are discussed. White and colleagues discuss the clinical usefulness of CK-MB for both infarct diagnosis and size estimation. Warner and colleagues present the recently developed data confirming the ability of quantitative criteria on the standard 12-lead ECG to indicate accurate location of the infarct and the possible estimate of its extent. Radionuclide techniques are being used more commonly for both diagnosis and sizing of infarcts, as indicated by Wackers. During the past several years, the common occurrence of right ventricular involvement accompanying left ventricular involvement has been documented for many patients with inferior infarcts. Harrison discusses the new clinical techniques for diagnosis of right ventricular involvement, and the important differences in therapy for hemodynamic

compromise due to right versus left ventricular infarction.

Methods for monitoring the patients with acute myocardial ischemia are presented in the next section. It is often difficult to determine the optimal time for inserting a flow-directed right heart catheter (Swan-Ganz) in patients wth acute myocardial infarction. Robert and Richard Stack present a rationale for this decision and guidelines for using the hemodynamic data. Echocardiographic techniques have become sufficiently sophisticated to quantify wall motion abnormalities as well as the status of valves, the interventricular septum, and the pericardium, as indicated by Martin. Doppler ultrasound has been developed more recently and Teague provides information concerning its value in measuring the contractile function of both ischemic and nonischemic myocardium. Radionuclide angiography is primarily useful for describing global ventricular function and Palmeri discusses the sequential changes in function documented during the course of acute myocardial infarction. Often, tachyarrhythmias appear in patients with acute myocardial infarction for which an accurate diagnosis cannot be made using either standard CCU monitoring or 12-lead electrocardiograms. In these instances, other techniques may be required, as indicated by Broughton, to both determine the diagnosis and, at times, actually revert the arrhythmia.

The prehospital phase of coronary care becomes even more important as techniques are developed for acute intracoronary or intravenous clot lysis, since time of persistence of the clot is a most important variable. Eisenberg and his colleagues describe the three-tiered system for prehospital intensive care. Adgey and Webb provide insights into the characteristics of patients within the first hour of acute myocardial infarction. Cost-effectiveness of medical care is becoming increasingly more important and Goldstein discusses this aspect of mobile intensive care as it relates to an entire community.

As more sophisticated methods for attempting to reverse the natural history of this process are developed, the phase in coronary care immediately after admission to the hospital becomes critical. Selker and co-workers present guidelines for optimal identification of the patient who has acute myocardial ischemia, versus that patient with other forms of "noncardiac" chest pain. Lester provides a rationale for physiologic management of the acute chest pain rather than reliance solely on analgesic agents.

Stargel and co-workers review the various antiventricular arrhythmic agents and indicate protocols for their use and methods to evaluate their effectiveness. Since the thrombolytic agents are capable of providing either great benefits or significant complications of patients with acute infarction, Grierson and co-workers give current guidelines for their clinical use. Success of thrombolytic therapy requires both removal of the thrombus and salvage of ischemic myocardium. Richard and Robert Stack present a ventriculographic method for quantifying the effect of thrombolytic agents on regional myocardial performance. De Wood and his colleagues present results of using urgent coronary artery bypass grafting to maximize myocardial perfusion in both unstable angina and acute myocardial infarction.

The coronary care unit has changed medical care in many ways and has led to the development of many other specialty intensive care units. Nurses were given more independence on coronary care units than in other more general areas of the hospital. Many lessons were learned from coronary care that have been transferred both appropriately and inappropriately to other areas of management of patients with ischemic heart disease. Thomas presents a perspective of the evolution of care during the past 20 years. Bride and colleagues provide insight into the organization and administration of a modern coronary care unit and emphasize the important role of the CCU nurse. Coronary care is expensive and therefore a discussion by Goldman and Fineberg of the cost-effectiveness of CCUs is most important.

There are many aspects of coronary care as practiced on a coronary care unit. Hauer and Lie review indications for use of temporary pacemakers. With the large variety of drugs available, it is important, as Stargel points out, to be aware of the common drug–drug interactions and also of the clinical situations that predispose a patient to experiencing adverse side effects from even the

usual doses of these drugs. Prolonged bed rest is no longer practiced on coronary care units, but "resting" the myocardium with either beta-adrenergic or calcium-channel-blocking drugs has become important, as indicated by Stiles. Patients with acute coronary insufficiency can develop the complication of pulmonary congestion or may have coexisting chronic obstructive pulmonary disease. Hughes and Rubin present the pulmonologists' view of respiratory care for patients with acute myocardial ischemia. Previously, direct stimulation of myocardial contractility via agents such as digoxin and isoproterenol was commonly employed. More recently, our understanding of the effects of preload and afterload on myocardial function have directed care away from the direct agent and toward means of optimizing both the ventricular filling and the resistance to emptying, as discussed by Chatterjee. When infarction is extensive or when mechanical defects occur, cardiogenic shock may be produced. Norris discusses the medical management and Radford and Phillips the surgical management, and Norris concentrates on shock due to myocardial necrosis and Radford and Phillips on shock due to mechanical defects. Once an initial infarct has occurred, it may heal in a variety of ways, as indicated by Hochman and Bulkley. Infarct "expansion" is a very different event that infarct "extension." Pericarditis is a common problem and causes symptoms that may be confused with threatened infarct extension, as discussed by Floyd. Medical care should be aimed at patient comfort as well as at prolongation of life. When it becomes clear that the patient is likely to die despite all available methods of care, the comfort of both the patient and the family becomes the only goal of coronary care. Ferszt and Taylor discuss methods for preparation of the patient, the family, and the CCU staff.

Follow-up data from patients after discharge from the CCU and from the hospital have indicated that significant numbers die within a relatively short period of time. It is becoming more common, therefore, to perform predischarge evaluations on all patients to determine those at particularly high risk. Pryor indicates the methods for determining the optimal time of patient mobilization and discharge based upon the clinical parameters observed. Certain patients are at extremely high risk of sudden death in the weeks following CCU discharge, and their identification and prophylaxis is indicated by Lie. Several noninvasive methods have emerged for assessing subsequent risk in individual patients: Gibson describes the use of exercise thallium-201 scintigraphy; Morris, radionuclide angiography; Moss, ambulatory ECG monitoring; and Prystowsky, electrophysiologic testing. Califf and coworkers then present an overview of strategies for assessing risk, and indicate a two-step process: the first step prior to CCU discharge, and the second step prior to hospital discharge.

The special consideration of the patient with acute ischemia or infarction during the convalescent phase is considered in the final section It is often a difficult transition from the hospital to the home environment. David and Kaplinsky discuss the role of outpatient transtelephonic ECG monitoring and self-medication for these patients. The acute event is certain to be a psychological stress for both the patient and the family, and Rotman discusses the ways in which the physician can work to minimize this stress. Many patients will have continuing disability, particularly after an acute infarction. Williams indicates ways to minimize disability and to optimize return to work and function during the convalescent phase.

Coronary care is changing rapidly, both in our understanding of the basic pathophysiology and in the availability of new methods of therapy. If we are to care optimally for patients with acute myocardial ischemia and infarction, we must work to understand the pathophysiology and to anticipate the natural history for each individual patient. We should retain the working principle, "Do no harm." It is tempting to consider the acute event to be the entire illness. Rather, we need to realize that it is just one manifestation of a very chronic illness that has a prolonged time course in most patients. The multiple variables associated with acute myocardial ischemia and infarction dictate that no single treatment could ever be optimal for all patients. Not all patients should be resuscitated when they arrest, not all patients with heart block should receive temporary pacemakers, not all patients should receive thrombolytic therapy, not all patients should have Swan-Ganz catheters inserted, and not all patients should have cardiac catheterizations before hospital discharge. Coronary care will continue to be practiced by generalists as well as specialists because family practitioners and general internists will not wish to move totally aside during a single acute phase of an illness in a patient for whom they are responsible during the full course of the chronic illness. Therefore it is important that volumes such as this appear periodically that attempt to present clearly and comprehensively an understanding of the many aspects of care for the patient with acute myocardial ischemia and infarction.

Robert M. Califf
Galen S. Wagner

I. PATHOPHYSIOLOGY OF ISCHEMIC HEART DISEASE

1. FACTORS THAT REGULATE TRANSMURAL MYOCARDIAL BLOOD FLOW DISTRIBUTION

Joseph C. Greenfield, Jr.

Judith C. Rembert

This chapter describes the mechanical factors that regulate transmural myocardial blood flow distribution in hearts (a) with normal coronary circulation, (b) with coronary stenosis, and (c) in those having functional collateral vasculature. The control of coronary vasomotion during normal and pathologic states by both metabolic and neurogenic mechanisms is not discussed. In the past five years, there have been two excellent review articles [1, 2] and one monograph [3] that describe in detail the coronary circulation. The reader is referred to these sources for material not covered in this chapter. The physiologic data presented will be of necessity from animal models, but the principles outlined probably are applicable to the human coronary circulation. The importance of perfusion pressure in maintaining transmural myocardial blood flow distribution will be emphasized. The factors that make the endocardial layers especially vulnerable to hypoperfusion will be stressed.

Characteristics of Normal Coronary Circulation

The myocardium is perfused by two arteries that originate in the coronary sinuses of the aortic valve and traverse the surface of the heart. These large epicardial arteries give off two types of branches: one which perfuses the epicardial layers, and the other the penetrating arteries, which traverse the myocardium and give off branches near the endocardial surface supplying blood to the endocardial layer (figure 1-1). In general, these penetrating arteries do not branch until the endocardial layers are reached.

The metabolic demands of the myocardium are exquisitely coupled to the volume of myocardial blood flow. Since arterial-venous (AV) extraction of oxygen is quite high during resting conditions, increasing AV extraction provides only a minimal mechanism for augmenting myocardial oxygen supply in response to increased demands. The left ventricular myocardium has a high flow requirement relative to other organs (~0.8 cm^3/min/g under resting conditions). Right ventricular blood flow and atrial blood flow per gram are approximately 60% and 40% respectively, of the left ventricular flow. The entire organ receives approximately 5% of the cardiac output. When the requirement for flow is increased during stressful situations, flow to the myocardium can be augmented extremely rapidly, i.e., within a given heartbeat. Flow increases to meet precisely a wide range of metabolic needs. During exercise, flows in the range of $3-5$ cm^3/min/g, and during maximum coronary vasodilation, flows of $6-8$ cm^3/min/g, have been recorded. The transmural blood flow distribution in the left ventricle is such that flow

R.M. Califf and G.S. Wagner (eds.), ACUTE CORONARY CARE: Principles and Practice. Copyright © 1985. Martinus Nijhoff Publishing, Boston/Dordrecht/Lancaster.

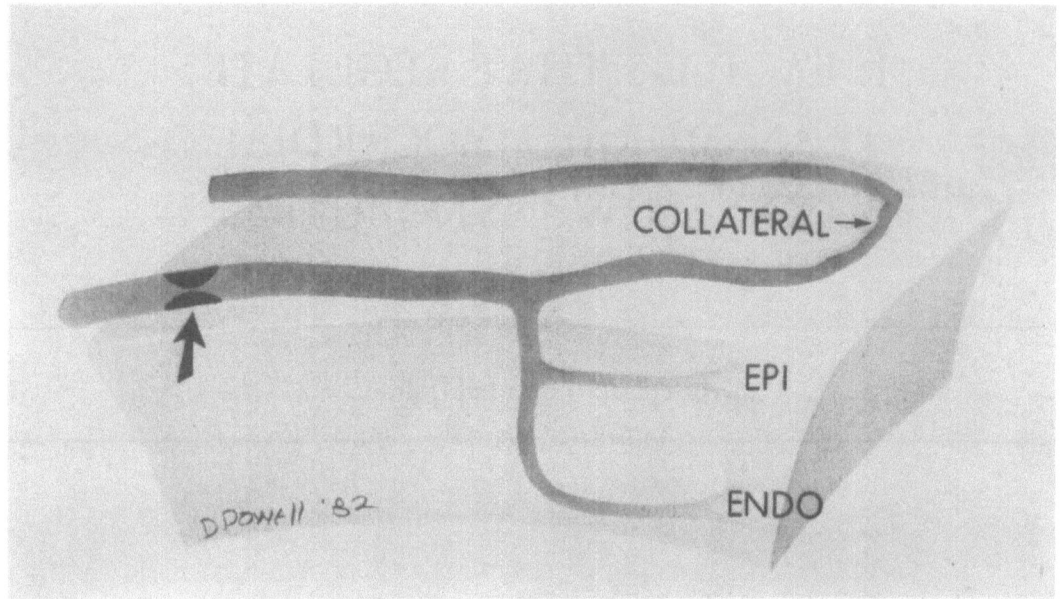

to the inner layers of the myocardium is approximately 10−30% higher than flow to the outer layers, i.e., the ratio of endocardial to epicardial (endo/epi) flow under physiologic conditions is in the range of 1.1−1.4. During marked increases in flow, a similar myocardial blood flow distribution is maintained (figure 1-2). Three factors are primarily responsible for maintaining the normal transmural myocardial blood flow distribution: (a) vasomotion of the resistance vessels, (b) the magnitude of the perfusion pressure, and (c) the duration of diastole.

Effect of Perfusion Pressure on Coronary Flow

Perfusion pressure has two components: the driving pressure and the back pressure. In the coronary circulation, the *driving pressure* usually is considered to be the mean diastolic pressure. This approximation is reasonably accurate for the endocardial layers, since perfusion of the endocardium occurs only during diastole. In the normal coronary circulation there is a minimal pressure drop (2−3 mmHg), which occurs from the coronary ostia to the origin of the penetrating arteries. This fall in driving pressure is of minimal significance.

As in most of the circulations of the body, it is probable that the major pressure drop occurs in

FIGURE 1-1. Schematic diagram of the coronary arterial circulation. A large epicardial coronary artery, having a significant stenosis and joined by an epicardial collateral vessel, is depicted. Note that arteries branch from this epicardial vessel to perfuse the epicardial layers of the myocardium and a penetrating artery traverses the transmural thickness of the myocardium, giving off branches that perfuse the endocardial layers. It is this transmural or penetrating artery that may provide the resistance leading to endocardial underperfusion when perfusion pressure in the epicardial vessels is significantly decreased.

the resistance coronary vessels located just proximal to the capillaries. These resistance vessels, which are controlled by neurogenic, myogenic, and metabolic mechanisms, provide the main loci of resistance in the normal coronary circulation. The pressure drop that does exist across the penetrating coronary vessels from the epicardial surface to the origin of the resistance vessels in the endocardial layers has not been quantitated. If the driving pressure in the epicardial arteries is in the physiologic range, e.g., 75 mmHg, the pressure drop in these penetrating vessels does not provide any significant hindrance to normal flow to the endocardial layers except with maximal vasodilation (figure 1-2). Since flow is somewhat higher (at least under resting conditions) at the endocardial layers, and myocardial perfusion to the inner layers occurs only during diastole, it

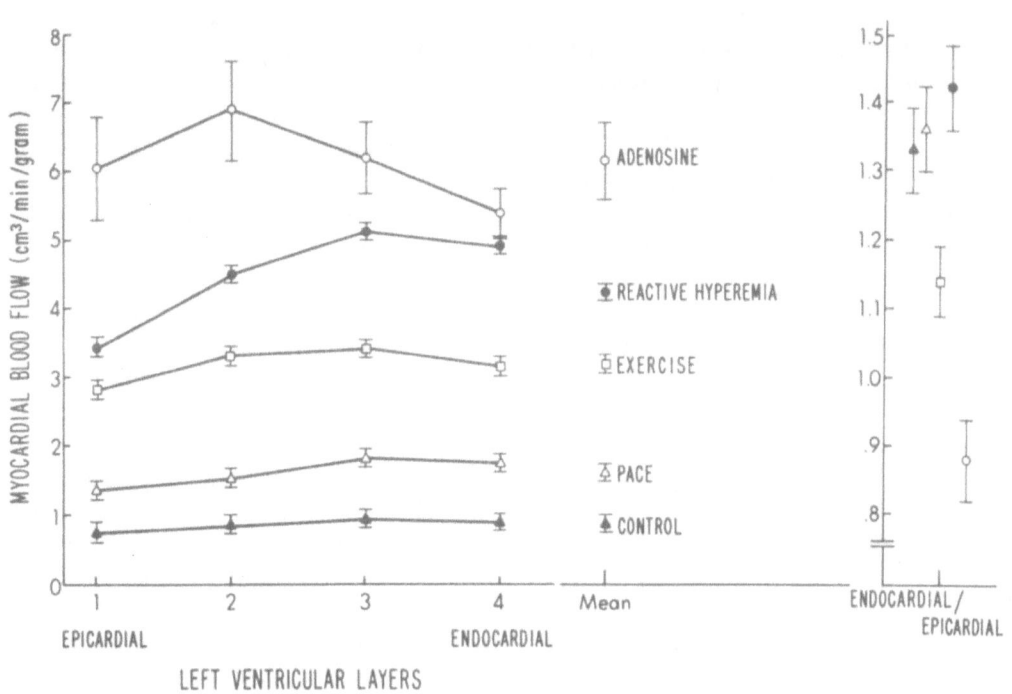

FIGURE 1-2. Myocardial blood flow obtained in the awake dog. Myocardial blood flow in cm³/min/g is given on the ordinate and the layers of the myocardium: the mean flow and the endocardial–epicardial flow ratio are given on the abscissa. The bars indicate the standard deviation. Flows were obtained during a variety of conditions as illustrated. Note that, during the control state, endocardial flow is slightly higher than epicardial flow, resulting in an endocardial–epicardial ratio greater than 1.0. This is maintained during increases in coronary flow. With maximum dilation induced by adenosine, the ratio is slightly less than 1.0. It should be noted that these flows are higher than are found under physiologic conditions.

however, it has been shown that other factors are operative so that a *vascular waterfall* phenomenon is present in the myocardium due to the combined effects of tissue pressure and intracavitary pressure [2]. It is likely that this effect is more pronounced at the endocardial layers and thus a gradient of back pressure highest at the endocardial layer is present. This effect will reduce the perfusion pressure more at the endocardial layer, and may be an important factor in making the endocardial layers more vulnerable to hypoperfusion.

Effect of Diastolic Duration on Coronary Flow

Perfusion of the epicardial layers may occur during both systole and diastole, whereas the endocardial layer is perfused only during diastole. Tachycardia would have the effect of shortening the period of diastole and, theoretically, endocardial underperfusion might occur. If normal vasomotion is present and the perfusion pressure is adequate, however, transmural blood flow to the endocardial layer is maintained during periods of

is evident that the resistance vessels must be more dilated at the endocardial region. If the vasodilating capacity or "reserve" of these resistance vessels is exceeded, then abnormal blood flow distribution with endocardial underperfusion may occur.

The other component of the myocardial perfusion pressure is the *back pressure*, which for the entire coronary circulation is the right atrial pressure. Thus, the perfusion pressure for the heart is calculated as the mean diastolic arterial pressure minus the mean right atrial pressure. Recently, rapid tachycardia. In studies in which maximum coronary vasodilation has been produced and the period of diastolic perfusion markedly shortened by increasing heart rate, the endocardial layers become hypoperfused. In these circumstances, both the occurrence of flow to the epicardial layers during systole and the additional resistance provided by the penetrating vessels become operative, and the endocardial layers receive less blood.

From the above discussion, it is clear that there are a variety of conditions that appear to make the endocardial layer vulnerable to hypoperfusion. In spite of these adverse factors, however, normal transmural blood flow distribution generally occurs unless the epicardial coronary arteries become stenotic.

Effect of Coronary Stenosis on Coronary Flow

It is well recognized that when significant stenoses of the large epicardial coronary arteries are present, as in the atherosclerotic process, augmented demands for flow (such as exercise) result in hypoperfusion of the endocardial layers of the myocardium, and the patient develops the symptoms of angina pectoris. In addition, when coronary occlusion leads to myocardial infarction, the endocardial layers are likely to be more extensively involved than those of the epicardium. These findings are true whether or not the myocardium has a poorly or a well-developed collateral circulation.

It is generally accepted that under resting conditions 75% of the cross-sectional area of the lumen of a coronary vessel must be obstructed before a pressure drop occurs across the stenosis. In situations such as exercise or with a markedly hypertrophied ventricle, however, in which the requirement for flow per gram stays the same and hence the overall flow needs are markedly increased, a stenosis of less than 75% may produce a pressure drop. Thus, the magnitude of the pressure drop depends upon both the percent of the lumen obstructed and the volume of flow across the stenosis. With critical stenosis, a marked pressure drop across the obstruction may occur. If, for example, mean diastolic perfusion pressure is in the range of 75 mmHg and the pressure drop across the stenosis is 50 mmHg,

then the driving pressure in the large epicardial arteries, at the point of origin of both the arteries that perfuse the epicardial layers and the penetrating arteries, will be only 25 mmHg. Assuming a pressure drop across the penetrating arteries of only 10 mmHg, it is obvious that there will be considerably less perfusion pressure at the endocardial layers. In addition, as noted above, the back pressure is greater at the endocardial layer and thus the effective perfusion pressure to the endocardial layer may be quite low.

The effects on transmural flow secondary to a coronary stenosis are readily apparent in figure 1-3, a stenosis of the coronary artery produced a marked pressure drop with a poststenotic mean diastolic perfusion pressure of 25 mmHg. This condition was associated with a marked maldistribution of flow, so that the epicardial layers were overperfused and the endocardial layers hypoperfused [4].

The analogous situation occurs in patients with coronary artery disease who have normal blood flow distribution at rest but develop angina pectoris during exercise. Under resting conditions, the vasodilation of the resistance vasculature compensates for the pressure drop across the stenosis. With exercise and the augmented demand for flow, however, the resistance vessels dilate, and the proximal stenosis becomes the primary locus of resistance. Pressures distal to stenoses in man have been measured during both angioplasty and surgery, and mean diastolic pressures in the range of 25−30 mmHg have been recorded. Thus, the clinical situation is analogous to that described above and is depicted in figure 1-3. Obviously, the stenosis can be secondary to a fixed lesion, vasospasm, or a combination of both.

That the resistance in the penetrating artery contributes markedly to the above conditions can be supported by the finding after administration of nitroglycerin in dogs. In similar experiments to that described in figure 1-3, pretreatment with nitroglycerin markedly reduces the endocardial underperfusion [5]. In these studies, before and after nitroglycerin administration, both the heart size and the mean coronary blood flow were unchanged. Therefore, the only effect that nitroglycerin could have had was to dilate the penetrating arteries, thus reducing the pressure

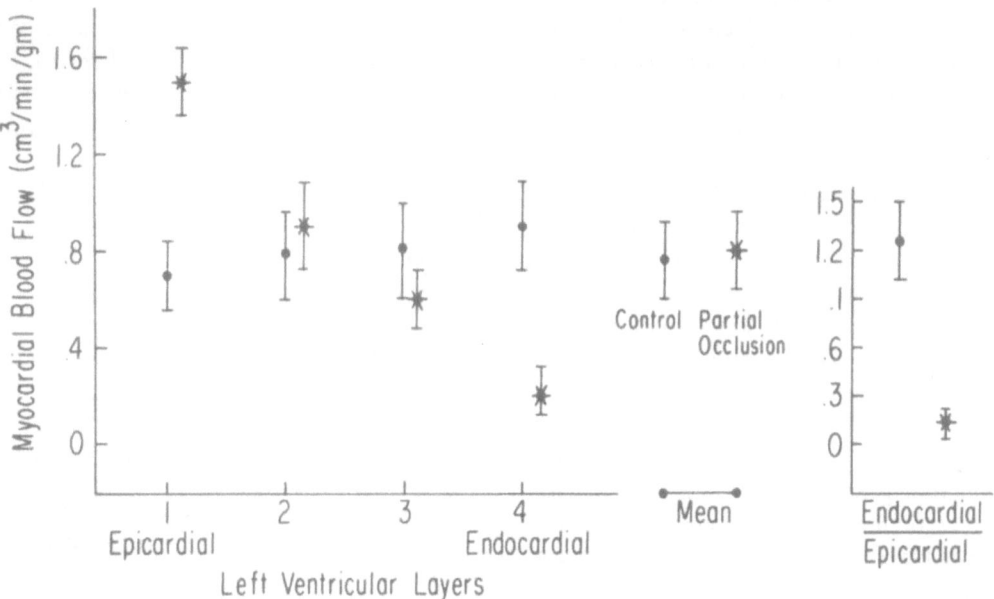

FIGURE 1-3. Myocardial blood flow distribution during ischemia with a flow-limited stenosis. The format is similar to that of figure 1-2. Flow was measured in the control state and after a brief period of ischemia following transient coronary occlusion. An artificial stenosis was utilized so that the hyperemic flow could not increase above the level present during the control state, i.e., the two mean flows are equal. During the partial occlusion state, the mean diastolic pressure distal to the occlusion was approximately 25 mmHg. Note that the epicardial flow is higher than control while endocardial flow is markedly reduced.

drop in these vessels. Therefore, a major factor responsible for endocardial underperfusion when a marked decrease in perfusion pressure occurs secondary to a pressure drop across a coronary stenosis is the resistance provided by the penetrating arteries. This situation may be worsened if the heart is dilated or if the left ventricular end-diastolic pressure is increased. In these situations, the back pressure at the endocardial layers will be elevated and will provide an additional hindrance to perfusion of the endocardial layers.

The pathophysiology described above also may be used to explain the endocardial underperfusion leading to angina pectoris in patients with aortic stenosis without coronary artery disease. If the myocardial wall is markedly thickened sec-

ondary to the pressure overload, but the cross-sectional area of the penetrating vessels does not increase concomitantly, the pressure drop across the vessel will become marked. These vessels may provide a significant enough resistance to flow so that endocardial underperfusion will occur during periods of augmented need, i.e., exercise.

Effect of Collateral Vessels on Coronary Flow

The effects on transmural perfusion when the heart is perfused through collateral vessels also may be somewhat analogous to the situation with a fixed coronary stenosis (figure 1-1). Collateral vessels on the surface of the heart that arise from a coronary artery and then perfuse another coronary vessel distal to a point of complete obstruction provide a resistance that may result in the development of a pressure drop. It has been shown both in experimental animals and in man that the pressure drop across an epicardial collateral bed can be significant. This pressure drop will result in abnormal transmural blood flow distribution when the pressure drop reaches a critical level by the same mechanisms described above for a localized coronary stenosis. In the dog, the collateral vessels are located primarily on the epicardial surface, whereas in man they may be both epicardial and transmural. There have been no studies defining the pressure—flow characteristics across transmural or endocardial collateral vessels, but it would seem reasonable that the same factors would be operative, and a pressure drop across the collateral vessels could result. If this is the case, then flow would be distributed away from the endocardial layers. With total coronary occlusion, the myocardium is dependent entirely on the collateral vasculature. If the perfusion pressure is low enough, then obviously no flow will occur and a transmural infarction will result. However, since myocardial infarction generally involves the deeper layers of the myocardium to a greater extent, it is evident that when flow occurs through collateral vessels the endocardial layers are not as well perfused as the epicardial layers.

Summary

The primary factor resulting in malperfusion of the endocardial layers in hearts with either a proximal coronary stenosis or collateral vasculature, or both, appears to be the lower perfusion pressure that is secondary to the pressure drop across either the stenosis or the collateral vessels. If the resulting perfusion pressure is low enough, then the two other factors, the resistance of the penetrating arteries and the gradient of back pressure, will impede flow to the endocardial layer still further and will result in decreased endocardial perfusion.

References

1. Berne RE, Rubio R: Coronary circulation. In: Handbook of physiology, sect 2, vol 1. Bethesda, MD: American Journal of Physiology, 1979, pp. 873—952.
2. Feigl E: Coronary physiology. In: Physiological reviews, vol 63 no. 1. Bethesda, MD: American Journal of Physiology, 1983.
3. Marcus ML: The coronary circulation in health and disease. New York: McGraw-Hill, 1983.
4. McHale PA, Greenfield JC Jr: Use of radioactive microsphere technique for determination of transmural distribution of coronary blood flow in conscious dogs. Ann Biomed Eng (in press).
5. Swain JL, Parker JP, McHale PA, Greenfield JC Jr: Effects of nitroglycerin and propranolol on the distribution of transmural myocardial blood flow during ischemia in the absence of hemodynamic changes in the unanesthetized dog. J Clin Invest 63:947—953, 1979.

2. THE RELATIONSHIP BETWEEN CORONARY BLOOD FLOW AND REVERSIBLE AND IRREVERSIBLE ISCHEMIC INJURY

Keith A. Reimer

Abrupt coronary occlusion results in acute myocardial infarction. However, the precise interrelationships between myocardial blood flow, the time at which ischemic cell injury becomes irreversible, and the ultimate infarct size remain incompletely understood. These interrelationships have been difficult to evaluate in patients and must be inferred in large part from animal studies. This chapter considers collateral coronary blood flow as a determinant of the time course of ischemic cell death and of ultimate infarct size in experimental animals and then considers the importance of collateral blood flow in patients with acute myocardial infarction.

The Transmural "Wavefront" of Ischemic Cell Death

When myocardial ischemia is induced by the occlusion of a coronary artery, a complex sequence of metabolic changes is initiated within the region supplied by the artery which, if the ischemia is sustained, results in the structural disintegration and death of the affected myocytes, i.e., a myocardial infarct. For a period of time, however, all of the ischemic myocytes re-

main viable [1]. If blood flow is restored during this time, infarction can be prevented and cellular metabolism [2−4], ultrastructure [5], and contractile function [4, 6] slowly recover. This time period of reversible injury is about 15 min in anesthetized dogs studied experimentally [1, 7]. Thereafter, some of the ischemic myocytes will enter a state of irreversible injury so that an infarct will occur even if coronary arterial flow is restored. However, not all of the ischemic cells become irreversibly injured simultaneously. Much of the subendocardial zone is dead by about 40 min of ischemia, but the mid- and subepicardial zones are still reversibly injured at this time and can be salvaged by reperfusion [8−14]. With increasing duration of coronary occlusion in dogs, a transmural wavefront of cell death progresses from the subendocardium to the subepicardium [8, 9] (figure 2-1) that, uninterrupted, eventually results in an infarct involving an average of 80% of the ischemic region. Reperfusion at 3 h can still limit the transmural extent of the infarct by about 10%, but by 6 h the infarct has reached its full size. Infarct size is not influenced by reperfusion at 6 h in either anesthetized [8, 9] or awake canine models [15].

The transmural progression of ischemic cell death may be related either to transmural differences in collateral blood flow, to intrinsic meta-

This work was supported in part by grant HL 27416.

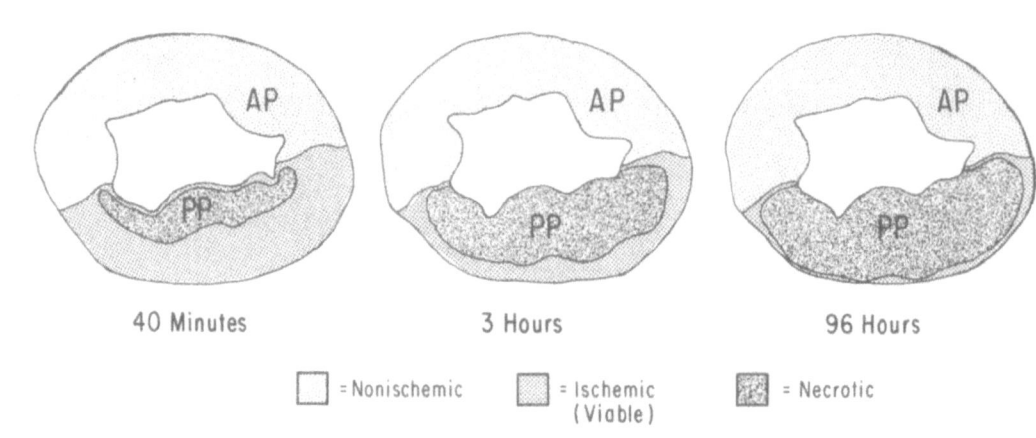

FIGURE 2-1. Progression of cell death versus time after left circumflex coronary artery occlusion. Necrosis occurs first in the subendocardial myocardium. With longer occlusions, a wavefront of cell death moves from the subendocardial zone across the wall to involve progressively more of the transmural thickness of the ischemic zone. In contrast, the lateral margins in the subendocardial region of the infarct are established as early as 40 min after occlusion and are sharply defined by the anatomic boundaries of the ischemic bed. AP, anterior papillary muscle; PP, posterior papillary muscle. Reimer and Jennings [9], with permission.

bolic properties of the tissue, or to both. Dogs often have substantial native collateral arterial anastomoses that can supply, on average, 10% − 15% of normal coronary flow to an ischemic region. This collateral flow is not uniformly distributed, but, for complex reasons that involve transmural differences in coronary perfusion pressure [16], is preferentially directed to the subepicardial region [17 − 19] (figure 2-2).

It is logical to reason (a) that the transmural wavefront of ischemic cell death is related to this transmural gradient of collateral blood flow, (b) that the subendocardial zone dies quickly because it is severely ischemic (flow ≤0.15 ml/min/g), and (c) that the subepicardial region either dies more slowly because it is moderately ischemic (flow = 0.15 − 0.30 ml/min/g) or else survives because it is mildly ischemic (flow >0.30 ml/min/g) [20]. There is some direct evidence to support a relationship between the amount of collateral blood flow and the speed at which cell death occurs. For example, among dogs with temporary 40-min coronary occlusions, those with very severe subendocardial ischemia have larger subendocardial infarcts than those with only mild subendocardial ischemia (K.A. Reimer, unpublished observations). Thus, small amounts of collateral flow can delay cell death in the subendocardial region.

On the other hand, several studies indicate that transmural differences in collateral blood flow are not the sole explanation for the transmural wavefront of cell death. In both pigs [21] and primates [12], there is virtually no native collateral blood flow to the ischemic region and the subepicardial zone is as severely ischemic as the subendocardial region. Nevertheless, analyses of both ultrastructure and infarct location in reperfusion studies in these species indicate the existence of a transmural wavefront of irreversible cellular injury despite the absence of a blood flow gradient [12, 21]. Also, in studies in which dog myocardium has been made totally ischemic in vivo or in vitro, ATP depletion and ultrastructural features of lethal cell injury have occurred more quickly in the subendocardial region than the subepicardial region, despite the transmural absence of blood flow [22 − 24]. Thus, there is considerable evidence for transmural differences in the cellular reponse to myocardial ischemia, independent of differences in collateral perfusion.

From the foregoing, it seems most likely that the *existence* of transmural progression of cellular injury is related to both intrinsic metabolic differences between subendocardial and subepicardial regions, and to preferential perfusion of the

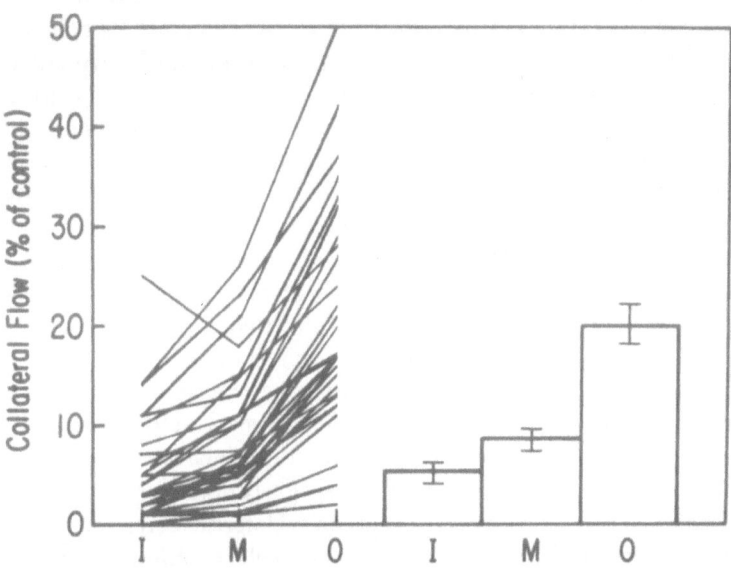

FIGURE 2-2. The transmural distribution of collateral flow found 20 min after circumflex occlusion in 31 dogs. Flow was measured with 9±1 μm microspheres before and after coronary occlusion. Collateral flow is expressed as a percentage of preocclusion flow to the same samples. The individual dogs are illustrated on the left and the group means ±SEM are shown on the right. I, M, and O represent inner, middle, and outer thirds of the transmural wall in the circumflex bed. Subendocardial flow was almost always severely depressed (< 15%) and averaged 4.5% of control. Subepicardial flow was greater (averaged 20% of control) and much more variable than subendocardial flow. From Reimer et al. [19], with permission.

subepicardial region via collateral flow. The *speed* at which the wavefront of cell death traverses the myocardium is variable among individual dogs and may be influenced both by variation in the amount of collateral blood flow and by variation in metabolic rate (MVO_2).

The speed of movement and indeed the very existence of a transmural wavefront of ischemic cell death have not been documented in patients and can only be inferred from animal studies such as those described above. The slow or intermittent release of cardiac proteins, such as myoglobin [25] or creatine kinase [26], to the bloodstream during infarction is consistent with a gradual evolution of human infarcts, but could also be explained on the basis of slow washout from the poorly perfused infarcted tissue.

Determinants of Ultimate Infarct Size

In dogs with experimental coronary occlusions, the final size of an infarct is related primarily to two factors—the anatomic size of the occluded vascular bed, and the amount of collateral blood flow provided to the ischemic region [9, 15, 27 – 30]. Although the nature of the lateral interface between ischemic and nonischemic myocardium has been the subject of considerable scientific controversy, current evidence seems to favor the concept that there is a rather sharp transition between ischemic and nonischemic myocardium in both experimental animals [9, 31, 32] and man [33, 34]. The anatomic basis for this sharp transition is that the important collateral anastomoses between major coronary arteries are on the epicardial surface of the heart and the smaller penetrating arteries are essentially end arteries with few or no interconnections between adjacent capillary beds [31, 34]. This sharp transition probably explains why, even when ischemic myocardium is reperfused as early as 40 min after occlusion, the resulting subendocardial infarct usually extends to within 1 or 2 mm of the edge of the ischemic vascular bed [9]. Nevertheless, even with permanent coronary ligations, there usually is some subepicardial sparing, averaging 20% of the ischemic vascular bed in dogs with circumflex occlusions [9]. Furthermore, the transmural extent of these infarcts was inversely related to the amount of collateral flow to the subepicardial region (figure 2-3). Other canine studies have also shown a correlation between collateral blood flow and the amount of myocardial necrosis in individual samples of ischemic myocardium [35].

In contrast to dogs, baboons have few native coronary collateral anastomoses and coronary occlusion is followed by severe transmural ischemia and by solid, transmural infarcts [12]. The size of infarcts in this species is determined primarily by the size of the occluded vascular bed.

The importance of collateral anastomoses in patients with ischemic heart tissue has been the subject of scientific controversy in recent years. It is now generally accepted that collateral anastomoses in normal human hearts are minimal, but that many patients with long-standing atherosclerotic coronary heart disease have developed extensive collateral anastomoses that often are sufficiently large to be visualized by coronary angiography [36–41]. Postmortem studies of hearts of patients with coronary heart disease frequently reveal total occlusion by atheromatous plaque of one or more coronary arteries, associated with either no infarct or a small subendocardial infarct in the myocardium supplied by the occluded artery [33, 42]. Furthermore, few myocardial infarcts, including those that are fatal, are transmural if a transmural infarct is rigidly defined as a solid, full-thickness infarct (see chapter 10). As with experimental canine infarcts, human infarcts are typically solid in the subendocardial region with irregular projection into the subepicardial region [33]. (In this regard the literature is confusing because there has been no standard definition of "transmural.") The incidence of "transmural infarcts" becomes greater when the definition is either an infarct involving more than half the myocardial wall or an infarct with focal projection to the epicardial surface [43–45].

To the clinician who has observed and treated many patients with myocardial infarcts superimposed on long-standing ischemic heart disease, the importance of induced coronary collateral anastomoses for myocardial survival may be inapparent. However, to the anatomic pathologist who commonly observes minimal myocardial scarring or at least partial subepicardial sparing in the vascular region of a previously completely occluded coronary artery, the critical role of collateral blood flow in limiting infarct size is strikingly clear. It is indeed fortunate that most infarcts are not completely transmural; such infarcts provide the anatomic substrate for serious complications of infarction, including myocardial rupture and aneurysm formation.

Thus, from purely anatomic observations, it is evident that collateral flow is sufficient to prevent or limit myocardial infarct size in many patients with either slowly developing or sudden coronary occlusion. Unfortunately, no techniques currently available permit quantitative mapping of collateral blood flow in subendocardial versus subepicardial zones of ischemic myocardium in clinical studies. Because of this technical limitation, the relationship between blood flow and extent of myocardial infarction observed in dogs cannot be studied in humans.

Given the apparent value of collateral blood flow in limiting infarct size, the ideal means to prevent or limit myocardial infarct size would be the prophylactic induction of coronary collaterals. Unfortunately, the mechanisms through which collateral growth is induced are not well understood and the principal, well-documented means of inducing collateral growth are chronic myocardial ischemia and/or anemia (hypoxia?) [36, 46, 47]. In the remaining sections we consider the possibility of limiting infarct size, after the acute onset of ischemia, with reference to the foregoing relationships between myocardial perfusion and infarction.

Therapeutic Limitation of Infarct Size

Much experimental effort has been devoted to the search for therapeutic interventions that could be applied in the acute phase of myocardial infarction to limit ultimate infarct size. Of the many interventions that have been studied, some have been selected for improving, or at least preserving, perfusion of the ischemic region [47]. Other interventions have been selected with the

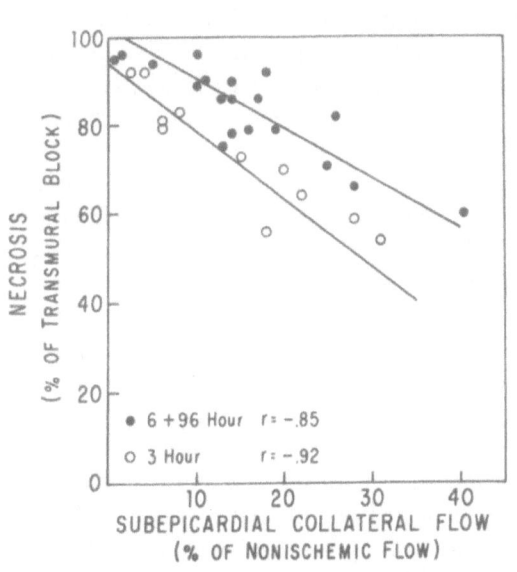

FIGURE 2-3. Relation between transmural necrosis and subepicardial collateral flow. Regression lines for permanent infarcts (96 h) and infarcts reperfused at 6 h were not significantly different and were combined. Infarcts reperfused at 3 h are indicated by the open circles. In both groups, the transmural extent of necrosis was inversely related to subepicardial flow measured at 20 min after left circumflex coronary occlusion. However, the 3-h regression line was shifted downward, indicating that reperfusion at 3 h limited infarct size. From Reimer and Jennings [9], with permission.

aim of delaying either the metabolic or structural consequences of ischemia on the affected myocytes [48]. It is assumed that some myocytes in the "border zone" between nonischemic and severely ischemic myocardium might have sufficient collateral blood flow to survive a relatively prolonged period of ischemia. Therapy that protected ischemic myocardium might further delay cell death in this zone and could limit ultimate infarct size if collateral flow improved or if arterial reperfusion ensued before infarction was complete. It is unlikely that any therapy could delay cell death indefinitely if the severe ischemia persisted. The possibility of acutely restoring perfusion through the occluded artery by either thrombolytic agents or emergency coronary bypass surgery is considered elsewhere in this volume (see chapters 22, 34, and 35).

Evolution of Collateral Blood Flow Following Coronary Occlusion

If the aim of therapy is to delay ischemic cell death until collateral blood flow improves, the crucial questions are "How long does it take for the caliber of collateral vessels to increase?" and "Can cell injury be sufficiently delayed with therapy?" These questions have been studied most extensively in dogs where some collateral blood flow is present immediately after occlusion and changes very little during the first 6 h (figure 2-4). In the subendocardial region, where both myocytes and the microvasculature often undergo infarction, collateral flow may be further depressed for days. In the subepicardial region, however, collateral flow begins to increase as early as 6−8 h and is markedly increased by four days [49] (figure 2-4). The earliest increases in collateral flow may be due to simple dilation of

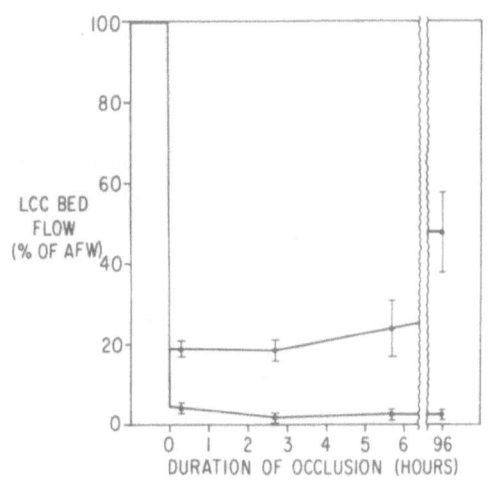

FIGURE 2-4. Collateral blood flow versus duration of left circumflex coronary (LCC) occlusion in dogs. Data are expressed as a percentage of coronary blood flow to the subepicardial anterior free wall (AFW) in the same hearts. The upper curve is flow to the subepicardial zone and the lower curve is flow to the much more severely ischemic subendocardial zone. Compared with collateral flow 20 min after occlusion, subendocardial flow was further depressed by 3 h and remained less than 5% of control even 96 h later. This graph is based on data from 13 dogs with 96-h occlusions. This group of dogs was part of the study published in Reimer and Jennings [9].

collateral anastomoses, but vascular growth, documented by DNA synthesis, is readily measurable by the fourth day [50].

The time course of collateral enlargement following acute coronary occlusion in patients is not well documented. In one isolated case study, extensive collaterals were observed nine days after formation of a traumatic right coronary to right atrial fistula and occlusion of the distal segment of the right coronary artery in a young boy with previously normal coronary arteries [51]. This suggests that collateral growth in humans may follow a time frame similar to that documented in dogs. Whether cellular injury can be sufficiently delayed with any intervention to limit ultimate infarct size via maximal collateral development in humans has not been determined.

Therapeutic Augmentation of Collateral Blood Flow

The major determinants of blood flow through preformed collateral vessels are (a) coronary perfusion pressure, (b) extravascular compressive forces, and (c) resistance of the collateral vessels themselves [52, 53]. Thus, collateral blood flow could potentially be improved by raising perfusion pressure, by minimizing left ventricular end-diastolic wall tension, and by dilating the collateral vessels. Various vasodilators may increase coronary blood flow either by direct coronary vasodilation or by reduction of extravascular compressive forces via peripheral vasodilation and reduced ventricular volume. The effect of vasodilators on coronary collateral flow is further dependent on the predominant site of action. Certain drugs, such as the nitrates, act primarily on larger arteries feeding the smaller collateral vessels and in theory should improve collateral flow. Other vasodilators such as adenosine or dipyridamole might actually reduce collateral blood flow because they dilate the small resistance vessels of the heart. This could cause a drain of flow through nonischemic microvasculature away from collateral connections (a "coronary steal" phenomenon) [52].

Direct experimental measurement of the magnitude of change in collateral blood flow with various vasodilators has been performed in many

studies with contradictory results. Some erroneous conclusions have been derived because of inadequacies in experimental design. For example, it has been reported in several studies [54–57] that calcium antagonists, which dilate both large and small coronary arteries, increase coronary flow to ischemic regions of myocardium. In these studies, however, the interface between ischemic and nonischemic regions was not accurately identified and the apparently higher collateral flows after therapy were most likely observed because the measurements were made in samples of "ischemic myocardium" contaminated with some nonischemic myocardium. Other studies, in which the interface between the ischemic and nonischemic regions has been carefully identified and the latter avoided during postmortem sampling, have demonstrated no increase in collateral flow to the ischemic regions after administration of calcium antagonists [58–62].

The effect on collateral flow to acutely ischemic myocardium of agents, such as nitroglycerin, that affect predominantly the large coronary arteries [63–73] has also been variable.

Acute Reperfusion of Ischemic Myocardium

In recent years, much attention has been devoted to the feasibility of early restoration of coronary blood flow by using either emergency surgical revascularization [74–79], or thrombolytic therapy [80–100] (see chapters 22, 34, and 35).

Thrombolytic therapy could potentially be beneficial in many patients because both postmortem and intraoperative studies [101, 102] have recently indicated that the frequency of acute occlusive thrombi during "transmural" ischemia approaches 90%. This frequency is much higher than had been generally accepted based on older autopsy studies that often failed to distinguish between hypotension-induced subendocardial injury versus solid infarcts, or between sudden arrhythmic deaths versus true myocardial infarcts (see chapter 6). From the rapidly growing number of recent reports [80–100], it is clear that (a) thrombi can by lysed by either intracoronary or intravenous administration of thrombolytic agents such as streptokinase, and (b) serious morbidity or mortality due to complications of thrombolytic therapy, such as hemorrhage or reperfusion arrhythmias, have been rare. However, the question of whether restoration of coronary blood flow significantly limits ultimate infarct size in patients has not been answered, despite the large number of studies published to date. No method of accurately predicting ultimate infarct size prior to reperfusion in an individual patient has been established. An additional complicating factor is that reperfusion may alter the relationship between actual infarct size and the clinical parameters used to estimate infarct size, such as plasma time—activity curves of creatine kinase.

If results from experimental studies described earlier in this chapter are applicable to man, one would predict that any intervention to limit infarct size might be of little benefit if it were begun after more than 3−6 hr of ischemia. However, because more gradual mechanisms of coronary occlusion and/or greater variation in collateral flow, patients may comprise a much more heterogeneous group regarding time course of infarction. Thus, it is not possible to conclude whether or not later intervention might limit infarct size in some individuals. As more and more clinical trials are completed, the effect of reperfusion on long-term mortality and on morbidity from cardiac dysfunction and arrhythmias will be established, but the specific question of whether reperfusion in the early phase of infarction in a given patient can limit the size of the developing infarct will be difficult to answer.

In a relatively small subset of patients, myocardial infarction may be initiated by dynamic coronary events such as vasospasm [103−107] (see chapter 5). In this group of patients, early intervention with calcium antagonists might relieve vasospasm and restore myocardial perfusion.

If infarct size is to be limited in patients, the ideal approach to treatment may be to combine pharmacologic therapy to relieve possible vasospasm and/or to delay the cellular consequences of ischemia (e.g., calcium antagonists [108,109]) with thrombolytic or surgical reperfusion. Immediate pharmacologic protection of ischemic myocardium might expand the window of time within which development of collateral flow or reperfusion could be achieved with beneficial effects on infarct size.

Summary

From experimental studies in dogs, the importance of collateral blood flow as a modifying influence in myocardial infarction is clear. Preferential perfusion of the subepicardial versus the subendocardial region may contribute to the slower time course of ischemic cellular injury in the subepicardial region. Furthermore, the amount of collateral blood flow to the subepicardial region is the single most important known determinant of the transmural extent of the ultimate infarct. In humans, even fatal infarcts studied at autopsy often do not involve the entire transmural thickness of an ischemic region, demonstrating the importance of preformed collateral vessels and/or spontaneous reperfusion in man as well as in experimental animals. Much effort has been devoted to the concept that it is possible to limit infarct size with appropriate intervention. It seems likely that any intervention that delays the cellular consequences of ischemia, but does not improve myocardial perfusion, will not limit ultimate infarct size. Such therapy may be beneficial, however, by providing a longer window of time within which myocardial perfusion can be restored by growth of new collaterals, by thrombolytic therapy, or by surgical revascularization.

References

1. Jennings RB, Reimer KA: Factors involved in salvaging ischemic myocardium: effect of reperfusion of arterial blood. Circulation 68:I-25−36, 1983.
2. Reimer KA, Hill ML, Jennings RB: Prolonged depletion of ATP and of the adenine nucleotide pool due to delayed resynthesis of adenine nucleotides following reversible myocardial ischemic injury in dogs. J Mol Cell Cardiol 13:229−239, 1981.
3. Swain JL, Sabina, RL, McHale PA, Greenfield JC Jr, Holmes EW: Prolonged myocardial nucleotide depletion after brief ischemia in the open-chest dog. Am J Physiol 242:H818−826, 1982.
4. Kloner RA, De Boer LWV, Darsee JR, Ingwall JS, Hale S, Tumas J. Braunwald E: Prolonged

abnormalities of myocardium salvaged by reperfusion. Am J Physiol 241:H591−H599, 1981.

5. Reimer KA, Jennings RB, Tatum AH: Pathobiology of acute myocardial ischemia: metabolic, functional and ultrastructural studies. Am J Cardiol 52: 72A−81A, 1983.

6. Weiner, JM, Apstein CS, Arthur JH, Pirzada FA, Hood WB Jr: Persistence of myocardial injury following brief periods of coronary occlusion. Cardiovasc Res 10: 678−686, 1976.

7. Jennings RB, Sommers HM, Smyth GA, Flack HA, Linn H: Myocardial necrosis induced by temporary occlusion of a coronary artery in the dog. Arch Pathol 70: 68−78, 1960.

8. Reimer KA, Lowe JE, Rasmussen MM, Jennings RB: The wavefront phenomenon of ischemic cell death. 1. Myocardial infarct size vs. duration of coronary occlusion in dogs. Circulation 56:786−794, 1977.

9. Reimer, KA, Jennings RB: The "wavefront phenomenon" of myocardial ischemic cell death. II. Transmural progression of necrosis within the framework of ischemic bed size (myocardium at risk) and collateral flow. Lab Invest 40:633−644, 1979.

10. Hofmann M, Hofmann M, Genth K. Schaper W: The influence of reperfusion on infarct size after experimental coronary artery occlusion. Basic Res Cardiol 75: 572−582, 1980.

11. Baughman, KL, Maroko PR, Vatner SF: Effects of coronary artery reperfusion on myocardial infarct size and survival in conscious dogs. Circulation 63:317−323, 1981.

12. Geary GG, Smith GT, McNamara JJ: Quantitative effect of early coronary artery reperfusion in baboons: extent of salvage of the perfusion bed of an occluded artery. Circulation 66:391−396, 1982.

13. Connelly C, Vogel WM, Hernandez YM, Apstein CS: Movement of necrotic wavefront after coronary artery occlusion in rabbit. Am J Physiol 243:H682−690, 1982.

14. Kloner RA, Ellis SG, Lange R, Braunwald E: Studies of experimental coronary artery reperfusion: effects on infarct size, myocardial function, biochemistry, ultrastructure and microvascular damage. Circulation 68:I-8−15, 1983.

15. Jugdutt BI, Hutchins GM, Bulkley BH, Becker LC: Myocardial infarction in the conscious dog: three-dimensional mapping of the infarct, collateral flow and region at risk. Circulation 60:1141−1150, 1979.

16. Hoffman, JIE: Determinants and prediction of transmural myocardial perfusion. Circulation 58:381−391, 1978.

17. Becker LC, Ferreira R, Thomas M: Mapping of left ventricular blood flow with radioactive microspheres in experimental coronary artery occlusion. Cardiovasc Res 7:391−400, 1973.

18. Wusten B, Flameng W, Schaper W, Carl M: The distribution of myocardial flow. I. Effects of experimental coronary occlusion. Basic Res Cardiol 69:422−434, 1974.

19. Reimer KA, Lowe JE, Jennings RB: The wavefront phenomenon of ischemic cell death. In: Hjalmarson A, Wilhelmsen L (eds) Acute and long-term medical management of myocardial ischemia. Molndal, Sweden: A Lindgren and Soner AB, 1978, pp. 75−82.

20. Jennings RB, Ganote CE, Reimer KA: Ischemic tissue injury. Am J Pathol 81: 179−198, 1975.

21. Fujiwara H, Ashraf M, Sato S, Millard RW: Transmural cellular damage and blood flow distribution in early ischemia in pig hearts. Circ Res 51:683−693, 1982.

22. Dunn, RB, Griggs DM Jr: Transmural gradients in ventricular tissue metabolites produced by stopping coronary blood flow in the dog. Circ Res 37:438−445, 1975.

23. Lowe JE, Cummings RG, Adams DH, Hull-Ryde EA: Evidence that ischemic cell death begins in the subendocardium independent of variations in collateral flow or wall tension. Circulation 68:190−202, 1983.

24. Eng C, Cho S, Kirk ES: The wavefront pattern of necrosis occurs despite uniform blood flow conditions [abstr]. Circulation 66:II-66, 1982.

25. Kagen L, Scheidt S, Butt A: Serum myoglobin in myocardial infarction: the 'staccato phenomenon'. Is acute myocardial infarction in man an intermittent event? Am J Med 62:86−92, 1977.

26. Mathey D, Bleifeld W, Buss, H, et al: Creatine kinase release in acute myocardial infarction: correlation with clinical, electrocardiographic, and pathological findings. Br Heart J 37:1161−1168, 1975.

27. Lowe, JE, Reimer KA, Jennings RB: Experimental infarct size as a function of the amount of myocardium at risk. Am J Pathol 90:363−379, 1978.

28. Reimer KA: Myocardial infarct size: measurements and predictions. Arch Pathol Lab Med 104:225−230, 1980.

29. Schaper W: Residual perfusion of acutely ischemic heart muscle. In: Schaper W (ed) The pathophysiology of myocardial perfusion. New York: Elsevier/North-Holland Biomedical, 1979, pp. 345−378.

30. Gottwik M, Zimmer P, Wusten B, Hoffmann M, Winkler B, Schaper W: Experimental myocardial infarction in a closed-chest canine model: observations of temporal and spatial evolution over 24 hours. Basic Res Cardiol 76: 670–680, 1981.
31. Factor SM, Okun EM, Kirk ES: The histological lateral border of acute canine myocardial infarction: a function of microcirculation. Circ Res 48:640–649, 1981.
32. Murdock RH, Harlan DM, Morris JJ III, Pryor WW Jr, Cobb FR: Transitional blood flow zones between ischemic and non-ischemic myocardium in the awake dog: analysis based on distribution of the intramural vasculature. Circ Res 52: 451–459, 1983.
33. Lee JT, Ideker RE, Reimer KA: Myocardial infarct size and location in relation to the coronary vascular bed at risk in man. Circulation 64:526–534, 1981.
34. Factor SM, Okun EM, Minase T, Kirk ES: The microcirculation of the human heart: end-capillary loops with discrete perfusion fields. Circulation 66:1241–1248, 1982.
35. Rivas F, Cobb FR, Bache RJ, Greenfield JC Jr: Relationship between blood flow to ischemic regions and extent of myocardial infarction: serial measurement of blood flow to ischemic regions in dogs. Circ Res 38:439–447, 1976.
36. Schaper W, Wusten B: Collateral circulation. In: Schaper W (ed) The pathophysiology of myocardial perfusion. New York: Elsevier/North Holland Biomedical, 1979, pp. 415–470.
37. Williams DO, Amsterdam EA, Miller RR, Mason DT: Functional significance of coronary collateral vessels in patients with acute myocardial infarction: relation to pump performance, cardiogenic shock and survival. Am J Cardiol 37:345–351, 1976.
38. Hemby RI, Aintablian A, Schwartz A: Reappraisal of the functional significance of the coronary collateral circulation. Am J Cardiol 38: 305–309, 1976.
39. Plotnick GD, Fisher ML, Lerner B, Carliner NH, Peters RW, Becker LC: Collateral circulation in patients with unstable angina. Chest 82:719–725, 1983.
40. Rowe GG: An angiographic and clinical study of coronary collateral circulation. Basic Res Cardiol 73:131–141, 1979.
41. Kuo PT, Kostis JB, Moreyra AE: Protection of myocardium by the compensatory mechanism of coronary collaterals after total occlusion of major coronary arteries shown in patients with familial hypercholesterolemia. Am Heart J 104: 36–43, 1982.
42. Roberts WC: Coronary artery pathology in fatal ischemic heart disease. In: Braunwald E (ed) The myocardium: failure and infarction. New York: HP Publishing, 1984, pp. 194–204.
43. Ideker RE, Wagner GS, Ruth WK, Alonso DR, Bishop SP, Bloor CM, Fallon JT, Gottlieb GJ, Hackel DB, Phillips HR, Reimer KA, Roark SF, Rogers WJ, Savage RM, White RD, Selvester RH: Evaluation of a QRS scoring system for estimating myocardial infarction size. II. Correlation with quantitative anatomic findings for anterior infarcts. Am J Cardiol 49: 1604–1614, 1982.
44. Freifeld AG, Schuster EH, Bulkley BH: Nontransmural versus transmural myocardial infarction: a morphologic study. Am J Med 75:423–432, 1983.
45. Cook RW, Edwards JE, Pruitt RD: Electrocardiographic changes in acute subendocardial infarction. Circulation 28: 603–612, 1958.
46. Abrams HL: The collateral circulation: response to ischemia. Am J Radiol 140: 1051–1063, 1983.
47. Bloor CM: Functional significance of the coronary collateral circulation. Am J Pathol 76: 562–588, 1974.
48. Reimer KA: Overview of potential mechanisms. In: Wagner GS (ed) Myocardial infarction: measurement and intervention. Boston: Martinus Nijhoff, 1982, pp. 387–395.
49. Bloor CM, White FC: Functional development of the coronary collateral circulation during coronary artery occlusion in the conscious dog. Am J Pathol 67:483–500, 1972.
50. Pasyk S, Schaper W, Schaper J, Pasyk K, Miskiewicz G, Steinseifer B: DNA synthesis in coronary collaterals with coronary artery occlusion in conscious dog. Am J Physiol 242: H1031–1037, 1982.
51. Seipser SL, Kaltman AJ, Mills N, Pughkem T, Fox AC: Coronary collateral flow after traumatic fistula between right coronary artery and right atrium. N Engl J Med 287:754–756, 1972.
52. Schaper W: Experimental coronary artery occlusion. III. The determinants of collateral blood flow in acute coronary occlusion. Basic Res Cardiol 73:584–594, 1978.
53. Becker LC: Increasing coronary blood flow. In: Wagner GS (ed) Myocardial infarction: measurement and intervention. Boston: Martinus Nijhoff, 1982, pp. 415–456.
54. Berdeaux A, Coutte R, Giudicelli J-F, Boissier

J-R: Effects of verapamil on regional myocardial blood flow and ST segment: role of the induced bradycardia. Eur J Pharmacol 39:287−294, 1976.

55. Henry PD, Shuchleib R, Borda LJ, Roberts R, Williamson JR, Sobel BE: Effects of nifedipine on myocardial perfusion and ischemic injury in dogs. Circ Res 43: 372−380, 1978.

56. Da Luz PL, De Barros LFM, Leite JJ, Pileggi F, Decourt LV: Effect of verapamil on regional coronary and myocardial perfusion during acute coronary occlusion. Am J Cardiol 45:269−275, 1980.

57. Jolly SR, Hardman HF, Gross GJ: Comparison of two dihydropyridine calcium antagonists on coronary collateral blood flow in acute myocardial ischemia. J Pharmacol Exp Ther 217:20−25, 1981.

58. Karlsberg, RP, Henry PD, Ahmed SA, Sobel BE, Roberts R: Lack of protection of ischemic myocardium by verapamil in conscious dogs. Eur J Pharmacol 42: 339−346, 1977.

59. Nakamura M, Koiwaya Y, Yamada A, Kikuchi Y, Senda Y, Ikeo T, Sunagawa K, Mori M, Kanaide H: Effects of diltiazem, a new antianginal drug, on myocardial blood flow following experimental coronary occlusion. In: Winbury MM, Abiko Y (eds) Ischemic myocardium and antianginal drugs. New York: Raven, 1979, pp. 129−142.

60. Sherman LG, Liang C, Boden WE, Hood WB Jr: The effect of verapamil on mechanical performance of acutely ischemic and reperfused myocardium in the conscious dog. Circ Res 48:224−232, 1981.

61. Weintraub WS, Hattori S, Agarwal J, Bodenheimer MM, Banka VS, Helfant RH: Variable effect of nifedipine on myocardial blood flow at three grades of coronary occlusion in the dog. Circ Res 48:937−942, 1981.

62. Zyvoloski MG, Brooks HL, Gross GJ, Warltier DC: Myocardial perfusion distal to an acute or chronic coronary artery occlusion: effects of diltiazem and nifedipine. J Pharmacol Exp Ther 222:494−500, 1982.

63. Bache RJ: Effect of nitroglycerin and arterial hypertension on myocardial blood flow following acute coronary artery occlusion in the dog. Circulation 57:557−562, 1978.

64. Becker LC: Effect of nitroglycerin and dipyridamole on regional left ventricular blood flow during coronary artery occlusion. J Clin Invest 58:1287−1296, 1976.

65. Capurro N, Kent KM, Epstein SE: Effects of intracoronary and intravenous nitroglycerin on coronary collateral function. J Pharmacol Ther 199:262−268, 1976.

66. Mathes P, Rival J: Effect of nitroglycerin on total and regional coronry blood flow in the normal and ischaemic canine myocardium. Cardiovasc Res 5:54−61, 1971.

67. Horwitz LD, Gorlin R, Taylor WJ, Kemp HG: Effects of nitroglycerin on regional myocardial blood flow in coronary artery disease. J Clin Invest 50:1578−1584, 1971.

68. Weisse AB, Senft A, Kahn MI, Regan TJ: Effect of nitrate infusions on the systemic and coronary circulations following experimental myocardial infarction in the intact dog. Am J Cardiol 30:362−370, 1972.

69. Chiariello M, Gold HK, Leinbach RC, Davis MA, Maroko PR: Comparison between the effects of nitroprusside and nitroglycerin on ischemic injury during acute myocardial infarction. Circulation 54:766−773, 1976.

70. Capurro NL, Kent KM, Smith HJ, Aamodt R, Epstein SE: Acute coronary occlusion: prolonged increase in collateral flow following brief administration of nitroglycerin and methoxamine. Am J Cardiol 39:679−683, 1977.

71. Jugdutt BI, Becker LC, Hutchins GM, Bulkley BH, Reid PR, Kallman CH: Effect of intravenous nitroglycerin on collateral blood flow and infarct size in the conscious dog. Circulation 63:17−28, 1981.

72. Fukuyama T, Schectman KB, Roberts R: The effects of intravenous nitroglycerin on hemodynamics, coronary blood flow and morphologically and enzymatically estimated infarct size in conscious dogs. Circulation 62:1227−1237, 1980.

73. Pearlman AS, Engler RL, Goldstein RA, Kent KM, Epstein SE: Relative effects of nitroglycerin and nitroprusside during experimental acute myocardial ischemia. Eur J Cardiol 11:295−313, 1980.

74. Dubost C, Carpentier A, Sellier P, Piwnica A, Deloche A, Relland J, Vial F, Fabiani JN: Emergency myocardial revascularization. Postgrad Med J 52:743−748, 1976.

75. Richmond DR, Baird DK: Coronary bypass grafting in the early stages of acute myocardial infarction. Med J Aust 1:203−206, 1979.

76. Selinger SL, Berg R, Leonard JJ, Grunwald RP, O'Grady WP: Surgical treatment of acute evolving anterior myocardial infarction. Cardiovasc Surg 64:II-28−33, 1981.

77. Phillips SJ, Zeff RH, Kongtahworn C, Skinner

JR, Iannone L, Brown TM, Wickemeyer W, Gordon DF: Surgery for evolving myocardial infarction. JAMA 248:1325–1328, 1982.

78. De Wood MA, Spores J, Berg R Jr, Kendall RW, Grunwald RP, Selinger SL, Hensley GR, Sutherland KI, Sheilds JP: Acute myocardial infarction: a decade of experience with surgical reperfusion in 701 patients. Cardiovasc Surg 68:II-8–16, 1983.

79. De Wood MA, Heit J, Spores J, Berg R Jr, Selinger SL, Rudy LW, Hensley GR, Shields JP: Anterior transmural myocardial infarction: effects of surgical coronary reperfusion on global and regional left ventricular function. J Am Coll Cardiol 1:1223–1234, 1983.

80. Rentrop P, Blanke H, Karsch KR, Kaiser H, Kostering H, Leitz K: Selective intracoronary thrombolysis in acute myocardial infarction and unstable angina pectoris. Circulation 63:307–317, 1981.

81. Kennedy JW, Fritz JK, Ritchie JL: Streptokinase in acute myocardial infarction: Western Washington randomized trial—protocol and progress report. Am Heart J 104:899–911, 1982.

82. Smalling RW, Fuentes F, Freund GC, Reduto LA, Wanta-Matthews M, Gaeta JM, Walker W, Sterling R, Gould KL: Beneficial effects of intracoronary thrombolysis up to eighteen hours after onset of pain in evolving myocardial infarction. Am Heart J 104:912–920, 1982.

83. Lee G, Low RI, Takeda P, Joe P, DeMaria AN, Amsterdam EA, Lui H, Dietrich P, Lee K, Mason D: Importance of follow-up medical and surgical approaches to prevent reinfarction, reocclusion, and recurrent angina following intracoronary thromblysis with streptokinase in acute myocardial infarction. Am Heart J 104:921–924, 1982.

84. Timmis GC, Gangadharan V, Hauser AM, Ramos RG, Westveer DC, Gordon S: Intracoronary streptokinase in clinical practice. Am Heart J 104:925–938, 1982.

85. Spann JF, Sherry S, Carabello BA, Mann, RH, McCann WD, Gault JH, Gentzier RD, Rosenberg KM, Maurer AH, Denenberg BS, Warner HF, Rubin RN, Malmud LS, Comerota A: High-dose, brief intravenous streptokinase early in acute myocardial infarction. Am Heart J 104:939–945, 1982.

86. Vetrovec GW, Leinbach RC, Gold HK, Cowley MJ: Intracoronary thrombolysis in syndromes of unstable ischemia: angiographic and clinical results. Am Heart J 104:946–952, 1982.

87. Hermens WT: Enzyme analysis in a multicentre trial on streptokinase treatment in acute myocardial infarction. Acta Med Scand 648:85–95, 1981.

88. Willems JL, Theiss W, Lubcke P: Arrhythmias in patients of a multicenter trial on streptokinase treatment in acute myocardial infarction. Acta Med Scand Supp 648:75–84, 1981.

89. Mathey DG, Kuck KH, Tilsner V, Krebber HJ, Bleifeld W: Nonsurgical coronary artery recanalization in acute transmural myocardial infarction. Circulation 63:489–497, 1981.

90. Ganz, W, Buchbinder N, Marcus H, Mondkar A, Maddahi J, Charuzi Y, O'Connor L, Shell W, Fishbein MC, Kass R, Swan HJC: Intracoronary thrombolysis in evolving myocardial infarction. Am Heart J 101:4–13, 1981.

91. Schwarz F, Schuler G, Katus H, Mehmel HC, Von Olshausen K, Hofmann M, Herrmann HJ, Kubler W: Intracoronary thrombolysis in acute myocardial infarction: correlations among serum enzyme, scintigraphic and hemodynamic findings. Am J Cardiol 50:32–38, 1982.

92. Meltzer RS, Van den Brand M, Serruys PW, Fioretti P, Hugenholtz PG: Sequential intracoronary streptokinase and transmural angioplasty in unstable angina with evolving myocardial infarction. Am Heart J 104:1109–1111, 1982.

93. Cowley MJ, Hastillo A, Vetrovec GW, Fisher LM, Garrett R, Hess ML: Fibrinolytic effects of intracoronary streptokinase administration in patients with acute myocardial infarction and coronary insufficiency. Circulation 67:1031–1038, 1983.

94. Khaja F, Walton JA Jr, Brymer JF, Lo E, Osterberger L, O'Neill WW, Colfer HT, Weiss R, Lee T, Kurian T, Goldberg AD, Pitt B, Goldstein S: Intracoronary fibrinolytic therapy in acute myocardial infarction: report of a prospective randomized trial. N Engl J Med 308:1305–1311, 1983.

95. Blanke H, Scherff F, Karsch KR, Levine RA, Smith H, Rentrop P: Electrocardiographic changes after streptokinase-induced recanalization in patients with acute left anterior descending artery obstruction. Circulation 68:406–412, 1983.

96. Stack RS, Phillips, HR III, Grierson DS, Behar VS, Kong Y, Peter RH, Swain JL, Greenfield JC Jr: Functional improvement of jeopardized myocardium following intracoronary streptokinase infusion in acute myocardial infarction. J Clin Invest 72:84–95, 1983.

97. De Feyter PJ, Van Eenige MJ, Van der Wall

EE, Bezemer PD, Van Engelen CLJ, Funke-Kupper AJ, Kerkkamp HJJ, Visser FC, Roos JP: Effects of spontaneous and streptokinase-induced recanalization on left ventricular function after myocardial infarction. Circulation 67: 1039–1044, 1983.

98. Smalling RW, Fuentes F, Matthews MW, Freund GC, Hicks CH, Reduto LA, Walker WE, Sterling RP, Gould KL: Sustained improvement in left ventricular function and mortality by intracoronary streptokinase administration during evolving myocardial infarction. Circulation 68:131–138, 1983.

99. Anderson JL, Marshall HW, Bray BE, Lutz JR, Frederick PR, Yanowitz FG, Datz FL, Klausner SC, Hagan AD: A randomized trial of intracoronary streptokinase in the treatment of acute myocardial infarction. N Engl J Med 308: 1312–1318, 1983.

100. Sheehan FH, Mathey DG, Schofer J, Krebber H-J, Dodge HT: Effect of interventions in salvaging left ventricular function in acute myocardial infarction: a study of intracoronary streptokinase. Am J Cardiol 52:431–438, 1983.

101. Davies MJ, Woolf N, Robertson WB: Pathology of acute myocardial infarction with particular reference to occlusive coronary thrombi. Br Heart J 38:659–664, 1976.

102. De Wood MA, Spores J, Notske R, Mouser LT, Burroughs R, Golden MS, Lang HT: Preva-lence of total coronary occlusion during the early hours of transmural myocardial infarction. N Engl J Med 303:897–902, 1980.

103. Oliva PB: What is the evidence for and the significance of spasm in acute myocardial infarction? Chest 80:730–735, 1981.

104. Dalen JE, Ockene IS, Alpert JS: Coronary spasm, coronary thrombosis and myocardial infarction: a hypothesis concerning the pathophysiology of acute myocardial infarction. Am Heart J 104:1119–1124, 1982.

105. Maseri A, Chierchia S: Coronary artery spasm: demonstration, definition, diagnosis, and consequences. Prog Cardiovasc Dis 25:169–192, 1982.

106. Gorlin R: Dynamic vascular factors in the genesis of myocardial ischemia. J Am Cell Cardiol: 897–906, 1983.

107. Cipriano PR, Koch FH, Rosenthal SJ, Baim DS, Ginsberg R, Schroeder JS: Myocardial infarction in patients with coronary artery spasm demonstrated by angiography. Am Heart J 105:542–547, 1983.

108. Henry PD: Comparative pharmacology of calcium antagonists: nifedipine, verapamil and diltiazem. Am J Cardiol 46:1047–1058, 1980.

109. McAllister RG Jr: Clinical pharmacology of slow channel blocking agents. Prog Cardiovasc Dis 25:83–102, 1982.

3. ENERGY METABOLISM AND TRANSPORT IN THE ISCHEMIC AND POSTISCHEMIC MYOCARDIUM

Judith L. Swain

Richard L. Sabina

The primary energy source for basic cell processes and contractile activity in the myocyte is the purine nucleoside triphosphate ATP. ATP is hydrolyzed to ADP by energy-consuming reactions, and the ADP thus formed can either be rephosphorylated to ATP or can be metabolized to nucleosides and bases that can diffuse out of the myocyte. A constant supply of purine substrate is necessary to ensure that ADP is available for phosphorylation either by oxidative processes in the mitochondria or through glycolytic reactions in the cytoplasm. The high-energy phosphate bond formed by the energy-generating processes must then be transported from the sites of energy production to the sites of energy utilization.

Thus, energy production and consumption can be viewed as comprising these steps: (a) generation of purine substrate (specifically ADP), (b) formation of high-energy phosphate bonds (by oxidative phosphorylation and glycolysis), and (c) transport of energy-containing compounds to the sites of energy consumption. Much has been written concerning the second step, the regulation of oxidative phosphorylation and glycolysis in the myocardium. This chapter deals with the first process in energy production, the synthesis and degradation of purine compounds in the myocardium, and the third step, the intracellular transport of energy.

Myocardial Adenine Nucleotide Metabolism

SYNTHESIS OF PURINE NUCLEOTIDES

Myocardial purine nucleotides are synthesized in two ways (figure 3-1): (a) de novo synthesis from glutamine and 5-phosphoribosyl-1-pyrophosphate (PRPP) via a series of small carbon and nitrogen additions, and (b) salvage synthesis from preformed purine bases and nucleosides. The activity of de novo synthesis depends on the availability of PRPP and the concentration of nucleotide end products [1, 2]. Salvage synthesis of purine bases is also regulated by the concentration of PRPP and purine nucleotides [3, 4], and depends on the availability of preformed purine substrate [5, 6].

In normoxic myocardium, which contains high concentrations of ATP ($5-6$ mM), the rate of de novo synthesis is reportedly only $6-12$ nmol/g wet tissue weight/h [7, 8]. Similarly, the rate of salvage synthesis is estimated to be $6-30$ nmol/g wet tissue weight/h at physiologic (i.e., submicromolar) concentrations of preformed purine substrate [5, 6]. Since the normoxic myocardial consumption of ATP is approximately 15 μmol/g wet tissue weight/min [9, 10], and is over 20,000-fold greater than the combined de novo

R.M. Califf and G.S. Wagner (eds.), ACUTE CORONARY CARE: Principles and Practice. Copyright © 1985. Martinus Nijhoff Publishing, Boston/Dordrecht/Lancaster.

21

and salvage synthetic rates, it is apparent that under normoxic conditions ADP is conserved and can be repeatedly rephosphorylated to ATP. The mechanisms responsible for the phosphorylation of ADP are discussed next.

ENERGY METABOLISM OF THE NORMOXIC MYOCARDIUM

Energy demands of the myocardial cell [11] are primarily satisfied (i.e., 70%) by aerobic lipid metabolism. Free fatty acids (FFA), derived from long-chained fatty acids in plasma, diffuse across the cell membrane and bind to coenzyme A (CoA) as acyl derivatives. Transfer into the mitochondria is accomplished via the acyl-transferase system where the resulting acyl-CoA enters the tricarboxylic acid (TCA) cycle.

Carbohydrates participate, to a lesser degree (i.e., 30%), in maintaining the aerobic energy status of the myocardium. Glucose crosses the cell membrane and is either preferentially stored as glycogen or remains in the cytoplasm where it feeds the glycolytic pathway via the hexokinase and phosphofructokinase reactions.

Oxidative phosphorylation and aerobic glycolysis, through their ADP-phosphorylating reactions, fuel the energy requirements of the myocardium by maintaining a high ATP−ADP ratio that also conserves the total adenine nucleotide pool. Since the rate of ATP consumption by normoxic myocardium is essentially balanced by the activity of these two energy-producing pathways, the combination of purine de novo and salvage synthesis functions to retard any net purine loss from the heart [5, 12].

ENERGY METABOLISM IN ISCHEMIC MYOCARDIUM

It is apparent from the preceding section that the supply of energy needed for normal contractile activity of the myocardium is dependent upon (a) sufficient transfer of oxygen to the respiratory chain in the mitochondria, and (b) the availability of oxidizable substrate from exogenous sources. During an ischemic insult when these two criteria for normal metabolism are not met, deleterious metabolic consequences ensue.

Ischemia results in inhibition of fatty acid oxidation at the level of β oxidation, and is associated with increased levels of long-chain acyl-

CoA and acyl-carnitine [13]. In contrast, ischemia initially stimulates glycolysis and glycogen stores are rapidly depleted, resulting in a maximal rate of lactate production in 1 min [14]. While briefly compensatory, the glycolytic rate decreases after about 4 min of ischemia, presumably due to the inhibition of glyceraldehyde-3-phosphate dehydrogenase [15]. Therefore, ischemia results in a change in the energy metabolism of the cell. Myocardial energy demand exceeds energy production due to the limited ability of oxidative phosphorylation and glycolysis to generate ATP. Consequently, high-energy phosphate levels begin to decline. A rapid drop in ATP is initially prevented at the expense of myocardial creatine phosphate stores [9]. By 12−15 min of ischemia, however, there is a 30%−50% reduction in ATP content [16−18]. A transitory increase in ADP and AMP results but, due to high levels of cardiac 5′-nucleotidase activity [19], dephosphorylated catabolites of purine nucleotides (i.e., adenosine, inosine, and hypoxanthine) begin to accumulate [17, 18]. Decreased levels and/or availability of high-energy phosphate stores in turn may be responsible for impaired mechanical function observed during ischemia [20].

ENERGY METABOLISM IN POSTISCHEMIC MYOCARDIUM

With restoration of blood flow after a brief ischemic insult, the return of oxygen and substrate availability should be rapid. However, it reportedly takes several minutes to reverse the inhibition of glycolysis and oxidative phosphorylation [21], indicating that the synthesis of ATP during the first few minutes of recovery could be limited by the rate of these pathways rather than by availability of oxygen and substrate. Nevertheless, in post ischemic myocardium, mitochondrial function returns rapidly, as evidenced by elevated creatine phosphate pools within minutes of reperfusion [16, 18].

Several studies have documented prolonged contractile dysfunction following brief periods of ischemia [22−24]. In addition, it is well established that the myocardial content of adenine nucleotides remains depressed long after perfusion has been restored [16−18]. This has led to the hypothesis that post ischemic myocardial dysfunction and prolonged depletion of ATP pools are causally related.

Since the mechanisms required to phosphorylate ADP to ATP are operational shortly after the ischemic insult, it is generally accepted that the prolonged return of myocardial ATP pools is due to a limited availability of purine substrate [6, 17, 18, 20]. With reperfusion, the purine nucleosides and bases that accumulate during ATP catabolism rapidly diffuse from the cell and are carried away in the blood. The limited availability of the salvage pathways to reuse these catabolites, combined with the relatively slow rate of purine de novo synthesis, contribute to a prolonged purine debt.

METABOLIC INTERVENTIONS FOR ENHANCING PURINE NUCLEOTIDE CONTENT IN POST ISCHEMIC MYOCARDIUM

Since it is well established that purine substrate is lost from myocardium during reperfusion after an ischemic insult, it can be concluded that the prolonged return of intracellular ATP content in postischemic tissue is due to the limited availability of purine substrate. Two basic approaches have been examined to eliminate this purine debt: (a) increasing the availability of precursors for de novo synthesis, and (b) supplying exogenous preformed purine to enhance salvage synthesis.

The release of feedback inhibition of purine de novo synthesis by a reduction in purine nucleotide levels and/or an increase in availability of PRPP results in a two- to sixfold increase in this pathway in postischemic myocardium [12]. Nevertheless, even at this accelerated rate of de novo synthesis, it would take days to replenish the lost purine substrate since PRPP availability still limits the rate at which this pathway can operate. Therefore, interventions have been designed to enhance the production of PRPP in post ischemic myocardium. PRPP is synthesized by the hexose monophosphate shunt, which limits its production. This pathway can be effectively stimulated by supplying pentoses and pentitols [25]. Ribose is particularly effective since it actually bypasses the initial and rate-limiting step of the hexose monophosphate shunt, and is directly converted to ribose-5-phosphate, the immediate precursor to PRPP (figure 3-1). As a

result, purine de novo synthesis can be stimulated an additional 3.5-fold in postanoxic myocardium [26]. While this approach accelerates the return of purine nucleotide levels, its effectiveness is governed by the initial, rate-limiting step of purine de novo synthesis [1, 2].

Because of the inherent limitations in PRPP availability, and because the initial step of purine de novo synthesis is rate limiting, more attention has been focused on the salvage pathways of purine nucleotide synthesis for repletion of post ischemic myocardial purine nucleotide pools. These include salvage of the purine bases, adenine and hypoxanthine, and the purine nucleosides, adenosine and inosine. Salvage of the preformed purines adenine and hypoxanthine requires PRPP, which results in the phosphoribosylation of these bases to the purine nucleotides AMP and IMP, respectively (figure 3-1). The nucleoside adenosine is phosphorylated to AMP using ATP as the phosphate donor. Inosine, although a nucleoside, cannot be directly phosphorylated to IMP due to the absence of significant inosine kinase activity in mammalian myocardium [5, 27]. Instead, this preformed purine substrate undergoes phosphorolysis to hypoxanthine and ribose-1-phosphate, and then is phosphoribosylated to IMP utilizing PRPP (figure 3-1).

Adenine, hypoxanthine, and inosine are incorporated into myocardial adenine nucleotides at lower rates than that observed for adenosine [5], presumably due to the limited availability of PRPP for salvage synthesis. Interventions using inosine have the additional complication that this preformed purine substrate can act as a positive inotropic agent [28, 29], which can complicate any interpretations as to its metabolic effectiveness in postischemic myocardium.

Salvage of adenosine, unlike the above-mentioned substrates, can be dramatically augmented by increasing its concentration in the myocardium. There is a dose-dependent increase in the incorporation of adenosine into myocardial nucleotides from 0.01 to 20 μM [5], reaching rates of $500-600$ nmol/g wet tissue weight. However, this effect becomes saturated at adenosine concentrations greater than 20 μM [6]. Presumably this reflects a lower Km of adenosine for myocardial adenosine kinase than for adenosine

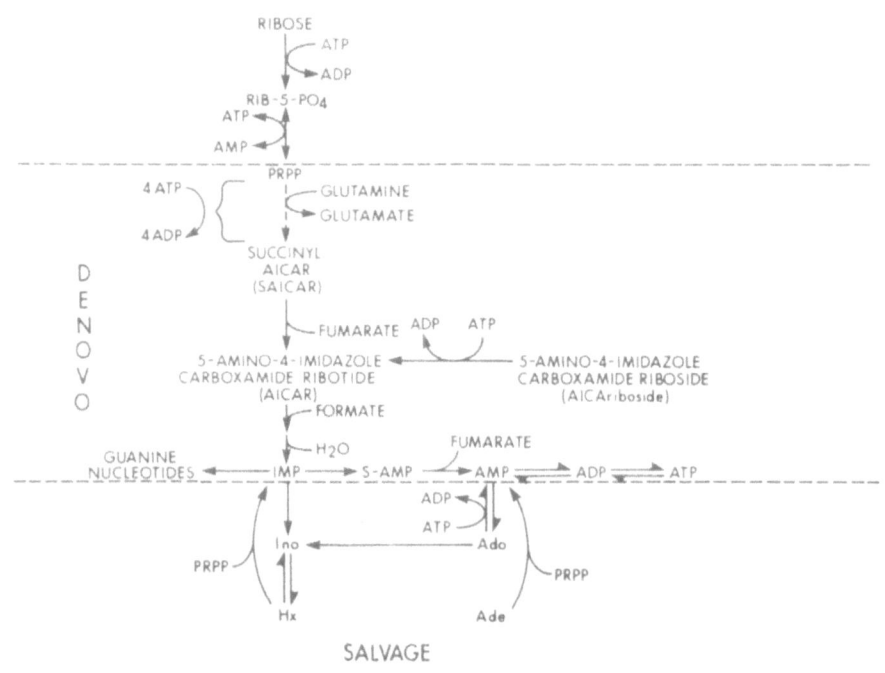

FIGURE 3-1. Schematic of purine de novo and salvage synthesis in myocardium. ATP, adenosine 5'-triphosphate; ADP, adenosine 5'-diphosphate; AMP, adenosine 5'-monophosphate; PRPP, 5'-phosphoribosyl-1-pyrophosphate; IMP, inosine 5'-monophosphate; S-AMP, succinyladenosine 5'-monophosphate; Ado, adenosine; Ade, adenine; Ino, inosine; Hx, hypoxanthine.

deaminase [30]. At lower concentrations, adenosine is preferentially phosphorylated to AMP, but at higher concentrations of adenosine the balance shifts toward deamination to inosine. This latter reaction can be effectively suppressed by the simultaneous administration of erythro-9(2-hydroxy-3-nonyl)-adenine hydrochloride (ENHA), a potent reversible inhibitor of adenosine deaminase. This results in a further enhancement of postischemic nucleotide levels over that observed with adenosine alone [31, 32]. EHNA itself has no therapeutic efficacy [31, 32].

Due to its more rapid salvage over that of other preformed purines, adenosine intervention has received the largest attention to date. While it is well documented that adenosine pretreatment can preserve adenine nucleotides in ischemic myocardium [31–33] and can lead to a rapid return of postischemic purine nucleotide pools [6], there are drawbacks to this approach. Infusion of adenosine results in reduced peripheral vascular resistance with a subsequent decrease in systemic blood pressure [34]. In addition, adenosine has been shown to decrease myocardial oxygen consumption [35], to slow atrioventricular conduc-

tion [34], and to be a potent renal vasoconstrictor [32, 36]. These additional effects, which may be independent of the nucleotide-repleting effect of adenosine, could all be detrimental to the recovery of the post ischemic heart.

Recently, an effective intervention has been reported for restoring post ischemic myocardial nucleotide pools that combines purine de novo and salvage synthesis. 5-Amino-4-imidazolecarboxamide riboside (AICAriboside) is a nucleoside precursor to the purine de novo intermediate 5-amino-4-imidazolecarboxamide ribotide (AICAR) (figure 3-1). This metabolite enters the de novo pathway distal to the rate-limiting and energy-consuming steps, but prior to the closure of the six-membered purine ring. AICAriboside is phosphorylated in an ATP-requiring reaction catalyzed by adenosine kinase, and the metabolism of this compound is not limited by the availability of PRPP. Unlike adenosine, however, AICAriboside administration is not accompanied by confounding hemodynamic effects [37].

The maximal rate of purine nucleotide synthesis achieved with this intervention has yet to be determined, but a 340 nmol/g wet wt increase in normoxic ATP levels was observed after only 30 min of administration to open-chest dogs [38], indicating that this approach may be as effective as any to date. This agent has subsequently been shown to effectively replete post ischemic purine nucleotide pools when administered in appropriate concentrations [37].

As observed with other interventions, however, the administration of high doses of AICAriboside may have several deleterious metabolic effects [38, 39]. The purine intermediate AICAR accumulates rapidly, presumably as a result of a limitation in formylation [38]. This purine de novo intermediate is a potent inhibitor of the bifunctional enzyme adenylosuccinate lyase [38, 40]. The accumulation of AICAR can result in a decrease in the rate of metabolism of IMP to AMP, effectively defeating the original purpose of the intervention. In addition, AICAR accumulation produces a reversal of flux in the de novo pathway, resulting in net succinyl-AICAR (SAICAR) synthesis and fumarate consumption [39]. High-dose AICAriboside administration also results in the accumulation of AICAriboside triphosphate in the myocardium [38]. The formation of this metabolite appears to require PRPP, and may have deleterious effects on myocardial function. The metabolic effects of SAICAR and AICAriboside triphosphate accumulation are unknown, but should be considered in evaluating high-dosage regimens of AICAriboside administration. It should be stressed, however, that these metabolic consequences can be avoided if care is taken to use a low enough dosage of AICAriboside. All indications are that low dosages are extremely effective in stimulating purine de novo synthesis, especially in postischemic myocardium [37]. Through the monitoring of AICAR and SAICAR in experimental models, an effective dose can be chosen that results in a rapid recovery of postischemic nucleotide pools.

Intracellular Energy Transport

The synthesis of ATP from ADP has been discussed in the previous section and in other reviews [10, 11, 41–46]. The ATP thus formed must be transported to sites of energy utilization. The important ATP-utilizing sites in the myocyte are: (a) the myosin ATPase, (b) the sarcoplasmic reticulum, (c) the calcium pump, and (d) the sarcolemmal $-Na^+$-K^+ ATPase. Cytoplasmically generated ATP may play a specific role in supplying energy at the sarcolemma and the sarcoplasmic reticulum. ATP generated in the mitochondria also may supply energy to membrane sites, but in addition supplies the majority of the energy requirements of the myofibril. The transduction of energy from the mitochondria to the myofibril, and the use of the energy for myofibrillar contraction, are discussed in this section.

TRANSDUCTION OF ENERGY WITHIN THE MITOCHONDRIA

Mitochondrial energy production in the heart is tightly coupled to energy demand as demonstrated by the linear relationship between oxygen consumption and mechanical performance [47]. Changes in energy demand produce very little change in either adenine nucleotide or creatine phosphate content of the myocyte, suggesting that an efficient feedback mechanism exists to link energy production with energy consumption. The first step in the transduction of energy from the matrix space to the myofibril is the transport of newly synthesized ATP out of the mitochondria (figure 3-2). The matrix space is separated from the intramembrane space by the inner membrane of the mitochondria. A transport system referred to as adenine nucleotide translocase is highly specific for ATP–ADP and excludes AMP as well as nucleotides with other bases (i.e., GTP–GDP) from transport [48]. ATP synthesized in the mitochondria is transported by the translocase to the intramembrane space. The previously accepted view was that ATP synthesized in the mitochondria and transported across the inner membrane by the translocase was used directly by the myofibril for contraction, and also used directly by the sarcolemma and the sarcoplasmic reticulum. This view also holds that creatine phosphate acts as a reser-

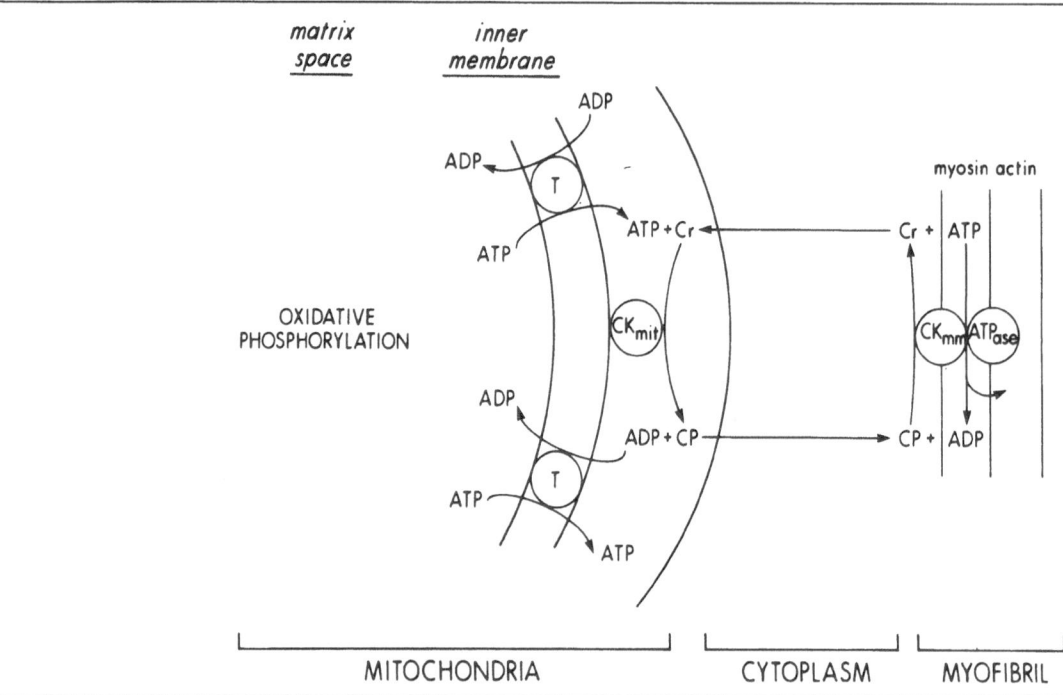

FIGURE 3-2. The creatine phosphate shuttle. T, adenine nucleotide translocase; CK_{mit}, mitochondrial isozyme of creatine kinase; CK_{MM}, myofibrillar isozyme of creatine kinase.

voir of high-energy phosphate bonds, but does not have a direct role in providing energy for myofibrillar contraction. This concept of creatine phosphate as a buffer has been challenged by newer data that indicate that creatine phosphate may play a primary role in the transduction of energy out of the mitochondria [49−51].

Jacobs and co-workers first identified a specific isozyme of creatine kinase localized to the mitochondria [52]. This isozyme is localized to the outer side of the inner mitochondrial membrane and may represent 30%−40% of the total creatine kinase activity of the myocyte [53]. This isozyme of creatine kinase appears to be functionally coupled to the adenine nucleotide translocase and ultimately to the rate of oxidative phosphorylation [54−56]. The ATP transported out of the matrix space by the translocase is channeled to the mitochondrial creatine kinase to be used as substrate for creatine phosphate synthesis. Previous studies have demonstrated close functional coupling between adenine nucleotide translocase and mitochondrial creatine kinase. It has also been estimated that the molar content of creatine kinase is nearly equivalent to the molar content of adenine nucleotide translocase [51].

The ADP produced by the phosphorylation of creatine is then channeled back into the matrix space by the translocase. The forward creatine kinase reaction (ATP + CR → ADP + CP) is kinetically less favorable than the reverse reaction, as evidenced by the high Km values for ATP (0.7 mM) and creatine (5.0 mM) compared with the Km values for ADP (0.05 mM) and CP (0.05 mM) [49]. The maximal velocities of the reactions are also different, with a velocity of the reverse reaction four times greater than that of the forward reaction. The mitochondrial creatine kinase reaction is able to proceed in the forward direction because of the high local concentration of ATP at the inner membrane supplied by the adenine nucleotide translocase, and because of the efficient removal of ADP also by the translocase. Mitochondrial creatine kinase has been demonstrated to preferentially use ATP generated by oxidative phosphorylation, and the rate of CP synthesis exceeds that which occurs when only extramitochondrial ATP is supplied [57]. Because of the high affinity of the translocase for adenine nucleotides, ADP is rapidly transported back into the matrix. Thus the nucleotide translocase is able to keep the mitochondrial creatine kinase reaction at steady state, but with an equilibrium shift in the direction of creatine phosphate synthesis.

TRANSDUCTION OF ENERGY WITHIN THE CYTOPLASM

The diffusion constant of creatine phosphate is greater than that of ATP, thus making creatine phosphate a more likely candidate for diffusion from the mitochondria to provide energy for reactions in the cytoplasm. In order for the creatine phosphate synthesized in the mitochondria to provide energy for ATP-consuming processes, creatine kinase must also be present at sites in the cytoplasm. The binding of the MM isozyme of creatine kinase to both sarcoplasmic reticulum [58] and plasma membrane [59, 60] has been demonstrated, as well as binding to myofibrils [61−63]. In the sarcoplasmic reticulum, the creatine kinase appears to be located on the reticular membrane in close proximity to the Ca^{2+}-dependent ATPase. There is also evidence that the ADP generated by the Ca^{2+}-ATPase is rephosphorylated by creatine phosphate through the creatine kinase reaction in preference to ATP provided in the medium [58].

The plasma membrane of the myocyte contains the Na^+,K^+-ATPase pump necessary to maintain the ionic balance of the cell. The plasma membrane also contains channels for the slow inward movement of Ca^{2+} that regulates the interaction of actin and myosin. Both the Na^+,K^+ pump and the slow calcium channels appear to be energy dependent. The MM isozyme of creatine kinase has been localized to the plasma membrane, and the ADP provided by the Na^+,K^+-ATPase reaction is rapidly rephosphorylated at the expense of creatine phosphate [59]. With respect to Ca^{2+}, the slow channels are activated by phosphorylation of proteins by a protein kinase reaction that utilizes ATP [64]. Myocardial ischemia and anoxia appear to alter the transport of Ca^{2+} in these slow channels, and these changes occur during a period of rapid decline in creatine phosphate before a decrease in the ATP content of the cell can be detected. Thus, creatine phosphate and the creatine kinase

reaction may play a role in regulating the slow calcium channel.

The largest proportion of the energy generated by oxidative phosphorylation is used to provide energy for myofibrillar contraction. The concept that ATP provides the immediate source of energy for the interaction of myosin and actin was first suggested by the discovery of ATPase activity associated with myosin. It was not until the work of Cain and Davis [65] that ATP was conclusively demonstrated to be the primary energy source for myofibrillar contraction. They demonstrated that the primary energy source for muscle contraction was ATP but, unless creatine phosphate was provided, muscle contraction ceased after only a small decrease in the ATP content. Other studies demonstrated that exogenously administered creatine could stimulate oxidative phosphorylation and promote the formation of creatine phosphate in muscle [66, 67]. The importance of creatine phosphate was further suggested by studies demonstrating that a portion of the MM isozyme of creatine kinase is bound to the myofibril [61, 62]. Creatine kinase has been further localized to the M line of muscle and interacts with myosin [63]. Since ATPase is also localized to the myosin molecule, this suggests that a functional coupling between creatine kinase and ATPase may occur. This association was first suggested by studies utilizing purified myofibrils with both the creatine kinase and ATPase activities intact. These studies indicated that ATP generated from creatine phosphate by the creatine kinase reaction is used in preference to free ATP in the ATPase reaction [68]. Thus, functional coupling of the myofibrillar creatine kinase and ATPase reactions was demonstrated. The low diffusion coefficient for ATP compared with creatine phosphate, and the preference of the myosin ATPase for ATP generated from creatine phosphate by the creatine kinase reaction, suggest that the transduction of energy from the intramembrane space of the mitochondria to the myofibril occurs via creatine phosphate, and the creatine liberated at the myofibril is the intermediate that links energy utilization at the myofibril with energy production in the mitochondria.

The concept of the creatine phosphate shuttle as a mechanism of energy transduction in the myocyte can be summarized as follows (figure 3-2). ATP synthesized in the matrix of the mitochondria is transported across the inner membrane by adenine nucleotide translocase. The translocase is functionally coupled to a specific isozyme of creatine kinase localized on the outer surface of the inner mitochondrial membrane. The ATP transported from the matrix is used to synthesize creatine phosphate, and ADP thus generated is transported back into the matrix by the translocase. The translocase allows high ATP concentrations and low ADP concentrations at the site of creatine kinase binding, and thus the creatine kinase reaction is pulled in the direction of creatine phosphate formation. The newly synthesized creatine phosphate diffuses to the myofibril, where an isozyme of creatine kinase is bound to myosin and is used to phosphorylate ADP. The ATP thus formed provides substrate for the myosin ATPase. The creatine generated diffuses back to the mitochondria to modulate respiration and to provide substrate for further creatine phosphate formation.

ALTERATIONS IN THE COMPONENTS OF ENERGY TRANSPORT DURING ISCHEMIA AND REPERFUSION

Myocardial ischemia has been postulated to produce alterations in each step of energy transduction from the mitochondria to the myofibril. Adenine nucleotide translocase is inhibited during myocardial ischemia [69]. This inhibition may be due to the accumulation of long-chained fatty acids, or may be secondary to depletion of intramitochondrial adenine nucleotides [70]. The next step in energy transduction, the phosphorylation of creatine by ATP, is catalyzed by the mitochondrial creatine kinase on the inner mitochondrial membrane. It has been shown in vitro that, under conditions that simulate ischemia, creatine kinase dissociates from the mitochondria [71]. It is unclear whether the in vitro dissociation is reversible when perfusion is restored, but in vivo studies indicate that reversible binding does not occur during reperfusion. Another observation made during reperfusion after brief ischemia is that the creatine phosphate content of the myocyte increases rapidly to above-normal levels [16, 18]. This rapid resynthesis of creatine phosphate indicates that the mitochon-

drial creatine kinase is at least partially functional, and suggests a defect in creatine phosphate utilization at the myofibril. The high-energy bond of creatine phosphate is transferred to free ADP by the creatine kinase on the myofibril and at other sites in the myocyte. If the ADP content were limiting, then creatine phosphate might be expected to accumulate.

Previous studies indicate that the total ADP content of the myocyte is decreased during the reperfusion period following reversible ischemia [18]. Less than 10% of the ADP of the cell is free while over 90% is bound to contractile proteins and thus unable to participate in the creatine kinase reaction [72]. It is unclear whether the decrease in ADP content seen in the post ischemic period occurs from changes in free ADP or from changes in the content of ADP bound to actin. A decrease in free-ADP content would not only account for the overshoot in creatine phosphate, but may also influence the contractile properties of the myocyte. The Km of ADP for myofibrillar creatine kinase has been estimated to be 77 μM [73, 74], greater than the estimated concentration of free ADP in the cell (40 μM). Myofibrillar creatine kinase has also been shown to be functionally coupled to the myosin ATPase. Thus, a decrease in the free-ADP concentration, such as may occur with ischemia, could slow the myofibrillar creatine kinase reaction and in turn decrease the ATPase reaction with a concomitant decrease in contractility. Another explanation for the rebound in creatine phosphate would be a dissociation of creatine kinase from the myofibril, similar to that seen in the mitochondria with ischemia. Dissociation of myofibrillar creatine kinase might also account for the contractile abnormalities seen in the reperfusion period.

References

1. Wyngaarden JB, Kelley WN: Gout. In: Stanbury JB, Wyngaarden JB, Fredrickson DS, Goldstein JL, Brown MS, (eds) The metabolic basis of inherited disease. New York: McGraw-Hill, 1983, pp. 1043–1114.
2. Holmes EW: Regulation of purine biosynthesis de novo. Handbook Exp Pharmacol 51:20–41, 1978.
3. Henderson JF: Kinetic properties of hypoxan-

thine—guanine and adenine phosphoribosyltrans-
ferases. Fed Proc 27:1053—1054, 1968.

4. Krenitsky TA, Papaioannou R, Elion GB:
Human hypoxanthine phosphoribosyltransferase.
I. Purification, properties, and specificity.
J. Biol Chem 244:1263—1270, 1969.

5. Namm DH: Myocardial nucleotide synthesis from
purine bases and nucleosides: comparison of the
rates of formation of purine nucleotides from
various precursors and identification of the enzymatic routes for nucleotide formation in the
isolated rat heart. Circ Res 33:686—695, 1973.

6. Reibel DK, Rovetto MJ: Myocardial adenosine
salvage rates and restoration of ATP content following ischemia. Am J Physiol 237:H247—252,
1979.

7. Goldthwait DA: Mechanisms of synthesis of purine nucleotides in heart muscle extracts. J Clin
Invest 36:1572—1578, 1957.

8. Zimmer HG, Ibel H, Steinhopff G, Korb G:
Reduction of the isoproterenol-induced alterations in cardiac adenine nucleotides. Science 207:
319—321, 1980.

9. Hearse DJ: Oxygen deprivation and early myocardial contractile failure: a reassessment of the
possible role of adenosine triphosphate. Am J
Cardiol 44:1115—1121, 1979.

10. Rovetto MJ: Energy metabolism in the ischemic
heart. Tex Rep Biol Med 39:397—407, 1979.

11. Neely JR, Morgan HE: Relationship between
carbohydrate and lipid metabolism and the energy balance of heart muscle. Annu Rev Physiol
36:413—459, 1974.

12. Zimmer HG, Trendelenburg C, Kammermeier
H, Gerlach E: De novo synthesis of adenine nucleotides in the rat: acceleration during recovery
from oxygen deficiency. Circ Res 32:635—642,
1973.

13. Whitmer JT, Idell-Wenger JA, Rovetto MJ,
Neely R: Control of fatty acid metabolism in
ischemic and hypoxic hearts. J Biol Chem 253:
4305—4309, 1978.

14. Siess M: Some aspects on the regulation of carbohydrate and lipid metabolism in cardiac tissue.
Basic Res Cardiol 75:47—56, 1980.

15. Rovetto MJ, Lamberton WF, Neely JR: Mechanisms of glycolytic inhibition in ischemic rat
hearts. Circ Res 37:742—751, 1975.

16. Vial C, Font B, Goldschmidt D, Pearlman AS,
Delaye J: Regional myocardial energetics during
brief periods of coronary occlusion and reperfusion: comparison with S-T segment changes.
Cardiovasc Res 12:470—476, 1978.

17. De Boer LWV, Ingwall JS, Kloner RA, Braun-

wald E: Prolonged derangements of canine myocardial purine metabolism after a brief coronary
artery occlusion not associated with anatomic
evidence of necrosis. Proc Natl Acad Sci USA
77:5471—5475, 1980.

18. Swain JL, Sabina RL, McHale PA, Greenfield JC
Jr, Holmes EW: Prolonged myocardial nucleotide depletion after brief ischemia in the open-
chest dog. Am J Physiol 242:H818—H826,
1982.

19. Arch JRS, Newsholme EA: Activities and some
properties of 5'-nucleotidase, adenosine kinase
and adenosine deaminase in tissues from verte-
brates and invertebrates in relation to the control
of the concentration and the physiological role of
adenosine. Biochem J 174:965—977, 1978.

20. Braunwald E, Kloner RA: The stunned myocardium: prolonged, postischemic ventricular dysfunction. Circulation 66:1146—1149, 1982.

21. Mochizuki S, Neely JR: Energy metabolism during reperfusion following ischemia. J Physiol
(Paris) 76:805—812, 1980.

22. Heyndrickx GR, Millard RW, McRitchie RJ,
Maroko PR, Vatner SF: Regional myocardial
function and electrophysiological alterations after
brief coronary artery occlusion in conscious dogs.
J Clin Invest 56:978—985, 1975.

23. Arentzen CE, Schneider JR, Ring WR, Visner
MS, Anderson RW: Prolonged alteration of myocardial material properties following transient
ischemia. Circulation (Suppl) 59:II-28, 1978.

24. Weiner JM, Apstein CS, Arthur JH, Pirzda FA,
Hood WB Jr: Persistence of myocardial injury
following brief periods of coronary occlusion.
Cardiovasc Res 10:678—686, 1976.

25. Zimmer HG, Gerlach E: Stimulation of myocardial adenine nucleotide biosynthesis by pentoses and pentitols. Pflugers Arch 376:223—
227, 1978.

26. Zimmer HG: Restitution of myocardial adenine
nucleotides: acceleration by administration of ribose. J Physiol (Paris) 76:769—775, 1980.

27. Wiedmeier VT, Rubio R, Berne RM: Inosine
incorporation into myocardial nucleotides. J Mol
Cell Cardiol 4:445—452, 1972.

28. Jones CE, Thomas JX, Devous MD, Norris CP,
Smith EE: Positive inotropic response to inosine
in the in situ canine heart. Am J Physiol 233:
H438—443, 1977.

29. Woollard KV, Kingaby RO, Lab MJ, Cole
AWG, Palmer TN: Inosine as a selective inotropic agent on ischaemic myocardium? Cardiovasc Res 15:659—667, 1981.

30. Olsson RA, Snow JA, Gentry MK, Frick GP:

Adenosine uptake by canine heart. Circ Res 31: 767–778, 1972.

31. Foker JE, Einzig S, Wang T: Adenosine metabolism and myocardial preservation. J Thorac Cardiovasc Surg 80:506–516, 1980.

32. Humphrey SM, Seelye RN: Improved functional recovery of ischemic myocardium by suppression of adenosine catabolism. J Thorac Cardiovasc Surg 84:6–27, 1982.

33. Silverman NA, Kohler J, Feinberg H, Levitsky S: Beneficial metabolic effect of nucleoside augmentation on reperfusion injury following cardioplegic arrest. Chest 83:787–792, 1983.

34. Rubio R, Belardinelli L, Thompson CI, Berne RM: Cardiac adenosine. In: Baer HP, Brummond GI (eds) Physiological and regulatory functions of adenosine and adenine nucleotides. New York: Raven, 1979, pp. 167–182.

35. Isselhard W, Eitenmuller J, Maurer W, De Vreese A, Reineke H, Czerniak A, Sturz J, Herb HG: Increase in myocardial adenine nucleotides induced by adenosine: dosage, mode of application and duration, species differences. J Mol Cell Cardiol 12:619–634, 1980.

36. Osswald H, Spillman WS, Knox FG: Mechanism of adenosine-mediated decrease in glomerular filtration rate in dogs. Circ Res 43:465–469, 1978.

37. Swain JL, Hines JJ, Sabina RL, Holmes EW: Accelerated repletion of ATP and GTP pools in postischemic myocardium using a precursor of purine de novo synthesis. Circ Res 51:102–105, 1982.

38. Sabina RL, Kernstine KH, Boyd RL, Holmes EW, Swain JL: Metabolism of 5-amino-4-imidazolecarboxamide riboside in cardiac and skeletal muscle: effects on purine nucleotide synthesis. J Biol Chem 257:10178–10183, 1982.

39. Sabina RL, Patterson D, Holmes EW: 5-amino-4-imidazolecarboxamide (z-base) metabolism in eukaryotic cells. J Biol Chem (In press).

40. Brox LW: The cleavage of adenylosuccinate and 5-amino-4-imidazole-N-succino-carboxamide ribonucleotide by an adenylosuccinate lyase from Ehrlich ascites tumor cells. Can J Biochem 51: 1072–1076, 1973.

41. Illingworth JA, Ford WCL, Kobayashi K, Williamson JR: Regulation of myocardial energy metabolism. In: Roy PE, Harris P (eds) Recent advances in studies on cardiac structure and metabolism, vol 8: the cardiac sarcoplasm. Baltimore: University Park Press, 1975, pp. 271–298.

42. Randle PJ: Regulation of glycolysis and pyruvate oxidation in cardiac muscle. Circ Res (Suppl 1) 38:I-8–15, 1976.

43. Shrago E, Shug AL, Sul H, Bittar N, Folts JD: Control of energy production in myocardial ischemia. Circ Res (Suppl 1) 38:I-75–79, 1976.

44. Opie, LH: Effects of regional ischemia on metabolism of glucose and fatty acids. Circ Res (Suppl 1) 38:I-52–74, 1976.

45. Vary TC, Reibel DK, Neely JR: Control of energy metabolism of heart muscle. Annu Rev Physiol 43:419–430, 1981.

46. Rovetto MJ: Myocardial metabolism. In: Cardiac pharmacology. New York: Academic, 1981, pp. 335–359.

47. Infante AA, Davies RE: The effect of 2,4-dinitrofluorobenzene on the activity of striated muscle. J Biol Chem 210:3996–4001, 1965.

48. Klingenberg M, Heldt HW: The ADP/ATP translocation in mitochondria and its role in intracellular compartmentation. In: Sies H (ed) Metabolic compartmentation. London: Academic, 1982, pp. 101–121.

49. Saks VA, Rosenshtraukh, Smirnov VN, Chazov EI: Role of creatine phosphokinase in cellular function and metabolism. Can J Pharmacol 56: 691–706, 1978.

50. Bessman SP, Geiger PJ: Transport of energy in muscle: the phosphorylcreatine shuttle. Science 211:448–452, 1981.

51. Saks VA, Kupriyanov VV: Intracellular energy transport and control of cardiac contraction. In: Chazov E, Smirnov V, Dhalla NS (eds) Advances in myocardiology, vol 3. New York: Plenum Medical, 1982, pp. 475–497.

52. Jacobs H, Heldt HW, Klingenberg M: High activity of creatine kinase in mitochondria from muscle and brain and evidence for a separate mitochondrial isozyme for creatine kinase. Biochem Biophys Res Commun 16:516–521, 1964.

53. Saks VA, Chernousova GB, Voronkov II, Smirnov VN, Chazov EI: Study of energy transport mechanism in myocardial cells. Circ Res (Suppl 3) 34:III-138–148, 1974.

54. Saks VA, Kupriyanov VV, Elizarova GV, Jacobus WE: Studies of energy transport in heart cells. J Biol Chem 255:755–763, 1980.

55. Moreadith RW, Jacobus WE: Creatine kinase of heart mitochondria. J Biol Chem 257:899–905, 1982.

56. Jacobus WE, Saks VA: Creatine kinase of heart mitochondria: changes in its kinetic properties induced by coupling to oxidative phosphorylation. Arch Biochem Biophys 219:167–178, 1982.

57. Yang WCT, Geiger PJ, Bessman SP, Bonrebaek B: Formation of creatine phosphate from creatine and ^{32}P-labelled ATP by isolated rabbit heart mitochondria. Biochem Biophys Res Commun 76:882–887, 1977.

58. Levitskii DO, Levchenko TS, Saks VA, Sharov VG, Smirnov WN: Functional coupling between Ca^{2+}-ATPase and creatine phosphokinase in sarcoplasmic reticulum of myocardium. Biokhimiya 42:1766–1773, 1977.

59. Saks VA, Lipina NV, Sharov VG, Smirnov VN, Chazov E, Grosse R: The localization of the MM isozyme of creatine phosphokinase on the surface membrane of myocardial cells and its functional coupling to ouabain-inhibited (Na^+,K^+)-ATPase. Biochim Biophys Acta 465:550–558, 1977.

60. Grosse R, Spitzer E, Kupriyanov VV, Saks VA, Repke KRH: Coordinate interplay between (Na^++K^+)-ATPase and creatine phosphokinase optimizes (Na^+/K^+)-antiport across the membrane of vesicles formed from the plasma membrane of cardiac muscle cell. Biochim Biophys Acta 603:142–156, 1980.

61. Turner DC, Wallimann T, Eppenberger HM: A protein that binds specifically to the M-line of skeletal muscle is identified as the muscle form of creatine kinase. Proc Natl Acad Sci USA 70:702–705, 1973.

62. Scholte HR: On the triple localization of creatine kinase in heart and skeletal muscle cells of the rat: evidence for the existence of myofibrillar and mitochondrial isoenzymes. Biochim Biophys Acta 305:413–427, 1973.

63. Mani RS, Kay CM: Physiochemical studies on the creatine kinase M-line protein and its interaction with the myosin and myosin fragments. Biochim Biophys Acta 453:391–399, 1976.

64. Sperelakis N, Schneider JA: A metabolic control mechanism for calcium ion influx that may protect the ventricular myocardial cell. Am J Cardiol 37:1079–1085, 1976.

65. Cain DF, Davis RE: Breakdown of adenosine triphosphate during a single contraction of working muscle. Biochem Biophys Res Commun 8:361–366, 1962.

66. Jacobus WE, Lehninger AL: Creatine kinase of rat heart mitochondria. J Biol Chem 248:4803–4810, 1973.

67. Seraydarian MW, Artaza L, Abbott BC: Creatine and the control of energy metabolism in cardiac and skeletal muscle cells in culture. J Mol Cell Cardiol 6:405–413, 1974.

68. Bessman SP, Yang WCT, Geiger PJ, Erickson-Virtanen S: Intimate coupling of creatine phosphokinase and myofibrillar adenosine triphosphatase. Biochem Biophys Res Commun 96:1414–1420, 1980.

69. La Noue KF, Watts JA, Koch CD: Adenine nucleotide transport during cardiac ischemia. Am J Physiol 241:H663–671, 1981.

70. Asimakis GK, Sordahl LA: Intramitochondrial adenine nucleotides and energy-linked functions of heart mitochondria. Am J Physiol 241:H672–678, 1981.

71. Jacobus WE, Bittl JA, Weisfeldt ML: Loss of mitochondrial creatine kinase in vitro and in vivo: a sensitive index of ischemic cellular and functional damage. In: Jacobus WE, Ingwall JS (eds) Heart creatine kinase. Baltimore: Williams and Wilkins, 1980, pp. 155–175.

72. McGilvery RW, Murry TW: Calculated equilibria of phosphocreatine and adenosine phosphates during utilization of high energy phosphate by muscle. J Biol Chem 249:5845–5850, 1974.

73. Saks VA, Lipina NV, Lyvlina NV, Chernousova GB, Fetter R, Smirnov VN, Chazov EI: Functional characterization of creatine phosphokinase reactions in heart mitochondria and myofibrils. Biokhimiya 41:1460–1470, 1976.

74. Saks VA, Chernousova GB, Vetter R, Smirnov WN, Chazov EI: Kinetic properties and the functional role of particulate MM-isoenzyme of creatine phosphokinase bound to heart muscle myofibrils. FEBS Lett 62:293–296, 1976.

4. THE PATHOPHYSIOLOGY OF ATHEROSCLEROSIS OF THE CORONARY ARTERIES AND THE CHANGES THAT PREDISPOSE TO ISCHEMIC HEART DISEASE

John T. Fallon

Each year, over a million Americans have myocardial infarctions and over a half a million die from ischemic heart disease and its complications. During the past decade, both the incidence of myocardial infarction and the mortality of ischemic heart disease have decreased. It is unclear why the former has occurred, although it is suggested to be a consequence of the recognition of the major risk factors of coronary artery disease and the public health measures applied to reduce these risk factors. The decline in mortality of acute myocardial infarction is partially explained by the introduction of new medical and surgical therapies directed toward its major complications. Despite these apparently successful interventions, ischemic heart disease remains the number one cause of mortality in Western man. Although a great deal has been learned about the major cause of ischemic heart disease, i.e., coronary atherosclerosis, this disease remains an enigma, both in its pathogenesis and in the biology of its complications [1].

Atherosclerosis of the major epicardial coronary arteries is responsible for 98% of all cases of ischemic heart disease by causing narrowing and occlusion of the arterial lumens, restricting or ceasing oxygen delivery to the myocardium [2]. Other causes of ischemic heart disease include aortic inflammatory diseases producing coronary ostial stenosis; dissecting aneurysm of the aorta, involving the ostia of the coronary arteries; embolism and thromboembolism; arteritis; "small vessel disease"; spasm; and anomalous or aberrant coronary arteries. Other factors contributing to ischemic heart disease include myocardial hypertrophy, valvular heart disease, hypotension or shock, anemia, and anoxia.

Coronary Arterial Anatomy and Function

The pathogenesis of atherosclerosis lies in the response of the vascular wall and its interaction with the blood-borne elements. To understand the process of atherosclerosis it is important to review the known structure and function of the components of the coronary arterial wall. The normal coronary arteries are highly compliant, distensible vessels. Microscopically, there are three layers: intima, media, and adventitia. The intima consists of a continuous layer of endothelial cells lying on a thin layer of extracellular matrix. The media consists of circumferentially oriented smooth muscle cells, collagen, and small amounts of elastic tissue. The adventitia contains a loosely arranged collagen network, a moderate amount of lamellar elastic tissue, a few fibroblasts and smooth muscle cells, and the vasa vasorum. Distinct internal and external elastic

R.M. Califf and G.S. Wagner (eds.), ACUTE CORONARY CARE: Principles and Practice. Copyright © 1985. Martinus Nijhoff Publishing, Boston/Dordrecht/Lancaster.

lamina separate intima from media and media from adventitia, respectively.

The endothelium of the coronary arteries consists of a single layer of flattened, fairly uniform, polygonal and elongated cells, 1–3 microns thick, 25–50 microns long, and 10–15 microns wide. The long axis of the endothelial cells is oriented in the direction of blood flow. The intercellular space is closed by special membrane structures. Endothelial cells contain the usual compliment of cell organelles and in addition contain a large number of micropinocytotic vesicles, many of which open onto the luminal and abluminal surfaces. One organelle called the Weibel-Palade body is distinctive for endothelial cells. Endothelial cells turn over slowly. Growth is stringently controlled by "contact inhibition," that is, once confluent, endothelial cells cannot be stimulated to make DNA or replicate. The endothelium functions as a barrier between the blood elements and the medial components of the arterial wall. Selective permeability is a function of the intercellular junctions for small molecules and the micropinocytotic vesicles for large molecules. Nonthrombogenicity is a passive property of the luminal "glycocalyx" composed of acidic glycoproteins, including heparin, which form a blood-compatible surface shielding the blood from tissue elements capable of activating coagulation. The endothelium actively inhibits clotting through synthesis and release of prostacyclin and plasminogen activator and also by binding activated coagulation factors and degrading potentially thrombogenic substances such as thromboxane and ADP. The endothelium also synthesizes factor VIII, the collagen and elastin of the subendothelial space, and factors that control medial smooth muscle cell growth and proliferation.

The medial smooth muscle cells are spindle shaped, 75–100 microns long, and up to 25 microns in diameter. They are arranged circumferentially in layers with a slight spiraling angle. Smooth muscle cells contain a central elongated nucleus with the usual cell organelles located at or near the nuclear poles. The cytoplasm or sarcoplasm is filled by thin actin filaments and dense bodies, the latter corresponding to the Z bands of striated muscle. Smooth muscle cell myosin is in a soluble nonfibrillar form. The plasma membrane or sarcolemma contains numerous micropinocytotic vesicles. A prominent basement membrane is also present. The functions of the smooth muscle cell include contraction, to maintain active compliance of the arterial wall, synthesis and maintenance of the extracellular connective tissues of the media, and a variety of quasi-macrophagic activities. Growth and proliferation of smooth muscle cell are under hormonal control. Substances produced by the endothelial cells inhibit proliferation, whereas several serum factors, including platelet-derived growth factor (PDGF), are stimulatory to the smooth muscle cells.

The extracellular matrix of the intima and the media is composed of collagen (types I, III, and IV), elastin, and various glycoconjugates. The matrix serves as a scaffolding for the cellular elements, a permeability filter, and as a potential reservoir for binding of blood components. The matrix is responsible for the passive compliance of the arterial wall.

Risk Factors for Atherosclerosis

In general, coronary artery disease increases in severity with age. It is not simply the result of unmodified intrinsic biologic aging processes, however, since most mammalian species age without spontaneously developing the disease-producing lesions of atherosclerosis. Males are affected more frequently than females with the differences tending to diminish with increasing age. Hereditary factors influence the severity of coronary atherosclerosis, directly by affecting arterial wall structure and function and indirectly via such factors as hypertension, hyperlipidemia, diabetes, and the environment. The severity of clinically apparent ischemic heart disease due to coronary atherosclerosis is influenced by a number of associated risk factors. The risk for developing clinical ischemic heart disease is increased by high-fat diets, hypertension, and smoking. It is potentially increased in patients with diabetes mellitus, gout, hypothyroidism, renal disease, and a familial history of premature atherosclerosis. Other factors with an uncertain role include sedentary life style, obesity, and emotional tension. It is now felt that the risk for developing clinical disease is potentially decreased with low-fat diets (see chapter 15), increased levels of exercise (see chapter 58), and increased levels of high-density lipoproteins.

Pathogenesis and Development of Coronary Atherosclerosis

Atherosclerosis is characterized by thickening of the intima due to smooth muscle cell proliferation and degeneration, and the deposition of abundant lipid, extracellular matrix proteins, necrotic debris, and calcium. The pathogenesis of atherosclerosis is complicated by the many factors that are involved: aging, hemodynamics, lipids, thrombi, and the cells of the arterial wall. Each of these major factors forms the basis of a theory of atherogenesis. However, atherogenesis clearly involves all of these factors to varying degrees and each is important in the genesis of the three types of morphologically distinct atherosclerotic plaques: the fibromuscular plaque, the simple atherosclerotic plaque (atheroma), and the complicated atherosclerotic plaque.

The intima of the coronary arteries is essentially devoid of smooth muscle cells in early life. With age, the subendothelial space is increasingly populated with smooth muscle cells and extracellular matrix. The process of intimal thickening as well as the genesis of the early atherosclerotic plaque is initiated by injury to the endothelium resulting in its physical or functional disruption [3]. The loss of the selective permeability function of the endothelium provides a point of entry for blood plasma constituents such as low-density lipoproteins (LDL). The loss of the nonthrombogenic and antithrombogenic functions results in the attachment of formed blood elements such as platelets and leukocytes to the luminal surface of the arterial wall and the formation of platelet-rich mural thrombi. Adherent platelets release PDGF, which induces the proliferation of smooth muscle cell and initiates their migration into the intima. There, these "modified" smooth muscle cells produce connective tissue in a fashion reminiscent of a healing wound and actively take up lipids and proteins that continue to infiltrate and accumulate in the intima. Monocytes migrate into the intima and also take up lipids, further stimulating plaque formation. The endothelium is slowly replaced in

normal adjacent areas by migration and mitosis. Once the endothelium is replaced, the stimulus to intimal plaque formation is reduced and regression ensues by resorption and reorganization, but the intimal thickening remains.

The normal aging process of intimal thickening is accentuated at sites of predilection for the occurrence of atherosclerotic lesions. These sites are located at bifurcations, branchings, curves, and points of widening where "hemodynamic stress" is maximal. At these sites, the endothelium is continually overstressed and this process of injury and repair is accentuated. This results in the formation of the earliest form of the atherosclerotic plaque, the fibromuscular plaque. These are localized, often eccentric, intimal lesions consisting of smooth muscle cells, monocytes, connective tissue, and variable amounts of intracellular and extracellular lipid. Normally such plaques do not significantly obstruct luminal blood flow. However, because of their position in the intima and the presence of large amounts of connective tissue, these lesions reduce the normal compliance of the coronary arteries by restricting the local arterial wall from expanding. The fibromuscular plaque is an area of altered permeability and intimal change predisposing to further endothelial injury, smooth muscle cell proliferation, connective tissue production, and lipid accumulation.

The progression from a fibromuscular plaque to an atheroma is a prolonged process that probably takes many years and is likely linked to the presence of the positive risk factors, e.g., elevated blood cholesterol. The fibromuscular plaque is converted into an atheroma by the process of combined endothelial injury, smooth muscle proliferation, the incorporation of both cellular and soluble blood components and cell necrosis. Morphologically, the atheroma is characterized by a central core of necrotic debris and lipids, mostly cholesterol, that is encased by a thin fibrous cap on the luminal surface and by the media below. In contrast to the fibromuscular plaques, atheroma may cause significant luminal stenosis and are often responsible for the earliest clinical symptoms of ischemic heart disease: angina pectoris, acute myocardial infarction, and sudden death [4–7].

Atheroma are converted into complicated atherosclerotic plaques as a result of necrosis, vascularization, hemorrhage, ulceration, thrombosis, and calcification. Progression from an atheroma to a complicated plaque is also a protracted process. Histologically, the complicated plaque appears similar to the atheroma (figure 4-1). There is a central core of cholesterol and necrotic debris, but in addition there is ingrowth of small endothelial-lined vessels from the vasa vasorum, destruction of the internal elastic lamina and thinning of the underlying media, and calcification of the base of the plaque. An inflammatory infiltrate composed of lymphocytes, plasma cells, macrophages, and multinucleated giant cells is often evident. Areas of hemorrhage are commonly present within the plaque (figure 4-2). Once formed, the complicated plaque is the underlying cause of events responsible for the rapid and unpredictable occurrence of unstable angina [8, 9] and acute myocardial infarction [4].

Pathology of Coronary Thrombosis

It is currently well appreciated that coronary thrombosis is the direct cause of most acute myocardial infarcts (see chapter 6). Furthermore, our own studies [10, 11] and those of others [12 − 16] indicate that the underlying cause of coronary thrombosis is ulceration of a complicated atherosclerotic plaque. The sequence of events leading to plaque ulceration is still obscure although several factors are implicated by pathologic and angiographic studies: neovascularization [13, 17], intraplaque hemorrhage [18 − 21], and spasm [22 − 26]. The following is a probable scenario of the role these three factors play. Due to their fragile makeup, the neovascular channels are the source of intraplaque hemorrhage, which itself has the untoward effect of adding substance to the plaque [27]. Extensive intraplaque hemorrhage results in localized spasm (by increasing the local concentration of circulating vasospastic substances) of the adjacent uninvolved artery (see chapter 5) and/or the frank ulceration of the plaque (figure 4-3). Plaque ulceration, in turn, results in either the release of the necrotic atheromatous debris or, more commonly, the rapid

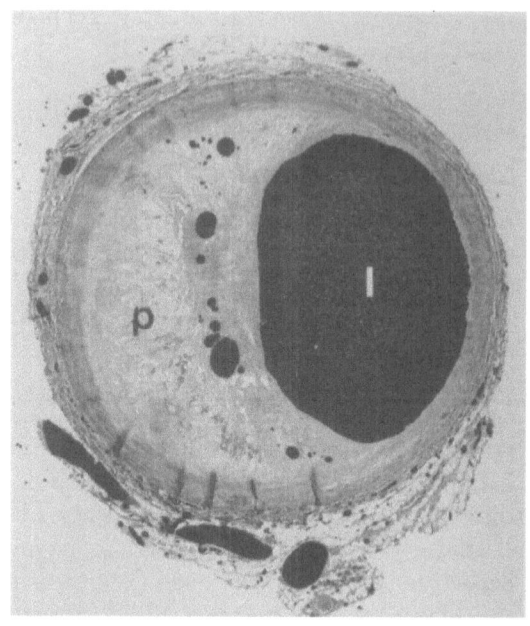

FIGURE 4-1. Photomicrograph of a human coronary artery containing a typical, eccentric complicated atherosclerotic plaque. The lumen (1) is filled by postmortem angiography dye as are the numerous neovascular channels in the plaque (p). Original magnification ×16.

formation of a platelet-rich thrombus on the ulcerated surface [28]. This mural thrombus is stabilized by fibrin and undergoes varying degrees of thrombolysis and/or incorporation into the plaque. Organization of the thrombus further increases plaque size and the degree of luminal plaque stenosis (figure 4-4). This process of intraplaque hemorrhage, plaque ulceration, mural thrombosis, and incorporation of the thrombus into the plaque continues cyclically [29, 30]. Eventually, when the degree of luminal stenosis is great enough to effect a decrease in luminal blood flow, the mural thrombus propagates and an occlusive thrombus results (figure 4-4).

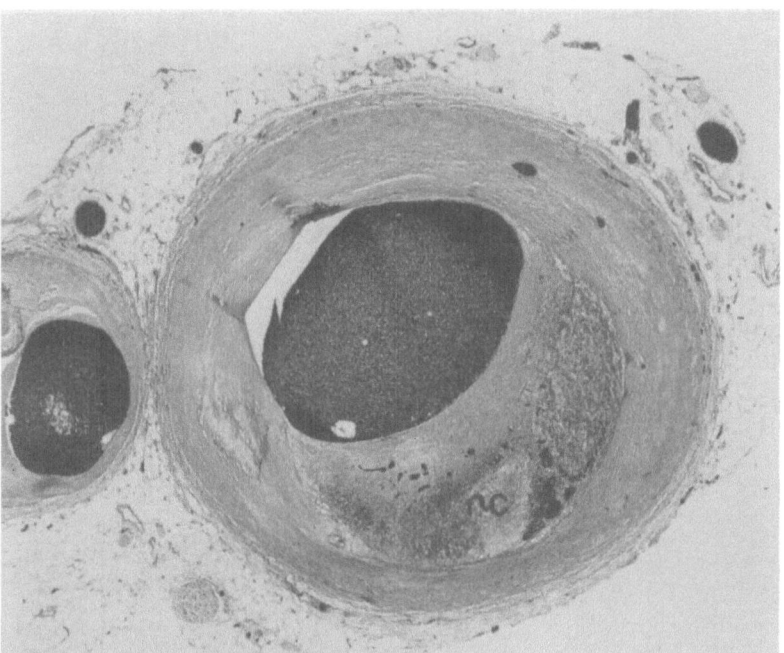

FIGURE 4-2. Another section of coronary artery showing a complicated plaque with intraplaque hemorrhage seen here as a darker staining of the necrotic
center (nc). Note also the presence of neovascular
channels. Original magnification ×16.

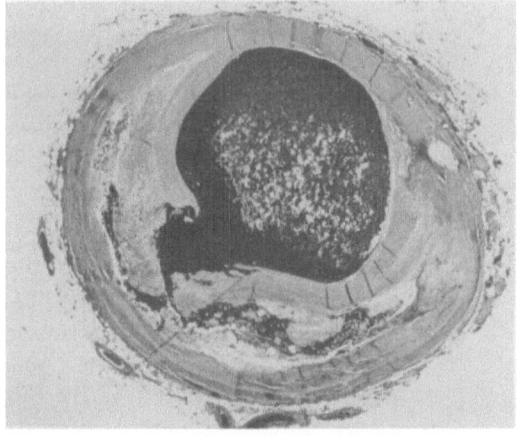

FIGURE 4-3. This section reveals rupture of the fibrous
cap of a complicated atherosclerotic coronary lesion.
The angiographic dye is clearly seen to penetrate the
plaque and is mixed with platelet-rich thrombus
within the plaque. Original magnification ×16.

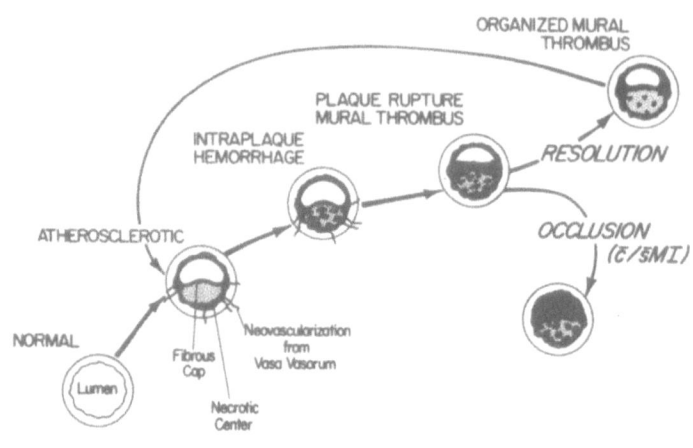

References

1. Friedman M: The pathogenesis of coronary plaques, thromboses, and hemorrhages: an evaluative review. Circulation (Suppl 3) 51−52: 34−40, 1975.
2. Roberts CS, Roberts WC: Cross-sectional area of the proximal portions of the three major epicardial coronary arteries in 98 necropsy patients with different coronary events: relationship to heart weight, age and sex. Circulation 62:953−959, 1980.
3. Ross R, Glomset JA: The pathogenesis of atherosclerosis. N Engl J Med 285:369−377 and 420−425, 1976.
4. Edwards JE: Correlations in coronary arterial disease. Bull NY Acad Med 33:199−217, 1957.
5. Fuchs RM, Becker LC: Pathogenesis of angina pectoris. Arch Intern Med 142:1685−1692, 1982.
6. Roberts WC: The coronary arteries and left ventricle in clinically isolated angina pectoris: a necropsy analysis. Circulation 54:388−390, 1976.
7. Vlodaver Z, Neufeld HN, Edwards JE: Pathology of angina pectoris. Circulation 46:1048−1064, 1972.
8. Horie T, Sekiguchi M, Hirosawa K: Case reports: relationship between myocardial infarction and preinfarction angina—a histopathological study of coronary arteries in two sudden death cases employing serial section. Am Heart J 94:81−88, 1978.
9. Roberts WC, Virmani R: Quantification of coronary arterial narrowing in clinically-isolated unstable angina pectoris: an analysis of 22 necropsy patients. Am J Med 67:792−799, 1979.
10. Fallon JT: Pathology of arterial lesions amenable to percutaneous transluminal angioplasty. Am J Radiol 135:913−916, 1980.
11. Levin DC, Fallon JT: Significance of the angiographic morphology of localized coronary stenoses: histopathologic correlations. Circulation 66:316−320, 1982.
12. Friedman M, Van Den Bovenkamp GL: The pathogenesis of a coronary thrombus. Am J Pathol 48:19−44, 1966.
13. Ridolfi RL, Hutchins GM: The relationship between coronary artery lesions and myocardial infarcts: ulceration of atherosclerotic plaques precipitating coronary thrombosis. Am Heart J 93:468−486, 1977.
14. Constantinides P: Plaque fissures in human coronary thrombosis. J Atheroscler Res 6:1−17, 1966.
15. Bouch DC, Montgomery GL: Cardiac lesions in fatal cases of recent myocardial ischemia from a coronary care unit. Br Heart J 32:795−803, 1970.
16. Chapman I: Morphogenesis of occluding coronary artery thrombosis. Arch Pathol 80: 256−261, 1965.
17. Barger AC, Beeuwkes R, Lainey LL, Silverman KJ: Hypothesis: vasorum and neovascularization of human coronary arteries—possible role in the

FIGURE 4-4. Diagramatic representation of the process of neovascularization, intraplaque hemorrhage, and plaque rupture leading to mural thrombosis with subsequent resolution or occlusion.

pathophysiology of atherosclerosis. N Engl J Med 310:175−177, 1984.

18. Paterson JC: Capillary rupture with intimal hemorrhage as a causative factor in coronary thrombosis. Arch Pathol 25:474−487, 1938.

19. Horn H, Finkelstein LE: Arteriosclerosis of the coronary arteries and the mechanism of their occlusion. Am Heart J 19:655−682, 1940.

20. Wartman WB: Occlusion of the coronary arteries by hemorrhage into their walls. Am Heart J 15:459−470, 1938.

21. Freidman M, Van den Bovenkamp GJ: The pathogenesis of coronary intramural heomorrhages. Br J Exp Pathol 47:347−355, 1966.

22. Oliva PB: Pathophysiology of acute myocardial infarction, 1981. 94:236−250, 1981.

23. Maseri A, Chierchia S, L'Abbate A: Pathogenetic mechanisms underlying the clinical events associated with atherosclerosis heart disease. Circulation (Suppl 5) 62:3−13, 1980.

24. De Wood MA, Spores J, Notske R, Mouser LT, Burroughs R, Golden MS, Lang HT: Prevalence of total coronary occlusion during the early hours of transmural myocardial infarction. N Engl J Med 303:897−902, 1980.

25. Zelinger AB, Abramowitz BM, Schick EC, Ryan TJ: Variant angina culminating in coronary thrombosis and myocardial infarction. Chest 82: 188−190, 1982.

26. MacAlpin RN: Relation of coronary arterial spasm to sites of organic stenosis. Am J Cardiol 46:143−153, 1980.

27. Lusby RJ, Ferrell LD, Ehrenfeld WK, Stoney RJ, Wylie EJ: Carotid plaque hemorrhage. Arch Surg 117:1479−1488, 1982.

28. Harker LA, Ritchie JL: The role of platelets in acute vascular events. Circulation (Suppl 5) 62: 13−18, 1980.

29. Chandler AB: Mechanisms and frequency of thrombosis in the coronary circulation. Thromb Res (Suppl 1) 4:3−23, 1974.

30. Neill WA, Ritzmann LW, Selden R: The pathophysiologic basis of acute coronary insufficiency: observations favoring the hypothesis of intermittent reversible coronary obstruction. Am Heart J 94:439−444, 1977.

5. THE ROLE OF CORONARY ARTERY SPASM IN ACUTE ISCHEMIC SYNDROMES

Robert A. Chahine

Our concepts of the pathophysiology of myocardial ischemia have oscillated over the years like a pendulum. For more than a century since Allan Burns in 1809 [1] suspected coronary artery spasm as a cause of angina pectoris, until Sir William Osler in 1910 stated that he could not think of a better explanation of anginal pain [2], coronary artery spasm was believed to be the primary mechanism underlying acute myocardial ischemia. The pendulum began to swing away from spasm under the influence of Keefer and Resnik, who in the 1920s questioned the ability of rigid atherosclerotic coronary arteries to constrict or go into spasm [3]. Shortly after, Blumgart and co-workers focused attention on the association between the clinical history of angina and the finding of coronary atherosclerosis at autopsy [4]. Subsequently, the failure to find coronary artery spasm with any significant frequency during the first decade of coronary arteriography helped to shift thinking further away from spasm.

In the early 1970s, the documentation of coronary artery spasm as the etiologic mechanism underlying the chest-pain attacks in patients with Prinzmetal's variant angina reinitiated the movement of the pendulum again toward spasm [5–10]. Shortly after, the appearance of some evidence suggesting a role for spasm in myocardial infarction [11–14], unstable angina [15, 16], classic angina [17, 18], and sudden death [19, 20] added momentum to the swing, and it seemed for a moment that spasm had regained a primary role in the pathophysiology of ischemic heart disease. However, the introduction of intracoronary thrombolysis during the acute phase of myocardial infarction, which provided an opportunity to document the presence of a fresh thrombus in more than 90% of patients studied [21–23], reversed the direction of thinking away from spasm [24]. Nonetheless, in view of the evidence accumulated during the past decade, the role of coronary artery spasm in the production of myocardial ischemia has become well established. It is now believed that the whole spectrum of ischemic heart disease may be accounted for by various combinations of fixed coronary obstruction secondary to atherosclerosis and transient dynamic narrowing due to spasm [25, 26]. The interrelationship between spasm and the atherosclerotic process and the relative role of each in specific clinical syndromes remain yet to be determined.

Definition of Coronary Artery Spasm

Coronary artery spasm has been defined as a reversible segmental or diffuse narrowing of a coronary artery secondary to constriction of its smooth muscle coat. A purist's definition would insist that the vascular smooth muscle contraction should be localized and be much more forceful than the normal generalized vasoconstriction that involves the rest of the vessel [27] (figures 5-1A and 5-2). It is now well recognized that vasoconstriction in response to pharmacologic or reflex stimuli may increase partial narrowings and result in complete obstruction of a segment of the

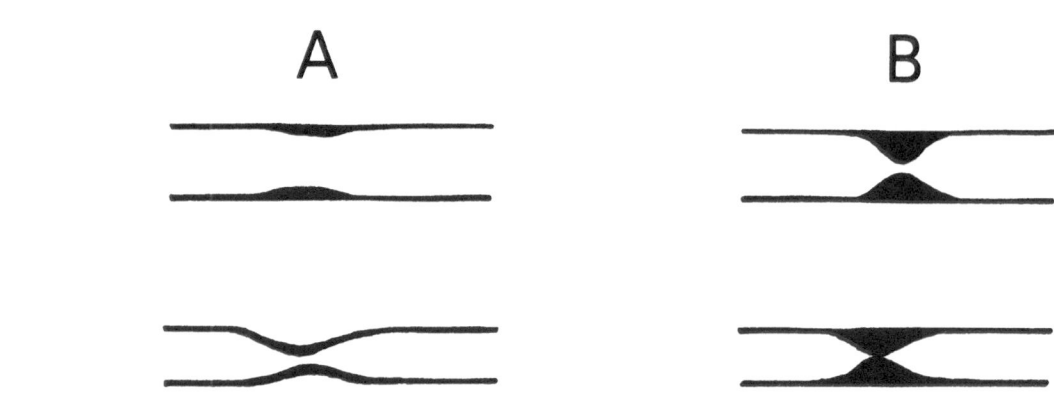

FIGURE 5-1. Types of coronary vasomotility resulting in transient coronary narrowing: (A) hypermotility of a coronary artery segment producing significant narrowing in the absence of critical atherosclerotic narrowing, and (B) diffuse vasoconstriction producing total obstruction at the site of a critical atherosclerotic lesion.

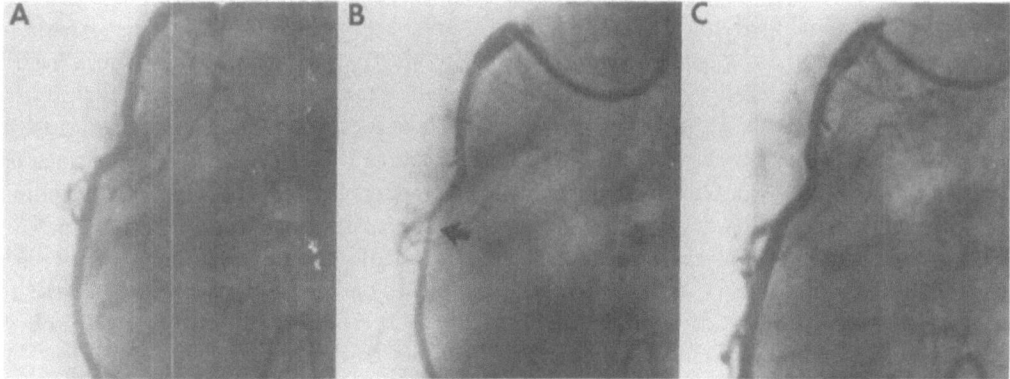

FIGURE 5-2. Cineframes of an angiographically normal or near-normal right coronary artery: (A) before the spasm and in the absence of chest pain, (B) during coronary artery spasm (arrow), and (C) after administration of nitroglycerin and relief of the spasm. From Chahine [26], with permission.

of the coronary tree (figures 5-1B and 5-3). Such a phenomenon would satisfy a broad definition of spasm as a reversible segmental narrowing of a coronary artery, but not the purist's definition. Since our current angiographic techniques do not provide enough resolution to differentiate reliably between the two mechanisms and since there is yet no clear practical value to such differentiation, the term coronary artery spasm may justifiably be utilized to encompass both situations. Therefore, a discussion of coronary artery spasm at this time would include both instances of focal hypermotility involving an angiographically normal coronary segment or a segment with minimal atherosclerosis, as well as instances of generalized coronary vasoconstriction resulting in increased focal narrowing in a coronary segment with severe or critical atherosclerotic lesion.

Some investigators have added to the definition of coronary artery spasm the necessity of evidence of myocardial ischemia resulting from the transient coronary narrowing [28]. This limi-

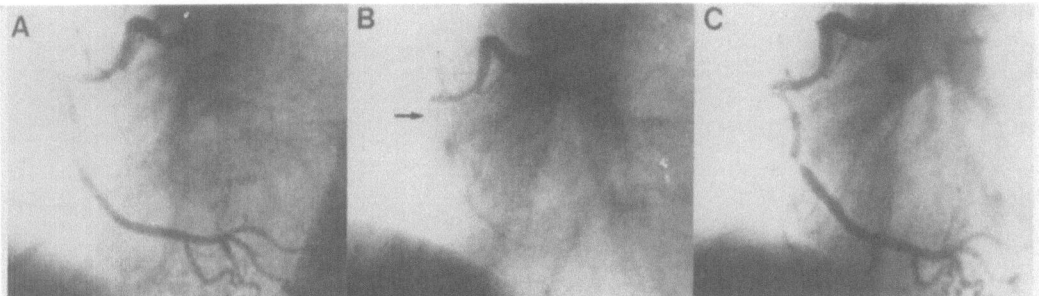

FIGURE 5-3. Cineframes of a right coronary artery with spasm occurring at the site of a significant atherosclerotic lesion: (A) coronary injection before the spasm, (B) during the spasm (arrow), and (C) after administration of nitroglycerin and relief of the spasm. From Chahine [26], with permission.

tation is also unnecessary, since it is well known that fixed obstruction may be present without manifest evidence of ischemia. Further, the clinical, biochemical, or electrocardiographic evidence of ischemia secondary to spasm depends on the severity and duration of the obstruction. Therefore, mild coronary spasm may not be associated with demonstrable ischemia.

Etiology and Pathophysiology of Coronary Artery Spasm

The mechanism of coronary artery spasm unfortunately remains largely unknown, but the great interest and extensive studies during the past decade have helped identify a number of factors that play a role in the production of spasm [29–49]:

A. Neurogenic factors (see chapter 36)
1. Parasympathetic influences
2. Alpha-adrenergic stimulation
3. Beta-adrenergic blockade
4. Reflex mechanisms
5. Corticothalmic influences

B. Intraluminal factors
1. Platelet aggregates
2. Endogenous vasoconstrictors (thromboxane A_2)
3. Metabolic or ionic factors ($Ca^{2+} \uparrow$, $H^+ \downarrow$)
4. Mechanical factors (microemboli?)

C. Other important factors
1. Atherosclerotic changes in coronary intima
2. Stress (physical or emotional)
3. Exogenous pharmacologic influences (ergot derivatives)
4. Miscellaneous exogenous factors (alcohol, smoking?)

Considering the possibility that any or all of these factors may play a role in a given instance of spasm, one could formulate a scheme as presented in figure 5-4. The neural influences may facilitate or neutralize each other; the intraluminal factors may also enhance or balance each other and may in turn be exaggerated or inhibited by the resultant effect of the neural influences. At the center of all these factors the atherosclerotic plaque appears to play an important role in predisposing a given segment of the coronary tree to spasm. It could constitute the roughened area where platelets are damaged, aggregate, and release the potent vasoconstrictor thromboxane A_2 (see chapter 4).

That a possible relationship may exist between coronary artery spasm and atherosclerosis is suggested by the high incidence of atherosclerotic findings in the majority of patients with Prinzmetal's variant angina, where clinically important spasm is well documented [42, 43, 49]. Although a small series of patients with Prinzmetal's variant angina have been reported to have angiographically normal coronary arteries [50], such cases constitute only a small minority of the overall Prinzmetal's angina population [51]. In a recent review [51] of the available series of patients with variant angina where cardiac catheterization findings were reported [29, 41, 52–55], 78% of the patients had a significant atheroscle-

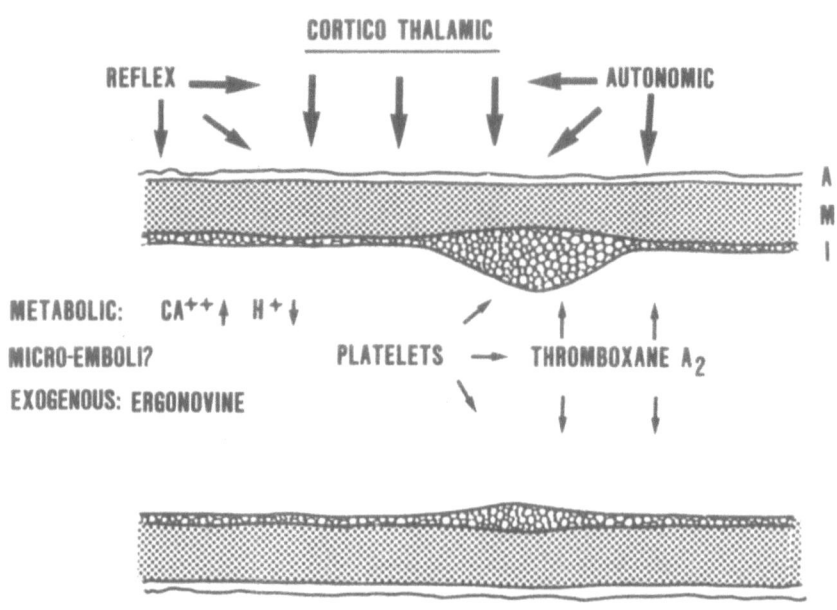

FIGURE 5-4. Schematic display of the various factors that are known to play a role in the production of coronary artery spasm. For details please see the text.

rotic lesion in one or more of the major coronary arteries (table 5-1). Of the remaining 22%, about half had evidence of minimal disease or nonobstructive plaquing. It should also be stressed that, even in those with angiographically normal coronary arteries, the possibility of small plaques that cannot be detected on routine coronary cineangiography cannot be excluded with certainty. More importantly, in 88% of the cases where an episode of coronary artery spasm was witnessed and documented, the spasm seemed to occur consistently in the vicinity of an atherosclerotic lesion [49].

Diagnosis of Coronary Artery Spasm

Coronary arteriography is the best available technique for the diagnosis of coronary artery spasm [56]. Despite some important limitations, it remains the standard to which all over diagnostic modalities are compared. Because of the prevailing skepticism about coronary spasm in the early 1970s, rigid criteria were proposed for its unequivocal documentation [30]. Two of the following three criteria must be present: (a) appearance of transient narrowing in a coronary segment that initially or subsequently appeared to be angiographically normal; (b) occurrence of transient total obstruction in a normal coronary segment or at the site of partial narrowing due to an atheromatous lesion; (c) prompt response of the narrowing or obstruction to the administration of nitroglycerin or other vasodilators or its spontaneous relief documented upon subsequent injections of the same coronary artery. These criteria, although widely used for the definitive diagnosis of severe vasospastic episodes, also have some inherent imperfections: (a) they do not include recognition of milder episodes of spasm, and (b) they do not differentiate obstruction caused by excessive focal vasomotility from generalized vasoconstriction resulting in total obstruction at the site of an atheromatous narrowing.

Radionuclide techniques have recently become popular for the diagnosis of coronary artery spasm. Thallium-201 scintigraphy is utilized to demonstrate myocardial perfusion defects in the area supplied by the artery involved with the spasm [56, 57], and radionuclide angiography is used

TABLE 5-1. Coronary anatomy in Prinzmetal's angina [51]

Author	No. of patients	Normal or minimal disease	One-vessel disease	Two-vessel disease	Three-vessel disease	Left main disease
MacAlpin et al., 1973 [52]	19	2	14	0	1	2
Shubrooks et al., 1975 [53]	20	3	5	9	2	1
Endo et al., 1975 [29]	35	19	9	7	0	—
Higgins et al., 1976 [54]	17	8	4	3	2	—
Johnson et al., 1978 [55]	42	11	16	5	10	—
Maseri et al., 1978 [14]	107	9	38	34	26	—
Total	240	52	86	58	41	3
Percent		22	35	24	17	1

to demonstrate the consequent segmental wall motion abnormalities [56, 58]. Neither of these techniques, however, differentiates with certainty transient obstruction from fixed disease. Radionuclide techniques are therefore more useful in the diagnosis of spasm in patients known to have angiographically normal coronary arteries. Coronary artery spasm may also be diagnosed by documentation of the electrocardiographic ST-segment elevation accompanying the Prinzmetal's anginal episodes and other noninvasive approaches.

Whether one attempts to diagnose the spasm by imaging techniques or other means, an attack must occur at the time of study to permit such documentation. A major advance in this perspective has been achieved by the introduction of spasm provocation techniques [59–63]. These include reflex, metabolic, and pharmacologic modalities, the latter being the most popular and ergonovine maleate being the agent of choice for this purpose. Extensive experience has now accumulated with ergonovine testing to demonstrate that this technique is highly sensitive and specific for the documentation of spasm in Prinzmetal's variant angina. Although in experienced hands this technique is reasonably safe, some rare catastrophic complications have been described [64]. Other pharmacologic agents such as methylergometrine, methacholine, epinephrine, and propranolol have also been used for spasm provocation [33, 34, 65] as well as reflex stimulation such as the cold pressor test [46] and

metabolic interventions such as hyperventilation with tris-buffer administration [39].

Electrocardiographic, Hemodynamic, and Angiographic Consequences

It is now well established that coronary artery spasm produces acute myocardial ischemia. This may be accompanied by a variety of electrocardiographic, hemodynamic, and angiographic consequences [66]. Transient, reversible ST-segment elevation in electrocardiographic leads corresponding to ischemic myocardium is now considered a hallmark for the diagnosis of coronary artery spasm. This usually reflects the transmural ischemia that is seen during Prinzmetal-type anginal episodes secondary to total or near-total obstruction of a major coronary artery. It is also well documented, however, that spasm may be accompanied by ST-segment depression or T-wave or U-wave changes. The latter ECG changes may reflect lesser degrees of spasm. All types of arrhythmias have also been documented in conjunction with severe vasospastic episodes. The most serious include severe bradyarrhythmias, ventricular tachycardia, and ventricular fibrillation.

Hemodynamically, coronary spasm may be accompanied by increases in the left and right ventricular end-diastolic pressures and by decreases in arterial pressure, cardiac output, and indices of left ventricular contractility. Contrast and radionuclide angiograms performed during acute episodes of spasm have also demonstrated transient severe alterations of segmental wall motion secondary to the spasm.

Clinical Expressions of Coronary Artery Spasm

PRINZMETAL'S VARIANT ANGINA

Prinzmetal's variant angina is characterized by attacks of chest pain occurring usually at rest with accompanying electrocardiographic ST-segment elevation corresponding to the ischemic area [67, 68]. Extensive studies during the past decade have demonstrated a definite etiologic relationship between the chest-pain attacks and the underlying coronary artery spasm [5, 10, 41, 43, 69, 70]. While more than 75% of the patients may present significant atherosclerotic lesions in their coronary tree, the spasm appears to play the crucial role that results in the characteristic clinical syndrome [51].

The vasospastic episodes appear to satisfy the following criteria: (a) severity: severe enough to produce consequent total or near-total occlusion of the involved coronary artery, resulting in transmural ischemia of the corresponding myocardial segment; (b) duration: relatively short because, if prolonged, necrosis may occur, resulting in an infarction pattern; (c) frequency: recurrence often enough to permit documentation of the typical accompanying electrocardiographic changes; and (d) occurrence: the majority of the spasm attacks occur at rest.

During the phase of clinical activity, spontaneous attacks are frequently documented during routine coronary angiography. When patients are studied during episodes of relative inactivity of the clinical syndrome, however, in most instances the attack of spasm producing the typical clinical picture can be reproduced by various techniques of provocation.

CLASSIC AND UNSTABLE ANGINA

Spontaneous coronary artery spasm has been documented in some cases of classic angina pectoris [17, 18, 71, 72]. Provocative studies in large series of patients with coronary artery disease have also shown that spasm may be provoked in a small percentage of patients with chronic effort angina [73] (table 5-2). However, that spasm may play a role in classic exertional angina is also suggested by the documentation of exercise-induced spasm. Interestingly, the documentable spasm secondary to exercise is mostly accompanied by ST-segment elevation and attacks usually tend to resemble the resting episodes of Prinzmetal's variant angina [44, 48, 74–76]. However, some episodes of exercise-induced spasm have also been documented with accompanying ST-segment depression similar to the usual attacks of classic angina [71, 72].

The incidence of documented spasm in unstable angina is clearly higher than in patients with chronic effort angina, but is less than in patients with Prinzmetal's variant angina [77]. Considering the available information in that regard, it appears that the atherosclerotic process plays a more important role in the production of chest-pain attack in unstable angina patients than in those with Prinzmetal's variant angina. On the other hand, it appears that the vasospastic element has a more important role in unstable angina than in chronic stable angina. One is therefore tempted to look at angina as a spectrum consisting of one extreme represented by patients with classic angina and fixed exercise tolerance in whom the critical atherosclerotic lesion appears to dominate the mechanisms underlying the chest pain, and another extreme represented by the Prinzmetal's variant angina patients with angiographically normal coronary arteries or minimal plaquing, where the vasospastic element dominates the pathophysiology of the ischemia. Inbetween the two extremes, one can place the patients with unstable angina and the other acute ischemic syndromes (figure 5-5).

MYOCARDIAL INFARCTION AND SUDDEN DEATH

Logically, it should be no surprise that, if an episode of spasm in a patient with Prinzmetal's angina is prolonged, myocardial necrosis may ensue and the clinical picture of infarction would become apparent. Maseri et al. have convincingly demonstrated that such instances do occur [14]. They provided objective support for the hypothesis that spasm plays a role in the production of myocardial infarction. In addition, Oliva et al. demonstrated spasm in 40% of patients present-

TABLE 5-2. Incidence of provoked spasm in patients with significant atherosclerotic lesions in the absence of Prinzmetal's angina [73]

	No. of patients	Spasm	%
Exertional angina	94	2	2.1
Effort and rest angina	73	11	15.0
Rest angina	71	13	18.0
Recent myocardial infarction	109	23	21.0
Old myocardial infarction	61	4	6.6

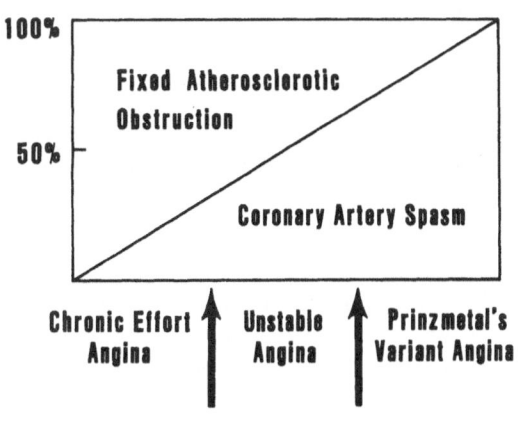

FIGURE 5-5. A theoretical display of the spectrum of angina pectoris with regard to the role of underlying fixed atherosclerotic obstruction and coronary artery spasm.

ing with acute myocardial infarction who were studied up to 12 h after the onset of the chest pain [12]. We also have our own small, unpublished series of cases where we believe that spasm was a key element in the production of infarction. Interestingly, in some patients the spasm may have triggered the formation of an occlusive thrombus, and in others the coronary artery was documented to be patent following the spasm and the acute transmural infarction. Unfortunately, we could not tell whether, in the latter situation, the spasm was the sole mechanism underlying the infarction process or whether a thrombus had formed and recanalized. It should therefore be kept in mind that the demonstration of a high incidence of coronary thrombosis during the early hours of acute myocardial infarction does not exclude the possibility of an important role for spasm in the process. It is very likely that the

spasm may be the starting phenomenon that initiates the thrombotic process. The new data from the thrombolysis studies should therefore not dampen enthusiasm for continued studies to pinpoint the exact role of coronary spasm in myocardial infarction. Further, it should be remembered that, without the current knowledge about coronary spasm, the new techniques of percutaneous transluminal coronary angioplasty and thrombolysis in acute myocardial infarction, involving intracoronary manipulation of catheters, may not have been possible. Most, if not all, of the protocols for these interventions include antispasm preparation of the patients with the administration of vasodilators such as the calcium antagonists and intracoronary nitroglycerin immediately before the procedure [21, 23, 78, 79].

It is generally believed today that the mechanisms of acute myocardial infarction include the establishment of a vicious cycle involving coronary atherosclerosis, coronary spasm, and coronary thrombosis [80–83] (figure 5-6), but the details of the interrelationships among these three elements remain to be determined.

There are also sparse reports of cases where the spasm may have been responsible for sudden death [19, 20, 77]. Documentation of the cause-and-effect relationship in such cases is not easy, but when ventricular fibrillation is documented on a 24-h Holter monitoring study following an episode of typical ST elevation of the Prinzmetal's angina type (figure 5-7), it should take extreme skepticism not to accept the hypothesis that the spasm was the trigger for the lethal arrhythmia. Further studies are definitely necessary to determine more accurately the potential role of spasm in sudden death.

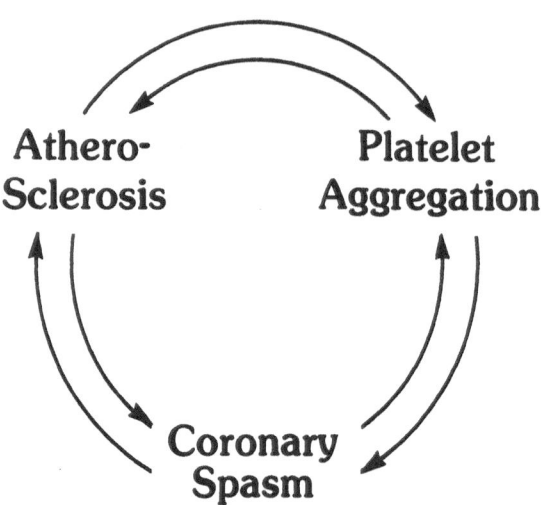

FIGURE 5-6. The vicious cycle underlying acute myocardial infarction.

Treatment of Coronary Spasm

The treatment of coronary spasm may be divided into two phases: (a) the treatment of the acute episode, and (b) the maintenance therapy oriented toward prevention of recurrent vasospastic episodes [84].

The treatment of the acute attack consists primarily of sublingual nitroglycerin, but in cases of resistant episodes, intravenous nitroglycerin should be utilized (see chapter 31). Intracoronary injections may also be considered if the episode is witnessed during cardiac catheterization. Other nitrates such as isosorbide dinitrate may also be utilized sublingually or parenterally. Nitroprusside intravenously and the calcium antagonist nifedipine sublingually, intravenously, or intracoronary may also be considered for the therapy of the acute episode.

Maintenance therapy for spasm at this time is largely utilized in the treatment of patients with Prinzmetal's variant angina, but such therapy may have future implications in the treatment of all types of angina as well as in the prevention of myocardial infarction and sudden death. The nitrates constitute the first line of management. Nitroglycerin used orally in the sustained-release form or transcutaneously constitutes the most popular choice. Isosorbide dinitrate administered sublingually or orally is also very popular. Other alternatives in the nitrate group are also available.

The beta-blockers, which are widely used in the treatment of classic exertional angina, were advocated in Prinzmetal's variant angina by Guazzi and co-workers [85]. However, more recent studies have shown that the number of resting angina attacks in patients with variant angina increased or were unchanged during propranolol therapy [86, 87]. There are also reports of coronary spasm being provoked by the administration of a beta-blocker [33]. This is not surprising since beta-blockers are known to be coronary vasoconstrictors. It is therefore recommended to avoid beta-blockers in patients where coronary spasm is believed to play an important role in the clinical syndrome.

The most important advance in the maintenance therapy of vasospasm has been the introduction of the calcium antagonists [88–93]. Of these, three agents—nifedipine, verapamil, and diltiazem—are now available for clinical use in the United States. Both open trials and double-blind, placebo-controlled investigations have confirmed the effectiveness of these agents in the prevention of coronary artery spasm. Other calcium antagonists such as bepridil, nicardipine, and many more are currently being evaluated. Also, other compounds such as amiodarone and alpha-sympathetic blockers have been reported

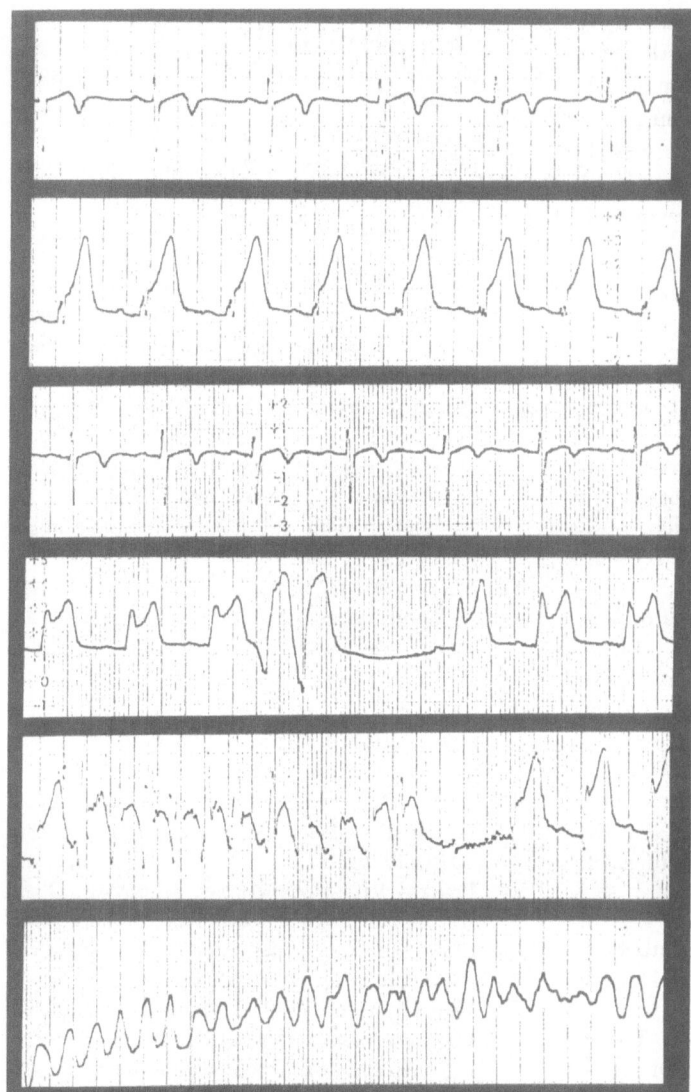

FIGURE 5-7. Holter monitor strips from a patient with Prinzmetal's variant angina and ventricular arrhythmias culminating in ventricular fibrillation. From Chahine [26], with permission.

to be valuable in the prevention of coronary spasm [18, 94].

There is therefore no question that an effective medical therapy is available to decrease or abolish the frequency of vasospastic episodes. Such therapy has found encouraging applications in patients with Prinzmetal's variant angina, particularly in those in whom no critical fixed lesion is found. The calcium antagonists are also effective in stable and unstable angina because of their afterload-reducing effect, regardless of whether spasm is present. However, the prophylactic therapy for spasm may still have further important and broader applications in the prevention of other more lethal ischemic clinical syndromes such as myocardial infarction and sudden death.

Surgical interventions have also been utilized in the therapy of Prinzmetal's angina. Such techniques are either directed toward bypassing an atherosclerotic lesion on which spasm is frequently superimposed [51] or aimed at prevention of recurrent spasm by interrupting the coronary nerve supply [37] or a combination of both [38, 95]. The exact and final role of surgery in vasospastic disease may not be completely established before further knowledge about the etiology and pathophysiology of spasm is acquired.

References

1. Burns A: Observations on some of the most frequent and important diseases of the heart; on aneurysm of the thoracic aorta; on preternatural pulsation in the epigastric region and on the unusual origin and distribution of some of the large arteries of the human body. London: Thomas Bryce and Co, 1809.

2. Osler W: Lumleian lectures on angina pectoris. Lancet 1:697, 1910.

3. Keefer CS, Resnick WH: Angina pectoris: a syndrome caused by anoxemia of the myocardium. Arch Intern Med 41:769, 1928.

4. Blumgart HL, Schlesinger MJ, David D: Studies on the relation of the clinical manifestations of angina pectoris, coronary thrombosis and myocardial infarction to the pathologic findings. Am Heart J 1:19, 1940.

5. Oliva PB, Potts DE, Plus RG: Coronary arterial spasm in Prinzmetal angina: documentation by coronary arteriography. N Engl J Med 288:745, 1973.

6. Dhurandar RW, Watt DL, Silver MD, Trimble AS, Adelman AG: Prinzmetal's variant form of angina with arteriographic evidence of coronary arterial spasm. Am J Cardiol 30:902, 1972.

7. King MJ, Zir LM, Kaltman AJ, Fox AC: Variant angina associated with angiographially demonstrated coronary artery spasm and REM sleep. Am J Med Sci 265:419, 1973.

8. Hart, NJ, Silverman ME, King SB: Variant angina pectoris caused by coronary artery spasm. Am J Med 56:269, 1974.

9. Kerin N, MacLeod GA: Coronary artery spasm associated with variant angina pectoris. Br Heart J 36:224, 1974.

10. Maseri A, Mimmo R, Chierchia S, Marchesi C, Pesola A, L'Abbate A: Coronary artery spasm as a cause of acute myocardial ischemia in man. Chest 68:625, 1975.

11. Cheng, TO, Bashour T, Singh BK, Kelser GA: Myocardial infarction in the absence of coronary arterosclerosis: result of coronary spasm? Am J Cardiol 30:680, 1972.

12. Oliva PB, Brenchkenridge JC: Arteriographic evidence of coronary arterial spasm in acute myocardial infarction. Circulation 56:366, 1977.

13. Johnson AD, Detwiler JH: Coronary spasm, variant angina, and recurrent myocardial infarctions. Circulation 55:947, 1977.

14. Maseri A, L'Abbate A, Varoldi G, Chierchia S, Marzilli M, Ballestra AM, Severi S, Parodi O, Biagini A, Distante A, Pesola A: Coronary vasospasm as a possible cause of myocardial infarction: a conclusion derived from the study of preinfarction angina. N Engl J Med 299:1271, 1978.

15. Maseri A, Pesola A, Marzilli M, Severi S, Parodi O, L'Abbate A, Ballestra AM, Maltinti G, De Nes DM, Biagini A: Coronary vasospasm in angina pectoris. Lancet 1:713, 1977.

16. Marzilli, M, L'Abbate A, Ballestra AM, Maseri A: Coronary angiographic findings during angina at rest with ST-depression. Circulation (Suppl 2) 55 and 56:83, 1977.

17. Chahine RA, Raizner AE, Luchi RJ: Coronary arterial spasm in classic angina pectoris. Cathet Cardiovasc Diagn 1:337, 1975.

18. Levene DL, Freeman MR: Alpha-adrenoceptor mediated coronary artery spasm. JAMA 236:1018, 1976.

19. Prchkov VK, Mookherjee S, Schiess W, Obeid AI: Variant anginal syndrome, coronary artery spasm, and ventricular fibrillation in absence of chest pain. Ann Intern Med 81:858, 1974.

20. Wei JY, Genecin A, Greene HL, Achuff SC: Coronary spasm with ventricular fibrillation during thyrotoxicosis: response to attaining euthyroid state. Am J Cardiol 43:335, 1979.

21. Rentrop KP, Blanke H, Karsch KR, Wiegand V, Kostering G, Oster H, Leitz K: Acute myocardial infarction: intracoronary application of nitroglycerin and streptokinase. Clin Cardiol 2:354, 1979.

22. De Wood MA, Spores J, Notske R: Prevalence of coronary occlusion during the early hours of transmural myocardial infarction. N Engl J Med 303:897, 1980.

23. Ganz W, Buchbinder N, Marcus H, Mondkar A, Maddahi J, Charuzi Y, O'Connor L, Shell W, Fishbein MC, Kass R, Miyamoto A, Swan HJC: Intracoronary thrombolysis in evolving myocardial infarction. Am Heart J 101:4, 1981.

24. Ganz W: Coronary spasm in myocardial infarc-

tion: fact or fiction? Circulation 63:487, 1981.

25. Chahine RA: Pathophysiology of ischemic heart disease. In: Blocker WP, Cardus D (eds) Rehabilitation in ischemic heart disease. SP Medical and Scientific Books, 1982.

26. Chahine RA: Coronary artery spasm. Mt Kisco NY: Futura, 1983.

27. MacAlpin RN: Terminology and classification in coronary artery spasm. Chahine R (ed). Mt Kisco NY: Futura, 1983.

28. Conti CR, Pepine CJ, Feldman RL: Coronary artery spasm. Baylor College of Medicine Cardiology Series vol 4#2, McIntosh HD (ed), 1981.

29. Endo M, Kanda T, Hosoda S, Mayashi H, Hirosawa H, Kono S: Prinzmetal's variant form of angina pectoris: re-evaluation of mechanisms. Circulation 52:33, 1975.

30. Chahine RA, Raizner AE, Ishimori T, Luchi RJ, McIntosh HD: The incidence and clinical implications of coronary artery spasm. Circulation 52: 972, 1975.

31. Fernandez D, Rosenthal JE, Cohen LS, Hammond G, Wolfson S: Alcohol-induced Prinzmetal variant angina. Am J Cardiol 32:238, 1973.

32. Ellis EF, Oelz O, Roberts LJ, Payne NA, Sweetman BJ, Nies AS, Oates JA: Coronary arterial smooth muscle contraction by a substance released from platelets: evidence that it is thromboxane A_2. Science 193:1135, 1976.

33. Yasue H, Touyama M, Kato H, Tanaka S, Akiyama F: Prinzmetal's variant form of angina as a manifestation of alpha-adrenergic receptor-mediated coronary artery spasm: documentation by coronary arteriography. Am Heart J 91:148, 1976.

34. Endo M, Kirosawa K, Kaneko, N, Hase K, Inoue Y, Konno S: Prinzmetal's variant angina: coronary arteriogram and left ventriculogram during angina attack induced by methacholine. N Engl J Med 294:252, 1976.

35. Schroeder JS, Bolen JL, Quint RA, Clark DA, Hayden WG, Higgins CB, Wexler L: Provocation of coronary spasm with ergonovine maleate: new test with results in 57 patients undergoing coronary arteriography. Am J Cardiol 40:487, 1977.

36. Raizner AE, Ishimori T, Chahine RA: Recurrent catheter-induced coronary artery spasm. Cathet Cardiovasc Diagn 3:187, 1977.

37. Clark DA, Quint RA, Mitchell RL, Angell WW: Coronary artery spasm: medical management, surgical denervation, and autotransplantation. Thorac Cardiovasc Surg 73:332, 1977.

38. Grondin CM, Limet R: Sympathetic denervation in association with coronary artery grafting in patients with Prinzmetal's angina. Ann Thorac Surg 23:111, 1977.

39. Yasue H, Nagao M, Omoto S, Takizawa A, Miwa K, Tanaka S: Coronary arterial spasm and Prinzmetal's variant form of angina induced by hyperventilation and tris-buffer infusion. Circulation 58:56, 1978.

40. Heupler FA, Proudfit WL, Razavi M, Shirey EK, Greenstreet R, Sheldon WC: Ergonovine maleate provocative test for coronary arterial spasm. Am J Cardiol 41:631, 1978.

41. Maseri A, Severi A, De Nes M, L'Abbate A, Chierchia S, Marzilli M, Ballestra AM, Parodi A, Distante A: Variant angina: one aspect of a continuous spectrum of vasospastic myocardial ischemia—pathogenetic mechanisms, estimated incidence and clinical and coronary arteriographic findings in 138 patients. Am J Cardiol 42:1019, 1978.

42. Zacca N, Chahine RA, Raizner AE, Ishimori T, Luchi RJ, Miller RR: The angiographic spectrum of coronary artery spasm. Clin Res 27: 218A, 1979.

43. Chahine RA: Prinzmetal's variant angina: a syndrome apart or another clinical presentation of atheromatous heart disease. Arch Intern Med 139: 26, 1979.

44. Waters DD, Chaitman BR, Dupras G, Theroux P, Mizgala HF: Coronary artery spasm during exercise in patients with variant angina. Circulation 59:580, 1979.

45. Lewy RI, Wiener L, Smith JB, Walinsky P, Silver MJ, Saia J: Comparison of plasma concentration of thromboxane B_2 in Prinzmetal's variant angina and classical angina pectoris. Clin Cardiol 2:404, 1979.

46. Raizner AE, Chahine RA, Ishimori T, Verani MS, Zacca N, Jamal N, Miller RR, Luchi RJ: Provocation of coronary artery spasm by the cold pressor test: hemodynamic, arteriographic and quantitative angiographic observations. Circulation 62:925, 1980.

47. Dalal JJ, Sheridan DJ, Bloom AL, Henderson AH: Platelet aggregates and coronary artery spasm. Lancet 2:1146, 1980.

48. Fuller CM, Raizner AE, Chahine RA, Nahormek P, Ishimori T, Verani MS, Nitishin A, Mokotoff D, Luchi RJ: Exercise-induced coronary arterial spasm: angiographic demonstration, documentation of ischemia by myocardial scintigraphy and results of pharmacologic intervention. Am J Cardiol 46:501, 1980.

49. MacAlpin RN: Relation of coronary arterial spasm to sites of organic stenosis. Am J Cardiol 46:143, 1980.

50. Cheng TO, Bashour T, Kelser GA, Weiss L, Bacos J: Variant angina of Prinzmetal with normal coronary arteriogram: a variant of the variant. Circulation 47:476, 1973.

51. Raizner AE, Chahine RA: The treatment of Prinzmetal's variant angina with coronary bypass surgery. In: Hurst JW (ed) Update II to The Heart. New York: McGraw-Hill, 1979, p. 85.

52. MacAlpin RN, Kattus AA, Alvaro AB: Angina pectoris at rest with preservation of exercise capacity: Prinzmetal's variant angina. Circulation 47:946, 1973.

53. Shubrooks SJ, Bete JM, Hutter AM, Block PC, Buckley MH, Daggett WM, Mundth ED: Variant angina pectoris: clinical and anatomic spectrum and results of coronary bypass surgery. Am J Cardiol 36:142, 1975.

54. Higgins CB, Wexler L, Silverman JF, Schroeder JS: Clinical and arteriographic features of Prinzmetal's variant angina: documentation of etiologic factors. Am J Cardiol 37:831, 1976.

55. Johnson AD, Stroud HA, Vieweg VR, Ross J: Variant angina pectoris: clinical presentations, coronary angiographic patterns, and the results of medical and surgical management in 42 consecutive patients. Chest 73:786, 1978.

56. Chahine RA, Verani MS: Diagnosis and documentation. In: Chahine RA (ed) Coronary artery spasm. Mt Kisco NY: Futura, 1983.

57. Maseri A, Parodi D, Severi S, Pesola A: Transient transmural reduction of myocardial blood flow, demonstrated by thallium-201 scintigraphy, as a cause of variant angina. Circulation 54:280, 1976.

58. Chahine RA, Verani MS, Zacca NM, et al: Reversible segmental contraction abnormalities during exercise-induced coronary artery spasm and their effect on global left ventricular function. Am J Cardiol 47:451, 1981.

59. MacAlpin RN: Provoking variant angina. N Engl J Med 294:277, 1976.

60. Nelson C, Nowak B, Childs H, Weinrauch L, Forwand S: Provocative testing for coronary arterial spasm: rationale, risk and clinical illustrations. Am J Cardiol 40:624, 1977.

61. Helfant R: Coronary arterial spasm and provocative testing in ischemic heart disease. Am J Cardiol 41:787, 1978.

62. Bertrand ME, Rousseau MJ, Lablanche JM, Warembourg H, Carre AG, Lekieffre JP: La detection du spasme des arteres coronaires par le test a la methylergometrine. Arch Mal Coeur 72:123, 1979.

63. Chahine RA: The provocation of coronary artery spasm. Cathet Cardiovasc Diagn 6:1, 1980.

64. Buxton A, Goldberg S, Hirshfeld JW, Wilson J, Mann F, Williams DO, Overlie P, Oliva P: Refractory ergonovine-induced coronary vasospasm: importance of intracoronary nitroglycerin. Am J Cardiol 46:329, 1980.

65. Bertrand ME, Lablanche JM, Tilmant PY: Frequency of provocated coronary artery spasm in 273 patients with chest pain. Am J Cardiol 45:390, 1980.

66. Yasue H: Electrocardiographic, hemodynamic and angiographic consequences. In: Chahine RA (ed) Coronary artery spasm. Mt Kisco NY: Futura, 1983.

67. Prinzmetal M, Ekmekci A, Kennamer R, Kwoczynski JK, Shubin H, Toyoshima H: Variant form of angina pectoris: previously undelineated syndrome. JAMA 174:1794, 1960.

68. Prinzmetal M, Kennamer R, Merlis R, Wada T, Bor N: Angina pectoris: a variant form of angina pectoris. Am J Med 27:375, 1959.

69. Chahine RA, Raizner AE: Another look at Prinzmetal's variant angina. Eur J Cardiol 6:71, 1977.

70. Meller J, Pichard A, Dack S: Coronary arterial spasm in Prinzmetal's angina: a proven hypothesis. Am J Cardiol 37:938, 1976.

71. Yasue H, Omote S, Takizawa A, Nagao M, Miwa K, Tanaka S: Exertional angina pectoris caused by coronary arterial spasm: effects of various drugs. Am J Cardiol 43:647, 1979.

72. Boden WE, Bough EW, Korr KS, Benham I, Gheorghiade M, Caputi A, Shulman RS: Exercise-induced coronary spasm with S-T segment depression and normal coronary arteriography. Am J Cardiol 48:193, 1981.

73. Bertrand ME, Lablanche JM, Tilmant PY, Thieuleux F, Chahine RA: Ergometrine provocation in patients with significant atherosclerotic coronary lesions in the absence of Prinzmetal's angina. Circulation (Suppl 4) 64:244, 1981.

74. Specchia G, Servi S, Falcone C, Braumucci E, Angoli L, Mussine A, Marinoni GP, Montemartini C, Bobba P: Coronary arterial spasm as a cause of exercise-induced S-T segment elevation in patients with variant angina. Circulation 59:948, 1979.

75. Yasue H, Omote S, Takizawa A, Nagao M, Miwa K, Tanaka: Circadian variation of exercise capacity in patients with Prinzmetal's variant angina: role of exercise-induced coronary arterial spasm. Circulation 59:938, 1979.

76. Chaitman BR, Waters DD, Theroux P, Hanson JS: S-T segment elevation and coronary spasm in response to exercise. Am J Cardiol 47:1350, 1981.
77. Verani MS, Kinney EL, Chahine RA: The role of coronary artery spasm in other clinical ischemic syndromes. In: Chahine RA (ed) Coronary artery spasm. Mt Kisco NY: Futura, 1983.
78. Gruntzig AR, Senning A, Siegenthaler WE: Nonoperative dilatation of coronary-artery stenosis: percutaneous transluminal coronary angioplasty. N Engl J Med 301:61, 1979.
79. Simpson JB, Baim DS, Robert EW, Harrison DC: A new catheter system for coronary angioplasty. Am J Cardiol 49:1216, 1982.
80. Oliva PB: Pathophysiology of acute myocardial infarction. Ann Intern Med 94:236, 1981.
81. Luchi RJ, Chahine RA: Coronary artery spasm, coronary artery thrombosis and myocardial infarction. Ann Intern Med 95:502, 1981.
82. Gertz SD, Uretsky G, Wajnberg RS, Navot N, Gotsman MS: Endothelial cell damage and thrombus formation after partial arterial constriction: relevance to the role of coronary artery spasm in the pathogenesis of myocardial infarction. Circulation 63:476, 1981.
83. Oliva PB: The role of coronary artery spasm in acute myocardial infarction. In: Chahine RA (ed) Coronary artery spasm. Mt Kisco NY: Futura, 1983.
84. Chahine RA: Coronary artery spasm: current therapy. Primary Cardiol 8:60, 1982.
85. Guazzi M, Fiorentini C, Polese A, et al: Treatment of spontaneous angina pectoris with beta blocking agents: a clinical, electrocardiographic, and hemodynamic appraisal. Br Heart J 37:1235, 1975.
86. Yasue H: Pathophysiology and treatment of coronary arterial spasm. Chest (Suppl) 78:216, 1980.
87. Robertson RM, Wood AJ, Vaughn WK, Robertson D: Exacerbation of vasotonic angina pectoris by propranolol. Circulation 65:281, 1982.
88. Stone PH, Antman EM, Muller JE, Braunwald E: Calcium channel blocking agents in the treatment of cardiovascular disorders. II. Hemodynamic effects and clinical applications. Ann Intern Med 93:886, 1980.
89. Kimura E, Kishida H: Treatment of variant angina with drugs: a survey of 11 cardiology institutes in Japan. Circulation 63:844, 1981.
90. Antman E, Muller JE, Goldberg S, et al: Nifedipine therapy for coronary artery spasm: experience with 127 patients. N Engl J Med 302:1269, 1980.
91. Rosenthal SJ, Ginsberg R, Lamb I, Baim D, Schroeder J: Efficacy of diltiazem for control of symptoms of coronary arterial spasm. Am J Cardiol 46:1027, 1980.
92. Johnson SM, Mauritson DR, Willerson JT, Hillis LD: A controlled trial of verapamil for Prinzmetal's variant angina. N Engl J Med 304:862, 1981.
93. Waters DD, Theroux P, Szlachcic J, Dauwe F: Provocative testing with ergonovine to assess the efficacy of treatment with nifedipine, diltiazem, and verapamil in variant angina. Am J Cardiol 48:123, 1981.
94. Fauchier JP, Charbonnier B, Brochier R, Raynaud R: Amiodarone injectable et par voie orale dans le traitement de l'angor de Prinzmetal severe et syncopal. Ann Cardiol Angeiol 27:193, 1978.
95. Bertand ME, Lablanche JM, Rousseau MF, Warembourg H, Stankowiak C, Soots G: Surgical treatment of variant angina: use of plexectomy with aortocoronary bypass. Circulation 51:877, 1980.

6. THE ROLE OF THROMBOSIS IN ACUTE MYOCARDIAL ISCHEMIC SYNDROMES

David C. Hueter

Coronary Artery Thrombosis and Acute Myocardial Infarction: Causation vs Correlation

The association between thrombosis of the coronary arteries and myocardial infarction was originally reported over a century ago [1, 2], but the exact role of the thrombotic process in the pathophysiology of acute myocardial infarction has remained a source of debate and active investigation to the present day. In Herrick's original description of the clinical features of acute myocardial infarction [3], he was careful to attribute the cause of this syndrome to any sudden obstruction of a coronary artery, though he surmised that the nature of the obstruction is often thrombotic. In a subsequent report of further clinicopathologic correlations on this syndrome [4], he found an occlusive intracoronary thrombus in each case, and directed his discussion to the thrombotic nature of the acute obstruction, carefully noting that the thrombus generally occurred in a region of significant underlying atherosclerosis.

There have been numerous pathologic studies over the subsequent years, using a variety of clinical definitions and pathologic techniques, correlating the occurrence of coronary thrombosis in acute fatal ischemic heart disease syndromes. Although coronary thromboses were found in all studies, the correlation was by no means perfect, and there has been considerable variability between studies in the incidence with which thrombi were found. The observation has been made [5] that most of the disparity between

studies is resolved when distinction is made between subendocardial and transmural infarction. It has been uniformly found that the incidence of thrombosis in subendocardial infarction is much less than that in transmural infarctions. Most studies of transmural myocardial infarctions have found associated occlusive thrombi in more than 90% of cases.

Some careful studies attempting to focus on patients dying in the acute stages of infarction, including sudden death, reported recent thrombus in only 46%–66% of cases of acute transmural myocardial infarction [6–9]. These reports sparked an important controversy in recent years by bringing into question the causal relationship between coronary thrombosis and myocardial infarction. These studies suggested that coronary thrombosis occurred during the myocardial infarction secondary to the stasis of coronary flow in the setting of shock and hypotension, and was not, therefore, the principle trigger of vascular occlusion and subsequent infarction. This view was supported by studies in which radiofibrinogen injected into patients shortly after myocardial infarction was found to be diffusely taken up in coronary thrombi when subsequently examined postmortem [10, 11]. This latter evidence was later refuted, however, by experimental studies showing that fibrinogen is avidly incorporated into preexistent coronary arterial thrombi in experimental animals [12, 13]. More recent studies have reported that the core of most postinfarct radiolabeled coronary thrombi in humans is free of tracer [14], indicating the presence of thrombus in the early phases of infarction.

A recent meticulous clinicopathologic study sought to resolve this controversy in light of our current improved understanding of the various clinical syndromes of acute cardiac ischemia [15]. Their findings corroborated the majority view of earlier studies by finding recent occlusive coronary lesions in 90% of patients with recent transmural infarcts, in 35% with recent subendocardial infarcts, and in 10% with acute coronary insufficiency. Of the total of 61 patients with acute coronary occlusions, 57 had in situ thrombi, two had thromboembolic, and two had isolated hemorrhage into a plaque.

Over the past five years, new information bearing on the frequency and nature of acute coronary occlusion in acute myocardial ischemia syndromes has begun to emerge from the clinical studies of aggressive new diagnostic and therapeutic management of these conditions (see chapter 35). Arising as they do from a population of well-defined clinical subsets of surviving inpatients, these findings are particularly relevant to issues of patient management that confront the clinical cardiologist.

Coronary arteriography in patients studied within 24 h of acute transmural myocardial infarction [16, 17] has shown a high incidence of total coronary occlusion. A report of 322 patients studied within the first 24 h of transmural myocardial infarction [17] demonstrated total occlusion in 87% and subtotal occlusion in an additional 10% of patients studied within 4 h of infarction. The incidence fell to total occlusion in 65% and subtotal occlusion in 16% in those patients studied 12–24 hr after infarction, indicating resolution of some obstructions with time. Although a component of spasm can be demonstrated by reduction from total to subtotal occlusion with intravenous nitroglycerin in a minority of patients [16], fresh proximal thrombus was recovered with a Fogarty catheter from the involved coronary artery in 64 of 79 patients [17] undergoing emergency revascularization for acute myocardial infarction. Importantly, the distal portion of the removed thrombus was consistently found to be a thickened layer of fibrin and platelets, suggestive of an early platelet thrombus. Red thrombus more proximally indicated incorporation of red cells as the thrombus propagated retrograde from the point of initial occlusion, presumably due to stasis of coronary flow after the primary occlusion by the platelet–fibrin plug.

Perhaps the most compelling evidence supporting the view that arterial thrombosis has a central role in the pathogenesis of acute myocardial infarction comes from the clinical experience with thrombolytic therapy in acute myocardial infarction (see chapter 33). The first trials of thrombolytic therapy in the treatment of acute myocardial infarction were reported in 1959 [18]. These initial studies used systemic lytic therapy administered intravenously, and a number of large multicenter clinical trials using a variety of experimental designs were carried out in Europe over the next two decades. Though some showed encouraging reductions in mortality, others showed no benefit; hence no overall consensus could be reached.

Successful nonsurgical recanalization of totally obstructed coronary arteries during acute myocardial infarction by direct intracoronary administration of thrombolytic therapy was first reported in 1979 [19]. In contrast to the earlier studies of intravenous therapy, excellent results using the intracoronary route have been uniformly reported by many centers over the past few years [19–25]. Most of the patients were found to have total, and the rest near-total, major coronary obstructions, and the thrombosis occurred at the site of significant underlying atherosclerotic disease. Intracoronary nitroglycerin will convert only a small minority from total to near-total obstruction. Thrombolytic recanalization can be achieved in 75%–80% of cases [25] with resultant reduction in infarct size as judged by myocardial perfusion [20, 23], global and segmental wall motion [20], and ECG when recanalization is achieved in the first 4 h after onset of infarction [24]. Recurrent thrombosis at the same site has been documented in about 20% of patients within two weeks. The ability to recanalize an obstructed major coronary artery with a specific thrombolytic agent and to thereby reduce the resultant infarct size is a compelling argument for a causal role of thrombosis in myocardial infarction.

Factors Affecting Arterial Thrombosis

The clinicopathologic studies and the more recent clinical studies of coronary arteriography and intracoronary thrombolysis in acute myocardial infarction make a compelling argument that thrombogenesis plays an important role in the early development and ultimate severity of acute myocardial infarction. An understanding of the factors influencing thrombogenesis in a coronary artery will be crucial to the development of effective preventive and interventional therapy. These factors are multiple, and of variable importance to the thrombogenic process, but are presently incompletely understood.

It has been recognized for some time that arterial thrombi tend to occur where nonlaminar flow occurs, at branch points and vessel orifices [26]. In a porcine extracorporeal shunt model, platelet thrombi occurred at the bifurcation of the shunt and could be prevented by thrombocytopenia but not by dicoumarol [27]. Platelet aggregation and early intimal damage can be seen to occur within minutes of creation of a coronary arterial stenosis using an external constricting ligature in a rabbit preparation [28], presumably secondary to the resultant turbulence and increase in shear forces. The exact mechanism of how turbulence leads to platelet thrombi remains unclear. Rheologic studies in vitro have demonstrated an increase in platelet aggregability and adhesivity when shear rates are increased to levels found in arteries in vivo [29]. It has been postulated that, in the setting of flow separation and vortex formation, vortices can alter the physical surface of the intima [30], that potentially injurious substances can accumulate next to the intima because of the altered flow [31], and that an increased diffusion of platelets toward the vessel wall occurs [32].

A central role for platelet aggregation in the pathogenesis of acute myocardial ischemia and infarction has been emerging from recent experimental work in animals. In a series of animal experiments using a constricting external ring to produce a controlled degree of coronary stenosis, cyclic alterations in flow have been reported [33]. Typically this cycle consists of a gradual fall in flow over a period of minutes with an abrupt return to baseline, but occasionally it progresses to total cessation of flow with arrhythmic sudden death. This cyclic fall in flow is abolished by ibuprofen or indomethacin, but unaffected by papaverine or nitroglycerin, which indicates that recurrent spontaneous platelet aggregation rather than coronary spasm is occurring. Arteriographic demonstration of thrombotic occlusion coincident with flow reduction and retrieval of discrete platelet thrombi from the effluent blood when the flow rebounded to baseline [34] was further proof that recurrent occlusive platelet aggregates were the source of the obstruction. Cigarette smoke and nicotine infusion were tested in this same preparation [35] and found to potentiate the frequency, severity, and rapidity of recurrent coronary flow reductions. This appears to represent an alpha-adrenergic-mediated activation of platelet aggregability, since the potentiation is blocked by phentolamine. In another experimental preparation, electrically induced injury of the intimal surface of a coronary artery consistently produced a thrombotic occlusion, but this occlusion could be prevented by continuous infusion of prostacyclin, a potent inhibitor of in vivo platelet aggregation [36] (see chapter 16).

There is now ample evidence that platelet aggregation is a key step in the formation of an arterial thrombus, but it is not yet clear that platelet aggregation by itself without fibrin deposition results in ischemia. It is the formation of fibrin from the action of thrombin on fibrinogen and incorporation of the fibrin into the platelet aggregate that produces the stable platelet—fibrin occlusion.

Normal endothelium possesses potent antithrombogenic properties, allowing neither coagulation nor platelet adherence to occur on its surface, although the mechanisms remain poorly understood. This property does not appear to be primarily due to endothelial prostacyclin for it is not affected by aspirin inhibition of prostacyclin production [37]. The finding that endothelial cells that have been virally transformed in tissue culture lose this property suggests that the mechanism is related to surface properties of the cell itself [38] rather than to humoral factors.

Pathologic studies have shown that thrombi in coronary arteries occur only in areas of intimal damage, and almost always at a point of disruption of the intima over an atherosclerotic plaque

[39] (see chapter 4). When the endothelium is damaged, platelets adhere to the endothelial surface. Experimental evidence suggests that the platelets are bound to the surface by polymerizing fibrin [40], perhaps from fibrinogen released by the activated platelets themselves. Exposure of the subendothelium by disruption of the endothelium provides multiple potent stimuli to thrombus formation. The intrinsic coagulation pathway is triggered by contact of factor XII with fibrillar and vascular basement membrane collagen [41]. The extrinsic coagulation pathway is triggered by exposure of tissue thromboplastin either from the injured endothelium or from white cells [42] that have been stimulated, probably activated by the complement system [43]. Platelets adhere to exposed subendothelial collagen via the glycoproteins of the platelet surface [44]. They then spread, and undergo a reaction that releases fibrinogen and vasoactive amines, furthering the thrombotic process. These platelets release ADP [45] and thromboxane A_2 [46], both of which alter nonadhesive platelets to become adhesive and enter into the process. Local generation of thrombin polymerizes fibrinogen into fibrin, stabilizing the platelet aggregate and also stimulating further platelet release of ADP and thromboxane A_2.

Many of the factors released from platelets, including thromboxane A_2, ADP, and serotonin, possess potent vasoconstrictive properties. Coronary arteriography in patients with acute myocardial infarction has revealed that, in six of the 15 patients studied, total occlusions were reduced to subtotal occlusions after nitroglycerin [16]. It has been suggested that these vasoactive amines contribute to the thrombotic process by producing local vasospasm resulting in more turbulence and/or stagnation of flow.

Conclusion

Based upon the body of evidence presently available then, coronary thrombosis is more than a secondary finding in myocardial infarction, and most likely represents the primary final occlusive process resulting in the acute event. At the least it is a major modifier of the severity and extent of ischemic damage in acute myocardial infarction. It now appears likely that platelet aggregation at the intimal surface of a stenotic atherosclerotic plaque represents the key initial pathophysiologic step in the occlusive process resulting in infarction. It is also clear, however, that this process of platelet aggregation is involved in a complex interplay with other factors such as coronary flow dynamics, vascular tone, intimal damage, coagulation factors, and circulating humoral factors. As discussed in chapter 4, there is some evidence to support the view that these same factors, occurring repeatedly over a period of years, play a major role in atherogenesis. Viewed in this light, acute myocardial ischemic syndromes represent merely the transition from nonocclusive to occlusive thrombotic involvement in the ongoing atherosclerotic process. Research to elucidate the complex interplay between these and yet to be discovered factors represents the most promising direction to further our understanding, prevention, and management of acute myocardial ischemia and infarction, and perhaps atherogenesis in general.

References

1. Putney GE: Extracts from the records of the Middlesex East District Medical Society, Boston Med Surg J 103:398−400, 1880.
2. Weigert C: Uber die pathologischen gerinnungsvorgange. Virchows Arch [Pathol Anat] 79:87−123, 1880.
3. Herrick JB: Clinical features of sudden obstruction of the coronary arteries. JAMA 59:2015−2020, 1912.
4. Herrick JB: Thrombosis of the coronary arteries. JAMA 72:387−390, 1919.
5. Oliva PB: Pathophysiology of acute myocardial infarction, 1981. Ann Intern Med 94:236−250, 1981.
6. Baroldi F: Acute coronary occlusion as a cause of myocardial infarct and sudden coronary heart death. Am J Cardiol 16:859−880, 1965.
7. Roberts WC, Buja LM: The frequency and significance of coronary arterial thrombi and other observations in fatal acute myocardial infarction: a study of 107 necropsy patients. Am J Med 52:425−443, 1972.
8. Baroldi G, Radice F, Schmid G, Leone A: Morphology of acute myocardial infarction in relation to coronary thrombosis. Am Heart J 87:65−75, 1974.

9. Walston A, Hackel DB, Estes EH: Acute coronary occlusion and the "power failure" syndrome. Am Heart J 79:613−619, 1970.

10. Erhardt LR, Lundman T, Mellstedt H: Incorporation of 125I-labeled fibrinogen into coronary arterial thrombi in acute myocardial infarction in man. Lancet 1:387−390, 1973.

11. Erhardt LR, Unge G, Boman G: Formation of coronary arterial thrombi in relation to onset of necrosis in acute myocardial infarction in man: a clinical and autoradiographic study. Am Heart J 91:592−598, 1976.

12. Moschos CB, Oldewurtel HA, Haider B, Regan TJ: Effect of coronary thrombus age on fibrinogen uptake. Circulation 54:653−656, 1976.

13. Salimi A, Oliver GC Jr, Lee J, Herman LA: Continued incorporation of circulating radiolabeled fibrinogen into preformed coronary artery thrombi. Circulation 56:213−217, 1977.

14. Fulton WFM, Summer DJ: Causal role of coronary thrombotic occlusion in myocardial infarction: evidence of stereo-arteriography serial sections and autoradiography [abstr]. Am J Cardiol 39:322, 1977.

15. Buja LM, Willerson J: Clinicopathologic correlates of acute ischemic heart disease syndromes. Am J Cardiol 47:343−356, 1981.

16. Oliva PB, Breckenridge JC: Arteriographic evidence of coronary arterial spasm in acute myocardial infarction. Circulation 56:366−374, 1977.

17. DeWood MA, Spores J, Notske R, Mouser LT, Burroughs R, Golden MS, Lang HT: Prevalence of total coronary occlusion during the early hours of transmural myocardial infarction. N Engl J Med 303: 897−902, 1980.

18. Fletcher AR, Sherry S, Alkjaersig N, Smyrniotis FE, Jick S: The maintenance of a sustained thrombolytic state in man. II. Clinical observations on patients with myocardial infarction and other thrombo-embolic disorders. J Clin Invest 38: 1111−1119, 1959.

19. Rentrop KP, Blanke H, Karsch KR, Wiegand V, Kostering H, Oster H, Leitz K: Acute myocardial infarction: intracoronary application of nitroglycerin and streptokinase. Clin Cardiol 2:354−363, 1979.

20. Ganz W, Buchbinder N, Marcus H, Mondkar A, Maddahi J, Charuzi Y, O'Connor L, Shell W, Fishbein MC, Kass R, Miyamoto A, Swan HJC: Intracoronary thrombolysis in evolving myocardial infarction. Am Heart J 101:4−13, 1981.

21. Mathey DG, Kuck KH, Tilsner V, Krebber HJ, Bleifeld W: Non-surgical coronary artery recanalization in acute transmural myocardial infarction. Circulation 63:489−497, 1981.

22. Rentrop P, Blanke H, Karsch KR, Kaiser H, Kostering H, Leitz K: Selective intracoronary thrombolysis in acute myocardial infarction and unstable angina pectoris. Circulation 63:307−317, 1981.

23. Markis JE, Malagold M, Parker JA, Silverman KJ, Barry WH, Als AV, Paulin S, Grossman W, Braunwald E: Myocardial salvage after intracoronary thrombolysis with streptokinase in acute myocardial infarction assessment: by intracoronary thallium-201. N Engl J Med 305:777−782, 1981.

24. Schwartz F, Schuler G, Katus H, Hofmann M, Manthey J, Tillmanns H, Mehmel H, Kubler W: Intracoronary thrombolysis in acute myocardial infarction: duration of ischemia as a major determinant of late results after recanalization. Am J Cardiol 50: 933−937, 1982.

25. Weinstein J: Treatment of myocardial infarction with intracoronary streptokinase: treatment and safety data from 209 United States cases in the Hoechst-Roussel registry. Am Heart J 104: 894−898, 1982.

26. Murphy EA, Rowsell HC, Downie HG, Robinson GA, Mustard JF: Encrustation and atherosclerosis: the analogy between early in vivo lesions and deposits which occur in extracorporeal circulations. Can Med Assoc J 87:259−274, 1962.

27. Mustard JF, Jorgensen L, Hovig T: Role of platelets in thrombosis. In: Koller F (ed) Pathogenesis and treatment of thromboembolic diseases. Stuttgart: Schattauer, 1966, p. 131.

28. Gertz SD, Uretsky G, Wajnberg RS, Navot N, Gotsman MS: Endothelial cell damage and thrombus formation after partial arterial constriction: relevance to the role of coronary artery spasm in the pathogenesis of myocardial infarction. Circulation 63:476−486, 1981.

29. Grabowski EF: Role of blood flow in platelet adhesion and aggregation. In: Day HJ (ed) Thrombosis: animal and clinical models. New York: Plenum, 1977, p. 73.

30. Svendsen E, Jorgensen L: Intimal pits of aorta in rabbits: imprints of vortices of blood flow? Acta Pathol Microbiol Scand [A] 85:25−32, 1977.

31. Kniker WT, Cochrane CG: The localization of circulating immune complexes in experimental serum sickness: the role of vasoactive amines and hydrodynamic forces. J Exp Med 127:119−136, 1968.

32. Mustard JF, Kinlough-Rathbone RL, Packam

MA: The vessel wall in thrombosis. In: Colman RW, Hirsh J, Marder VJ, Salzman EW (eds) Hemostasis and thrombosis: basic principles and clinical practice. Philadelphia: JB Lippincott, 1982, pp. 703–715.

33. Folts JD, Crowell EB, Rowe GG: Platelet aggregation in partially obstructed vessels and their elimination with aspirin. Circulation 54:365–370, 1976.

34. Folts JD, Gallagher K, Rowe GG: Blood flow reductions in stenosed canine coronary arteries: vasospasm or platelet aggregation? Circulation 65:248–255, 1982.

35. Folts JD, Bonebrake FC: The effects of cigarette smoke and nicotine on platelet thrombus formation in stenosed dog coronary arteries: inhibition with phentolamine. Circulation 65:465–470, 1982.

36. Romson JL, Haack DW, Abrams GD, Luchessi BR: Prevention of occlusive coronary artery thrombosis by prostacyclin infusion in the dog. Circulation 64:906–914, 1981.

37. Dejana E, Cazenave JP, Groves HM, Kinlough-Rathbone RL, Mustard JF: The effect of aspirin inhibition of PGI_2 production on platelet adherence to normal and damaged rabbit aortae. Throm Res 17: 453–464, 1980.

38. Curwen KD, Gimbrone MA Jr, Handin RI: In vitro studies of thromboresistance: the role of prostacyclin (PGI_2) in platelet adhesion to cultured normal and virally transformed human vascular endothelial cells. Lab Invest 42:366–374, 1980.

39. Constantinides P: Plaque fissure in human coronary thrombosis. J Atheroscler Res 6:1–17, 1966.

40. Czervionke RL, Hoak JC, Fry GL: Effect of aspirin on thrombin-induced adherence of platelets to cultured cells from the blood vessel wall. J Clin Invest 62:847–856, 1978.

41. Wilner GD, Nossel HL, Le Roy EC: Activation of Hageman factor by collagen. J Clin Invest 47: 2608–2615, 1968.

42. Niemetz J, Fani K: Thrombogenic activity of leukocytes. Blood 42:47–59, 1973.

43. Muhlfelder TW, Niemetz J, Kreutzer D, Beebe D, Ward PA, Rosenfeld SI: C5 chemotactic fragment induces leukocyte production of tissue factor activity: a link between complement and coagulation. J Clin Invest 63:147–150, 1979.

44. Nurden AT, Caen JP: Specific roles for platelet surface glycoproteins in platelet function. Nature 255: 720–722, 1975.

45. Baumgartner HR, Muggli R, Tschopp TB, Turitto VT: Platelet adhesion, release and aggregation in flowing blood: effects of surface properties and platelet function. Throm Haemost 35:124–138, 1976.

46. Hamberg M, Svensson J, Samuelsson B: Thromboxanes: a new group of biologically active compounds derived from prostaglandin endoperoxides. Proc Natl Acad Sci USA 72:2994–2998, 1975.

7. THE BIOCHEMISTRY OF THROMBOLYTIC AGENTS

Louis Summaria

The use of thrombolytic agents for the treatment of acute myocardial infarction has recently received new impetus. There are two major reasons for this. First is the development and perfection of coronary angiography, which allows direct visualization of the acutely thrombosed coronary artery and subsequent administration of thrombolytic agents in proximity to the clot [1, 2]. Second, a highly purified streptokinase preparation is now available that is less allergenic than earlier preparations. This chapter reviews the biochemical and physiological properties of the therapeutic agents that promote thrombolysis by "activation," or conversion of plasminogen into plasmin. There are two available thrombolytic agents, urokinase and streptokinase, and another tissue plasminogen activator that has recently been isolated, purified, characterized, and resynthesized through recombinant DNA technology.

Urokinase and Streptokinase

Human urokinase exists as either a high molecular weight (54,000 daltons) or low molecular weight (32,000 daltons) form and can be isolated from urine, cultured kidney cells, or tumor tissues [3, 4]. Various types of urokinase preparations have been studied and used as thrombolytic agents. The mechanism by which all urokinase activators function is a direct enzymatic cleavage of the Arg-560-Val peptide bond in plasminogen to form the fibrinolytic enzyme plasmin [5]. Kinetic analyses have shown that all urokinase preparations have similar catalytic rate constants

of activation, but their binding constants of activation vary severalfold, producing approximately a fivefold variation in their catalytic efficiencies. The primary advantage of urokinase as a thrombolytic agent is the lack of antigenicity because of its human origin. This enzyme is in short supply, however, and consequently is more expensive than streptokinase.

Streptokinase is a bacterial protein that, by itself, has no biologic activity. It functions as an "activator" by combining with plasminogen in a 1:1 ratio to form a plasminogen−streptokinase complex (figure 7-1). This binding produces a conformational change in the plasminogen that creates an active site (without the cleavage of any peptide bond), which allows it to function as an activator of free circulating plasminogen [6]. This activation without bond cleavage is unique and poorly understood even though the complete amino acid sequences of both streptokinase and plasminogen are known [7, 8]. The plasminogen−streptokinase complex can convert to a plasmin−streptokinase complex [9−11] via the cleavage of a peptide bond. While this interaction is occurring, some of the plasminogen−streptokinase complex is cleaved to form plasminogen−streptokinase fragments 1 and 2 [12]. These fragments can be converted to plasmin−streptokinase fragments 1 and 2 [13]. All of these complexes can serve as activators of free circulating plasminogen.

Streptokinase activator complexes can be prepared with a variety of forms of plasminogen and plasminogen derivatives. The native form of

R.M. Califf and G.S. Wagner (eds.), ACUTE CORONARY CARE: Principles and Practice. Copyright © 1985. Martinus Nijhoff Publishing, Boston/Dordrecht/Lancaster.

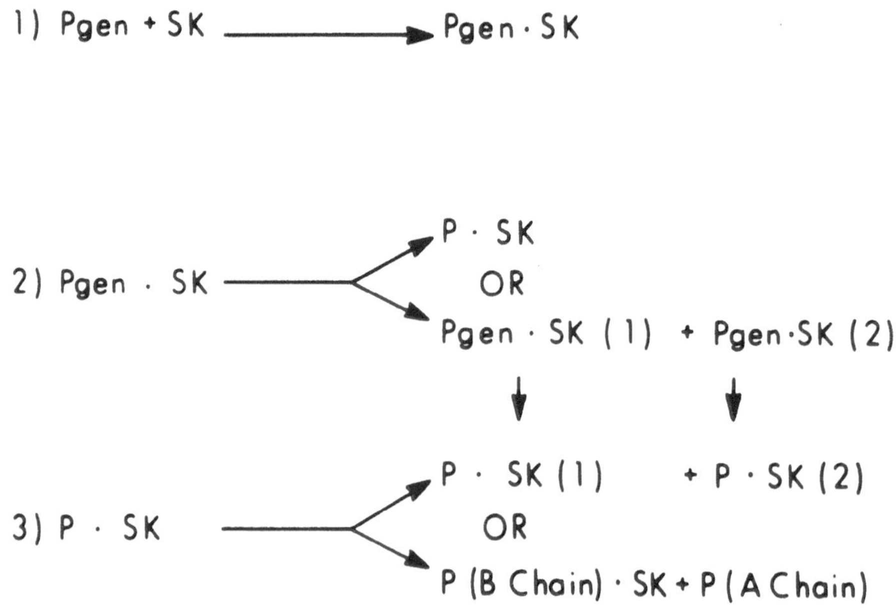

1) Pgen + SK ⎯⎯⎯⎯⎯⎯→ Pgen · SK

2) Pgen · SK ⎯⎯⎯⎯⎯
$$
\begin{array}{l}
\text{P · SK} \\
\text{OR} \\
\text{Pgen · SK (1)} \quad + \quad \text{Pgen · SK (2)} \\
\qquad\qquad\downarrow \qquad\qquad\qquad\qquad \downarrow \\
\end{array}
$$

3) P · SK ⎯⎯⎯⎯⎯
$$
\begin{array}{l}
\text{P · SK (1)} \quad + \quad \text{P · SK (2)} \\
\text{OR} \\
\text{P (B Chain) · SK + P (A Chain)}
\end{array}
$$

FIGURE 7-1. The various compounds that form as the result of the interaction between plasminogen and streptokinase are indicated. Initially a plasminogen—streptokinase complex is formed. This complex can then convert to a plasmin—streptokinase complex via the cleavage of a peptide bond. However, some of the plasminogen—streptokinase complex is cleaved to form plasminogen—streptokinase fragments 1 and 2. These fragments can in turn be converted to plasmin—streptokinase fragments 1 and 2. Also, the plasmin—streptokinase complex can be broken into the fragments of plasmin—streptokinase (1) or plasmin—streptokinase (2), or it can be converted to the extremely active plasmin (B chain)—streptokinase complex and the inactive plasmin (A chain).

human plasminogen is glu-plasminogen with a molecular weight of 88,000 daltons. Cleavage of a peptide bond by plasmin at the amino-terminal portion of this molecule produces lys-plasminogen. Two subforms of each of these two plasminogens, and at least 12 isoelectric forms of plasminogen, have been isolated [14]. Incubation of either form of plasminogen with the enzyme elastase causes specific peptide bond cleavages that result in the formation of a smaller plasminogen form, Val-442-plasminogen [8].

The smallest form that can be isolated and still function as an enzyme is the plasmin (B) chain (figure 7-1) with a molecular weight of 25,700 daltons [15]. Streptokinase complexes have been prepared with each of these forms of plasminogen and plasmin, and the kinetic parameters of activation of human glu-plasminogen with each complex have been determined (table 7-1) [16]. The catalytic efficiency by which the plasmin (B) chain—streptokinase complex converts plasminogen to plasmin is 169.0 $UM^{-1} min^{-1}$, which is the highest value ever determined for a plasminogen activator: 2.3 times as great as that of the glu-plasminogen—streptokinase complex, 4.3 times as great as the lys-plasmin—streptokinase complex, and nearly seven times as great as any form of urokinase. The plasmin (B)

chain—streptokinase complex is also a potent fibrinolytic enzyme. It is not inhibited by plasma antiplasmin, alpha-2-macroglobulin, or other plasma inhibitors. It is not inhibited by plasma antistreptokinase antibodies nor is it as antigenic as streptokinase. The complex has a longer half-life (in the dog) than either streptokinase or urokinase (4h compared with 20−30 min) and has a very high affinity for free circulating plasminogen forming a plasmin (B) chain—streptokinase—plasminogen complex [17]. The plasmin (B) chain—streptokinase complex has been evaluated as a fibrinolytic agent in in vitro clot lysis sys-

TABLE 7-1. Steady-state kinetic parameters of activation of human glu-plasminogen by various activator species at pH 7.4 and 37°C

Activator species	Activation parameters		
	K_{plg} (μM)	k_{plg} (min^{-1})	k_{plg}/K_{plg} (μM^{-1} min^{-1})
Streptokinase			
Glu-Plg·SK	0.12 ± 0.01	8.97 ± 0.53	74.8
Val-442 Plg·SK	0.25 ± 0.01	25.53 ± 1.92	102.1
Lys-Pln·SK	0.23 ± 0.02	8.97 ± 1.18	39.0
Val-442·PLN·SK	1.94 ± 0.32	28.71 ± 2.91	14.8
B·SK	0.15 ± 0.03	25.33 ± 2.51	169.0
SK	0.12 ± 0.02	8.21 ± 0.94	68.4
Urokinase			
UK-HMW	1.72 ± 0.12	47.06 ± 1.25	27.4
UK-LMW	2.64 ± 0.23	63.00 ± 4.50	23.9

tems, but it has never been evaluated as a thrombolytic agent in either man or animal models.

One possible limitation of either urokinase or streptokinase therapy is the plasminogen depletion that occurs during the prolonged administration of these agents. At low plasminogen levels, urokinase possesses minimal catalytic efficiency and will not effectively activate the residual circulating plasminogen. A new approach using small doses of either of these lytic agents in combination with infusion of plasminogen would prevent plasminogen depletion and allow the activator to function continually at a higher catalytic efficiency. Kakkar has used this approach in an attempt to determine the optimal regimen for streptokinase treatment in patients with deep-vein thrombosis [18]. Four groups of patients received intravenous streptokinase and/or lys-plasminogen in varying doses and sequences over a five-day treatment period. The streptokinase was infused over 30 min and the lys-plasminogen over 4–6 h. Thrombolysis was determined by pre- and posttreatment venograms. Group I (15 patients) received streptokinase (600,000 U [units]) once daily. Group II (29 patients) received 90–120 mg of lys-plasminogen followed by 600,000 U of streptokinase once daily. Group III (26 patients) received 600,000 U of streptokinase, followed by 90 mg of lys-plasminogen once daily. Group IV (18 patients) received 500,000 U of streptokinase followed by 45 mg of lys-plasminogen, followed by 250,000 U of

streptokinase on day 1; then only the latter two during the remaining four days. Complete clot lysis occurred in 20% of Group I, 55% of Group II, 27% of Group III, and 44% of Group IV patients. These results indicate that intermittent streptokinase in combination with lys-plasminogen has advantages over the use of intermittent streptokinase alone. The optimal sequence of administration and doses of plasminogen and streptokinase may not be determined until clinical tests are developed that give a better assessment of the hematologic changes that occur in the patient during the period of therapy. Although much more is known about the biochemistry of streptokinase than is known about any other activator, many of the physiologic changes occurring during and after the administration of streptokinase are still unknown.

Tissue Plasminogen Activator

A third type of plasminogen activator is the class described as "tissue activators." This class historically precedes both urokinase and streptokinase since the presence of plasminogen activators in tissue cultures was first demonstrated nearly 70 years ago. It is believed that most tissues synthesize plasminogen activators, but in considerably varying amounts. The uterus, adrenal glands, and lymph nodes produce the largest quantities of tissue activators, whereas the liver and spleen produce the least amount, if any. Very few tissue activators have been isolated from normal human tissue. Highly purified tissue activators have been isolated from pig heart tissue and human uterine tissue, and these have been partially characterized [19, 20]. Most tissue activators that have been isolated and characterized, however, have been derived from malignantly transformed cell lines.

In 1974, Reich and co-workers were the first to describe in detail the production of tissue plasminogen activators by mammalian fibroblasts that were transformed in vitro by oncogenic viruses or chemical carcinogens [21]. Since then, numerous malignantly transformed cell lines have been shown to produce a significantly increased level of plasminogen activator compared with their normal counterparts [22]. The potential importance of the production of this enzyme to the understanding of neoplasia lies in the observation that the expression of plasminogen activator activity is one of the earliest observable events associated with transformation of cell lines. This may serve a regulatory function, but it remains to be determined whether plasminogen activator activity is necessary for the establishment of tumorigenicity or whether it represents a function that is causally unrelated to malignancy.

Several tissue activators have been partially or completely purified from either transformed cell lines or human melanoma cells [23]. They are all serine proteases with molecular weights between 40,000 and 50,000 daltons. Other tissue activators have been isolated with molecular weights reported to be 70,000 daltons, 100,000 daltons, and some as high as several hundred thousand daltons. Besides having a greater molecular weight, these tissue activators differ in several other ways from urokinase or streptokinase. They show different binding affinities toward certain synthetic substrates, different binding properties toward fibrin, and different immunochemical reactivity [24].

The exact relationship of tissue activators to the vascular plasminogen activator has not been determined. It has been shown that postmortem blood contains an increased amount of vascular plasminogen activator activity, and it is believed that the source of this activator is the endothelial cell. Vascular plasminogen activators have been isolated by arterial perfusion of the lower ex-

tremeties of human cadavers. They have been purified by several different methods [25, 26], and their apparent molecular weight is 70,000 – 75,000 daltons. There was debate about whether the vascular plasminogen activator was, in fact, urokinase, but this was resolved when it was found to be unreactive with a urokinase-specific antibody. The ability of the vascular activator to convert free plasminogen to plasmin is considerably less than that of either urokinase or the streptokinase – plasminogen complexes. However, its affinity for fibrin is much higher than that of urokinase or the tissue activators isolated from melanoma cultures. Since it is believed that the regulation of physiologic fibrinolysis depends on the interaction of activators and plasminogen with fibrin [27], the enhanced binding capabilities of the vascular plasminogen activator to fibrin could be of paramount importance.

One difficulty with all tissue plasminogen activators has been the small amounts that can be isolated, since the source of starting material is a limiting factor. Collen et al., however, have isolated and purified the activator from melanoma cell lines [28] and the cloning and expression of the gene in *Escherichia coli* have been successfully accomplished [29]. Tissue plasminogen activator has been shown in the dog model of acute myocardial infarction to be an effective thrombolytic agent [30]. Clinical trials with tissue plasminogen activator are currently being organized. The major benefits of tissue plasminogen activator are the lack of systemic hyperplasminemia with its attendant effects on the coagulation system and its rapid elimination half-life, which should allow for safer invasive procedures after administration.

Monitoring Thrombolytic Therapy

New techniques for monitoring and evaluating thrombolytic therapy are now being developed using chromogenic substrates. Synthetic substrate assay methodology for determining plasminogen, antiplasmin, activator, plasmin, and plasmin generation rates in plasma has been recently published [31]. These tests have made it possible to detect and to kinetically characterize "variant" plasminogens in individual patients [32]. Thus far, more than ten variant plasminogens have been detected in patients with a history

TABLE 7-2. Catalytic efficiencies of activators on variant plasminogens

Activator	Plasminogen	k_{plg}/K_{plg} glu-plg	lys-plg	Ratio lys/glu
SK	Normal	68.4	404.1	5.9
SK	Chicago I	9.3	162.7	17.5
SK	Chicago II	24.6	184.0	11.5
B·SK	Normal	169.0	423.7	2.5
B·SK	Chicago I	1.2	415.8	347.0
B·SK	Chicago II	1.5	432.6	289.0
HMW-UK	Normal	27.4	26.5	1.0
HMW-UK	Chicago I	9.4	15.5	1.6
HMW-UK	Chicago II	10.5	25.9	2.5

of recurrent thrombotic disorders. The primary defect in many of these patients is the decreased catalytic efficiency of presently available activators to activate their variant form of plasminogen (table 7-2). In patients with variant plasminogens, preinfusion of normal plasminogen, followed by intermittent administration of the activator, would appear to be a viable therapeutic approach. The plasmin generation rate assay, developed by Wohl et al. [31] now permits one to determine the sensitivity of a patient's plasminogen to different activator species before treatment. Even though there is high antiurokinase inhibitor activity and high antistreptokinase antibody activity in plasma, this plasmin generation rate assay is sufficiently sensitive to measure the rate at which the patient's plasminogen is activated. This method allows one to select the most efficient activator for a particular patient, and will prove to be more valuable when the number of available activators increases.

The ability to specifically measure the activator activity in patients undergoing thrombolytic therapy with either urokinase or streptokinase will permit clinicians to regulate the dose and regimen with a much higher degree of efficiency, rather than relying on empirical factors to determine the treatment schedule. In addition to the high degree of sensitivity of each of these chromogenic substrate assays, two other distinct advantages are (a) that only a small sample of plasma is used for each assay (0.2—0.5 ml), and (b) that the battery of five assays can be performed in less than 1 h. In the near future, when these assays have been shown to be clinically useful, laboratory monitoring will be a more important factor in thrombolytic therapy for determining the type of activator and the dosing regimen, and may provide a more rational relationship between laboratory analyses and thrombolytic efficacy.

References

1. Rentrop P, Blanke H, Karsch KR, Kaiser H, Kostering H, Leitz K: Selective intracoronary thrombolysis in acute myocardial infarction and unstable angina pectoris. Circulation 63:307–317, 1981.
2. Ganz W: Intracoronary thrombolysis in evolving acute myocardial infarction. Am Heart J XX: 101–104, 1981.
3. Barlow GH: Urinary and kidney cell plasminogen activator (urokinase). Methods Enzymol 45: 239–244, 1976.
4. Markus G, Takita H, Camiolo SM, Corasanti JG, Evers JL, Hobika GH: Content and characterization of plasminogen activators in human lung tumors and normal lung tissue. Cancer Res 40:841–848, 1980.
5. Summaria L, Hsieh B, Robbins KC: The specific mechanism of activation of human plasminogen to plasmin. J Biol Chem 242:4279–4287, 1967.
6. McClintock DK, Bell PH: Mechanism of activation of human plasminogen by streptokinase. Biochem Biophys Res Commun 43:694–702, 1971.
7. Jackson KW, Tang J: Complete amino acid sequence of streptokinase and its homology with serine proteases. Biochemistry 21:6620–6625, 1982.
8. Sottrup-Jensen L, Claeys H, Sajdel M, Petersen RE, Magnusson S: The primary structure of

human plasminogen. Prog Chem Fibrinolysis 3:191–199.

9. Reddy KNN, Markus G: Mechanism of activation of human plasminogen by streptokinase: presence of an active center in streptokinase–plasminogen complex. J Biol Chem 247:1683–1691, 1972.

10. Markus G, Evers JL, Hobika GH: Activator activities of the transient forms of the human plasminogen–streptokinase complex during its proteolytic conversion to the stable activator complex. J Biol Chem 251:6495–6504, 1976.

11. Gonzalez-Gronow M, Siefring CE, Castellino FJ: The mechanism of activation of human plasminogen by the activator complex streptokinase–plasmin. J Biol Chem 253:1090–1094, 1978.

12. Summaria L, Arzadon L, Bernabe P, Robbins KC: The interaction of streptokinase with human, cat, dog and rabbit plasminogens: the fragmentation of streptokinase in the equimolar plasminogen–streptokinase complexes. J Biol Chem 249:4760–4769, 1974.

13. Summaria L, Robbins KC, Barlow GH: Dissociation of the equimolar human plasmin–streptokinase complex: partial characterization of the isolated plasmin and streptokinase moieties. J Biol Chem 246:2136–2142, 1971.

14. Summaria L, Arzadon R, Bernabe P, Robbins KC: Characterization of the NH$_2$-terminal glutamic acid and NH$_2$-terminal lysine forms of human plasminogen isolated by affinity chromatography and isoelectric focusing methods. J Biol Chem 248:2984–2991, 1973.

15. Summaria L, and Robbins KC: Isolation of a human plasmin-derived, functionally active, light (B) chain, capable of forming with streptokinase an equimolar light (B) chain–streptokinase complex with plasminogen activator activity. J Biol Chem 251:5810–5813, 1976.

16. Wohl RC, Summaria L, Arzadon L, Robbins KC: Steady state kinetics of activation of human and bovine plasminogens by streptokinase and its equimolar complexes with various activated forms of human plasminogen. J Biol Chem 253:1402–1407, 1978.

17. Summaria L, Boreisha I, Barlow GH, Robbins KC: The isolation and characterization of an equimolar human light (B) chain–streptokinase plasminogen complex. Circulation (Suppl 2) 66:II-179, 1982.

18. Kakkar VV: Intermittent plasminogen–streptokinase treatment of deep-vein thrombosis. Prog Fibrinolysis 5:420–431.

19. Cole ER, Bachmann FW: Purification and prop-

erties of plasminogen activator from pig heart. J Biol Chem 252:3729–3737, 1977.

20. Kok P, Astrup T: Isolation and purification of a tissue plasminogen activator and its comparison with urokinase. Biochemistry 8:79–86, 1969.

21. Unkelless J, Dano K, Kellerman GM, Reich E: Fibrinolysis associated with oncogenic transformation: partial purification and characterization of the cell factor, a plasminogen activator. J Biol Chem 249:4295–4305, 1974.

22. Rifkin DB, Loeb JN, Moore G, Reich E: Properties of plasminogen activators formed by neoplastic human cell cultures. J Exp Med 139:1317–1325, 1974.

23. Christman JK, Acs G, Silagi S, Silverstein SC: Plasminogen activator: biochemical characterization and correlation with tumorigenicity. Proteases Biol Control XX:827–839, 1975.

24. Aasted B: Immunochemical characterization of human plasminogen activators. Biochim Biophy Acta 668:339–348, 1981.

25. Binder BR, Spragg J, Austen KF: Purification and characterization of human vascular plasminogen activator derived from blood vessel perfusates. J Biol Chem 254:1998–2003, 1979.

26. Allen RA, Pepper DS: Isolation and properties of human vascular plasminogen activator. Thromb Haemost 45:43–50, 1981.

27. Collen D: On the regulation and control of fibrinolysis. Thromb Haemost 43:77–89, 1980.

28. Collen D, Rijken DC, Van Damme J, Billiau A: Purification of human tissue-type plasminogen activator in centigram quantities from human melanoma cell culture fluid and its conditioning for use in vivo. Thromb Haemost 48:294–296, 1982.

29. Pennica D, Holmes WE, Kohr WJ, Harkins RN, Vehar GA, Ward CA, Bennett WF, Yelverton E, Seeburg PH, Heyneker HL, Goeddel DV, Collen D: Cloning and expression of human tissue-type plasminogen activator CDNA in E. coli. Nature 301:214–221, 1983.

30. Bergmann SR, Fox KAA, Ter-Pogossian MM, Sobel BE, Collen D: Clot selective coronary thrombolysis with tissue type plasminogen activator. Science 220:1181–1183, 1983.

31. Wohl RC, Sinio L, Robbins KC: Methods for studying fibrinolytic pathway components in human plasma. Thromb Res 27:523–535, 1982.

32. Wohl, RC, Summaria L, Chediak J, Rosenfeld S, Robbins KC: Human plasminogen variant, Chicago III. Thromb Haemost 48:146–152, 1982.

8. CLINICAL PHARMACOLOGY
OF STREPTOKINASE

David S. Grierson

Streptokinase is a 47,000 molecular weight antigenic bacterial protein produced by Lancefield group-C beta-hemolytic streptococci. Since its discovery in 1933 by Tillett and Garner [1], it has been used as a thrombolytic agent in man. Despite extensive knowledge of the in vitro biochemistry of streptokinase (see chapter 7) [2, 3], few studies have specifically addressed its clinical pharmacology. Optimal dosing regimens and routes of administration, local or systemic, have not clearly been determined [4–8]. The lack of firm recommendations for its clinical use is related to two fundamental issues. First, the precise mechanism of clot lysis in vivo during streptokinase administration remains unclear [9, 10]. Second, the pharmacokinetics of streptokinase elimination have not been resolved [5]. Only by further knowledge in these two areas can clinical therapy with streptokinase be optimized. This chapter considers the three major theories of the mechanism of clot lysis [10] (see table 8-1) and reviews the available studies addressing the pharmacokinetics of streptokinase in man.

Theories on the Mechanism of Clot Lysis

The first comprehensive theory on the mechanism of clot lysis was proposed in 1959 by Alkjaersig and co-workers [11], based on a series of in vitro experiments and supported by assays of patients' plasma. This theory has been termed the "intrinsic activation theory" [10, 13], because it suggests that lysis occurs due to activation of plasminogen to plasmin within a formed

clot. Alkjaersig et al. showed that, upon addition of streptokinase to plasma, two measurable activities occurred: a proteolytic activity on casein substrates (a measure of the plasmin formed) and a plasminogen activator activity. (The terms "plasminogen activator" and "activator" will be used to refer to the streptokinase–plasminogen complex, which converts the proenzyme, plasminogen, to the active enzyme, plasmin.) They prepared plasma clots with ^{131}I fibrinogen and various amounts of plasminogen and measured clot lysis rates by release of ^{131}I into the supernatant. Several observations were made that supported this "intrinsic lysis theory" to explain the action of streptokinase.

With a fixed activator concentration in either buffer or plasma in which the ^{131}I clots were immersed, thrombolysis rates were linearly related to the logarithm of the clot plasminogen concentration [11]. Similarly, with clots of fixed plasminogen concentration, thrombolysis rates were linearly related to the logarithm of the activator concentration in the plasma bathing the clot. Also, the addition of an antithrombolytic agent (epsilon aminocaproic acid) to streptokinase in plasma, in amounts sufficient to prevent plasminogen activation, but insufficient to inhibit plasmin, markedly reduced the rate of thrombolysis. When clots of varying plasminogen content were immersed in a plasmin-containing solution, the thrombolysis rates were relatively slow and were unrelated to the clot plasminogen content. Thus, this "intrinsic lysis theory" suggests (a) that thrombolysis occurs by

R.M. Califf and G.S. Wagner (eds.), ACUTE CORONARY CARE: Principles and Practice. Copyright © 1985. Martinus Nijhoff Publishing, Boston/Dordrecht/Lancaster.

TABLE 8-1. The three major theories of the mechanism of clot lysis

Authors	Theory	Implied maintenance Dosing schedule
Alkjaersig et al. [11] "intrinsic activation theory"	Clot lysis depends on activator diffusing into thrombi activating entrapped plasminogen	High amounts of streptokinase
Ambrus and Markus [12] "extrinsic activation theory"	Clot lysis depends on high circulating plasmin and plasmin−antiplasmin complexes	Low amounts of streptokinase
Chesterman et al. [13] "surface activation theory"	Clot lysis depends on binding of activator to thrombi and activation of nearby plasminogen at the surface	High amounts of streptokinase with plasminogen supplementation or intermediate amounts of streptokinase in an attempt to prevent plasminogen depletion

diffusion of the activator into the thrombus with conversion of plasminogen entrapped within the fibrin to plasmin, and (b) that circulating plasmin has a minimal capacity to lyse thrombi. Important therapeutic principles emerge if one extends this theory to the clinical situation: (a) a very high dose of streptokinase would be required to overcome antibody resistance and maximally complex the circulating plasminogen into the activator form, and (b) the degree of systemic hyperplasminemia and attendant fibrinogenolysis should be minimized because of depletion of circulating free plasminogen available for conversion to plasmin.

The second theory of clot lysis was proposed by Ambrus and Markus in 1960 and has been termed the "extrinsic activation theory" [10, 12], because it suggests that lysis is caused by plasmin produced via activation of circulating plasminogen. In a series of in vitro experiments, they mixed plasmin (from activation of plasminogen either spontaneously or via streptokinase, urokinase, or chloroform) with human and bovine antiplasmin and tested the relative caseinolytic and fibrinolyic activities of the plasmin−antiplasmin mixtures. They showed that there was a linear relation between the caseinolytic effects and the fibrinolytic effects of plasmin in solutions free of antiplasmin. In the presence of antiplasmin, however, the caseinolytic effects were more completely inhibited than the fibrinolytic effects.

This observation supported the argument that the plasmin−antiplasmin complex could serve as a reservoir of fibrinolytic activity. Upon contact with fibrin in the circulation, the complex would dissociate, due to plasmin's higher affinity for its substrate (fibrin) than for its inhibitor (antiplasmin). Based on this theory, an initial dose of streptokinase sufficient to neutralize antibody should be given, followed by a low dose of streptokinase. Thereby, a small fraction of the total plasminogen would be complexed into the activator form, leaving substantial quantities of free circulating plasminogen available as substrate for activator. This dosing regimen would create a state of hyperplasminemia in which free plasmin along with the dissociable plasmin−antiplasmin complexes could produce "extrinsic lysis" of thrombi.

The third theory, the "surface activation theory" based on the work of Chesterman and co-workers, was proposed in 1972 [13]. It suggests that lysis occurs when activator, which is bound to the surface of the formed clot, converts plasminogen in the surrounding circulation into plasmin. In a first set of experiments, they prepared plasminogen-free ^{125}I fibrin clots by clotting ^{125}I fibrinogen in buffer solution. These clots were placed onto Pasteur pipettes and then incubated for 15 min in a solution of pooled normal plasma with streptokinase concentrations varying from zero to 10^5 U (units)/ml. Lysis was assessed by release of ^{125}I into the medium. This initial incubation produced $< 10\%$ clot lysis. The clots were removed, washed, and then reimmersed in normal plasma without streptokinase. Those clots, which had been preincubated in plasma containing streptokinase $(10^3-10^4$ U/ml), showed 70% lysis over 15 min of incubation. In a second set of experiments, tubes of whole blood with added ^{125}I fibrinogen were clotted and the clots were then removed and placed in multichannel perfusion chambers at 37°C with pressures of $100-120$ mmHg. The clots were perfused with various solutions and the lysis rates were monitored by measuring the ^{125}I released into the perfusate. Perfusion with streptokinase (100 U/ml) in saline produced only 19% lysis over 24 h. Similarly prepared ^{125}I whole blood clots were preincubated in streptokinase (1000 U/ml) in saline at 37°C for 1 h, washed, and placed in the perfusion apparatus. When the perfusion fluid was *streptokinase (100 U/ml) in saline*, only $< 15\%$ clot lysis occurred over 6 h. When perfused instead with *streptokinase (100 U/ml) in plasma*, the perfusate developed activator activity and plasminogen depletion occurred, but still only $< 15\%$ of the clot lysed over 6 h. When the clots were perfused with *normal plasma* (containing normal amounts of plasminogen and without streptokinase), 50% lysis occurred over 6 h. There was little additional lysis after this time and the perfusate showed neither activator activity nor plasminogen depletion. Thus, these investigators showed (a) that streptokinase could bind to whole blood clots, and (b) that clot lysis was a function of the plasminogen content of the perfusate. Extrapolation from this theory might then suggest two possible clinical dosing strategies. First, administer a very high initial dose of streptokinase to form high activator levels so that activator can bind to the thrombus, and follow this with plasminogen supplementation to ensure a high ambient plasminogen content. Second, a lower dose of streptokinase could be given, sufficient to form activator, but insufficient to cause plasminogen depletion.

In summary, the "intrinsic activation theory" indicates maintenance of high activator concentrations and avoidance of systemic hyperplasminemia, the "extrinsic activation theory" indicates maintenance of systemic hyperplasminemia, and the "surface activation theory" indicates maintenance of high plasminogen concentrations. Regardless of the dose of streptokinase that is given, as antibody resistance is overcome, plasminogen depletion will tend to occur, either because it is complexed into the activator form (by high doses) or because it is converted to plasmin (by lower doses).

Effects of Various Dosing Regimens

Clinical studies were performed to analyze the fibrinolytic effects that various dosing regimens produced. Johnson and McCarty produced thrombi in the forearm veins of volunteers and studied the thrombolysis of these clots assessed by venography with three different streptokinase infusion regimens [14]. The dosing regimens were described as "regimen P" (small intermittent doses of $25,000-50,000$ U of streptokinase/day after an initial antibody neutralization dose), designed to give the maximal attainable plasminemia; "regimen SK" $(45,000-60,000$ U/h by continuous infusion), designed to give the highest activator and free streptokinase concentrations and the lowest plasminogen; and "regimen SK-P" $(20,000-45,000$ U/h by continuous infusion), designed to give activator concentrations without plasminogen depletion. Regimen SK-P required frequent infusion rate adjustments that usually consisted of decreasing the infusion rate to prevent further lowering of plasminogen. With regimen P in seven subjects, partial clot lysis occurred in three, complete clot lysis occurred in one, but clots reformed in all four. With regimen SK in seven subjects, two had complete clot lysis, three had partial clot lysis but recurrent thrombus formation, and two had no lysis. In all 11 instances in which method SK-P was used to form activator but to avoid plasminogen depletion (by intermittent decrease of the infusion), complete and persistent clot lysis occurred. Thus, it appeared that maintaining sufficient circulating activator without severe plasminogen depletion was most efficacious. Fletcher et al. administered streptokinase to 50 patients with thromboembolic diseases and regulated the rate of infusion with the goal of maintaining a low plasminogen and a high activator concentration [15]. Data were presented from 21 patients who received intravenous streptokinase for 30 h after a loading infusion derived from the predicted dosage test (this was the dose equal to the amount of streptokinase per milliliter of plasma required to lyse a test clot in 20 min multiplied by the estimated plasma volume). The initial dose varied from 35,000 to 1,500,000 U. Thereafter the infusion rate was from 35,000 to 150,000 U/h. When plasminogen values were not "sufficiently lowered," the infusion rates were increased. Close analysis of the lysis zones on unheated fibrin plates and lysis rates of radio-labeled test clots (both measures of activator) showed that both of these measures decreased over the period of 14−32 h of the infusion.

After the studies of Alkjaersig et al. had clearly shown the need to give an initial dose of streptokinase to neutralize streptokinase antibody, subsequent studies used individualized dosing schemes based on in vitro measures of resistance [16]. Amery et al. standardized a method whereby resistance could be predicted [17]. Over the next few years, however, it was found that the individualization of therapy was unnecessary and fixed dose regimens were adopted. Standard loading doses designed to neutralize antibody rapidly in the majority of patients were followed by infusion rates of approximately 100,000 U/h to maintain circulating plasminogen at the lower levels endorsed by Alkjaersig et al. Verstraete and co-workers reported the use of a standardized dosing scheme [18]. They reviewed the prior published data quantifying streptokinase resistance, which had ranged from 25,000 to 1,500,000 U. Johnson et al. had found that 82% of a population of 149 patients had a resistance of less than 500,000 U [16]. Verstraete et al. found that, when combining his 132 patients to those reported in the literature, 97% of the patients had resistances of less than 1,250,000 U. They also found that a maintenance infusion of at least 70,000 U/h was required to maintain plasminogen values at less than 5% of baseline and that an infusion of 100,000 U/h reliably maintained plasminogen below this level. In treating 15 patients who had peripheral arterial occlusions, this standardized method was successful in lysing thrombi in 12. The point was made that with a standardized dosing regimen

"the laboratory control is greatly simplified and is not even essential."

Hirsh et al. evaluated a standard dosing regimen with a lower initial dose (250,000 U over 30 min) followed by 100,000 U/h for 24−48 h [19]. Of 80 patients studied, 50 received individualized loading doses based on their resistance. In these 80 patients, the mean resistance was 120,000 U and 92% had a resistance of less than 250,000 U. Four patients who had resistances of over 250,000 U received the standard dose. They had a delay in the onset of fibrinolytic activity of 4−8 h, but once the fibrinolytic state was achieved, it was similar regardless of the initial resistance. Amery et al. studied the changes in plasma plasminogen and fibrinogen in 71 patients receiving an initial dose of 1,200,000 U and 26 patients receiving an initial dose of 250,000 U with both groups receiving 100,000 U/h over 24−72 h [20]. The fibrinogen and plasminogen levels were significantly more depressed immediately after the initial high dose than after the lower dose. After 24 h of a maintenance infusion of 100,000 U/h in both groups, the number of patients with plasminogen levels below 5% of baseline was not significantly different. The plasminogen then remained depressed independent of the initial loading dose. After 24 h, the fibrinogen tended to rise in those receiving the higher initial dose while it was further depressed in those receiving the lower initial dose. At 48 and 72 h, there were no differences between the groups regarding either plasminogen or fibrinogen values.

During the 1970s, there were numerous trials comparing heparin and streptokinase therapy in patients with deep-vein thrombosis and pulmonary emboli. In the majority of these trials, the fixed regimen of a 250,000-U loading dose and maintenance with 100,000 U/h were used. A review of these trials is presented by Hirsh [21]. Investigators searched for correlations between thrombolytic efficacy and various coagulation tests, but no reliable correlations were evident between the clinical efficacy of streptokinase and measures of coagulation times, euglobulin lysis times, or plasma protein levels [22]. In the urokinase−streptokinase pulmonary embolism trial, there were no correlations between the coagulation and fibrinolytic measurements and angiographic resolution of pulmonary emboli [23]. The authors commented that "the age, size and composition of the pulmonary embolus and local pulmonary blood flow are probably more important determinants of successful thrombolysis" [24].

Pharmacokinetic Studies of Streptokinase Elimination in Man

As stated previously, the determination of specific values for the pharmacokinetic parameters of streptokinase elimination has been difficult because no direct assay for the protein exists. Even if such an assay did exist, the ability to distinguish free streptokinase from that in the multiple activator forms (see chapter 7) would be difficult and degradation products of the streptokinase protein molecule could be confounding. The half-lives of streptokinase elimination that are often quoted in the literature [5] come from the work of Fletcher et al., who studied the clearance rates of ^{131}I-labeled streptokinase in patients with a range of streptokinase resistances [25]. When doses of ^{131}I streptokinase were administered in amounts below the calculated resistance doses, the elimination half-lives ranged from 9 to 36 min, with an average of 17.5 min. When doses were administered in excess of the resistance dose, the elimination half-lives ranged from 62 to 110 min and averaged 83 min. In two representative patients who received ^{131}I streptokinase in a dose greater than their resistance, both phases of elimination were seen. In patients who had the clearance rates determined on the second day of continuous infusion, there was only one half-life of elimination, which ranged from 92 to 110 min. Apparently, the first and more rapid half-life represented elimination mediated by antigen–antibody complexes and this phase was absent after sufficient antigen (streptokinase) had been administered to neutralize antibody. The second half-life represented clearance by nonantibody-mediated mechanisms. During infusion, the plasma ^{131}I streptokinase concentration was correlated with the degree of lysis of in vitro test clots. One problem with the study was that, by 24 h, 40%–50% of the plasma ^{131}I was

free, not protein bound (as assessed by acid-precipitable radioactivity), so the ^{131}I counts may not have truly reflected streptokinase concentrations.

Amery [26] assessed the time course of the decrease in lysis zones on unheated fibrin plates as a measure of activator elimination in serial plasma samples taken after discontinuation of a streptokinase infusion. At an average of 18.5 min, the lysis zone areas had diminished by half. By 2 h, the remaining activity was less than 10% of the activity immediately before discontinuation of the infusion.

Martin used thromboelastographic measures of clot lysis times as an indirect method of determining streptokinase concentrations in plasma [27]. A standard curve of streptokinase concentration versus lysis time of standard clots was constructed. Plasma samples of patients undergoing streptokinase treatment were then used as the source of streptokinase in the assay and the clot lysis times were converted to plasma streptokinase concentrations. Unexpectedly, he found that, during constant-rate infusion of streptokinase at 100,000 U/h, there was a progressive fall in the plasma streptokinase concentration over three days in all 11 patients studied. A rise in antistreptokinase antibody during the infusion period was ruled out as an explanation for the decreasing levels over three days.

Recently, chromogenic peptide substrates susceptible to hydrolysis by specific activated coagulation factors, proteases, and plasminogen activators are finding increasing use in coagulation and fibrinolysis research [28–31]. The chromogenic substrate S-2251 is susceptible to amidolysis by both plasmin and the streptokinase plasminogen activator complex. In an in vitro buffer system of plasminogen and streptokinase, using hirudin as a plasmin inhibitor, Latallo et al. showed a linear relationship between amidolytic activity and streptokinase concentration [31]. Using this principle, we constructed standard linear curves of plasma amidolytic activity versus streptokinase concentration in pretreatment plasmas of patients who received intravenous streptokinase for myocardial infarction and venous thromboemoblism. During and after the loading and continuous infusions of streptokinase, amidolytic activity of plasma (activator complex activity) was determined and expressed as streptokinase units using pretreatment standard curves. With this method, the average elimination half-life of streptokinase was 85.7 min. During continuous infusion over 16–78 h, there was a progressive decline in streptokinase concentrations [32].

In summary, the studies by Fletcher et al. showed the average elimination half-life of antibody-bound streptokinase to be 17 min. The nonantibody-mediated elimination half-life averaged 83 min. From our studies, it appears that this half-life of approximately 90 min reflects the elimination of streptokinase in the activator form. Close analysis of the data of Fletcher et al. showed decreasing lysis zones on unheated fibrin plates (a measure of activator content of plasma) during streptokinase infusions; Martin showed decreasing streptokinase concentrations in the thromboelastographic assay during continuous infusions over three days, and our study showed a time-dependent decrease in amidolytic activator complex activity during continuous infusions for up to 78 h.

The following sequence of events during the administration of the loading dose and subsequent continuous infusion of streptokinase is supported by these studies. First, the loading dose will neutralize circulating antibody in a majority of patients. If this dose is insufficient to neutralize antibody, the resistance will be overcome during the first few hours of continuous infusion. As further streptokinase is administered, it will complex with plasminogen and, inevitably during the early period after antibody neutralization, the ratio of low levels of activator to high levels of uncomplexed plasminogen will create a degree of systemic hyperplasminemia and fibrinogenolysis. As plasminogen levels fall and streptokinase infusion continues, the ratio of plasminogen in the activator form to free plasminogen will reverse with very low levels of free plasminogen. Thereafter, with continued infusion of streptokinase, the free plasminogen availability becomes the limiting factor for activator formation and activator levels subsequently decline. It appears that thrombolytic therapy with streptokinase may become somewhat self-limiting even before the point at which antistreptokinase antibody levels rise. Thus, there are sound arguments

that can be advanced for using intermittent streptokinase doses, allowing plasminogen levels to rise between doses [33], or using streptokinase in combination with plasminogen [34, 35], especially in disease states such as venous thromboembolism that require sustained thrombolytic therapy.

Clinical Use in Acute Myocardial Infarction

Myocardial infarction presents a different clinical situation since the critical issue is rapid lysis of the intracoronary thrombus to potentially salvagable ischemic myocardium (see chapter 33). In initial studies, intracoronary streptokinase was used with the rationale that selective infusion of low doses of streptokinase would cause thrombolysis without producing a systemic lytic state. Some studies comparing intracoronary with intravenous streptokinase showed that the time to clot lysis after drug administration was shorter by the intracoronary route, and that intracoronary administration was sometimes more efficacious [36–38]. However, certain facts have now increased the interest in returning to intravenous streptokinase [39]. First, the number of patients with acute myocardial infarcts having rapid access to catheterization facilities is limited. Second, there is an irreducible time delay from identification of a thrombolytic therapy candidate to initial visualization of the infarct-related vessel in the catheterization laboratory; this time may range from 45 to 120 min during the initial period when myocardial necrosis is occurring rapidly. Administration of intravenous streptokinase can shorten this delay until initiation of thrombolytic therapy and would be applicable to larger numbers of patients. Third, recent studies have shown a strong correlation between the efficacy of intracoronary streptokinase and the development of fibrinolytic profiles reflecting a systemic lytic state [40, 41]. Some investigators have proposed that the systemic lytic state may be a necessary requirement for coronary thrombolysis [40]. In a review of the intracoronary dosing regimens, Cowley noted a trend toward higher success rates with higher infusion rates and higher total administered doses [42].

Until newer thrombolytic agents are available,

streptokinase is the thrombolytic agent of choice for patients with acute myocardial infarction. From the experimental and theoretical considerations in this chapter and the newer clinical studies [43], it appears that the higher doses of streptokinase, by either the intravenous or intracoronary methods, result in higher reperfusion rates. Future clinical studies will be required to determine whether further improvement can be achieved either by addition of plasminogen or by replacement of the streptokinase with specific tissue plasminogen activators [44]. Van de Werf et al. have recently shown that intravenous tissue plasminogen activator is an effective thrombolytic agent in patients with acute myocardial infarction, without induction of a systemic fibrinolytic state [45].

References

1. Tillet WS, Garner RL: The fibrinolytic activity of hemolytic streptococci. J Exp Med 58:485, 1933.
2. Castellino FJ, Sodetz JM, Brockway WJ, Siefring GE: Streptokinase. Methods Enzymol 45: 244−256, 1986.
3. Wohl RC, Summaria L, Arzadon L, Robbins KC: Steady state kinetics of activation of human and bovine plasminogens by streptokinase and its equimolar complexes with various activated forms of human plasminogen. J Biol Chem 253:1402−1407, 1978.
4. Marder VS: Pharmacology of thrombolytic agents: implications for therapy of coronary artery thrombosis. Circulation (Suppl 1) 68:2−5, 1983.
5. Bell WR, Meek AG: Guidelines for the use of thrombolytic agents. N Engl J Med 301:1266−1270, 1979.
6. Barlow GH: Pharmacology of fibrinolytic agents. Prog Cardiovasc Dis 21:315−326, 1979.
7. Sharma GVRK, Cella G, Parisi AF, Sasahara AA: Thrombolytic therapy. N Engl J Med 306: 1268−1276, 1982.
8. Marder VJ: The use of thrombolytic agents: choice of patient, drug administration and laboratory monitoring. Ann Intern Med 0:802−808, 1979.
9. Sasahara AA, Sharma GVRK, Tow D, McIntyre KM, Parisi AF, Cella G: Clinical use of thrombolytic agents in venous thromboembolism. Arch Intern Med 142:684−688, 1982.
10. Verstraete M: Biomedical and clinical aspects of thrombolysis. Semin Hematol 15:35−54, 1978.
11. Alkjaersig N, Fletcher AP, Sherry S: The mechanism of clot dissolution by plasmin. J Clin Invest 38:1086−1095, 1959.
12. Ambrus CM, Markus G: Plasmin−antiplasmin as a reservoir of fibrinolytic enzyme. Am J Physiol 199:491−494, 1960.
13. Chesterman CN, Allington MJ, Sharp AA: Relationship of plasminogen activator to fibrin. Nature [New Biol] 238:15−17, 1972.
14. Johnson AJ, McCarty WR: The lysis of artificially induced intravascular clots in man by intravenous infusions of streptokinase. J Clin Invest 38:1627−1643, 1959.
15. Fletcher AP, Alkjaersig N, Sherry S: The maintenance of a sustained thrombolytic state in man. I. Induction and effects. J Clin Invest 38:1096−1110, 1959.
16. Johnson AJ, Fletcher AP, McCarty WR, Tillett WS: The intravascular use of streptokinase. Ann NY Acad Sci 68:201, 1957.
17. Amery A, Maes H, Vermylen J, Verstraete M: The streptokinase reactivity test I. Standardization. Thromb Diath Haemorrh 9:175−188, 1963.
18. Verstraete M, Vermylen J, Amery A, Vermylen C: Thrombolytic therapy with streptokinase using a standard dosing scheme. Br Med J 1:454−456, 1966.
19. Hirsh J, O'Sullivan EF, Martin M: Evaluation of a standard dosage schedule with streptokinase. Blood 35:341−349, 1970.
20. Amery A, Donati MB, Vermylen J, Verstraete M: Comparison between the changes in plasma fibrinogen and plasminogen levels induced by a moderate or high initial dose of streptokinase. Thromb Diath Haemorrh 23:504−572, 1970.
21. Hirsh J: Venous thromboembolism. New York: Grune and Stratton, 1981.
22. Marder VJ, Soulen RL, Atichartakarn V, Budzynski AZ, Parulekar S, Kim JR, Edward N, Zahavi J, Algazy KM: Quantitative venographic assessment of deep vein thrombosis in the evaluation of streptokinase and heparin therapy. J Lab Clin Med 89:1018−1029, 1977.
23. Urokinase−streptokinase embolism trial: phase II results: cooperative study. JAMA 229:1606, 1974.
24. Urokinase pulmonary embolism trial: cooperative study. Circulation (Suppl 2) 47:73−80, 1973.
25. Fletcher AP, Alkjaersig N, Sherry S: The clearance of heterologous protein from the circulation of normal and immunized man. J Clin Invest 37:1306−1315, 1959.

26. Amery A: Changes in fibrinolytic parameters after prolonged streptokinase infusion. Thromb Diath Haemorrh (Suppl) 32:151−155, 1969.

27. Martin M: Indirect measurement of streptokinase concentration in the plasma of patients undergoing fibrinolytic treatment. Thromb Diath Haemorrh 32:633−650, 1974.

28. Friberger P: Chromogenic peptide substrates: their use for the assay of factors in the fibrinolytic and the plasma kallikrein−kinin system. Scand J Clin Lab Invest 162:1−298, 1982.

29. Wohl RC, Sinio L, Robbins KC: Methods for studying the fibrinolytic pathway components in plasma. Thromb Res 27:523−535, 1982.

30. Latallo ZS, Teisseyre E, Lopaciuk S: Evaluation of a fibrinolytic profile of plasma using chromogenic substrates: chromogenic peptide substrates. Scully and Kakkar (eds), 1979, pp. 262−268.

31. Latallo ZS, Teisseyre E, Raczka E: Activators of plasminogen, measurements using chromogenic substrates: chromogenic peptide substrates. Scully and Kakkar (eds), 1979, pp. 154−168.

32. Grierson DS, Bjornsson T: Pharmacokinetics of streptokinase in patients based on amidolytic activator complex activity. Circulation 68:39, (Suppl 2) 1983.

33. Verstraete M, Vermylen J, Schetz J: Biochemical changes noted during intermittent administration of streptokinase. Thromb Haemost 39:61−68, 1978.

34. Kakkar VV, Sagar S, Lewis M: Treatment of deep vein thrombosis with intermittent streptokinase and plasminogen infusion. Lancet 2:674−676, 1975.

35. Scully MF, Lane A, Sagar S, Thomas DP, Kakkar VV: Intermittent plasminogen−streptokinase treatment of deep vein thrombosis. Thromb Haemost 37:162−169, 1977.

36. Saltups A, Boxall J, Ho B: Intracoronary vs intravenous streptokinase in acute myocardial infarction. Circulation (Suppl 3) 68:119, 1983.

37. Berte LE, Jutzy KR, Alderman EL, Miller RG, Friedman JP, Creger WP, Eliastam M: Ran-domized trial of intravenous and intracoronary streptokinase early post-myocardial infarction. Circulation (Suppl 3) 68:119, 1983.

38. Saltups, A, Boxall J, Ho B, Bower S, Balazs N, Dennis P: Intracoronary vs intravenous streptokinase in myocardial infarction. JACC 3:525, 1984.

39. Spann JF, Sherry S, Carabello BA, Mann RH, McCann WD, Gault JH, Gentzler RD, Rosenberg KM, Maurer AH, Denenberg BS, Warner HF, Rubin RN, Malmud LS, Camerota, A: High dose, brief intravenous streptokinase early in acute myocardial infarction. Am Heart J 104:939−945, 1982.

40. Rothbard RL, Fitzpatrick PG, Caton DM, Francis CW, Hood WB, Marder VJ: Relationship of systemic lytic state to acute thrombolysis with standard and low dose intracoronary streptokinase. Circulation (Suppl 3) 68:38, 1983.

41. Jutzy KR, Berte LE, Alderman EL, Miller RG, Friedman JP, Creger WP, Eliastam M: Relation of systemic fibrinolytic state with route of streptokinase administration and recanalization. Circulation (Suppl 3) 68:39, 1983.

42. Cowley MS: Methodologic aspects of intracoronary thrombolysis: drugs, dosage and duration. Circulation (Suppl 1) 68:90−95, 1983.

43. Maddahi J, Weiss T, Geft I, Suah PK, Berman D, Swan HSC, Ganz W: Coronary thrombolysis with intravenous streptokinase salvages jeopardized myocardium in evolving myocardial infarction: assessment of quantitative thallium-201 imaging. Circulation (Suppl 3) 68:120, 1983.

44. Collen D, Verstraete M: Systemic thrombolytic therapy of acute myocardial infarction? Circulation 68:462−465, 1983.

45. Van de Werf F, Ludbrook PA, Bergmann SR, Tiefenbrunn AJ, Fox KAA, De Geest H, Verstraete M, Collen D, Sobel BE: Coronary thrombolysis with tissue-type plasminogen activator in patients with evolving myocardial infarction. N Engl J Med 310:609−613, 1984.

9. TERMINOLOGY FOR LOCATION OF ACUTE MYOCARDIAL INFARCTS

William C. Roberts

Julius M. Gardin

Among patients with clinical features suggesting acute myocardial infarction (AMI), the standard 12-lead electrocardiogram (ECG) has been extremely useful during the past 50 years in establishing the diagnosis of myocardial necrosis. In addition to indicating the presence of AMI, the ECG has provided certain information regarding the location of the AMI. This chapter, which is adapted from a previous report [1], reexamines the reliability of the ECG in predicting the anatomic location of AMI and suggests a common terminology for designating the location of AMI, applicable both electrocardiographically and morphologically.

Anatomic Approach to Terminology for Localization of AMI

The normal left ventricle at necropsy in essence is a *cone*. Proper description of the location of an AMI of the left ventricle necessitates designation of the portion(s) of involvement of each of the three dimensions of the cone, namely, (a) the *circle*, (b) the *thickness*, and (c) the *length* (top to bottom) (figure 9-1).

The circle includes the *anterior*, *posterior*, and *lateral* free walls and the *ventricular septum*. The thickness may be designated as *subendocardial*, meaning inner one-half; *subepicardial*, meaning outer one-half; and *transmural*, meaning involvement of both subendocardium and subepicardium. We prefer defining subendocardium as the

inner half of the myocardial wall, rather than just the inner third, because most subendocardial infarcts involve only the inner third, and, therefore, by using the half-way cutoff, a clear demarcation usually is present between subendocardial and transmural. Furthermore, most transmural infarcts involve >75% of the myocardial wall, and, consequently, they are clearly separable from infarcts limited to subendocardium (see chapter 10). The length or top-to-bottom dimension may be divided into basal third, middle third, and apical third, or simply into *basal half* ("high") and *apical half* ("low") (figure 9-2). We prefer the latter. The specific compartments of the walls of the cardiac ventricles are shown diagrammatically in figure 9-2. Designating each of the various compartments of the heart, obviously, is somewhat arbitrary. We include, for example, the anterolateral papillary muscle of the left ventricle in the anterior compartment, although it can just as easily be included in the lateral compartment. The portion of ventricle at each end of the ventricular septum, when viewed transversely, could be included in either the posterior or the anterior compartment, or in the ventricular septum. We prefer to include these junction points between right and left ventricular free walls as part of the ventricular septum. We divide the right ventricular free wall into two compartments (anterolateral and posterior) as contrasted to the three free-wall compartments of the left ventricle (anterior, posterior, and lateral).

R.M. Califf and G.S. Wagner (eds.), ACUTE CORONARY CARE: Principles and Practice. Copyright © 1985. Martinus Nijhoff Publishing, Boston/Dordrecht/Lancaster.

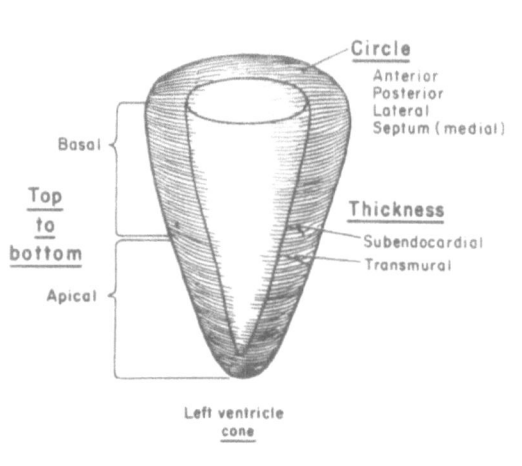

FIGURE 9-1. Diagram illustrating the three dimensions of the left ventricle as a cone, for localization of infarction.

Anatomic Compartments of the Heart Involved by AMI

To show the portion of cardiac ventricles involved by AMI, the ventricles are divided into basal and apical halves (figure 9-2). Three portions of the basal half infrequently are sites of myocardial necrosis—namely, the anterior and anteroseptal compartments of the left ventricle and the anterolateral compartment of the right ventricle. "Anterior" AMI spares the right ventricular free wall [2], whereas nearly 25% of patients with "posterior" left ventricular AMI have necrosis of all or portions of the posterior wall of the right ventricle. Most patients with "posterior" AMI have necrosis of portions or all of the posteromedial papillary muscle of the left ventricle. In contrast, many patients with "anterior" AMI have no involvement of the anterolateral papillary muscle of the left ventricle.

One problem in designating an AMI as "anterior" or "posterior" is that each may be only partially true. A large infarct, for example, may be limited to the posterior, posteroseptal, or posterolateral portion of the left ventricle in its basal half, whereas the area of myocardial necrosis may be completely circumferential in much or some of the apical half of the left ventricle. Likewise, an area of myocardial necrosis may be entirely subendocardial in one portion and transmural in another. The latter are classified as "transmural."

Terminology for Describing Sites of AMI

Certain terms used in designating AMI by electrocardiogram are not used for designating its location at necropsy. The terms "inferior," "diaphragmatic," and "true posterior," for example, are electrocardiographic terms, and they are poor ones because they break the principle of parallelism. Their opposites namely, "superior," "sternal," or "false posterior" (or indeed "true anterior" or "false anterior"), are never employed. Therefore, these terms might best be eliminated so that the same may be used both electrocardiographically and anatomically. "Inferior" and "diaphragmatic" AMI are simply those involving the "posterior" left ventricular wall, possibly primarily the "posteroapical" portion. "True posterior" generally has been considered "posterobasal," but evidence for this is not firm.

Electrocardiographic Patterns for Localizing AMI in the Three Dimensions of the Cone

The focus in this section centers on abnormalities in the QRS complex in AMI. Most but not all "QRS infarcts" are transmural, but some transmural infarcts occur without QRS changes (see chapter 10). Fatal AMI limited to the subendocardium, i.e, inner half of the left ventricular wall, is infrequent in our experience at necropsy and it has been observed by us, with rare exception, only in patients with left ventricular hypertrophy from another condition (systemic hypertension or left ventricular outflow obstruction) or prolonged shock (of any origin). Thus, opportunity for electrocardiographic—anatomic correlative studies among patients with isolated subendocardial AMI is limited.

ECG PATTERN IN "TRANSMURAL" AMI INVOLVING THE ANTERIOR WALL OF LEFT VENTRICLE

AMI at necropsy infrequently involves the more basal portion of the anterior wall of the left ventricle. Therefore, "anterior" AMI by ECG nearly always indicates necrosis of all or portions of the

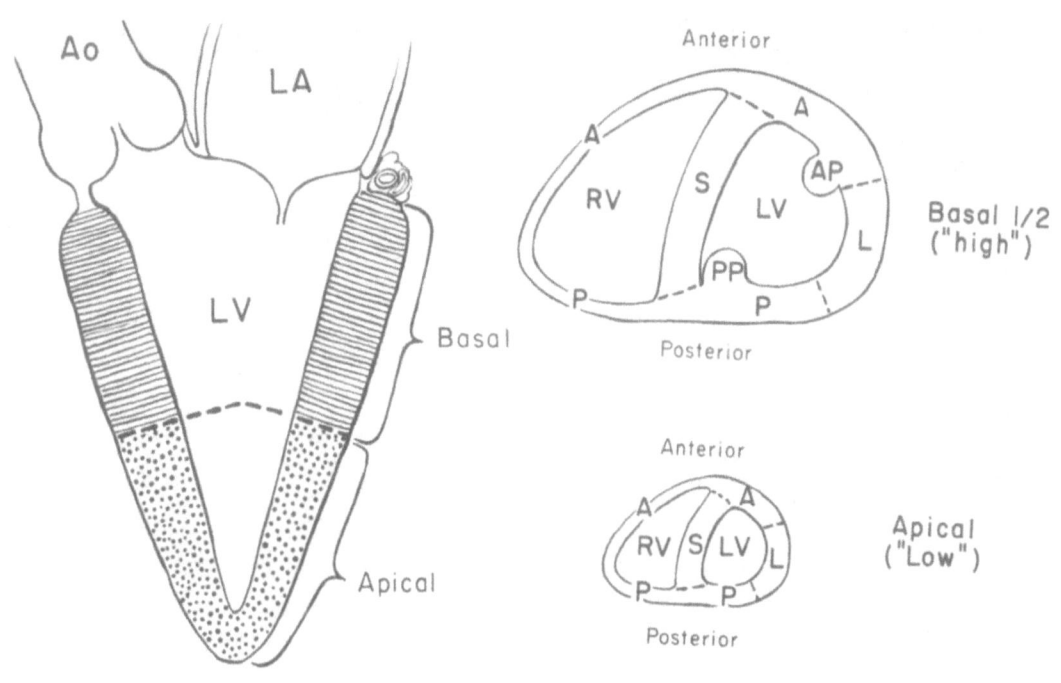

FIGURE 9-2. Diagrams showing the left ventricle (LV) illustrated as a cone (left) and transverse cuts across the right (RV) and left ventricles (LV) (right). The length of the ventricle is divided into basal and apical halves. The larger transverse slice (upper right) is from the basal half and the smaller transverse slice is from the apical half. The dotted lines serve to define the various compartments of the left ventricle. A, anterior wall of the left ventricle and anterolateral wall of the right ventricle; Ao, aorta; AP, anterolateral papillary muscle; L, lateral wall of left ventricle; LA, left atrium; P, posterior wall of the right and left ventricles; PP, posteromedial papillary muscle; S, ventricular septum.

apical half, and, in general, is characterized by the presence of Q waves of greater than 0.03 s in leads V_3 and/or V_4 (table 9-1). AMI, however, infrequently is limited to just the anterior wall of the left ventricle: the lateral or septal wall or both is (are) usually also involved. "Anteroseptal" AMI is characterized by the presence of Q waves in V_1 and V_2 in addition to the usual presence of Q waves in V_3 and/or V_4, and "anterolateral" AMI is characterized by the presence of Q waves in V_5 and/or V_6, sometimes in leads I and/or

aVL, in addition to the expected Q waves in V_3 and/or V_4.

ECG PATTERN IN "TRANSMURAL" AMI INVOLVING THE POSTERIOR WALL OF LEFT VENTRICLE

Although differences by ECG between "true posterior" ("plain posterior") and "inferior" ("diaphragmatic" or "inferoposterior") AMI have been described, the evidence is by no means convincing that "posterior" AMI involving the basal half of the left ventricle can be distinguished by ECG from "posterior" AMI involving the apical half of this ventricle. ("True posterior" AMI has been characterized by "tall" [R to S ratio ≥ 1] and "broad" [≥ 0.04-s duration] R waves in V_1 and/or V_2; "inferior" AMI, by Q waves of ≥ 0.04-s duration in leads II, III, and aVF.) Furthermore, although it has been suggested that the additional presence of Q waves in V_5 and V_6 denotes involvement (extension) of the "posterolateral" wall, AMI involving the "posterolateral" wall cannot be reliably differentiated from AMI involving the "posteroseptal" wall, and neither can be reliably delineated from AMI limited to the

TABLE 9-1. Electrocardiographic patterns of transmural AMI[a]

Anatomic site of left ventricular (LV) AMI	Electrocardiographic QRS changes
Anterior wall	Q V_3 and/or V_4
Anteroseptal	Q V_3 and/or V_4 + V_1 and V_2
Anterolateral	Q V_3 and/or V_4 + V_5 and/or V_6
Posterior wall	Q II, III and aVF and/or R $\geq$ S in V_1 and/or V_2 and $\geq$0.04 s
Posteroseptal	Unknown
Posterolateral	Unknown
Ventricular septum	
Lateral wall	Nothing specific
Papillary muscles	
Right ventricle	

[a]The electrocardiographic pattern shown here can be altered by abnormal cardiac position, cardiomegaly, bundle branch block, previous myocardial infarction, and, obviously, incorrect lead placement.

"posterior" free wall of the left ventricle. Thus, "posterior" AMI with or without involvement of the adjacent septal or lateral walls generally is characterized by Q waves in leads II, III, and aVF and/or the presence of broad ($\geq$0.04 s) and tall (R wave to S wave ratio $\geq$1) R waves in V_1 and/or V_2.

ECG PATTERN IN "TRANSMURAL" AMI INVOLVING ONLY VENTRICULAR SEPTUM, LATERAL WALL OF LEFT VENTRICLE, PAPILLARY MUSCLE, OR RIGHT VENTRICLE

In contrast to its ability to distinguish clearly between AMI involving the "anterior" wall from that involving the "posterior" wall of the left ventricle, the ECG provides no specific pattern to indicate necrosis of the ventricular septum, lateral wall of the left ventricle, papillary muscles, or right ventricle. AMI, however, is rarely, if ever, limited exclusively to the lateral wall of the left ventricle, to the ventricular septum, or to the right ventricle. Thus, whenever the ventricular septum or the left ventricular lateral wall is the site of AMI, either the anterior or the posterior wall also is involved. Furthermore, as mentioned, AMI secondary to coronary arterial narrowing and involving the right ventricle is always associated with "posterior" left ventricular AMI, never "anterior" left ventricular AMI [2]. Consequently, necrosis is never limited to the anterolateral wall of the right ventricle; when this portion is

necrotic, all or a portion of the posterior right ventricular wall is either necrotic or fibrotic or both. Also, necrosis of the posteromedial papillary muscle occurs in most patients with "posterior" AMI; therefore, involvement of this structure can be predicted simply by knowing that the AMI is "posterior." In contrast, most patients with left ventricular "anterior" wall AMI do not have involvement of the anterolateral papillary muscle and, therefore, involvement of this structure cannot be predicted reliably by knowing that the AMI involves the "anterior" wall.

Summary

The same terminology applicable for describing the location of an AMI at necropsy is applicable for defining its location by electrocardiogram. Certain terms used electrocardiographically, namely, "inferior," "diaphragmatic," and "true posterior," should be avoided because their opposites are not used. Ideally, a proper description of the location of an AMI should include defining its involvement in all the dimensions of the left ventricle (considered as a cone): the portion of the walls of the circle involved (anterior, posterior, lateral, and septal), the amount of the wall's thickness involved (transmural or nontransmural [subendocardial]), and the portions of the wall's length involved (basal half or apical half or both). Certain portions of the walls of both the left and right ventricles are rare sites of AMI, and knowing these sites helps in more precisely defining by ECG the location of the AMI. AMI involving the anterior wall of the left ventricle rarely is limited to just its basal half; and, therefore, anterior AMI, for practical purposes, indicates involvement of at least the apical half of the ventricle. AMI involving the basal half of the posterior left ventricular wall, in contrast, is common, but the ECG is not accurate in differentiating posterobasal from posteroapical AMI. Furthermore, the ECG provides no specific pattern to indicate AMI of the ventricular septum, lateral wall of the left ventricle, either posterior or anterolateral walls of the right ventricle, or papillary muscles. AMI of the right ventricle virtually never occurs with "anterior" AMI of the left ventricle. In contrast, nearly 25% of patients with "posterior" transmural AMI also have associated AMI involving at least the posterior wall of the right ventricle.

References

1. Roberts WC, Gardin JM: Location of myocardial infarcts: a confusion of terms and definitions. Am J Cardiol 42:868–872, 1978.
2. Isner JM, Roberts WC: Right ventricular infarction complicating left ventricular infarction secondary to coronary heart disease: frequency, location, associated findings and significance from analysis of 236 necropsy patients with acute or healed myocardial infarction. Am J Cardiol 42: 885–894, 1978.

10. SUBENDOCARDIAL VERSUS TRANSMURAL INFARCTION

Anatomic and Electrocardiographic Considerations

Raymond E. Ideker

Several recent editorials and reviews deal with the relationship between the transmural extent of an infarct in the left ventricle and the QRS and ST-T changes observed in the electrocardiogram [1−4]. This chapter supplements these publications by emphasizing anatomic and electrocardiographic aspects of subendocardial and transmural infarcts that have not been previously considered.

Anatomic Considerations

DESCRIPTION OF INFARCT ANATOMY
Infarcts vary in circumferential extent, base-to-apex extent, size, location, and degree of patchiness in addition to transmural extent. All of these factors may influence the electrocardiogram. Analysis of the electrocardiographic effect of each of these anatomic factors is complex because (a) the factors are continuous and not binary, and (b) the factors are not independent. For example, transmural infarcts tend to be larger and less patchy than subendocardial infarcts [5−7].

Supported in part by SCOR grant HL-17670 from the National Heart, Lung and Blood Institute. Dr. Ideker is the recipient of a Research Career Development Award (HL-00546) also from the National Heart, Lung and Blood Institute.

Most of these anatomic factors are not consistent throughout the infarct. The border regions of most solid infarcts are patchy (figure 10-1), i.e., containing peninsulas of viable myofibers interspersed within infarcted tissue [8]. Because of coronary anatomy, the circumferential extent of anterior infarcts is usually greater at the apex than at the base, while the opposite is true of inferior infarcts (figure 10-2) [9].

Transmural extent also varies throughout most infarcts (figure 10-1) [10]. Many anterior infarcts are subendocardial at the base and transmural at the apex of the left ventricle (figure 10-3) [5]. Some inferior infarcts are subendocardial at the base, transmural in the middle section, and intramural or subepicardial near the apex of the left ventricle [6]. These infarcts become intramural or subepicardial because they are in the distribution of the posterior descending coronary artery, which supplies the subepicardium of the inferior left ventricular apex. The subendocardium of the inferior apex is supplied by the distal portion of the left anterior descending coronary artery [11].

DEFINITIONS OF TRANSMURAL INFARCTION
There are no universally accepted definitions of subendocardial and transmural infarction. Different studies correlating anatomy and electrocardiography variously define a transmural infarct

R.M. Califf and G.S. Wagner (eds.), ACUTE CORONARY CARE: Principles and Practice. Copyright © 1985. Martinus Nijhoff Publishing, Boston/Dordrecht/Lancaster.

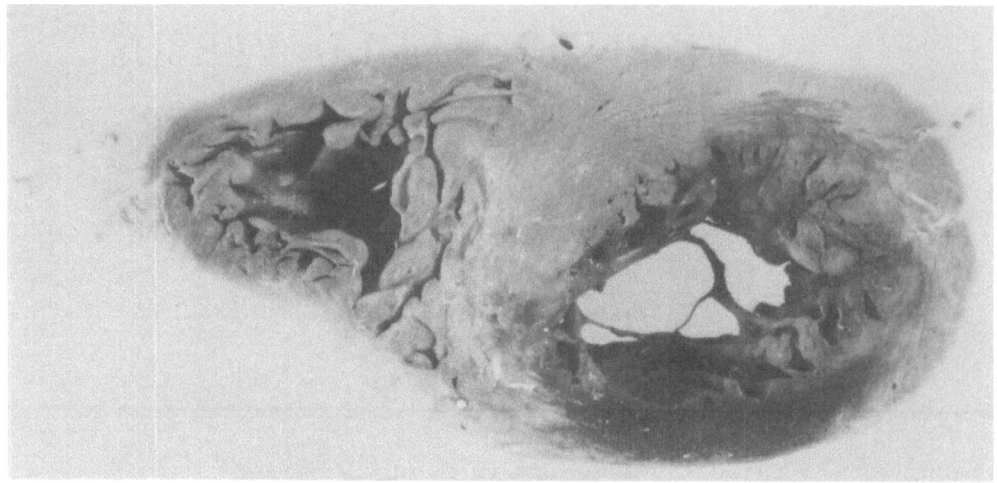

FIGURE 10-1. Photograph of the basal surface of a human heart slice showing an organizing infarct that is solid and transmural in the anterior left ventricular free wall (dark region at bottom of figure), but patchy and subendocardial in the anterior septum and posterolateral free wall.

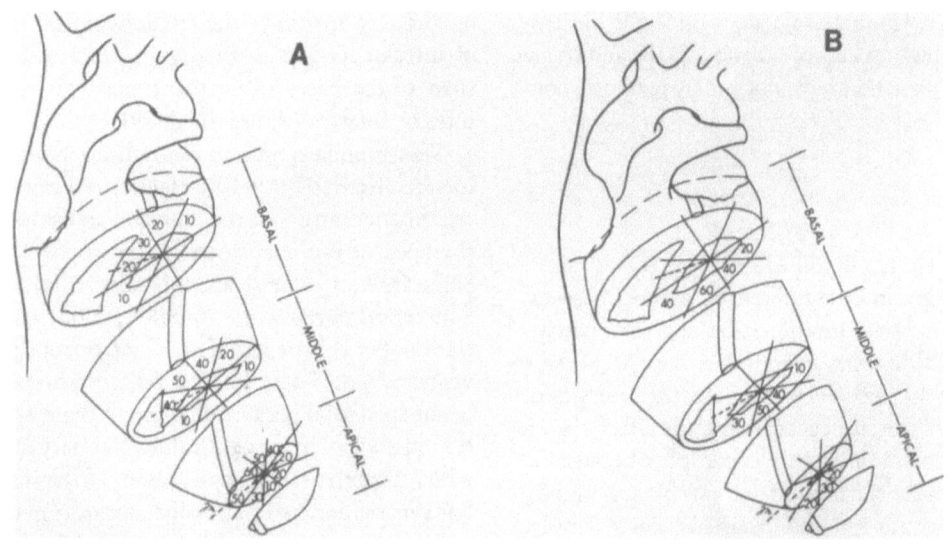

FIGURE 10-2. Mean size and location at autopsy of 26 anterior (A) and 26 inferior (B) infarcts. The left ventricle is divided into 24 parts, consisting of eight octants each in the basal, middle, and apical thirds. The average percent infarction for each octant is rounded to the nearest 10%. Circumferential extent is greater at the apex for anterior infarcts (A) and greater at the base for inferior infarcts (B). From Ideker et al. [8], with permission.

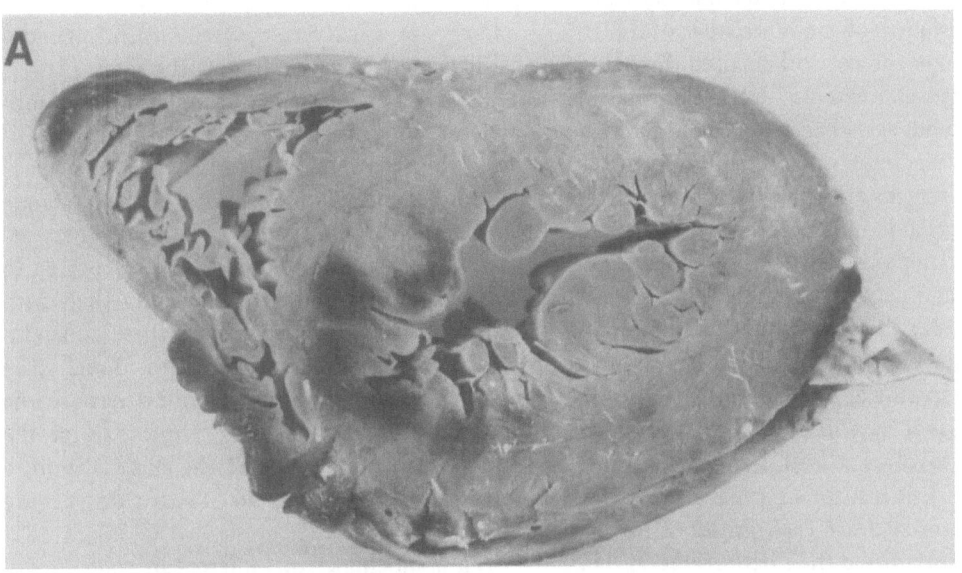

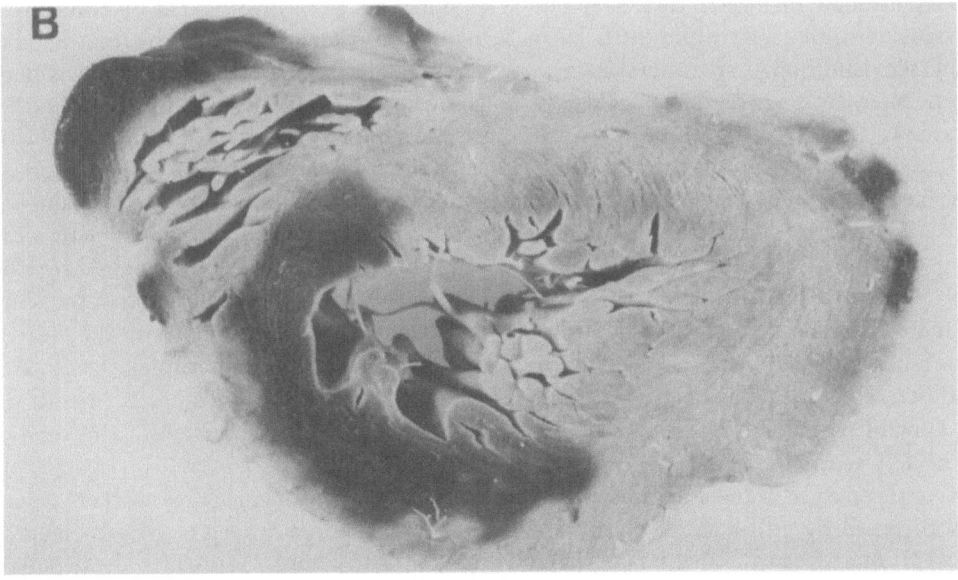

FIGURE 10-3. Photographs of the basal surface of two
human heart slices showing a recent anteroseptal infarct that is subendocardial at the base (A) and transmural at the apex (B). Hemorrhage within epicardial
fat is present in both slices and the basal slice (A)
contains a coronary artery bypass graft.

as one that extends to the outer one-half, one-third, or one-fourth of the ventricular wall [10]. Studies by Cook and co-workers used three divisions of transmural extent: "subendocardial infarction" extends less than halfway through the wall, "nontransmural infarction" extends one-half to three-fourths of the way; and "transmural infarction" extends more than three-fourths of the way through the wall [12]. In the studies from Duke, an infarct is considered to be "transmural" if it (a) extends from the endocardial surface to the epicardial surface except for a few cell layers of sparing at either surface, (b) is solid or, if patchy, is at least 50% infarcted within that area, and (c) involves at least 1 cm of the epicardial surface [5]. It is surprising that these definitions are so varied since each group of investigators apparently based their definitions on their concept of the natural grouping of infarcts into different classes, either anatomically or electrocardiographically. The stringent definition of the Duke group was chosen so that it means what the word implies: a transmural infarct extends through the wall.

The studies reporting that abnormal Q waves occur only with transmural infarction used a definition of transmural infarction that does not require extension to the epicardium [10]. Even when the Duke definition of transmural is met, there may be many areas where the infarct is only subendocardial. Thus, even the presence of abnormal Q waves does not rule out the possibility of salvageable myocardium in the infarcted region.

TYPES OF SUBENDOCARDIAL INFARCTS
There is more than one type of subendocardial infarct, each of which may affect the electrocardiogram differently. One type of subendocardial infarct is circumferential, involving all vascular beds of the left ventricle (figure 10-4). These infarcts were reported to occur after episodes of hypotension caused by either shock or any arrhythmia [13]. More recently, such infarcts have been reported after prolonged ischemia during cardiac surgery [14]. These infarcts are usually hemorrhagic and exhibit contraction band necrosis, signifying ischemia followed by reperfusion. Circumferential subendocardial infarcts are less common than other subendocardial infarcts in

postmortem studies [12, 15]. Circumferential infarcts are usually fatal, while other subendocardial infarcts are infrequently fatal [5−7]. Thus, the actual incidence of circumferential subendocardial infarcts is even less than that indicated from postmortem studies.

Most commonly, subendocardial infarcts are within the distribution of a single coronary artery. Coronary thrombosis has been reported to be less common with these infarcts than with transmural infarcts [10]. Even these subendocardial infarcts can be subdivided. Some spare only a few cell layers of myofibers next to the endocardium. Others spare almost all of the muscle in the trabeculae of the endocardium, a region that may be up to 5 mm thick (figure 10-5).

A few subendocardial infarcts are so heterogeneous that they do not fall into either of these categories (figure 10-6).

Electrocardiographic Considerations

EXPERIMENTAL STUDIES
The effect of subendocardial infarcts on the QRS complex has been investigated by clinicopathologic correlation [10, 12, 16], by recording body surface and cardiac potentials in humans undergoing cardiac surgery [17], by recording body surface and cardiac potentials in animals with subendocardial lesions produced by occluding a coronary artery [18], by injecting formalin [19], by electrocautery [20], and by simulation [21]. Much of this work has been reviewed by Pruitt [1]. Most early studies indicated that transmural infarction causes a QS complex in the overlying electrocardiographic leads while subendocardial infarction causes a QR complex, the R wave being generated by activation of the surviving epicardial muscle [22].

In 1954, Prinzmetal and co-workers reported that the subendocardium is electrically silent and that the QRS complex is produced by depolarization of the subepicardium [20]. Q waves were never seen in precordial and epicardial leads recorded directly over chronic subendocardial infarcts in seven dogs and acute subendocardial necrosis produced by burns in 12 dogs. They reported that unipolar intramural electrodes re-

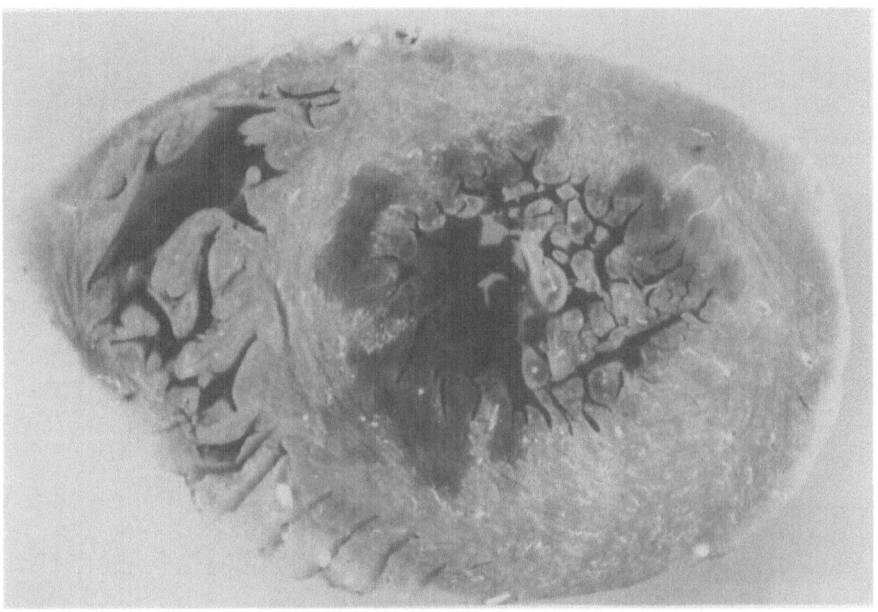

FIGURE 10-4. Photograph of the basal surface of a
human heart slice showing an acute, circumferential,
subendocardial infarct.

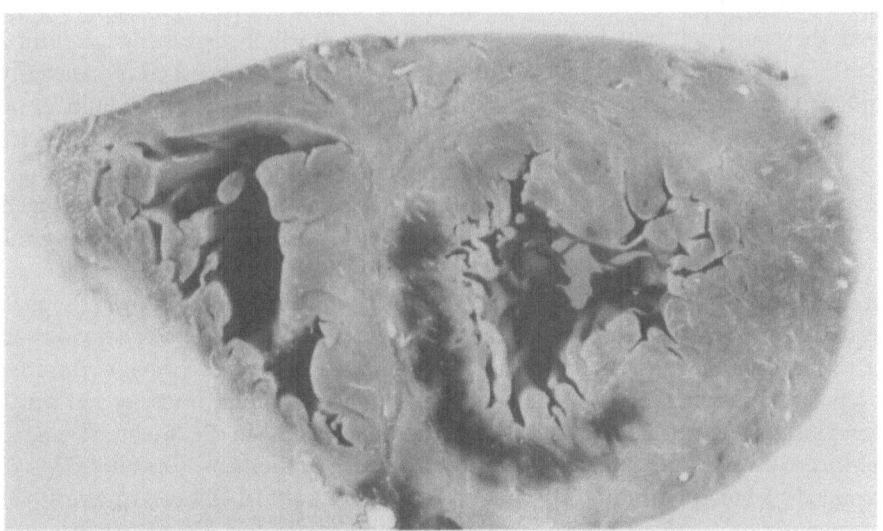

FIGURE 10-5. Photograph of the basal surface of a
human heart slice showing an organized anteroseptal
subendocardial infarct sparing the trabeculated portion of the subendocardium.

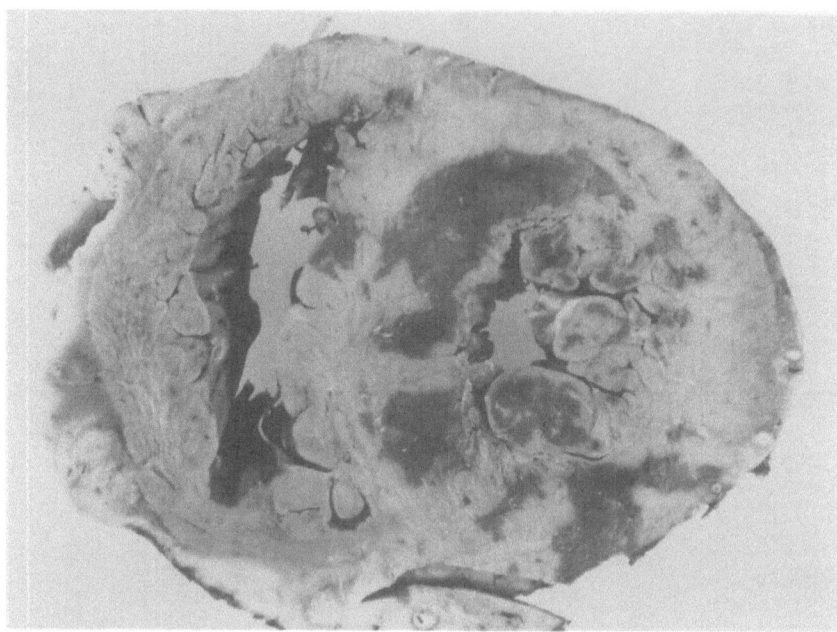

FIGURE 10-6. Photograph of the basal surface of a human heart slice showing an organizing infarct that is difficult to classify. It is in the distribution of more than one coronary artery. It is solid in some regions and patchy in others. While most of the infarct is subendocardial, one portion is transmural and another is subepicardial.

corded QS waves throughout the subendocardium, which activated almost simultaneously throughout its extent. Only in the subepicardium were R waves observed, caused by the spread of activation outward toward the epicardium. They explained these findings by hypothesizing that Purkinje fibers ramify throughout the subendocardium, causing the entire region to activate almost simultaneously. From these findings they concluded that pure subendocardial infarcts do not significantly alter the QRS complex [20]. This study appears to be the primary source of the concept that Q waves indicate transmural infarction.

These results have since been refuted by numerous studies. In 1957, after the development of more refined recording techniques, another report from Prinzmetal's laboratory indicated that the inner layers of the left ventricle accounted for part of the first third of the R wave, contradicting the earlier reports that these inner layers were electrocardiographically silent [23]. However, the conflict of this result with the previous findings from Prinzmetal's laboratory is not discussed in this later manuscript.

Durrer and co-workers found that subendocardial scars no larger than 1 cm in diameter produced abnormal Q waves in unipolar epicar-

dial recordings overlying the scar [18]. In agreement with Prinzmetal's findings, Durrer's group also found that much of the subendocardium in the dog was activated almost simultaneously. Thus, in the dog, the subendocardium is not silent, but exerts a smaller influence on the electrocardiogram than does the subepicardium.

Intramural recordings in human hearts made by both Boineau's group [24] and Durrer's group [25] indicate that most of the ventricular wall including the subendocardium activates sequentially by the outward spread of activation toward the epicardium. The only exceptions to this finding occurred in the papillary muscles and within large trabeculae. Thus, in the absence of conduction disturbances in humans, subendocardial infarcts can cause abnormal Q waves (figure 10-7).

CLINICOPATHOLOGIC STUDIES
Numerous clinicopathologic studies have also indicated that infarcts extending only part of the

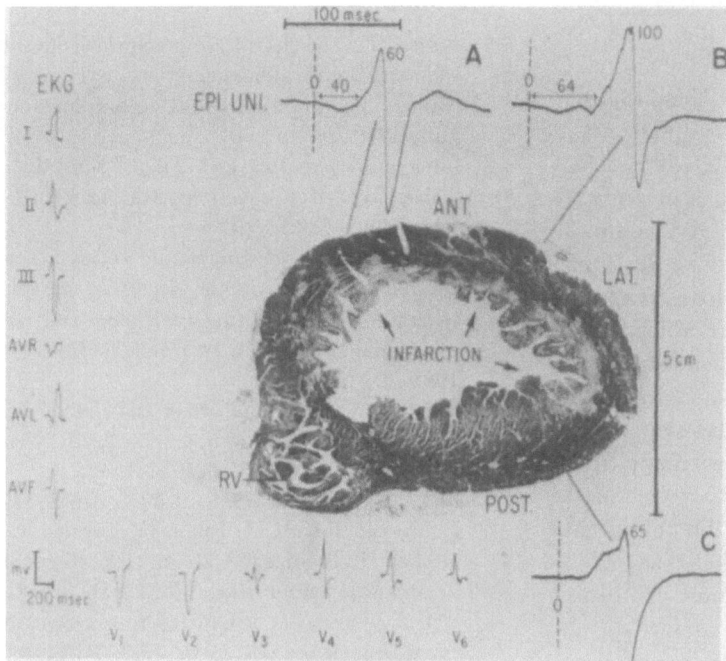

FIGURE 10-7. Human anterolateral subendocardial infarction in cross section. The preoperative electrocardiogram is on the left and below. Q waves of 40- and 64-ms duration are seen in epicardial unipolar complexes A and B over the infarct. No Q wave is present in complex C, which is not over the infarct. Numbers to the right of the complexes represent local activation times in milliseconds. EPI. UNI., epicardial unipolar complexes; RV, right ventricle; ANT., anterior; LAT., lateral; POST., posterior. From Daniel et al. [23], with permission.

infarcts of all ages are included, the average size of transmural infarcts is greater than that of subendocardial infarcts [5–7]. The average size of single infarcts with abnormal Q waves is larger than the average size of single infarcts without abnormal Q waves [28]. The presence of abnormal Q waves is more closely associated with infarct size than with the transmural extent of infarction [28].

way through the left ventricular wall frequently cause abnormal Q waves [5–7, 10, 12, 16, 26]. The incidence of this finding depends upon the definition used for an abnormal Q wave, being greater for Q waves of only 30 ms than for those of at least 40 ms. The Duke group defines an abnormal Q wave as one lasting at least 30 ms, based upon the high specificity of this definition [27]. In a study of 72 patients with a single infarct and in whom electrocardiographic signs of ventricular hypertrophy or conduction disturbances were absent, almost all transmural infarcts and the majority of subendocardial infarcts caused at least 30-ms Q waves [5–7]. Several other pertinent findings have been obtained by clinicopathologic study of these same patients. When

CLINICAL STUDIES

Some clinical studies find the prognosis after subendocardial infarction to be better than after transmural infarction while other studies find the prognosis to be worse [3, 4]. One explanation for this discrepancy is the inability to judge the transmural extent of infarction from the presence or absence of abnormal Q waves. Another explanation for this discrepancy has recently been advanced: the prognosis after subendocardial infarction is good over the short term (first two years after infarction), but is poor over the long term [29].

Complicating electrocardiographic factors of left bundle branch block or of left ventricular hypertrophy can obscure the abnormal Q waves of myocardial infarction [30]. If two or more infarcts are present within the same heart, one infarct can prevent the generation of abnormal Q waves by the other infarct [31]. These findings provide a third explanation for the differences in results of studies of prognosis after subendocardial infarction. In patients with acute infarcts who had a previously normal QRS complex, Mahony et al. found that those who developed abnormal Q waves had a greater long-term mortality rate than those who did not develop such Q waves [32]. Conversely, in patients sustaining infarction who had a previously abnormal QRS complex secondary to previous infarction, bundle branch block, or ventricular hypertrophy, those who developed new abnormal Q waves had a better prognosis than those who did not develop such new Q waves [32]. In studies that include patients with electrocardiograms exhibiting complicating factors, patients without new abnormal Q waves may have more than one infarct. Such patients may have more total infarction than patients with a single infarct exhibiting new abnormal Q waves, and total infarct size is a major determinant of prognosis [33].

Conclusions

There is no uniform definition of transmural infarction. Other anatomic characteristics of an infarct including infarct size, location, degree of patchiness, circumferential extent, and base-to-apex extent may exert at least as much influence on the presence and size of Q waves as does the transmural extent of the infarct. The transmural extent of infarction varies over the circumferential and base-to-apex extent of the infarct. There are several different kinds of subendocardial infarcts that may have different effects on the electrocardiogram.

If only a single infarct is present and electrocardiographic signs of bundle branch block or ventricular hypertrophy are absent, almost all transmural infarcts and most subendocardial infarcts cause significant Q waves. In the presence of left ventricular hypertrophy, left bundle branch block, or multiple infarcts, the abnormal Q waves of an infarct may be obscured. Thus, the terms abnormal Q wave and transmural infarct are not synonymous.

References

1. Pruitt RD: The electrocardiogram in acute subendocardial myocardial infarction. In: Hurst JW (ed) The heart, update IV. New York: McGraw-Hill, 1979, pp 55–70.
2. Pipberger HV, Lopez EA: "Silent" subendocardial infarcts: fact or fiction? Am Heart J 100: 597–599, 1980.
3. Spodick DH: Q-wave infarction versus S-T infarction: nonspecificity of electrocardiographic criteria for differentiating transmural and nontransmural lesions. Am J Cardiol 51:913–915, 1983.
4. Phibbs B: "Transmural" versus "subendocardial" infarction: an electrocardiographic myth. J Am Coll Cardiol 2:561–564, 1983.
5. Ideker RE, Wagner GS, Ruth WK, Alonso DR, Bishop SP, Bloor CM, Fallon JT, Gottlieb GJ, Hackel DB, Phillips HR, Reimer KA, Roark SF, Rogers WJ, Savage RM, White RD, Selvester RH: Evaluation of a QRS scoring system for estimating myocardial infarct size. II. Correlation with quantitative anatomic findings for anterior infarcts. Am J Cardiol 49:1604–1614, 1982.
6. Roark SF, Ideker RE, Wagner GS, Alonso DR, Bishop SP, Bloor CM, Bramlet DA, Edwards JE, Fallon JT, Gottlieb GJ, Hackel DB, Phillips HR, Reimer KA, Rogers WJ, Ruth WK, Savage RM, White RD, Selvester RH: Evaluation of a QRS scoring system for estimating myocardial infarct size. III. Correlation with quantitative anatomic findings for inferior infarcts. Am J Cardiol 51:382–389, 1983.
7. Ward RM, White RD, Ideker RE, Hindman NB, Alonso DR, Bishop SP, Bloor CM, Fallon JT, Gottlieb GJ, Hackel DB, Hutchins GM, Phillips HR, Reimer KA, Roark SF, Rochlani SP, Rogers WJ, Ruth WK, Savage RM, Weiss JL, Selvester RH, Wagner GS: Evaluation of a QRS scoring system for estimating myocardial infarct size. IV. Correlation with quantitative anatomic findings for posterolateral infarcts. Am J Cardiol (in press).
8. Factor SM, Okun EM, Kirk ES: The histological lateral border of acute canine myocardial infarction. Circ Res 48:640–649, 1981.
9. Ideker RE, Hackel DB, McClees E: Postmortem: anatomic quantitation. In: Wagner GS (ed) Myocardial infarction: measurement and intervention. The Hague: Martinus Nijhoff, 1982, pp 347–371.
10. Freifeld AG, Schuster EH, Bulkley BH: Nontransmural versus transmural myocardial infarc-

tion: a morphologic study. Am J Med 75:423–432, 1983.

11. James TN: Anatomy of the coronary arteries. New York: Harper and Row, 1961, pp 68–69.

12. Cook RW, Edwards JE, Pruitt RD: Electrocardiographic changes in acute subendocardial infarction. I. Large subendocardial and large non-transmural infarcts. Circulation 18:603–612, 1958.

13. Hackel DB, Ratliff N, Mikat E: The heart in shock. Circ Res 35:805–811, 1974.

14. Hassan N, Henson D, Dye WS, Javid H, Hunter JA, Callaghan R, Eisenstein R, Julian OC: Left ventricular hemorrhagic necrosis. Ann Thorac Surg 7:550–561, 1969.

15. Cook RW, Edwards JE, Pruitt RD: Electrocardiographic changes in acute subendocardial infarction. II. Small subendocardial infarcts. Circulation 18:613–622, 1958.

16. Raunio H, Rissanen V, Romppanen T, Jokinen Y, Rehnberg S, Helin M, Pyorala K: Changes in the QRS complex and ST segment in transmural and subendocardial myocardial infarctions: a clinicopathologic study. Am Heart J 98:176–184, 1979.

17. Boineau JP, Spach MS, Sabiston DC, Blumenschein SD, Gallie TM, Long EC: Body surface potentials and ventricular excitation in myocardial infarction. In: Manning GW, Ahuja SP (eds) Electrical activity of the heart. Springfield IL: Charles C Thomas, 1969, pp 83–97.

18. Durrer D, Van Lier AAW, Buller J: Epicardial and intramural excitation in chronic myocardial infarction. Am Heart J 68:765–776, 1964.

19. Abildskov JA, Boyle RS: Further studies of the electrodiographic effects of experimental myocardial lesions. Am Heart J 69:49–55, 1965.

20. Prinzmetal M, Shaw CMCK Jr, Maxwell MH, Flamm EJ, Goldman A, Kimura N, Rakita L, Borduas JL, Rothman S, Kennamer R: Studies of the mechanism of ventricular activity. Am J Med 16:469–489, 1954.

21. Toyama J, Mimi N, Ishikawa T, Wada M, Oguri H, Okajima M, Yamada K: Computational reconstruction of body surface isopotential maps in myocardial infarction: comparison between non-transmural and transmural infarction. Adv Cardiol 21:77–81, 1978.

22. Myers GB: The interpretation of the unipolar electrocardiogram. St Louis: CV Mosby, 1956, pp 145–155.

23. Pipberger H, Schwartz L, Massumi RA, Wenger SM, Prinzmetal M: Studies on the mechanism of ventricular activity. XXI. The origin of the depolarization complex with clinical applications. Am Heart J 54:511–530.

24. Daniel TM, Boineau JP, Sabiston DC: Comparison of human ventricular activation with a canine model in chronic myocardial infarction. Circulation 44:74–89, 1971.

25. Durrer D, Van Dam RT, Freud GE, Janse MJ, Meijler FL, Arzbaecher RC: Total excitation of the isolated human heart. Circulation 41:899–912, 1970.

26. Sullivan W, Vlodaver Z, Tuna N, Long L, Edwards JE: Correlation of electrocardiographic and pathologic findings in healed myocardial infarction. Am J Cardiol 42:724–32, 1978.

27. Wagner GS, Freye CJ, Palmeri S, Roark SF, Stack NC, Ideker RE, Harrell FE Jr, Selvester RH: Evaluation of a QRS scoring system for estimating myocardial infarct size. I. Specificity and observer agreement. Circulation 65:342–347, 1982.

28. Ideker RE, Wagner GS, Reimer KA, Alonso DR, Bishop SP, Bloor CM, Fallon JT, Gottlieb GJ, Hackel DB, Phillips HR, Roark SF, Rogers WJ, Ruth WK, Savage RM, Selvester RH, Ward RM: Q waves and transmural infarcts: the terms are not the same [abstr]. Am J Cardiol 47:464, 1981.

29. Krone RJ, Friedman E, Thanavaro S, Miller JP, Kleiger RE, Oliver GC: Long term prognosis after the first Q-wave (transmural) non-Q-wave (nontransmural) myocardial infarction: analysis of 593 patients. Am J Cardiol 52:234–239, 1983.

30. Horan LG, Flowers NC, Johnson JC: Significance of the diagnostic Q wave of myocardial infarction. Circulation 43:428–436, 1971.

31. Silverman ME, Silverman BD: The diagnostic capabilities and limitations of the electrocardiogram. In: Hurst JW (ed) The heart, update I, New York: McGraw-Hill, 1979, pp 13–45.

32. Mahony C, Hindman MC, Aronin N, Wagner G: Prognostic differences in subgroups of patients with electrographic evidence of subendocardial or transmural myocardial infarction. Am J Med 69:183–186, 1980.

33. Sobel BE: Infarct size, prognosis, and causal contiguity. Circulation (Suppl 1) 53:146–148.

11. HEMODYNAMIC ABNORMALITIES IN ACUTE MYOCARDIAL INFARCTION

John T. Baker

Normal Cardiovascular Hemodynamics

An interpretation of hemodynamic measurements in patients with acute myocardial infarction requires: (a) an understanding of the determinants of myocardial pump function and their relationship to the cardiac output, and (b) a thoughtful analysis of the parameters in the Fick equation and the definition of their normal values.

The cardiac output is the product of the heart rate and the stroke volume of the left ventricle with each cardiac contraction. The stroke volume is determined by (a) left ventricular filling or preload (clinically, the mean pulmonary capillary wedge pressure is considered an indirect measure of left ventricular filling), (b) systolic left ventricular wall tension or afterload, (c) myocardial contractility, and (d) the integrity of the cardiac valves and the interventricular septum.

The graphic relationship (figure 11-1, Control) between left ventricular filling pressure and stroke volume is called a ventricular function curve and is considered to be a manifestation of the Starling mechanism in the three-dimensional ventricle [1]. As diastolic filling pressure and end-diastolic volume are increased, stroke volume increases toward a maximum. The "failure limb" of the Starling curve in the laboratory probably does not manifest itself at physiologically obtainable filling pressures in the intact ventricle. Any observed decrease in stroke volume at high filling pressure is probably an indirect effect mediated through associated arterial hypoxemia, myocardial ischemia, systemic aci-

dosis, mitral regurgitation, and increased afterload [2].

Preload or left ventricular filling is the only diastolic determinant of the stroke volume and, therefore, is the most important of the four determinants of left ventricular pump function. If the ventricle is not adequately filled during diastole, then attempts to augment stroke volume by manipulating the other systolic determinants will be less effective. At any given filling pressure an increase in contractility or a decrease in afterload will tend to increase stroke volume and therefore cardiac output if heart rate remains constant. This effect is more prominent at high filling pressures (figure 11-1).

The Fick equation defines the steady-state relationship between tissue oxygen demand and oxygen delivery:

$$\dot{V} = \dot{Q} \times [\text{Hbg}] \times 1.39 \times (A \text{ sat} - V \text{ sat})$$

where

$\quad\quad V = $ oxygen consumption in cc/min
$\quad\quad Q = $ cardiac output in cc blood/min
$\quad[\text{Hbg}] = $ hemoglobin concentration in g%.
$\quad\quad 1.39 = $ oxygen carrying capacity of hemoglobin in cc/g
$\quad A \text{ sat} = $ arterial oxygen saturation (%)
$\quad V \text{ sat} = $ mixed venous (pulmonary arterial) oxygen saturation (%)

In the steady state this equation must balance so that oxygen supply and demand are equal. If the

R.M. Califf and G.S. Wagner (eds.), ACUTE CORONARY CARE: Principles and Practice. Copyright © 1985. Martinus Nijhoff Publishing, Boston/Dordrecht/Lancaster.

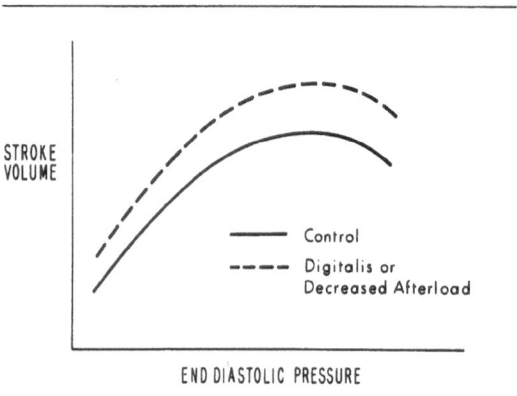

FIGURE 11-1. Examples of two left ventricular function curves are constructed by relating the parameters of stroke volume and end-diastolic pressure. An increase in contractility with digitalis or decreased afterload would result in greater stroke volume at the same end-diastolic pressure and would shift the curve upward and to the left.

delivery system on the right side of the equation is unable to supply oxygen demands, then a steady state no longer exists and anaerobic metabolism will result in systemic metabolic acidosis. Many pathologic conditions can disturb this equation, including fever, hyperthyroidism, heart failure of any cause, anemia, and hypoxemia with arterial desaturation. In each condition, one component of the equation is affected and must be compensated for by some change elsewhere to rebalance the equation.

Measurement of the cardiac output has fascinated investigators and clinicians for many years. With the incorporation of thermodilution techniques via the balloon flotation catheter, cardiac output measurement has become routine practice on intensive care units. However, interpretation of cardiac output measurements requires understanding of the differences between (a) normal values, (b) appropriate values, and (c) adequate values. Normal values (a) are determined by making resting or basal measurements of the cardiac output in large numbers of normal individuals and computing a mean and standard deviation. Two standard deviations above and below the mean are considered the "limits of normal." An appropriate value (b) of cardiac output is the level of flow that would be delivered by a normal cardiovascular system for a given patient

either with or without stresses such as exercise, fever, anemia, hypoxemia, or thyrotoxicosis. When the cardiac output is appropriate, the arteriovenous oxygen (AVO$_2$) difference may remain within the normal range or may be slightly elevated. Adequate values (c) of cardiac output are those sufficient to permit the body to maintain aerobic metabolism. When the cardiac output is inadequate, lactate is produced via anaerobic metabolism and metabolic acidosis may result.

The range of "normal" for cardiac output is quite wide, and remains wide despite correcting for body surface area (cardiac index). Values below the "lower limit" are clearly "abnormal," and this level has high specificity (minimal false positives) as a marker of an "inappropriately" low cardiac output. This "lower limit of normal" is, however, a relatively insensitive determinant of an "inappropriately" low cardiac output. An individual with a resting cardiac output in the upper range of normal may decrease the cardiac output significantly as a result of acute myocardial infarction to an "inappropriate" level without dropping below the "lower limit of normal."

In the presence of the numerous stresses to the oxygen delivery system mentioned above, the cardiac output will change. For example, what would be the lower limit of "appropriate" cardiac output for patients with fever of 103 degrees, an arterial saturation of 88%, a hemoglobin of 9g%, and a normal heart? Without this information, it is difficult to evaluate the "appropriateness" of the cardiac output in patients in intensive care units with abnormal hearts and multiple other medical problems.

Even for the vast majority of patients with acute myocardial infarction who do not have other medical problems, normal and appropriate levels of cardiac output may not be identical: for example, (a) arterial saturation may not be maintained in its normal range via oxygen administration in the presence of pulmonary congestion, and (b) oxygen consumption may be significantly increased by circulating catecholamines, anxiety, pain, and increased work of breathing. It is, therefore, important to identify the patient whose cardiac output is depressed relative to his "appropriate" level, but is still above the "lower limit of normal."

A precise determination of the "appropriateness" of the cardiac output is not possible. Examination of the Fick equation provides several other parameters, however, that are useful for managing the individual patient. The AVO_2 difference is calculated:

$$[Hbg] \times 1.39 \times (A\ sat - V\ sat)$$

This portion of the Fick equation can also be determined and compared with population limits. The value of the AVO_2 difference increases as the cardiac output falls because systemic extraction of oxygen is increased to compensate. The range of normal of AVO_2 difference is somewhat narrower than that for the cardiac output. An abnormally high value despite a "normal" cardiac output suggests a problem with pump function that was not indicated by that less-sensitive measurement. The "normal" cardiac output apparently was inappropriate; it did not meet systemic needs so more oxygen was extracted.

The mixed venous oxygen saturation is a useful (but often neglected) indirect measure of the adequacy of cardiac output. In a normal population it has the narrowest range of "normal" of any of the previously considered hemodynamic parameters, and it can be measured with a high degree of accuracy and reproducibility. When the cardiac output is reduced, the venous oxygen saturation must fall as peripheral extraction of oxygen is increased to compensate and preserve oxygen delivery. Normally this saturation is above 70% and, if the cardiac output falls to half normal, it will decrease to 50% or less. There is a limit to the extent to which increased oxygen extraction can compensate for a decreased cardiac output. When this limit is reached, any further decrease in blood flow will result in anaerobic metabolism and lactate production. This will result in metabolic acidosis (a nonsteady state) if compensatory alkalizing mechanisms are inadequate. Before this limit is reached the cardiac output is an "adequate value" although it may be neither appropriate nor normal. Excess of this limit may be identified on the admission arterial blood gases as an unexplained mild metabolic acidosis. A mixed venous oxygen saturation of 50% in the patient with acute myocardial ischemia and infarction indicates an inappropriate

cardiac output and should warn the physician that any additional decrease in the systemic flow of blood may result in an inadequate output and, thereby, a nonsteady state leading to acidosis and perhaps cardiac arrest.

Hemodynamic Alterations with Myocardial Infarction

PATHOPHYSIOLOGY OF HEMODYNAMIC ABNORMALITIES

Within minutes after the onset of ischemia, the involved segment of myocardium ceases to contract. If severe ischemia persists beyond a certain length of time, myocardial necrosis and, thereby, irreversible loss of function will ensue (see chapter 2). Global left ventricular ejection fraction is reduced, and stroke volume and cardiac output decreased, unless other determinants of the cardiac output are adjusted to maintain forward blood flow. Left ventricular filling pressure rises, which facilitates use of the Starling mechanism to preserve stroke volume by increasing end-diastolic volume. Two factors that may contribute to the increase in left ventricular filling pressure are a change in left ventricular compliance (increased stiffness requiring higher pressures to achieve any given end-diastolic volume) and mitral regurgitation resulting from malfunction of the mitral support apparatus.

An increase in heart rate may represent an attempt to preserve cardiac output via an increase in sympathetic tone, although it may also represent an inappropriate and potentially detrimental response to anxiety, fear, chest pain, or an autonomic reflex. Increased sympathetic tone, in addition to increasing heart rate, results in venoconstriction and increased venous pressure, enhanced contractility in uninvolved myocardial segments, and arteriolar constriction to maintain blood pressure and perfusion particularly to the brain. Arteriolar constriction may be excessive and result in hypertension, which augments myocardial oxygen demand unnecessarily but, even when not excessive, results in increased afterload (see chapter 43), which further decreases stroke volume.

An increase in left ventricular filling pressure associated with a decrease in stroke volume is indicative of depression of the left ventricular function curve downward and to the right [1]. In some patients an increase in filling pressure predominates and stroke volume is well preserved. In others both filling pressure and stroke volume become abnormal. The magnitude of the changes depends on multiple factors, including (a) the size of the necrotic and ischemic myocardial segments supplied by the occluded vessel, (b) the extent of disease in the other coronary arteries, (c) the state of the ventricle before the onset of infarction, including the degree of hypertrophy, dilatation, and scarring from previous infarctions, and (d) the presence and severity of mitral regurgitation. If one plots the pulmonary capillary wedge pressure against the stroke volume or cardiac output for a large number of patients with acute myocardial infarction, the result is a scatter diagram that represents the variability of the hemodynamic alterations that may occur. Each data pair represent a single point on a different left ventricular function curve, which is unique for each patient.

Infarction that involves the right ventricle as well as the left results in an interesting clinical syndrome that is different from the more common left ventricular infarction. Right ventricular infarction is discussed in detail in chapter 21.

CLINICAL CLASSIFICATION OF HEMODYNAMIC ABNORMALITIES

The clinical symptoms and signs of pulmonary congestion and cardiogenic shock are related to an elevated pulmonary capillary wedge pressure and a decreased cardiac output, respectively. They have been used to classify patients with acute myocardial infarction into categories that reflect the severity and pattern of the hemodynamic changes. The most commonly used classification system for many years was proposed by Killip and Kimball [4] and divided patients into four subgroups: class I—patients with no clinical evidence of pulmonary congestion or hypoperfusion; class II—patients with clinical evidence of mild pulmonary congestion; class III—patients with clinical evidence of severe pulmonary congestion or pulmonary edema; and class IV—patients with the clinical syndrome of cardiogenic shock. Using this classification system, Killip and Kimball reported the distribution of hemodynamic findings and the associated mortality in 250 patients with acute infarction [4]. Class-I patients constituted 33% of the group and had a mortality in hospital of 6%, class II were 38% with a 17% mortality, class III were 10% with a 38% mortality, and class IV were 19% with a 81% mortality. These figures are representative of many series published by investigators who used this or a similar clinical classification [5—10]. Although the distribution may be weighted in favor of more complicated patients, the mortality figures are typical and demonstrate the prognostic value of classifying patients according to the clinical severity of the hemodynamic alterations produced by acute infarction.

CLASSIFICATION BY HEMODYNAMIC MEASUREMENTS

The introduction of the balloon flotation catheter for continuous pulmonary arterial pressure measurement and the thermodilution method for measuring cardiac output in the early 1970s made hemodynamic monitoring in patients with acute myocardial infarction a relatively simple and safe procedure for use in the coronary care unit. Subsequently, numerous studies have documented the value of hemodynamic measurements for classifying patients into high-risk and low-risk mortality groups [7, 9, 11—14].

A pulmonary capillary wedge pressure above 18 was reported by Shell et al. to separate patients with acute myocardial infarction into high- and low-risk groups [12]. They reported a 10% mortality over 30 days in patients with an initial pulmonary capillary wedge pressure less than 18 mmHg compared with a 33% mortality if the wedge pressure was 18 mmHg or greater. None of these patients had clinical evidence of cardiogenic shock. Cohn et al. reported similar results using a wedge pressure of 20 mmHg. Mortality at 21 days was 5.1% for the low-wedge group and 19.5% for the high-wedge group [14].

Direct and indirect measurements of cardiac output have been reported to define high- and low-risk groups. In 200 patients reported by Forrester et al. the hospital mortality was 5% in 95 patients with a cardiac index greater than 2.2 l/min/m^2 and 42% in 105 patients with a cardiac index less than this value [11]. A low serum bicarbonate as a reflection of a metabolic acidosis from inadequate tissue oxygen delivery also identifies patients with a poor prognosis. Kirby and McNichol reported a 75% mortality from acute infarction if the admission bicarbonate concentration was 15 meq/l or less compared with 37% if the value was above this level [15].

Combinations of abnormal hemodynamic parameters can identify subgroups with an extremely poor prognosis that approaches a 100% mortality. In the 1977 series of Forrester et al. a pulmonary capillary wedge pressure greater than 18 mmHg and a cardiac index less than 2.2 l/min/m^2 was associated with a mortality of 51% [11], while in an earlier series reported in 1972 by Ratshin et al. these hemodynamic findings were associated with a 100% mortality [9]. The differences in reported mortality over time may reflect improvements in our understanding of hemodynamic alterations and in available forms of therapy between 1972 and 1977.

CORRELATION OF CLINICAL AND HEMODYNAMIC ABNORMALITIES

In general a correlation exists between clinically defined subsets of patients and the measured hemodynamic abnormalities. Although the mean values between groups may differ significantly, there is considerable overlap [16–18], and the ability of clinical parameters to predict hemodynamic abnormalities is relatively crude. Rotman et al. evaluated the predictive value of rales, a ventricular gallop, and an abnormal chest x-ray (hilar haze or alveolar fluid) with respect to left ventricular filling pressure (14 mmHg and below vs 15 mmHg and above). The overall predictive accuracy was 70% for a ventricular gallop, 75% for rales, and 79% for an abnormal chest x-ray [18]. Rales were the most sensitive but also the least specific parameter. Elevated left ventricular filling pressure was noted in 47% of patients without rales, 52% without a gallop, and 40% without an abnormal chest x-ray. Similarly, Riley et al. noted an overall predictive accuracy of 57% for a ventricular gallop. In their population, 58% of patients without a gallop had an elevated left ventricular filling pressure [6].

Forrester et al. reported similar diagnostic errors in predicting both an elevated left ventricular filling pressure and a depressed cardiac output

[11]: 33% of patients with a clinically uncomplicated myocardial infarction had either a wedge pressure greater than 18 mmHg or a cardiac index less than 2.2 l/min/m^2, 15% with no evidence of pulmonary congestion had an elevated filling pressure, and 24% with no clinical evidence of hypoperfusion had a depressed cardiac index. Perhaps their most important observation was that all deaths in the clinical subset of patients with isolated evidence of pulmonary congestion occurred in patients with clinically unsuspected depression of the cardiac index.

Hemodynamic Monitoring in Acute Myocardial Infarction

No study is available to measure the possible impact of hemodynamic monitoring on mortality from acute myocardial infarction. It is clear, however, from the available data that hemodynamic studies over the last 15 years have expanded the understanding of the clinical manifestations of myocardial infarction and have defined the limitations of bedside assessment of left ventricular dysfunction. Most clinical cardiologists would agree that hemodynamic monitoring has made the management of the complicated patient more precise, especially the critically ill patient with cardiogenic shock. Whether routine hemodynamic monitoring in clinically uncomplicated patients is indicated to identify the subset of patients with undetected hemodynamic abnormalities is, as yet, unanswered. Available data would suggest that this subset of patients has an increased risk, but very little data exist to demonstrate a beneficial effect of therapy. The recently reported Veterans Administration Cooperative Study of the use of nitroprusside suggests that patients with a persistently elevated wedge pressure (greater than 19 mmHg) beyond 9 h from the onset of symptoms benefit from vasodilator therapy [14]. Selection of patients for this study was based on hemodynamic findings, and many were clinically uncomplicated. These results, combined with knowledge that bedside assessment of the patient is often inaccurate, lend support to the argument for routine use of hemodynamic monitoring in patients with acute myocardial infarction.

References

1. Sarnoff JS, Berglund E: Ventricular function. I. Starling's law of the heart studied by means of simultaneous right and left ventricular function curves in the dog. Circulation 9:706−718, 1954.

2. MacGregor DC, Covell JW, Mahler F, Dilley RB, Ross J: Relations between afterload, stroke volume, and descending limb of the Starling's curve. Am J Physiol 227:884−890, 1974.

3. McDonough JR, Danielson RA: Variability in cardiac output during exercise. J Appl Physiol 37:579−583, 1974.

4. Killip T, Kimball JT: Treatment of myocardial infarction in a coronary care unit: a two year experience with 250 patients. Am J Cardiol 20:457−467, 1969.

5. Weber KT, Ratshin RA, Janicki JS, Rackley CE, Russell RO: Left ventricular dysfunction following acute myocardial infarction: a clinicopathologic and hemodynamic profile of shock and failure. Am J Med 54:697−705, 1973.

6. Riley CP, Russell RO, Rackley CE: Left ventricular gallop sound and acute myocardial infarction. Am Heart J 86:598−602, 1973.

7. Weber KT, Janicki JJ, Russell RO, Rackley CE: Identification of high risk subsets of acute myocardial infarction. Am J Cardiol 41:197−203, 1978.

8. Wolk MJ, Scheidt S, Killip T: Heart failure complicating acute myocardial infarction. Circulation 45:225−238, 1972.

9. Ratshin RA, Rackley CE, Russell RO: Hemodynamic evaluation of left ventricular function in shock complicating myocardial infarction. Circulation 45:127−139, 1972.

10. Hamosh P, Cohn JN: Left ventricular function in acute myocardial infarction. J Clin Invest 50:523−533, 1971.

11. Forrester JS, Diamond GA, Swan HJC: Correlative classification of clinical and hemodynamic function after acute myocardial infarction. Am J Cardiol 39:137−145, 1977.

12. Shell W, Peter T, Mickle D, Forrester JS, Swan HJC: Prognostic implications of reduction of left ventricular filling pressure in early transmural acute myocardial infarction. Am Heart J 102:334−340, 1981.

13. Rutherford BD, McCann WD, O'Donnovan TPB: The value of monitoring pulmonary artery pressure for early detection of left ventricular failure following myocardial infarction. Circulation 43:655−666, 1971.

14. Cohn JA, Franciosa JA, Francis GS, Archibald D, Tristani F, Fletcher R, Montero A, Cintron G, Clarke J, Hager D, Saunders R, Cobb F, Smith R, Loeb H, Settle H: Effects of short term infusion of sodium nitroprusside on mortality rate in acute myocardial infarction complicated by left ventricular failure: results of a Veterans Administration cooperative study. N Engl J Med 306:1129−1135, 1982.

15. Kirby BJ, McNichol MW: Acid−base status in acute myocardial infarction. Lancet 2:1054−1056, 1966.

16. Resnekov L: Hemodynamic effects of acute myocardial infarction. Med Clin North Am 57:243−257, 1973.

17. Ramo BW, Myers N, Wallace, AG, Starmer F, Clark DO, Whalen RE: Hemodynamic findings in 123 patients with acute myocardial infarction on admission. Circulation 42:567−577, 1970.

18. Rotman M, Chen JTT, Seningen RP, Hawley J, Wagner GS, Davidson RM, Gilbert MR: Pulmonary artery diastolic pressure in acute myocardial infarction. Am J Cardiol 33:357−362, 1974.

12. AUTONOMIC IMBALANCE DURING ACUTE MYOCARDIAL ISCHEMIA AND INFARCTION

Marc D. Thames

During the early minutes to hours of an acute myocardial infarction there are major changes in both parasympathetic and sympathetic outflow to the heart and peripheral circulation. These changes in autonomic outflow may be important in the pathogenesis of ventricular arrhythmias and of the hypotension and bradycardia that occur frequently in this setting.

The autonomic responses of patients with myocardial infarction may differ dramatically, depending on which region of the myocardium is rendered ischemic. Data to substantiate this impression recently have been provided by Webb and colleagues [1], who observed patients during the first few moments after the onset of acute myocardial infarction. They found that there was a marked difference in autonomic responses between patients with inferoposterior infarcts as opposed to those with anterior infarcts. Many patients with inferior infarcts (without a prior inferior infarct) had evidence of parasympathetic overactivity as indicated by bradycardia and hypotension. In contrast, patients with anterior infarcts rarely had evidence of parasympathetic overactivity, but over 50% had sympathetic overactivity as indicated by tachycardia and increased arterial pressure. Similar differential responses of heart rate and blood pressure to inferior versus anterior ischemia have been reported in patients with variant angina due to coronary artery spasm [2]. Finally, Wei and colleagues [3] have reported that lysis of an intracoronary thrombus

with intracoronary streptokinase in patients with acute inferior infarcts commonly resulted in bradycardia and hypotension. In contrast, those who were reperfused after occlusion of the anterior descending artery usually had tachycardia, hypertension, and increased ventricular ectopy. These observations confirm that the autonomic responses to acute myocardial ischemia or infarction are primarily dependent on the region of the myocardium involved.

These interesting clinical observations stimulate several fundamental questions:

1. Why are the responses to inferoposterior ischemia or infarction different from those with anterior ischemia or infarction?
2. Why is there bradycardia accompanying the hypotension despite the presence of arterial baroreceptor reflexes that would normally mediate reflex tachycardia?
3. What are the mechanisms for these differential autonomic responses to myocardial ischemia or infarction?

Cardiac Sensory Receptors Activated During Ischemia or Infarction

It has been established that there are sensory endings throughout the cardiopulmonary region [4−6]. Some of these endings are mechanoreceptors and respond to changes in stretch while others are chemically sensitive endings and re-

R.M. Califf and G.S. Wagner (eds.), ACUTE CORONARY CARE: Principles and Practice. Copyright © 1985. Martinus Nijhoff Publishing, Boston/Dordrecht/Lancaster.

spond instead to a variety of algesic or irritant substances [7, 8]. Others are polymodal and respond both to stretch and to chemical stimulation [9]. The impulses originating from sensory endings in the heart are transmitted to the central nervous system via afferent fibers that travel in either the vagal nerves to the brain stem or the cardiac sympathetic nerves to the spinal cord. Information traveling in these sympathetic afferents is then transmitted via the cord to higher centers.

There are many sensory endings with vagal or sympathetic afferent fibers that are located in the left ventricle [10–14]. During left ventricular ischemia or infarction these endings may be activated by bulging of the ischemic region (activation of mechanoreceptors), by release of potassium (activation of both mechanosensitive and chemosensitive endings), or by release of algesic substances such as bradykinin (activation of chemically sensitive endings). Both vagal and sympathetic left ventricular afferents are stimulated during coronary occlusion [15–17] and their discharge is increased as the result of both mechanical and chemical stimulation.

Reflex Responses to Stimulation of Cardiac Afferents

In experimental studies, activation of left ventricular receptors with vagal afferents by (a) chemical stimulation (with veratrum alkaloids, capsaicin, or bradykinin), (b) mechanical stimulation (with aortic occlusion or volume expansion), or (c) with experimental coronary occlusion results in reflex increases in efferent vagal and reduced sympathetic outflow to the heart and peripheral circulation [6]. These effects are particularly striking when the arterial baroreceptor reflexes have been ablated previously. Activation of similar receptors in the inferoposterior left ventricle during myocardial ischemia or infarction in humans may account for the bradycardia and hypotension commonly observed.

Activation of cardiac receptors with sympathetic afferents in anesthetized animals has been reported to result in (a) excitatory responses of tachycardia and increased arterial pressure, (b) reflex bradycardia and hypotension, or (c) biphasic responses [18]. Recent studies in conscious animals suggest that activation of these endings with bradykinin results solely in cardioaccelerator and vasopressor responses [19]. Reflex responses to activation of these sympathetic afferents by coronary occlusion are minimal in anesthetized dogs [20], larger in cats with intact spinal cords [21], but maximal in both dogs [22] and cats [23] with sectioned spinal cords. Many of these sympathetic afferents are pain fibers and their activation in conscious subjects may well give rise to responses mediated through higher centers. Thus, these reflex responses may be mediated either at the spinal level or at higher centers. The importance of the spinal component of these reflexes is unclear [22].

Responses to Regional Myocardial Ischemia

How could activation of vagal and sympathetic afferents account for the strikingly different cardiovascular responses to inferior versus anterior ischemia or infarction? One possible explanation is that the vagal afferents are located preferentially in the inferior wall of the left ventricle. Recent evidence in dogs strongly supports this view [20, 24, 25]. There is greater bradycardia, hypotension, and inhibition of sympathetic outflow to the skeletal muscle [24], kidney [25], and heart [20] during occlusion of the circumflex than during occlusion of the anterior descending coronary artery. The responses of heart rate, arterial pressure, and cardiac sympathetic nerve activity to circumflex versus anterior descending coronary occlusions are illustrated in figure 12-1. These differential responses are due to a preferential distribution of vagal receptors to the inferior wall of the left ventricle since the amounts of myocardium rendered ischemic by occlusion of each vessel were similar [24]. These inhibitory responses to coronary occlusions are abolished by vagotomy, indicating that the afferent pathways for these reflexes traverse the vagal nerves. A similarly preferential distribution of inhibitory cardiac receptors to the human inferior myocardium may account for the high incidence of bradycardia and hypotension when this area is rendered ischemic.

Another possible explanation for the differences in the cardiovascular responses to inferior versus anterior ischemia or infarction could be a prefer-

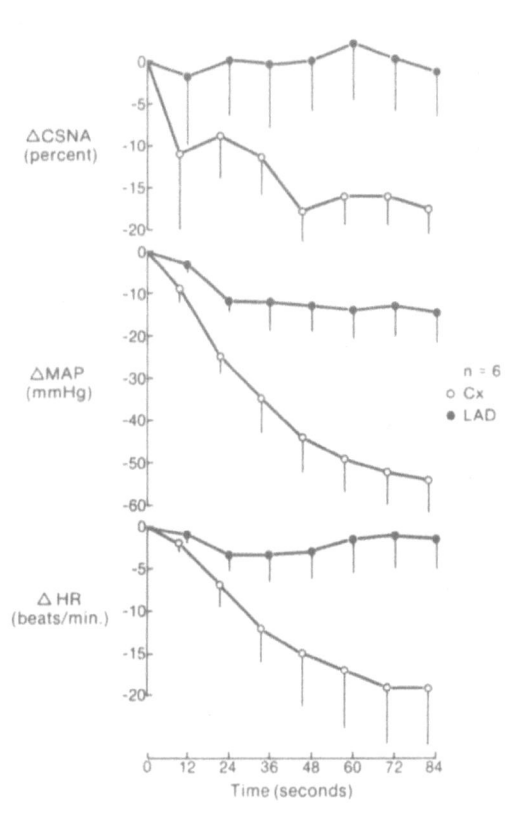

FIGURE 12-1. Time course and contrasting responses of (top to bottom) cardiac sympathetic nerve activity, mean arterial pressure, and heart rate to 90 s of circumflex (open symbols) or anterior descending (solid symbols) coronary occlusion in dogs with sinoaortic arterial baroreceptor denervation. Note the large inhibitory responses during circumflex (Cx) but not during anterior descending (LAD) occlusion. The peak responses of these dogs to coronary occlusion before and after arterial baroreceptor denervation are summarized in figure 12-2. From Felder and Thames [20], with permission.

ential distribution of cardiac sympathetic afferents to the anterior myocardium. Although the responses to activating these endings by coronary occlusion are small in anesthetized dogs [22], they are more prominent in cats [21] and may be prominent also in humans. It recently has been reported that, in cats with sinoaortic baroreceptor and vagal denervation, excitatory responses (increases in arterial pressure and renal nerve activity) to coronary occlusion are larger during anterior

descending than circumflex occlusion [21]. These responses were abolished by interrupting cardiac sympathetic afferent nerves. Occurrence of similar responses in humans might help to explain the tachycardia and increases in arterial pressure observed commonly during anterior infarction.

There is another explanation for the excitatory responses to anterior infarction observed in humans. Previous studies have suggested that a major function of cardiac sympathetic afferents may be to transmit the sensation of the pain of myocardial ischemia to higher centers [26]. The pain of myocardial ischemia can be eliminated in humans by removing the stellate ganglia and the first through fifth thoracic ganglia [26]. Increases in heart rate and blood pressure are common responses to pain. Why, then, don't patients with inferior infarcts also have excitatory responses since they also have pain? It is quite possible that activation of inhibitory cardiac receptors during inferior infarction results in such powerful cardioinhibitory and vasodepressor reflex responses that these overwhelm the response to pain. Since there are few of these receptors in the anterior myocardium, the pain response will be relatively unopposed during anterior infarction.

An additional factor is that activation of vagal afferent fibers may interfere with pain transmission in the spinal cord. Thies and Foreman [27] have shown that second-order neurons in the spinal pain pathways that are activated by cardiac sympathetic afferents can be inhibited by increased vagal afferent input. Thus, vagal afferents may not only have direct reflex cardioinhibitory and vasodepressor influences, but they also may reduce the input of pain information to the central nervous system.

Interaction of Cardiac and Arterial Baroreflexes during Myocardial Infarction

Figure 12-2 illustrates the afferent and efferent limbs of the major cardiovascular reflexes that may be involved in the integrated reflex responses to myocardial ischemia or infarction.

It seems somewhat puzzling that there should be bradycardia despite the hypotension of acute inferior myocardial infarction. Decreases in arterial pressure of similar magnitude resulting from

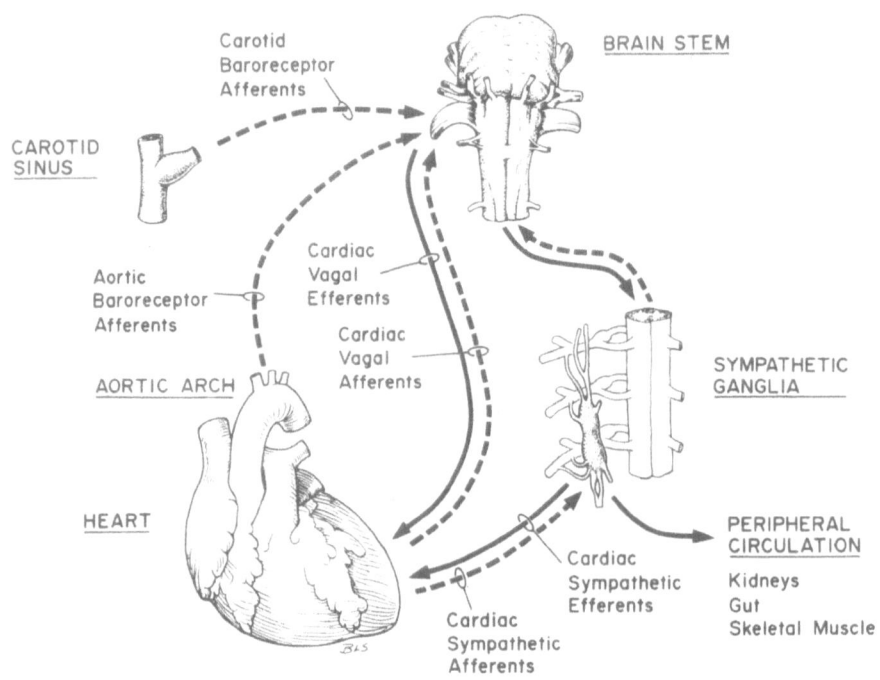

FIGURE 12-2. Schematic diagram illustrating efferent (solid lines) and afferent (dashed lines) pathways involved in reflex responses to myocardial ischemia or infarction.

hemorrhage or from hypotensive agents such as hydralazine result in striking reflex tachycardia. During inferior infarction there is a simultaneous increase in cardiac vagal afferent input and, because of hypotension, a decrease in arterial baroreceptor input to the central nervous system. The net reflex responses will depend on the magnitude of the change in the stimulus to each receptor group, the relative influence of each reflex on a given autonomic response, and the integration of these opposing sensory inputs within the central nervous system.

All of these factors probably account for the bradycardia observed in patients with inferior infarction and hypotension. These same factors influence the integrated reflex changes in sympathetic outflow to different regional circulations that have been examined in dogs during myocardial ischemia. During anterior descending occlusion, few inhibitory cardiac vagal afferents are stimulated so that the response is determined mainly by arterial baroreflexes (and possibly by sympathetic afferents). During circumflex occlusion and activation of many vagal afferents the response of sympathetic outflow is determined by

the factors outlined above. Thus, sympathetic outflow to skeletal muscle [24] is increased because of hypotension and the more dominant influence of arterial baroreflexes on sympathetic outflow to muscle. In contrast, there is no change in renal sympathetic nerve activity [25] because the influence of increased vagal afferent input (myocardial ischemia) and decreased baroreceptor input (hypotension) balance each other sufficiently to result in no net change. Changes in cardiac sympathetic nerve activity [20] are intermediate between those of kidney and skeletal muscle. The responses to coronary occlusion of gracilis perfusion pressure and of renal and cardiac sympathetic nerve activity and their dependence on the artery occluded and on the state of innervation are summarized in figure 12-3. The responses of regional circulations to myocardial ischemia or infarction in humans remain uninvestigated, but the presence of such striking hypotension in many patients with inferior infarc-

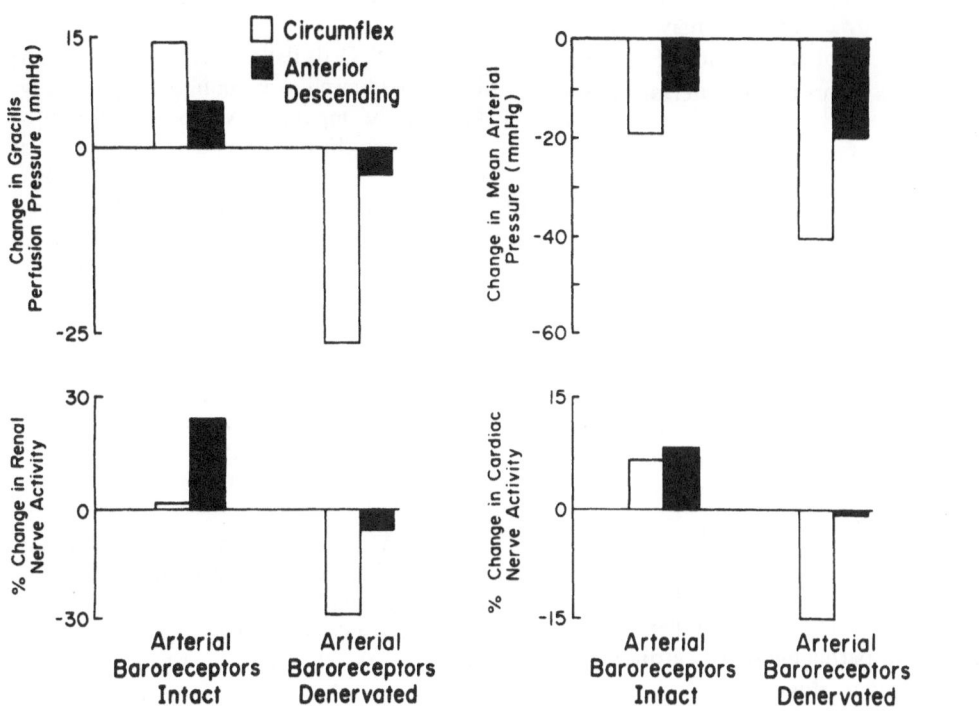

FIGURE 12-3. Responses of perfusion pressure in the isolated, constant-flow perfused gracilis muscle (top left), renal nerve activity (bottom right), and arterial pressure (top right) to circumflex (Cx) or anterior descending (LAD) coronary occlusion before and after baroreceptor denervation. Note similar responses after baroreceptor denervation. Nonuniform responses observed with baroreceptors intact are the result of the interaction between the left ventricular vagal reflex and arterial baroreflexes.

tion may result in part from reflexly mediated withdrawal of sympathetic outflow to the peripheral circulation due to activation of cardiac receptors in the inferior wall of the heart that mediate cardioinhibitory and vasodepressor reflex responses.

Integrated Responses to Myocardial Infarction

It should be apparent, based on the information reviewed to this point, that the autonomic responses to myocardial infarction are determined by many factors. They are highly dependent on the region of the myocardium that is rendered ischemic and thus on the magnitude of the stimu-

lus to inhibitory cardiac receptors. They are dependent on the blood pressure responses and thus on the stimulus to the arterial baroreceptors. Finally, they may depend on changing input from sympathetic afferents, many of which may serve as pain fibers. The net autonomic responses will depend on the integrated reflex responses to concomitant changes in input in these afferent pathways. The regional circulatory responses to myocardial ischemia or infarction are nonuniform. Thus, it is not possible to examine the response of a given vascular bed and assume that this response is representative of changes in other vascular beds.

Concluding Remarks

Based on this review we should be able to answer the three questions stated at the beginning of this chapter:

1. The responses to inferior or inferoposterior ischemia (or infarction) differ from those to anterior ischemia (or infarction) because of a preferential distribution of "inhibitory" car-

diac receptors to the inferoposterior left ventricular myocardium. They also may be due in part to a preferential distribution of "excitatory" cardiac receptors to the anterior myocardium.

2. The occurrence of bradycardia despite hypotension during inferior wall ischemia or infarction is the result of powerful activation of inhibitory cardiac reflexes that override the arterial baroreflex influence on heart rate.

3. The differential heart rate and regional circulatory responses to myocardial ischemia are the result of the magnitudes and directions of the changes in afferent input in the major cardiovascular afferent pathways to the central nervous system and on the central integration of these changing inputs.

It seems likely that the integrated autonomic reflex responses to coronary occlusion play a significant role in the pathogenesis of cardiac arrhythmias that occur in this setting.

References

1. Webb SW, Adgey AA, Pantridge JF: Autonomic disturbance at onset of acute myocardial infarction. Br Med J 3:89−92, 1972.

2. Perez-Gomez F, Matin Deios R, Rey J, Garcia Aguadi A: Prinzmetal's angina: reflex cardiovascular response during an episode of pain. Br Heart J 42:81−87, 1979.

3. Wei JY, Markis JE, Mulagold M, Braunwald E: Cardiovascular reflexes stimulated by reperfusion of ischemic myocardium in acute myocardial infarction. Clin Res 30:230A, 1982.

4. Paintal AS: Cardiovascular receptors. In: Neil E (ed) Handbook of sensory physiology. Berlin: Springer-Verlag, 1973, pp 1−45.

5. Paintal AS: Vagal sensory receptors and their reflex effects. Physiol Rev 53:159−227.

6. Toren P: Role of cardiac vagal C-fibers in cardiovascular control. Rev Physiol Biochem Pharmacol 86:1−94, 1979.

7. Baker DG, Coleridge HM, Coleridge JCG: Vagal afferent C-fibers from the ventricle. In: Hainsworth R, Kidd C, Linden RJ (eds) Cardiac receptors, Cambridge: Cambridge University Press, 1978, pp 117−137.

8. Kaufman MP, Baker DG, Coleridge HM, Coleridge JCG: Stimulation by bradykinin of afferent vagal C-fibers with chemosensitive endings in the heart and aorta of the dog. Circ Res 46:476−484, 1980.

9. Lombardi F, Della Bella P, Casati R, Malliani A: Effects of intracoronary administration of bradykinin on the impulse activity of afferent sympathetic nonmyelinated fibers with left ventricular endings in the cat. Circ Res 48:69−75, 1981.

10. Thames MD, Donald DE, Shepherd JT: Behavior of cardiac receptors with nonmyelinated vagal afferents during spontaneous respiration in cats. Circ Res 41:694−701, 1977.

11. Thoren P: Characteristics of left ventricular receptors with nonmedullated vagal afferents in cats. Circ Res 40:415−421, 1977.

12. Gupta BN, Thames MD: Behavior of left ventricular mechanoreceptors with myelinated and nonmyelinated afferent vagal fibers in cats. Circ Res 52, 1983.

13. Malliani A, Recordati G, Schwartz PJ: Nervous activity of afferent cardiac sympathetic fibers with atrial and ventricular endings. J Physiol (Lond) 229:457−469, 1973.

14. Hess GL, Zuperku EJ, Coon RL, Kampine JP: Sympathetic afferent nerve activity of left ventricular origin. Am J Physiol 227:543−546, 1974.

15. Uchida Y, Murao S: Excitation of afferent cardiac sympathetic nerve fibers during coronary occlusion. Am J Physiol 226:1094−1099, 1974.

16. Thoren PN: Activation of left ventricular receptors with nonmedullated vagal afferent fibers during occlusion of a coronary artery in the cat. Am J Cardiol 37:1046−1051.

17. Bosnjak ZJ, Zuperku EJ, Coon RL, Kampine JP: Acute coronary artery occlusion and cardiac sympathetic afferent nerve activity. Proc Soc Exp Biol Med 161:142−148, 1979.

18. Felder RB, Thames MD: Responses to activation of cardiac sympathetic afferents with epicardial bradykinin. Am J Physiol 242:H148−153, 1982.

19. Pagani M, Pizzinelli P, Furlan R, Guzzetti S, Rimoldi O, Malliani A: A sympathetic pressor reflex from the heart of conscious dogs. Circulation 66:II−35, 1982.

20. Felder RB, Thames MD: Interaction between cardiac receptors and sinoaortic baroreceptors in the control of efferent cardiac sympathetic nerve activity during myocardial ischemia in dogs. Circ Res 45:728−736, 1979.

21. Weaver LC, Danos LM, Oehl RS, Meckler RS: Contrasting reflex influences of cardiac afferent nerves during coronary occlusion. Am J Physiol 240:H620−629, 1981.

22. Felder RB, Thames MD: The cardiocardiac sympathetic reflex during coronary occlusion in anesthetized dogs. Circ Res 48:685−692, 1981.

23. Malliani A, Lombardi F: Neural reflexes associated with myocardial ischemia. In: Schwartz PJ, Brown AM, Malliani A, Zanchetti A (eds) Neural mechanisms in cardiac arrhythmias. New York: Raven, 1978, pp 209−219.

24. Thames MD, Klopfenstein HS, Abboud FM, Mark AL, Walker JL: Preferential distribution of inhibitory cardiac receptors with vagal afferents to the inferoposterior wall of the left ventricle activated during coronary occlusion in the dog. Circ Res 43:512−519, 1978.

25. Thames MD, Abboud FM: Reflex inhibition of renal sympathetic nerve activity during myocardial ischemia mediated by left ventricular receptors with vagal afferents in dogs. J Clin Invest 63:395−402, 1979.

26. White JC, Bland EF: The surgical relief of severe angina pectoris: methods employed and end results in 83 patients. Medicine 27:1−42, 1948.

27. Thies R, Foreman RD: Descending inhibition of spinal neurons in the cardiopulmonary region by electrical stimulation of vagal afferent nerves. Brain Res 207:178−183, 1981.

II. THE PREDICTION AND PREVENTION OF ACUTE MYOCARDIAL ISCHEMIA AND INFARCTION

13. THE CHANGING PROGNOSIS OF PATIENTS WITH UNSTABLE ANGINA AND ACUTE MYOCARDIAL INFARCTION

Robert M. Califf

The Changing Prognosis

The treatment of patients with acute manifestations of coronary artery disease in the 1970s was marked by a change in philosophy toward a more aggressive approach. Rather than treating complications of acute infarction as they occurred, many practitioners began to accept the concept of limitation of infarct size. In addition, the medical and surgical therapy of unstable angina became oriented toward the prevention of infarction (see chapters 8, 33, and 35). Simultaneously, the technology of monitoring devices was markedly improved so that complications could be detected earlier and more accurately, leading to more numerous interventions. Emergency medical services were expanded so that patients who might otherwise have gone untreated for a prolonged period of time were treated earlier (see chapters 27 and 28). In patients who survived their acute episodes, attempts were made to prevent future events with pharmacologic, behavioral, and surgical interventions [1].

As these changes in therapy for patients with established disease have occurred, a well-documented decline in mortality from ischemic heart disease in the United States has been observed [2]. The age-adjusted mortality dropped 25% from 1968 to 1978. Once these figures became known, a debate ensued over whether this decline was due to a change in the incidence of the disease with the implication that primary prevention resulted in the improvement, or whether a reduced mortality has occurred in patients with documented disease with the implication that improved medical care was responsible [3]. The purpose of this chapter is to review the evidence that the mortality and morbidity of patients with an established acute manifestation of ischemic heart disease have declined.

Methods for Detecting the Changes

When a randomized clinical trial is feasible, it is the method-of-choice to determine the efficacy of a particular therapy. Chapter 17 discusses the available evidence from randomized trials that particular therapies can affect mortality in patients with unstable angina or acute myocardial infarction (MI). However, the randomized trial cannot address the issue of the actual impact of the therapy on the entire population of patients who may be exposed to a variety of treatments. Only observational studies can provide this information.

When an apparent change over time in the outcome of a population is observed, the change may be due to one of two reasons: Either the prognosis of patients with the same degree of illness has changed (implying that treatment has resulted in the change) or the degree of illness in the population has changed. In patients with acute symptoms of coronary disease who come to

R.M. Califf and G.S. Wagner (eds.), ACUTE CORONARY CARE: Principles and Practice. Copyright © 1985. Martinus Nijhoff Publishing, Boston/Dordrecht/Lancaster.

medical care, a variety of reasons for a change in the degree of illness of the population may exist. Improved emergency medical services may lead to earlier treatment of acute MI before the infarction has progressed to the complicated stage. Patients with minimal disease, who previously may not have reported the symptoms to a physician, now may be treated in hospitals due to increased community awareness. Alternatively, patients with maximal disease may be salvaged in the field by emergency medical services or bystander-initiated CPR, potentially leading to "sicker" patients reaching the hospital.

The problem is further compounded by the dramatic change in diagnostic techniques and nomenclature over the past decade. Creatine kinase isoenzymes (CK-MB) for detecting acute MI are now available routinely in most hospitals and sophisticated myocardial imaging techniques are available in specialized centers. Thus, patients who might have been diagnosed as having an acute infarction in 1970 may not have met diagnostic criteria in 1984. Furthermore, the accuracy with which the degree of illness (routine coronary angiography and noninvasive techniques) can be characterized has changed dramatically in the last decade.

A similar change in the manner in which unstable angina patients have been characterized has occurred. A variety of definitions of this entity have been used [4]. Patients with chest pain and ST-T wave changes on the ECG who may have been classified as having unstable angina in the past may now be classified as having acute MI because of the detection of low levels of CK-MB. Referral patterns have also changed so that these patients are now more often admitted to hospitals where the degree of illness and clinical course can be characterized.

Given these problems with characterizing the population, several methods are available for making observations about the changing prognosis in patients with ischemic heart disease. Sequential compilations of results of randomized trials or observational studies may suggest a change in outcome [5]. Randomized trials are poorly suited for this purpose because the patients are usually carefully selected and have volunteered for randomization. For these reasons patients from randomized trials may not be rep-

resentative of the entire population. Most observational studies have not included enough detailed information about the severity of illness for comparisons to be made across reports. Nonetheless, rough observations about changes in prognosis can be made.

A second method for gauging changes in prognosis over time involves serial compilation of mortality and morbidity in the entire population of a specific geographic area. This method is well suited to the purpose when done prospectively using the same diagnostic criteria to ensure that patients are properly classified and that the same methods of characterizing the patients are used so that changes in the degree of illness can be recognized. Unfortunately, no such studies have been reported to date, but several well-done retrospective studies are now available.

Finally, advances in computer technology have enabled a number of centers to serially characterize in detail their patients with the diagnosis of unstable angina or acute infarction. These centers are now in a position to compare the prognosis of patients during one period of time to patients with the same degree of illness in another period of time. Statistical methods have been developed to control for differences in the severity of illness so that the importance of time trends can be studied in relative isolation [6].

Myocardial Infarction: Acute Phase

No clear trends are evident from the numerous reports from isolated centers and cooperative studies on the inhospital mortality from acute MI. In general, mortality from studies dating from 1970 to 1980 ranges from 8 to 25%, with no apparent change over time. However, since comparable sets of baseline characteristics have not been collected across studies, adequate comparisons of the degree of illness can not be made.

Connolly et al. [7] evaluated the hospital case/fatality rates for Rochester, Minnesota, for each five-year period between 1950 and 1975. No significant change in the case/fatality rate occurred until the 1970−75 period, when it dropped from 18% to 9%. Similar trends were observed in all age groups and in both sexes. A comparison of the case/fatality rates of 1966−67 to 1971 in metropolitan Baltimore was reported by Goldberg et al. [8]. The case/fatality rate dropped from 27.5% in 1966−67 to 20% in 1971. The difference remained significant after adjustment for 16 variables describing demographic factors and the degree of illness of the patients at baseline.

Two large-scale epidemiologic studies have recently been reported examining the issue of inhospital mortality from acute MI. Goldman et al. studied 63 acute-care hospitals in a defined geographic area around Boston [9] (see chapter 38]. Discharge diagnoses were registered in a prospective computerized system in 33 hospitals, while chart review was required in the other 30 hospitals. Inhospital mortality and length of stay were recorded in addition to secondary diagnoses, age, and sex. No information about severity of infarction was available. Outcome was compared in patients between 1973−74 and 1978−79. Gillum et al. evaluated a seven-county area involving Minneapolis-St. Paul [10]. Only one hospital in this area was not included in the study. Limited descriptors of the degree of illness were recorded prospectively (other discharge diagnoses, previous MIs, previous angina, and enzyme levels). Outcome was compared among patients admitted from 1970 to 1980.

The case/fatality rate in the study by Goldman et al. was 22% in 1973−74 and 23% in 1978−79. When age-specific rates were examined, no reduction in hospital mortality rates was seen, but an 11% reduction in hospital admissions for acute MI was observed in patients less than age 70. These results suggested that no measurable change in inhospital mortality occurred during this five-year period, but that the risk of having an MI declined in patients less than age 70. The inhospital mortality rate of 22%−23% is higher than usually reported. Since the baseline characteristics of the patient population are not available, reasons for this high mortality cannot be assessed.

In contrast, Gillum et al. found a reduction in case/fatality rate from 16.7% to 11.9% in men and from 16.6% to 12.2% in women. These changes represented a 28.7% decline for men and a 26.5% decline for women. They estimated that 27% of the decline in mortality due to coronary heart disease in men versus only 6% of the decline in women could be attributed to a lower inhos-

pital mortality rate for acute MI. The major methodologic problem with this study was the difference in diagnostic criteria for MI during the course of the study, primarily reflecting increased use of cardiac isoenzymes. A reduction in admission rates for acute MI was also found (18% for men and 13% for women). Furthermore, an increased rate of prehospital resuscitation with survival to hospitalization was documented. The authors concluded that the decline in mortality due to ischemic heart disease could be attributed to (a) better emergency medical care and (b) better inhospital care for patients with clinically manifest disease as well as (c) primary prevention of the disease.

Reasons for the differences in results between the study by Goldman et al. [9] and the other three studies [7, 8, 10] are not clear. Goldman et al. suggested that the majority of the change in mortality with improved inhospital care occurred prior to 1973, since the extensive uses of cardiac monitoring and prophylactic lidocaine were initiated prior to this time. This rationale is compatible with the other studies that encompassed an earlier time span. The large difference in overall case/fatality rates in the population reported by Goldman et al. [9] versus Gillum et al. [10] remains unexplained.

Myocardial Infarction: Convalescent Phase

Despite convincing evidence that specific medical and surgical interventions can prolong survival in selected groups of post-MI patients [1], little information is available from population studies about long-term survival trends. Weinblatt et al. compared the long-term outcome in 436 men who survived a first MI between 1961 and 1970 with the outcome in 697 men who survived a first MI between 1971 and 1978 [11]. No significant differences in survival with up to five years of follow-up were evident between the groups, even after age adjustment. Although more patients in the later group entered the study within three months after the initial MI, no difference in outcome could be found when this factor was adjusted for using the Cox model. Numerous other baseline characteristics were recorded in these patients, but differences were not found to affect the overall result. However, no documentation of the size of infarction or extent of anatomic disease was available. The major drawback of this study was that patients were not entered during the hospital phase of the acute MI. Since mortality is highest during the initial period after hospital discharge [12], important survival trends could have been missed.

Connolly et al. [7] and Goldberg et al. [8] also evaluated long-term prognosis in their populations. In the Rochester population, five-year survival was 60% in the 1965–69 cohort and 66% in the 1970–75 cohort. This difference was not statistically significant. Similarly, Goldberg et al. found no significant difference in five-year survival of the 1966–67 cohort compared with the 1971 cohort.

Pryor et al. reported 1911 consecutive medically treated patients who underwent cardiac catheterization between 1969 and 1982 [13]. A previous myocardial infarction had been documented in 54% of these patients. Detailed characterization of the risk factors, demographic characteristics, and symptoms was available as well as quantitative descriptors of the coronary anatomy and extent of left ventricular dysfunction resulting from previous infarction. Between 1971 and 1978, a decline of 1.9% in one-year mortality (9.75% to 7.84%) occurred in this population. Similar declines in the risk of recurrent nonfatal infarction were observed. After adjusting for differences in the degree of illness of these patients at baseline, the improvement in prognosis over time remained significant. Thus, a higher proportion of patients with the same amount of coronary disease, left ventricular dysfunction, and symptoms were alive with each passing year.

Although the report by Pryor et al. cannot characterize the effect of advances in therapy in a defined geographic region, it does provide documentation that the long-term prognosis of equally sick patients with coronary disease has changed during the 1970s. Similar changes have been found in the operative survival and even more dramatic changes are evident in the long-term survival of patients who survive the initial operation (DB Pryor, personal communication). This evidence strongly suggests that improvements in medical and surgical therapy have re-sulted in a changing prognosis of patients with well-defined disease.

Unstable Angina

The treatment of unstable angina has fluctuated substantially in the past decade. A lack of knowledge about the prognosis of the disorder has led to different opinions about therapy [14]. Early reports found a high rate of progression to acute MI and death. Later reports have found that more-symptomatic patients are at higher risk of ischemic events compared with less-symptomatic patients [15, 16], but the average absolute risk is lower than previously observed [17].

Serial studies cannot be used reliably to evaluate changes in the prognosis of unstable angina because its variable definitions have resulted in different patient populations and outcomes. In general, however, a trend toward better survival and lower infarction rates is evident, especially in surgically treated patients. The report by Mulcahy et al. is contrary to this trend [17]. These authors found comparable results to the National Unstable Angina trial [18] with a simple medical regimen consisting of bedrest and sublingual nitrates. No studies of entire populations in geographically defined areas are available.

The study by Pryor et al. included 732 patients with progressive angina and 109 patients with prolonged angina at rest ("preinfarction" angina), but it did not separate these patients for specific analysis of the changing prognosis of unstable angina. Both the National Cooperative Study of Unstable Angina and the report by Rahimtoola et al. [19] found a lower operative mortality over time in patients with unstable angina. Neither of these surgical reports included adjustments for the degree of illness in later patients compared with earlier patients. Thus, despite the large numbers of new treatments and technical advances in the treatment of patients with unstable angina, clear-cut evidence of a change in the prognosis of these patients is not available.

Conclusion: Perspectives for the Future

The 1980s will be characterized by more dramatic changes in therapeutic approaches. Direct revascularization with surgery or thrombolytic therapy is currently being applied to patients with acute MI. The routine use of beta-blocking agents in the convalescent phase should have a dramatic effect on survival if results in practice are as good as in the randomized trails. Trials to help delineate the roles of antiarrhythmic drugs and vasodilator therapy are planned or under way. New drugs and surgical techniques including percutaneous angioplasty have recently become available for unstable angina patients. The greater prevalence of computerized record-keeping systems should enable investigators to document more clearly the changing prognosis of future patients.

References

1. May GS, Eberlein KA, Fruberg CD, Passamani ER, De Mets DL: Secondary prevention after myocardial infarction: a review of long-term trials. Prog Cardiovasc Dis 25:331−352, 1983.
2. Stern MP: The recent decline in ischemic heart disease mortality. Ann Intern Med 91:630−40, 1979.
3. Walker WJ: Changing United States life-style and declining vascular mortality: cause or coincidence. N Engl J Med 297:163−165, 1977.
4. Fowler NO: "Preinfarctional" angina: a need for an objective definition and for a controlled clinical trial of its management. Circulation 44:755−757, 1971.
5. Braunwald E: Effects of coronary-artery bypass grafting on survival. N Engl J Med 309:1181−84, 1983.
6. Rosati RA, Lee KL, Califf RM, Pryor DB, Harrell FE Jr: Problems and advantages of an observational data base approach to evaluating the effect of therapy on outcome. Circulation 65:II-27−32, 1982.
7. Connolly, DC, Oxman HA, Nobrega FT, Kurland LT, Kennedy MA, Elveback ER: Coronary heart disease in residents of Rochester, Minnesota, 1950−1975. I. Background and study design. Mayo Clin Proc 56:661−672, 1981.
8. Goldberg R, Szklo M, Tonascia JA, Kennedy

HL: Time trends in prognosis of patients with myocardial infarction: a population-based study. Johns Hopkins Med J 144:73−80, 1979.
9. Goldman L, Cook F, Hashimoto B, Stone P, Muller J, Loscalzo A: Evidence that hospital care for acute myocardial infarction has not contributed to the decline in coronary mortality between 1973−1974 and 1978−1979. Circulation 65:936−942, 1982.
10. Gillum RF, Folsom A, Luepker RV, Jacobs DR, Kottke TE, Gomez-Marin O, Prineas RJ, Taylor HL, Blackburn H: Sudden death and acute myocardial infarction in a metropolitan area, 1970−1980. N Engl J Med 309:1353−1358, 1983.
11. Weinblatt E, Goldberg JD, Ruberman W, Frank CW, Monk MA, Chaudhary BS: Mortality after first myocardial infarction: search for a secular trend. JAMA 247:1576−1581, 1982.
12. Madsen EB, Hougaard P, Gilpin E: Dynamic evaluation of prognosis from time-dependent variables in acute myocardial infarction. Am J Cardiol 51:1579−84, 1983.
13. Pryor DB, Harrell FE Jr, Lee KL, Califf RM, Rosati RA: An improving prognosis over time in medically treated patients with coronary artery disease. Am J Cardiol 52:444−448, 1983.
14. Russell RO, Rackley CE, Kouchoukos NT: Unstable angina pectoris: do we know the best management? Am J Cardiol 48:590−591, 1981.
15. Chahine RA: Unstable angina: the problem of definition. Br Heart J 37:1246−1249, 1975.
16. Roberts KB, Califf RM, Harrell FE JR, Lee KL, Pryor DB, Rosati RA: The prognosis of patients with new onset angina undergoing cardiac catheterization. Circulation 68:970−978, 1983.
17. Mulcahy R, Daly L, Graham I, Hickey N, O'Donoghue S, Owens A, Ruane P, Tobin G: Unstable angina: natural history and determinants of prognosis. Am J Cardiol 48:525−528, 1981.
18. National Cooperative Study Group to Compare Surgical and Medical Therapy: In-hospital experience and initial follow-up results in patients with one, two and three vessel disease. Am J Cardiol 42:839−848, 1978.
19. Rahimtoola SH, Nunley D, Grunkemeier G, Tepley J, Lambert L, Starr A: Ten-year survival after coronary bypass surgery of unstable angina. N Engl J Med 308:676−81, 1983.

14. RISK FACTORS THAT PREDICT FATAL AND NONFATAL CARDIAC EVENTS

Phillip J. Harris

Robert A. Rosati

The basis for therapeutic decision making is the clinician's estimate of the risk of unwanted events using one therapy versus another. In the patient with ischemic heart disease the major adverse events that are difficult to anticipate are myocardial infarction (MI) and sudden death. Death from progressive heart failure can be predicted more easily and will not be discussed further. If a physician is to make a prediction of the patient's risk, an understanding of the factors associated with these events is necessary. Increasing insight into these factors has been gained by the recent development of statistical methods for predictive models based on pathophysiology. In ischemic heart disease one would hope that the factors predicting MI reflect the likelihood of coronary thrombosis, while the factors predicting sudden death reflect "electrical instability." If the risk factors for each end point were distinct, specific therapies could be designed to prevent particular events by altering those risk factors.

Unfortunately, the circumstances surrounding a fatal event are often not clear. Death may be unwitnessed or, when it is witnessed, the necessary information to distinguish sudden arrhythmic death in the absence versus the presence of an acute infarction may not be available. Because of the confusion engendered by this lack of clinical clarity, no entirely satisfactory method of distinguishing risk factors that predict these specific events has been developed.

Several different approaches to the evaluation of risk factors for events in patients with ischemic heart disease have been advocated: (a) Prediction of the risk of any event (fatal or nonfatal), then determining the risk factors that distinguish likelihood of a fatal versus a nonfatal event. The advantage of this approach is that events can be clearly demarcated, but the differing pathophysiologic mechanisms are not considered (i.e., sudden death in both the absence and presence of an acute infarct is considered a single "event"). (b) Prediction of the risk of sudden death versus MI (fatal or nonfatal), then identifying the risk factors that distinguish a fatal from a nonfatal infarct. This approach has the advantage of separating end points by presumed pathophysiology (arrhythmia versus infarction), but is limited by our inability to distinguish a sudden death from an acute infarct death. (c) Prediction of the risk of each event separately: nonfatal infarction, fatal infarction, and sudden death in the absence of infarction. This approach would seem to be the most logical since it separately considers both outcomes, which differ in pathophysiology (ischemic versus nonischemic) and in severity (fatal versus nonfatal). It may be both difficult and confusing, however, to consider the different risk factors for varying outcomes for the same pathophysiologic entity (MI). For example, the extent of coronary atherosclerosis is less in patients at risk for nonfatal infarction. Therefore, single-vessel stenosis might be a stronger risk factor than double- or triple-vessel stenosis for the outcome of nonfatal infarction, since most infarcts in patients with multivessel disease are fatal. This information does not lead to definition of an effective preventive strategy, since the strategy should be aimed at prevention of the pathophysiologic process of infarction rather than at a subgroup of patients who are at low risk overall. This chapter reviews the studies that have used each of these various approaches to determine the risk factors for these unfavorable events in patients with ischemic heart disease.

Myocardial Infarction in Asymptomatic Individuals

If a myocardial infarct causes significant left ventricular damage it dramatically worsens a patient's prognosis, and it is therefore an important event in the natural history of coronary artery disease (CAD). The factors that predict imminent acute MI have not been clearly identified.

The conventional risk factors for CAD do not distinguish between the various manifestations of the disease. However, the Framingham study identified an association between sex and the likelihood of a nonfatal MI as the first manifestation of CAD [1]. In men, nonfatal MI was the most common initial event, occurring in 45% of those who developed CAD. In women, angina pectoris was the most frequent initial event and nonfatal MI was the presenting event in only 32% of those who developed CAD.

Many smaller studies have reported associations between various characteristics and MI. Usually the other manifestations of CAD have not been considered as end points and it remains unknown whether the association is with MI in particular or CAD in general. Oral contraceptive use is one factor that does appear to be associated with an increased risk of fatal and nonfatal MI [2]. But because of the low incidence of MI in young women, the risk associated with oral contraceptive use is not clinically significant unless other risk factors such as smoking and hypertension are also present.

Nonfatal versus Fatal Events in Patients with CAD

In a Duke study [3] of 1214 patients with angiographically proven CAD the risk of nonfatal MI over seven years was 18%. This was half the risk of death, which was 35%. In the Cleveland Clinic series [4] and in an international study [5] there were also more deaths than nonfatal MIs, but in the HIP Study [6] there were more nonfatal MIs than deaths in patients with a diagnosis of CAD. Differences in definition and follow-up technique may account for these variations, but the weight of evidence indicates that, in an average population of patients with CAD, the risk of death is greater than the risk of nonfatal MI. This is in contrast to the situation in asymptomatic individuals [1].

The Duke study [3] demonstrated, however, that the risk of nonfatal MI is not uniform in patients with CAD. The pattern of chest pain, the extent of coronary disease, and the degree of impairment of left ventricular function were identified as the most important predictors of ischemic events, defined as death or nonfatal MI. These predictors defined subsets in which there was considerable variation in the relative frequency of nonfatal MI and death (figure 14-1).

In patients with single-vessel disease, the risk of nonfatal MI exceeded the risk of death. With increasing severity of coronary disease the risk of an event increased dramatically, but was almost entirely due to an increase in the risk of death. In patients with three-vessel disease the risk of nonfatal MI was similar to that in single-vessel disease, but in patients with left main disease the risk of a nonfatal infarct was actually less than in patients with single-vessel disease because virtually all the ischemic events were fatal.

Left ventricular function had a similar effect. With normal left ventricular function the risk of nonfatal MI exceeded the risk of death, but with severely impaired left ventricular function, although the risk of an event was dramatically increased, virtually all the events were fatal and the risk of nonfatal MI was less than with normal left ventricular function.

The prognostic significance of the pattern of chest pain was different from the other factors.

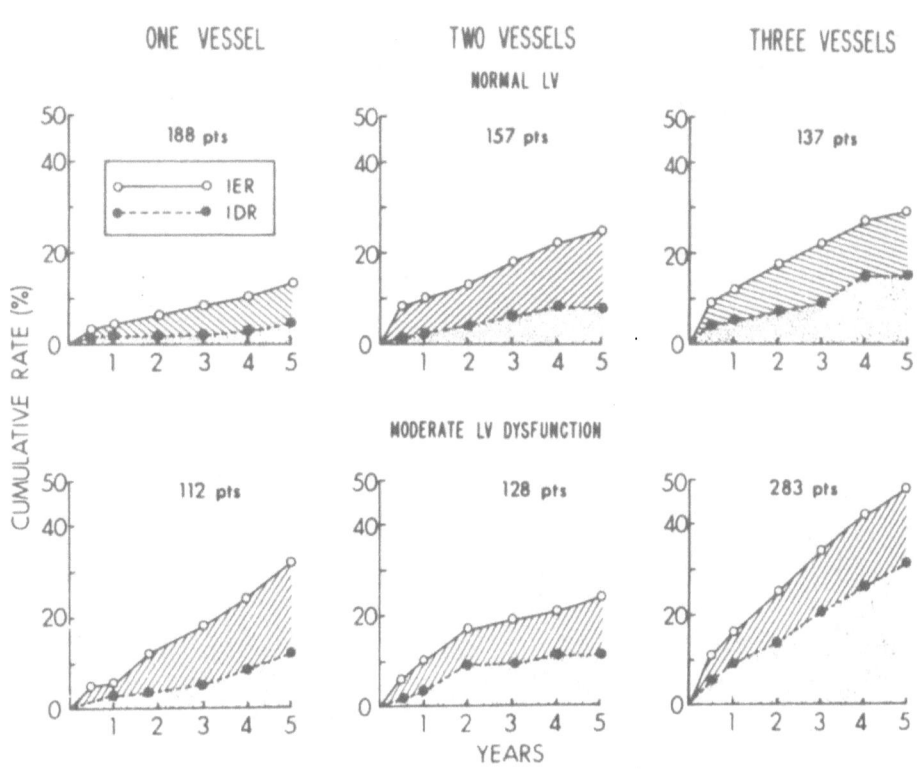

FIGURE 14-1. Event rates related to the presence of one-, two-, or three-vessel disease and normal left ventricular (LV) function or moderate left ventricular dysfunction. IER, initial event rate (nonfatal infarction or death); IDR, initial death rate (deaths that were the initial event). The nonfatal infarction rate is represented by the difference between the initial event rate and the initial death rate. From Harris et al. [3], with permission.

Progressive pain, which is the equivalent of accelerating angina, increased the risk of both nonfatal MI and death in most patients. Its effect in patients with three-vessel disease is illustrated in figure 14-2. At all levels of left ventricular function, progressive pain doubled or tripled the rate of nonfatal MI. Progressive angina is associated with a significantly increased risk of MI and whether the infarcts are fatal or nonfatal is probably determined by other factors such as left ventricular function.

In another Duke study [7], age, left ventricular function, a history of previous MI, and the presence of left main stenosis or total occlusion of the left anterior descending (LAD) or right coronary artery (RCA) were identified as the main factors that distinguished between the likelihood of nonfatal MI versus death as the next event in patients with CAD.

Together, the two Duke studies indicate that the risk of an event is related to the extent of coronary disease, impairment of left ventricular function and the severity of pain. In older patients and in patients with left main disease or severely impaired left ventricular function the majority of events are fatal. In patients with good left ventricular function, the risk of nonfatal MI is greater than the risk of death. The risk of nonfatal MI is highest in young patients with progressive chest pain, normal or near-normal left ventricular function, and three-vessel CAD involving subtotal stenoses of the RCA and LAD.

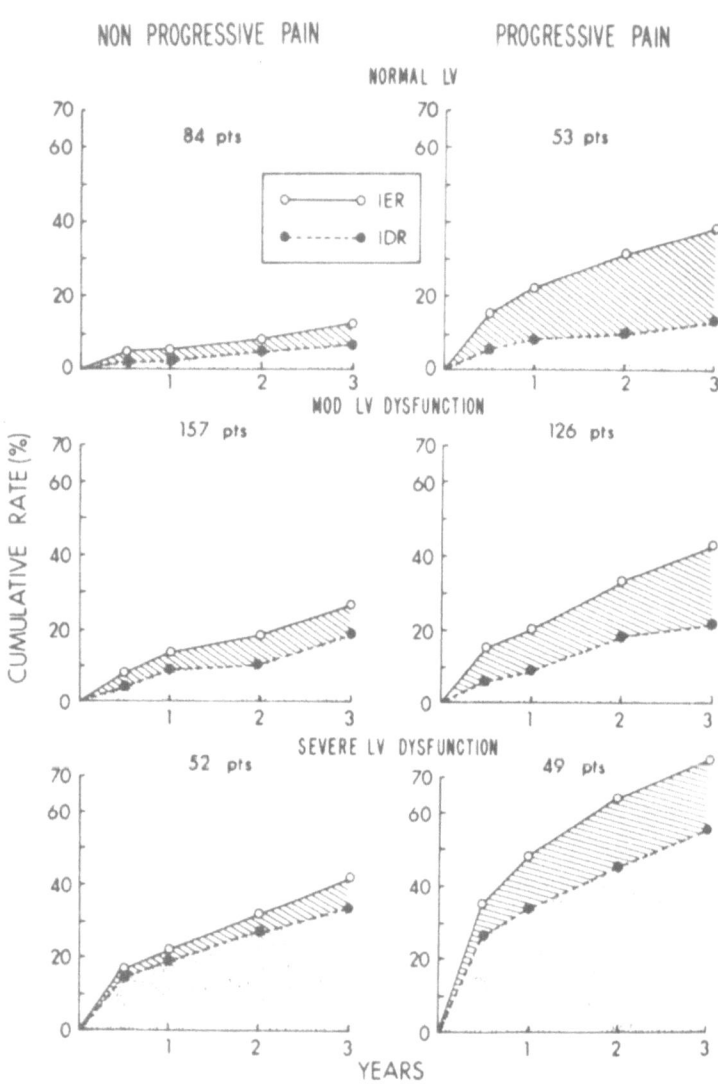

FIGURE 14-2. The effect of progressive pain on event rates in patients with three-vessel disease classified according to whether they had normal left ventricular (LV) function, moderate LV dysfunction, or severe LV dysfunction. IER, initial event rate (nonfatal infarction or death); IDR, initial death rate (deaths that were the initial event). The nonfatal infarction rate is represented by the difference between the initial event rate and the initial death rate. From Harris et al. [3], with permission.

Reinfarction in Postinfarct Patients

Several of the recently published secondary prevention trials have documented the incidence of reinfarction. Unfortunately there is wide variation in the reinfarction rates. The reasons for this variation have been discussed by Furberg and Bell [8]. Generally it appears that the rate of nonfatal reinfarction in the year after MI is increased to the same extent as the risk of death. For example, in the Norwegian timolol trial the cumulative nonfatal reinfarction rate in placebo-treated patients exceeded 10% in 12 months [9].

It has proven difficult to identify factors that predict reinfarction. In a Swedish study [10] there was no relationship between the characteristics that predicted survival and the incidence of nonfatal reinfarction. In fact, nonfatal reinfarction appeared to be a random event. One factor that may be associated with a high incidence of fatal and nonfatal reinfarction is the initial occurrence of a subendocardial MI. Hutter et al. [11] reported a 21% incidence of reinfarction in the nine months after subendocardial MI compared with only 3% after transmural MI.

Because of the difficulty in predicting nonfatal reinfarction it is argued that all post-MI patients should be treated with beta-blocking drugs (see chapter 55). More information is needed about the characteristics that predict reinfarction if beta-blocking drugs are to be used with discrimination in post-MI patients.

Sudden Death

Sudden death is the most common mode of death in males aged 20—64 years. It has been estimated that there are 1200 sudden cardiac deaths per day in the USA [12] and it has been reported that from 25% [12] to 50% [13] of those who die suddenly have no previous symptoms of heart disease. But despite the large number of sudden deaths that occur in the community, the problem for the epidemiologist trying to identify predictors of sudden death is that in asymptomatic individuals the risk of sudden death is low, and probably does not exceed 1% per year [14].

SUDDEN DEATH IN
ASYMPTOMATIC INDIVIDUALS
In the Framingham Study, sudden death was the initial manifestation of CAD in 11% of males and in 6% of females who developed CAD [1]. In patients aged 45—74 years with no history of heart disease, 56% of the coronary deaths were sudden.

Because sudden death is usually one of the end points in trials aimed at identifying risk factors for CAD, the characteristics that have been reported as risk factors for CAD are also predictors of sudden death. In the Framingham Study [13], none of the conventional risk factors could be identified as being specifically associated with sudden death as opposed to the other manifestations of CAD. In a univariate analysis, the proportion of sudden deaths decreased with increasing age and increased with obesity, smoking, and increasing physical activity, but, in a multivariate analysis, no risk factor distinguished accurately between candidates for sudden death and candidates for other forms of CAD.

Several abnormalities in the resting ECG, including ST-T wave changes, left ventricular hypertrophy, left bundle branch block, and intraventricular conduction defect, have been associated with an increased risk of death in asymptomatic individuals [15, 16]. While these abnormalities are associated with an increased risk of death from CAD there is little proof that they are specifically associated with sudden death.

The prognostic significance of ventricular premature beats (VPBs) in asymptomatic individuals is also an important question. In older patients, particularly in those with other risk factors for CAD, VPBs are associated with increased mortality from CAD [17]. Rabkin et al. [18] found that, particularly in older males, VPBs were more strongly associated with sudden death than with other manifestations of CAD. It is likely, however, that the prognostic significance of VPBs in these studies was due to an association between VPBs and undiagnosed CAD. Califf et al. [19] recently reported no deaths in up to five years of follow-up in 71 patients who had insignificant CAD, but who had high-grade ventricular arrhythmias, during Holter monitoring.

SUDDEN DEATH IN PATIENTS WITH
CORONARY ARTERY DISEASE
Although the risk of death is increased in patients with CAD, the proportion of deaths that are sudden appears to be the same (approximately 50%) as in asymptomatic individuals [19—21]. Characteristics associated with a high mortality rate are therefore associated with a high risk of sudden death. An interesting question is whether any characteristics distinguish the likelihood of sudden death from other modes of death.

Bruce et al. [22], investigating the role of exercise testing in predicting sudden death, found that cardiomegaly, an exercise duration of less than 3 min, and exertional hypotension were the best predictors of sudden death. The annual risk of sudden death was 12/1000 in the absence of these characteristics, increasing to 638/1000 in the presence of all three characteristics. Other modes of death were not considered in this study and it is therefore not known whether these characteristics specifically predicted sudden death as opposed to overall mortality.

The extent of coronary disease and the degree of impairment of left ventricular function are the most important predictors of overall survival in patients with CAD [23]. The clinician is aware that the risk of sudden death is ever-present in patients with left main disease and poor left ventricular function. However, there does not appear to be conclusive proof that in these patients the risk of sudden death is increased to a greater extent than the total risk of death.

The relationship between VPBs recorded on the resting ECG or during Holter monitoring and sudden death in patients with CAD has received a lot of attention (see chapter 53). Ventricular premature beats are prognostically significant and the mortality rate increases with complex VPBs [17, 19]. There is a close relationship, however, between the frequency and complexity of VPBs and the extent of coronary disease and severity of left ventricular dysfunction [19]. In addition, VPBs are not specifically associated with sudden death, but are associated with overall mortality. In the HIP study in patients with angina [21], the risk of sudden death in patients with VPBs was approximately 50% of the total risk of death, the same proportion of sudden deaths that has been recorded in asymptomatic individuals and patients with CAD in general. In a detailed multivariable analysis by Califf et al. [19], ventricular arrhythmias recorded during Holter monitoring were not independently predictive of either total mortality or sudden death when coronary anatomy and left ventricular function were taken into account.

SUDDEN DEATH AFTER
MYOCARDIAL INFARCTION
The mortality rate in the year after myocardial infarction is 10% − 15% compared with 4% − 5% per year in patients with angina. The prevailing concept is that the majority of these deaths are sudden. This concept was confirmed by Bigger et al. [24], who reported a one-year mortality rate of 19% with 80% of deaths in the first six months being sudden. However, when the definition is limited to deaths occurring within 1 or 2 h of the onset of symptoms, the proportion of deaths reported to be sudden is less. For example, in the placebo group in the Anturane Reinfarction Trial [25], only 37 of 62 deaths were classified as sudden; and in the placebo group in the timolol trial [26], only 38 of 113 deaths occurred within a few seconds. Finally, in the recently published results of the Multicenter Postinfarction Research Group [27], only 37% of the cardiac deaths were classified as sudden.

Although the proportion of sudden deaths in postinfarct patients may not exceed the 50% observed in other populations, the actual incidence of sudden death is high because of the increased mortality rate. Considerable effort has been expended in attempting to identify those specifically at risk of sudden death. Moss [28] has recently reviewed the significance of VPBs in postinfarct patients (see chapter 53). Initial results indicate that left ventricular dysfunction and complex ectopy may provide independent prognostic information [29, 30]. Several authors [31 − 33] have reported that a repetitive response to intracardiac electrical stimulation predicts subsequent mortality and that the proportion of instantaneous or sudden deaths is greater than 50% (see chapter 54). Thus, electrophysiology studies may specifically identify patients at risk of sudden death, but the relationship between electrophysiologic characteristics and other prognostic factors in postinfarct patients has not yet been determined.

SUDDEN DEATH IN SURVIVORS OF
CARDIAC ARREST
Patients who have survived a cardiac arrest undoubtedly have the highest risk of sudden death. The one-year mortality in patients discharged after resuscitation is 26% and three-quarters of the deaths are sudden [34]. The risk of subsequent death is further increased if the cardiac arrest did not occur in the context of a transmural MI or if there is a history of previous MI or heart failure. Electrophysiologic testing appears to be helpful in further defining the risk of recurrence and in selecting appropriate treatment in these patients [35], but there is not yet general agreement about the prognostic significance of certain electrophysiologic parameters such as the ability to induce ventricular fibrillation.

Summary

Nonfatal MI occurs more frequently than death in asymptomatic individuals and is more likely to be the initial manifestation of CAD in males than in females. Although the risk of dying from CAD is low in asymptomatic individuals, 50% of the deaths are sudden and there are no characteristics that indicate that a person is more prone to sudden death than the other manifestations of CAD.

As a general rule, in patients with CAD, the risk of death exceeds the risk of nonfatal MI. Approximately 50% of the deaths are sudden, the same as in asymptomatic individuals. However, there is considerable variation in the relative frequency of nonfatal MI and death in subsets defined by prognostic factors.

Young patients with normal left ventricular infarction are more likely to have a nonfatal MI than to die. The chance of a nonfatal MI is further increased if they have progressive angina or three-vessel disease with subtotal LAD and RCA stenoses. In patients with severely impaired left ventricular function or left main disease, the risk of an event is dramatically increased and virtually all of the events are fatal. It is unclear whether the proportion of deaths that are sudden is also increased.

The risk of sudden death is increased in post-infarct patients, but this is probably due to a general increase in the mortality rate rather than a specific increase in the risk of sudden death. Electrophysiologic testing may help to identify patients who are specifically at risk of sudden death.

Patients who have survived a cardiac arrest have the highest risk of sudden death. Electrophysiologic testing may also be of benefit in these patients in further defining the risk of recurrence and in selecting the appropriate treatment.

References

1. Kannel WB: Some lessons in cardiovascular epidemiology from Framingham. Am J Cardiol 37: 269–282, 1976.
2. Dalen JE, Hickler RB: Oral contraceptives and cardiovascular disease. Am Heart J 101:626–639, 1981.
3. Harris PJ, Lee KL, Harrell FE, Behar VS, Rosati RA: Outcome in medically treated coronary artery disease: ischaemic events—nonfatal infarction and death. Circulation 62:718–726, 1980.
4. Proudfit WL, Bruschke AVG, Sones FM: Natural history of obstructive coronary artery disease: ten-year study of 601 nonsurgical cases. Prog Cardiovasc Dis 21:53–78, 1978.
5. Keys A, Aravanis C, Blackburn H, Van Buchem FSP, Buzina R, Corcondilas A, Djordjevic BS, Dontas AS, Fidanza F, Imbimbo B, Karvonen MJ, Kimura N, Leko D, Menotti A, Mohacek I, Monti M, Puchner T, Puddu V, Punsar S, Parlin RW, Taylor HL, Vasquez C: Coronary heart disease in seven countries. Circulation (Suppl 1) 41:I-148–153, 1970.
6. Weinblatt E, Frank CW, Shapiro S, Sager RV: Prognostic factors in angina pectoris: a prospective study. J Chron Dis 21:231–245, 1968.
7. Harris PJ, Harrell FE, Lee KL, Rosati RA: Nonfatal myocardial infarction in medically treated patients with coronary artery disease. Am J Cardiol 46:937–942, 1980.
8. Furberg CD, Bell RL: Effect of beta-blocker therapy on recurrent nonfatal myocardial infarction. Circulation (Suppl 1) 67: I-83–85, 1983.
9. Pedersen TR: The Norwegian multicenter study of timolol after myocardial infarction. Circulation (Suppl 1) 67: I-49–53.
10. Vedin A, Wilhelmsen L, Wedel H, Pettersson B, Wilhelmsson C, Elmfeldt D, Tibblin G: Prediction of cardiovascular deaths and non-fatal reinfarctions after myocardial infarction. Acta Med Scand 201:309–316, 1977.
11. Hutter AM, De Sanctis RW, Flynn T, Yeatman LA: Nontransmural myocardial infarction: a comparison of hospital and late clinical course of patients with that of matched patients with transmural anterior and transmural inferior myocardial infarction. Am J Cardiol 48:595–602, 1981.
12. Lown B: Sudden cardiac death: the major challenge confronting contemporary cardiology. Am J Cardiol 43:313–328, 1979.
13. Kannel WB, Thomas HE: Sudden coronary death: the Framingham study. Ann NY Acad Sci 382:3–21, 1982.
14. Kuller LH: Sudden death: definition and epidemiologic considerations. Prog Cardiovasc Dis 23: 1–11, 1980.
15. Kannel WB, Doyle JT, McNamara PM, Quickenton P, Gordon T: Precursors of sudden coronary death. Circulation 51:606–613, 1975.
16. Rabkin SW, Mathewson FAL, Tate RB: The electrocardiogram in apparently healthy men and

the risk of sudden death. Br Heart J 47:546–552, 1982.

17. Moss AJ: Clinical significance of ventricular arrhythmias in patients with and without coronary artery disease. Prog Cardiovasc Dis 23:33–51, 1980.

18. Rabkin SW, Mathewson FAL, Tate RB: Relationship of ventricular ectopy in men without apparent heart disease to occurrence of ischemic heart disease and sudden death. Am Heart J 101:135–142, 1981.

19. Califf RM, McKinnis RA, Burks J, Lee KL, Harrell FE, Behar VS, Pryor DB, Wagner GS, Rosati RA: Prognostic implications of ventricular arrhythmias during 24 hour ambulatory monitoring in patients undergoing cardiac catheterization for coronary artery disease. Am J Cardiol 50:23–31, 1982.

20. Margolis JR, Hirshfeld JW, McNeer JF, Starmer CF, Rosati RA, Peter RH, Behar VS, Kong Y: Sudden death due to coronary artery disease: a clinical, hemodynamic and angiographic profile. Circulation (Suppl 3) 51 and 52:III-180–188, 1975.

21. Ruberman W, Weinblatt E, Goldberg JD, Frank CW, Shapiro S, Chaudhary BS: Ventricular premature complexes in prognosis of angina. Circulation 61:1172–1178, 1980.

22. Bruce RA, DeRouen T, Peterson DR, Irving JB, Chinn N, Blake B, Hofer V: Noninvasive predictors of sudden death in men with coronary heart disease. Am J Cardiol 39:833–840, 1977.

23. Harris PJ, Harrell FE, Lee KL, Behar VS, Rosati RA: Survival in medically treated coronary artery disease. Circulation 60:1259–1269, 1979.

24. Bigger JT, Heller CA, Wenger TL, Weld FM: Risk stratification after acute myocardial infarction. Am J Cardiol 42:202–210, 1978.

25. The Anturane Reinfarction Trial Research Group: Sulfinpyrazone in the prevention of sudden death after myocardial infarction. N Engl J Med 302:250–256, 1980.

26. The Norwegian Multicenter Study Group: Timolol-induced reduction in mortality and reinfarction in patients surviving acute myocardial infarction. N Engl J Med 304:14, 1981.

27. The Multicenter Postinfarction Group: Risk stratification and survival after myocardial infarction. N Engl J Med 309:331–336, 1983.

28. Moss AJ: Postinfarction PVBs: marker for sudden death? Primary Cardiol Clin 5:19–23, 1983.

29. Lesch M, Kehoe RF: Predictability of sudden cardiac death: a partially fulfilled promise. N Engl J Med 310:255–257, 1984.

30. The Multicenter Postinfarction Research Group: Risk stratification and survival after myocardial infarction. N Engl J Med 309:331–336, 1983.

31. Greene HL, Reid PR, Schaeffer AH: The repetitive ventricular response in man: a predictor of sudden death. N Engl J Med 299:729–734, 1978.

32. Hamer A, Vohra J, Hunt D, Sloman G: Prediction of sudden death by electrophysiologic studies in high risk patients surviving acute myocardial infarction. Am J Cardiol 50:223–229, 1982.

33. Richards DA, Cody DV, Denniss AR, Russell PA, Young AA, Uther JB: Ventricular electrical instability: a predictor of death after myocardial infarction. Am J Cardiol 51:75–80, 1983.

34. Cobb LA, Werner JA, Trobaugh GB: Sudden cardiac death. II. Outcome of resuscitation; management, and future directions. Mod Concepts Cardiovasc Dis 49:37–42, 1980.

35. Roy D, Waxman HL, Kienzle MG, Buxton AE, Marchlinski FE, Josephson ME: Clinical characteristics and long-term follow-up in 119 survivors of cardiac arrest: relation to inducibility at electrophysiologic testing. Am J Cardiol 52:969–974, 1983.

15. THE ROLE OF NUTRITION IN ATHEROGENESIS AND ACUTE MYOCARDIAL INFARCTION

Rudolph M. Ballentine

Atherosclerosis and its sequelae, principally coronary heart disease and cerebrovascular accidents, are easily credited with being the number one killer in the United States. While many factors have been identified in the process of atherosclerosis, nutrition is one which offers the most obvious potential for intervention. What is eaten is regularly chosen and, if there is any causal connection between diet and atherosclerosis, this choice would provide a simple and straightforward opportunity to deter or prevent atherogenesis.

The data available on the relationship between nutrition and atherogenesis fall into several areas. That which has received most attention deals with dietary fat (and cholesterol), and atherosclerosis. But there are other components of diet—fiber, protein, vitamins, and minerals—which seem to be of at least equal importance, even though they have attracted much less research effort. We will briefly survey the voluminous literature on dietary fat and atherosclerosis, and then turn to some of the promising new data on other dietary factors.

Dietary Fat and Atherogenesis

Perhaps discussions of diet and atherosclerotic diseases tend to focus on the intake of fats because the plaques that occur in the disease are predominantly lipid in composition. Though the cholesterol and fat theories of the etiology of atherosclerosis have served as fruitful hypotheses yielding a massive quantity of data, the conclusions that can be drawn are still modest in scope and the thinking underlying the research still bears critical reexamination. It may be helpful to remember that mainstream thinking about lipids and arterial disease is based on three separate propositions:

Proposition I. Dietary intake of lipids is *related to* blood lipids.

Proposition II. Blood lipids are *related to* atherosclerosis. What we really want to know, from a practical point of view, is how diet is related directly to atherosclerosis. Why confuse the issue by interposing blood lipid levels? More direct studies are done when possible but, with human subjects, assessing coronary heart disease (CHD) (and even atherosclerosis, in general) is difficult. Therefore the measure of blood cholesterol as an intervening variable and its use as an indicator of increased risk remains a valuable research and clinical tool.

Proposition III. Atherosclerosis is *related to* coronary heart disease and cerebrovascular accidents. While this might seem self-evident, there are good reasons for examining it and for qualifying it appropriately. For example, Massai tribesmen develop increasing atherosclerosis as they age, but the incidence of myocardial infarction is extremely low [1]. Unfortunately, a thorough exploration of this proposition is beyond the scope of this chapter.

R.M. Califf and G.S. Wagner (eds.), ACUTE CORONARY CARE: Principles and Practice. Copyright © 1985. Martinus Nijhoff Publishing, Boston/Dordrecht/Lancaster.

RELATIONSHIP OF DIETARY
TO BLOOD LIPIDS

In proposition I, "dietary intake of lipids" could refer to a number of different variables. The most obvious and widely studied is cholesterol. Does one's dietary intake of cholesterol affect its level in the blood? One is tempted to answer "of course," but actually the question is still being debated.

It has been correctly pointed out that endogenous cholesterol accounts for a large percentage of the cholesterol present in the body at any given time and that, if dietary cholesterol is reduced, synthesis is increased to some extent. However, research in animals shows a firm and conclusive correlation between the dietary intake of cholesterol and blood levels. Moreover, in humans, epidemiologic cross-cultural data support a similar clear correlation between dietary intake of cholesterol and blood levels. On the other hand, studies of homogeneous populations, where diets are similar (such as the Framingham and Tecumseh studies), have failed to show any difference in CHD between those persons consuming the most cholesterol and the least [2, 3]. In reporting the results of the Tecumseh study, the authors acknowledged: "The apparent independence of dietary habits and serum lipid levels suggested by this study does not mean that diet and lipid levels are unrelated." They note: "Diet—lipid relationships that are evident in comparisons of different populations apparently do not aply to ndividuals within a given population" [3].

Studying the etiology of atherosclerosis is difficult when research is carried out on populations where the disease is so prevalent. Trying to uncover causal factors is nearly impossible without clearly unaffected groups with which to compare those affected. There are two avenues of potentially valuable evidence. First are epidemiologic studies that examine other cultures with radically different dietary patterns. Second are studies of groups of Americans who have significantly and consistently altered their dietary patterns to follow some well-defined practice, such as vegetarianism. As an example of the latter, a large number of studies spanning the last two decades in eight different countries have found significantly lower serum cholesterol in groups of vegetarians than in controls in the same country [4—15]. Differences are appreciable as indicated by one of the more recent studies that showed a mean cholesterol in vegetarians of 126 mg%, compared to 184 in controls. Triglycerides were 59 for vegetarians and 86 for the controls [13]. LDL in vegetarians was 73 and in controls 118; HDL was also lower in vegetarians, but less so—42 as opposed to 49 in controls. Hypertension, which is a risk factor for CHD, is also much less frequent in vegetarians [16].

There is even some direct evidence that a vegetarian diet dramatically decreases CHD mortality. In one study, deaths from myocardial infarction among vegetarians were one-third that seen in a group of matched controls [17]. Since there are many different kinds of vegetarian diets it is difficult to generalize, or to deduce what characteristics of such diets might be responsible for the lower incidence of atherosclerotic disease. Vegetarians have a different kind of dietary fat (vegetable in origin and/or butterfat) and generally take in lower overall levels of fat [14, 15]. Those consuming as much fat as nonvegetarians do not show the favorable triglyceride, total cholesterol, and HDL levels of those who consume less fat [18].

Epidemiologic studies comparing various countries with radically different patterns of fat intake and atherosclerosis have also been important. The celebrated study of Japanese living in Japan, Hawaii, and finally California showed an increasing degree of heart disease as dietary patterns shifted progressively toward that typical of contemporary America [19]. While Americans consume an average of 40%—45% of their dietary calories in the form of fats and oils, the percentage for Chinese and Japanese is as low as 10% [20]. The incidence of atherosclerosis is quite low among these, as well as other, groups where dietary fats and oils comprise a small percentage of the caloric intake [20]. Dramatic exceptions to this rule have been noted. In North India where fat intake is 19 times that in South India, the incidence of ischemic heart disease was found to be only one-seventh of that in the South [21]. It is quite possible that other factors, even nutritional ones, are operating in such instances; e.g., a high percentage of the fat consumed by

North Indians was butterfat [22].

"Dietary intake of lipids" also includes (besides cholesterol) animal fats, fish oil, and hydrogenated vegetable fats, in various combinations. The effect of saturated fats versus the unsaturated vegetable oils on blood cholesterol has been widely studied. Generally, saturated fats have been found to raise blood cholesterol while unsaturated oils lower it [23]. The effects of one kind of fat or oil cannot be extrapolated to another: one vegetable oil may influence serum lipids differently from another [24]. Neither are all saturated fats the same. The chain lengths of the fatty acids of butterfat are quite different from those of beef suet and there is considerable evidence that their effects can be different, though in many studies they are lumped together. There is some evidence that indirectly supports the proposition that butterfat aids in calcium absorption [22], and also that "calcium may retard increases in cholesterol and other lipids in the blood and exert a protective action against the development of atherosclerosis" [25]. Only recently has there been a widespread recognition that each fat or oil in the diet can behave in a unique way. Many early works were based on assumptions that polyunsaturates were all alike, and that saturated fats had identical effects. These are probably reasons why the literature is so filled with paradoxes and contradictions.

Moreover, in proposition I, "serum lipid" can refer to total cholesterol, triglycerides, LDL, VLDL, HDL, etc. Even after the investigation has been narrowed to one dietary fat or oil, its effects in a number of serum lipids need to be explored. Actually proposition I should be even further refined. There are, in fact, two hypotheses involved. The first is that there is a *statistical correlation* between dietary intake and blood levels. The second is that there is a *causal relationship* between dietary intake and blood levels. The same is true for proposition II (table 15-1). These are really two quite distinct ideas. While the matter of correlation can be established with some degree of certainty through the careful analysis of data, the question of causality is more difficult. Unfortunately, we often tend, perhaps without realizing it, to move from statistical correlation to an assumption of causality.

RELATIONSHIP OF BLOOD LIPIDS TO ATHEROSCLEROSIS

Most studies agree that there is a strong correlation between serum cholesterol levels and both generalized atherosclerosis and coronary heart disease [20]. The correlation is significantly, though not dramatically, improved by dividing total cholesterol into groups based on its protein carrier. If low-density lipoprotein (LDL) cholesterol is measured separately and is compared with high-density lipoprotein (HDL) cholesterol levels, there is some improvement in statistical correlations. Some recent studies have begun to look at HDL fractions. Not only do patients with coronary artery disease also show elevated levels of cholesterol, they also have higher levels of triglycerdies (though the correlation is better with cholesterol). This is especially true in men and in cases of severe coronary artery disease [26].

While there is substantial consensus that blood lipid levels are positively correlated with atherosclerotic coronary artery disease and myocardial infarction, most of the data support a statistical correlation, but not necessarily a causal relationship. The simplest way to study *causality* is to lower blood lipids and see whether the incidence of CHD changes. Animal studies that have involved dietary changes that lower blood cholesterol levels have clearly reduced and, in some studies, even reversed atherosclerotic changes [27]. The several impressive studies done in patient populations have also shown a lowering of blood cholesterol through dietary change [28], and some reduction in CHD [29–31], but some authorities do not consider these data to be totally conclusive [32]. Therefore, for the most part, the evidence available suggests that a diet which lowers blood cholesterol will prevent coronary heart disease.

Despite the reduction in mortality from coronary heart disease in such studies, total mortality was often unchanged, and in one study there was an increase in deaths from malignancy [33]. In an attempt to examine the possibility that the cholesterol-lowering diets used in the studies might predispose to malignancy, the pooled data from the four major studies were analyzed [34]. It was concluded that the total data available do not indicate that the cholesterol-lowering diets

TABLE 15-1.

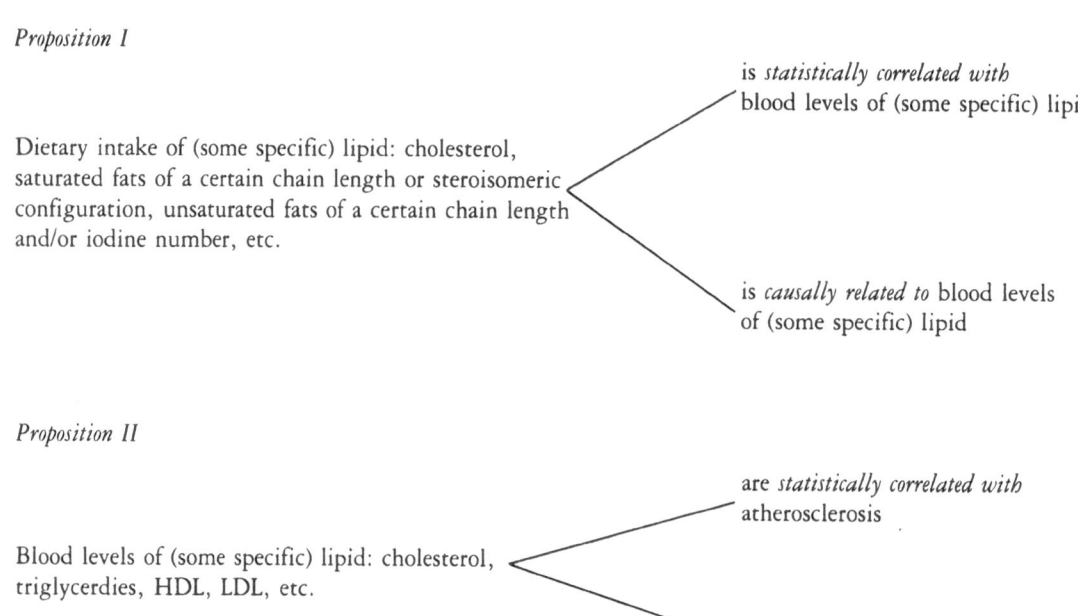

Proposition I

Dietary intake of (some specific) lipid: cholesterol, saturated fats of a certain chain length or steroisomeric configuration, unsaturated fats of a certain chain length and/or iodine number, etc.

is *statistically correlated with* blood levels of (some specific) lipid

is *causally related to* blood levels of (some specific) lipid

Proposition II

Blood levels of (some specific) lipid: cholesterol, triglycerdies, HDL, LDL, etc.

are *statistically correlated with* atherosclerosis

are *causally related to* atherosclerosis

will produce cancer. Nevertheless, the majority of these diets do entail an increase in polyunsaturated oils and there are data to support the hypothesis that the free radicals that inevitably result from peroxidation of such polyunsaturates are harmful [35–38].

SUMMARY

The above is only a brief overview of the data available. Sorting through these studies on dietary fats, oils, and cholesterol and their relationship to atherosclerosis, one might cautiously formulate a few practical guidelines: (a) Dietary cholesterol should probably be limited. (b) Dietary fats and oils are probably even more important, and lowering the total percentage of calories in the diet taken as fat from 40%–45% to 30% or less is probably helpful. As long as the reduction in cholesterol, fats, and oils is not at the expense of nutritious foods that are not properly replaced, such as eggs, milk products, and poultry, but is accomplished by eliminating added fat such as that found in spreads, dressings, sauces, fried foods, and high-fat snack and junk foods, then there is no danger of taking in too little fat. How the American diet can be modified to ac-

complish this has been detailed elsewhere [39]. (c) Raising polyunsaturate intake to increase the P/S ratio may not be wise [35–38]; reducing total fat intake is certainly safer.

Cholesterol and the Enterocolic Circulation

It is generally accepted that an increased "pool" of cholesterol in the body predisposes to plaque formation. Therefore a discussion of cholesterol would not be complete without mention of how it is removed from the body. The liver and biliary tree is the primary route for clearance of cholesterol. It is removed by the liver from the blood as it is converted to bile acids. Bile acids are released from the gallbladder into the small intestine and they either pass out with the stool or are reabsorbed. Those bile acids that exit with the stool effectively reduce the total pool of cholesterol in the body. Those which are reabsorbed (as much as 90%) return via the portal vein to the liver where they are recycled. Obviously those factors which promote the exit of bile salts with the stool could play an important role in decreasing cholesterol. Of central importance here is dietary fiber.

It is well established that bile acids are picked

up by dietary fiber and carried out with the feces [40, 41]. It is thought that this is due primarily to binding of the bile acids to the fiber (adsorption) [42]. The removal of bile acids by fiber has two desirable effects on lipid metabolism. First, and most obviously, bile acid excretion is enhanced. This reduces the amount of bile acids returning to the liver via the enterohepatic circulation and thus increases the conversion of cholesterol to bile acids there. The result is a net reduction of total cholesterol.

Second, the bile salts removed in this way are unavailable for the emulsification of fats. This reduces the absorption of cholesterol as well as the absorption of dietary fats and oils. The fecal content of fats and oils on a pectin-supplemented diet showed an increase in fecal fat excretion of 44% (fecal bile acids were increased by 33%) [43]. In another study, a diet high in fruits and vegetables, which are high in pectinaceous fiber, increased fecal fat by 30% [44]. Wheat bran, which has become increasingly accepted as a treatment for diverticular disease, dramatically increases stool bulk, but does *not* absorb bile acids to a significant extent [41]. Neither does wheat bran decrease blood cholesterol [45, 46] as do the pectinaceous types of fiber found in fruits and vegetables and the fiber of other whole grains and legumes [45, 47–50]. Not only does bran have a different effect from pectin, it has been shown that two different fibers extracted from the soybean have distinctly different effects in lipid metabolism [51]. It would appear that in the case of fiber, as in other areas in nutrition, we are only beginning to appreciate the uniqueness of each food or food constituent.

It is clear that blood cholesterol levels do drop significantly on a diet rich in the kind of fiber found in a diet of various fruits and vegetables, grains, and legumes. It is also obvious that total dietary fiber drops as one takes more fiber-free foods such as fats and oils or refined carbohydrates. More sophisticated food technology has made the extraction of such foods as sugars and oils from their fiber-rich vegetable sources more feasible economically and now these two items account for between 60% and 70% of the average American's caloric intake. The other 30%–40% of calories are supplied by a variety of foods—but

a number of these, such as bread made from refined flour, are also very low in fiber. It is estimated that the dietary fiber intake of the average person in the industrialized West is only one fifth what it was 100 years ago [52].

It is generally accepted that high-residue feeding also alters the microbial flora of the colon [53]. Since bacteria in the gut play some role in the metabolism of bile acids and cholesterol [54], it has been suggested that microbial alteration may be one way that fiber increases bile acid excretion and lowers serum cholesterol. Of even more direct relevance, it has been shown that high-fiber diets reduce plaque formation in the coronary arteries [55] and decrease coronary heart disease mortality [56–60].

Excretion of cholesterol through the biliary system also seems to be affected by dietary vitamin C. Experimental animals deficient enough in vitamin C to show decreased vitamin-C concentrations in the liver had a reduced rate of conversion of cholesterol to bile acids even though they did not have obvious scurvy. Aside from the reduced vitamin-C intake, they were eating normally and had a normal appearance. Cholesterol accumulated in the serum and in the liver of such experimental animals (guinea pigs). This brings up the possibility that mild, subclinical vitamin-C deficiency might play a role in inadequate cholesterol clearance. The conversion of cholesterol to bile acids involves several hydroxylation reactions on the cholesterol nucleus and on the side chain. Because of the known function of ascorbic acid in such hydroxylation reactions, it has been suggested that this accounts for the significant correlation between vitamin-C levels in the liver and the rate of cholesterol transformation to bile acids [61].

Another variable that may be important in the enterocolic excretion of cholesterol is the competition of plant sterols present in leguminous seeds with metabolized cholesterol for reabsorption [62]. A number of studies have shown that regular consumption of legumes (beans and peas) produced a significant lowering of serum cholesterol levels [62–64]. No such effect was seen when other vegetable foods, even those relatively high in bulk such as bread and potatoes, were substituted [65]. Legume feeding increased the fecal bile acid levels at the same time that it lowered cholesterol in the serum [62]. Another study showed that complex carbohydrate (starch), as compared with sucrose, increased fecal excretion of bile acids and lowered blood cholesterol [66, 67]. An even more direct correlation between higher starch intake and decreased coronary artery plaque formation has also been reported [53].

An appreciation of the role played by the enterocolic circulation in the clearance of cholesterol may be important in understanding how a widely diverse group of dietary variables such as vegetarianism [4−39], legumes [62−65], fiber-rich fruits and vegetables [40−43, 45, 47−50, 55−60], and a high intake of vitamin C [61] have been helpful in lowering serum cholesterol levels and, in some cases, even reducing the incidence of atherosclerotic coronary heart disease.

Protein Sources and Atherogenesis

Other studies suggest that the type of dietary protein consumed may play a role in atherogenesis and have explored the difference between vegetable and animal proteins as they correlated with serum cholesterol and triglycerides. Such studies have been conducted on a range of experimental animals as well as man and generally are in agreement, demonstrating that animal protein is more cholesteremic and atherogenic than is that from vegetable sources [53, 68, 69]. In experimental animals an extract of soy protein has repeatedly been shown to decrease both serum cholesterol and atherosclerotic lesions when compared with animal sources of protein such as casein or powdered-beef protein. This difference is accentuated if sugar (dextrose) [69] is included in the diet, but extinguished if a source of leafy plant fiber is included (alfalfa) [69, 70]. In humans with type-II hyperlipoproteinemia, already on a diet low in fats and oils, plasma cholesterol was lowered by 14%−21% by substituting vegetable for the usual variety of animal protein. This difference persisted unchanged even when 500 mg of cholesterol per day was added to the diet. Nor was this effect completely eliminated when saturated fats in the diet were increased [71]. Such improvement was not seen in a more recent study where the shift was from casein (which might be less cholesteremic than meat) to soy protein and where both diets were 30% lard (which may have interfered with the soy protein's effect) [72]. A review of the work in this area [69] concludes that dietary protein per se can significantly influence both blood cholesterol and atherosclerosis, but that the relation between protein and other components of the diet is important.

This is demonstrated in another study with a very interesting methodology that found strong correlations between kinds of protein and atherosclerosis. Most studies have correlated dietary patterns with serum levels of cholesterol, but this work looked directly at the relation between diet and coronary artery lesions. It was done on 253 patients who were examined at autopsy for the degree of atherosclerotic plaque formation in the coronary arteries. Subjects studied were limited to those who had shared a household for at least the last year of life with a woman who was available to give a detailed dietary history. Dietary patterns were then compared with degree of plaque in the coronaries. Correlations between fat or sugar intake and degree of atherosclerosis did not attain statistical significance, but there was a highly significant correlation between starch and protein intake and freedom from plaques. Those patients who had a typically high intake of vegetable protein and starch showed less atherosclerosis of the coronary arteries. There was a weaker correlation between dietary fiber and relative freedom from coronary atherosclerosis [53]. Subsequent study of these data revealed that the most likely explanation was that the patients who had relative freedom from coronary atherosclerosis were those who habitually consumed a combination of beans and rice [73], a common feature in traditional diets around the world, and one which provides a complementarity of amino acids so that the resulting vegetable protein is equivalent in value to that from animals. This grain−legume combination is a nearly universal and perhaps critical feature of vegetarian diets, which are found to be consistently correlated with low serum cholesterol and relative freedom from coronary atherosclerosis. There are a number of possible reasons that this dietary feature correlates so well with healthy coronary arteries: (a) It supplies a high-quality protein so that the nutritional need for high fat and cholesterol sources of protein such as meat or cheese is reduced. (b) It, itself, brings relatively little fat or cholesterol. (c) It supplies plant sterols that may compete with cholesterol for absorption. (d) It supplies ample fiber. (e) It supplies complex carbohydrate. (f) It is relatively rich in trace minerals.

The Significance of Trace Minerals in the Diet

As the critical role played by metalloenzymes in human metabolism has become more apparent, the significance of trace mineral nutriture has begun to be appreciated. Though only minute quantities of the trace minerals are needed to manufacture enzymes, without sufficient amounts these enzymes will not be readily available and the metabolic machinery will slow. Such impairments are increasingly suspected of playing a role in overall psychophysiologic dysfunction as well as in the origin of various degenerative diseases [74].

While deficiencies or imbalances in the ratios of a number of trace minerals have been implicated in the etiology of atherosclerosis [75−77], perhaps the most intriguing evidence to emerge is that in relation to chromium. Experimental animals put on a chromium-free diet develop severe diabetes and marked atherosclerosis. When chromium was returned to the diet the blood sugar normalized and the atherosclerotic plaques dissolved [78]. The symptoms of chromium deficiency can be exaggerated by subjecting experimental animals to some form of stress [79]. Chromium in aortic tissues was significantly lower in patients dying of coronary heart disease as compared with controls [78]. This was apparently not a simple dilution resulting from plaque, since the difference did not hold true for other minerals. Epidemiologic studies show that Americans have chromium tissue levels significantly lower than those of other populations [80]. Moreover, levels in Americans decline sharply with age [78, 81, 82]. It has been proposed that these declining levels with age might be a result of urinary losses that are due to a high intake of refined carbohydrate, since glucose loading increases chromium excretion [83].

Chromium is present in the body in the form of a complex molecule termed glucose tolerance factor (GTF). GTF is critical to the functioning of insulin and, when chromium is deficient, unphysiologically large concentrations of insulin are necessary to achieve a normal response [84]. An improvement in glucose tolerance in certain diabetics when chromium supplements were added to the diet has been demonstrated (though in 40%−60% of the cases it was of no benefit) [84]. Trials in which the supplementation was given for six weeks or less failed to show a response [85]. This suggests that in some diabetics chromium deficiency may contribute to the disorder. Involvement of chromium metabolism in insulin-mediated reactions is interesting in view of the association between diabetes and early, severe atherosclerosis. In addition to the fact that diabetics suffer inordinately from atherosclerosis, the reverse is also true: a substantial percentage of patients with atherosclerotic diseases show impaired glucose tolerance [86−88].

A similar striking relationship is found between exaggerated insulin response ("hyperinsulinemia") and both blood lipids and atherosclerosis. Patients with atherosclerosis show a hyperinsulinemic response to refined sugar. Moreover, hyperinsulinemic patients, not yet identified as atherosclerotic, show elevated levels of total cholesterol and LDL [89, 90]. Earlier studies that found a simple correlation between sugar consumption and atherosclerotic heart disease [91−94] were not confirmed by later work [95, 96]. Nevertheless, several impressive facts remain: (a) Hyperinsulinemic patients are more prone to atherosclerosis. (b) Insulin increases when chromium (GTF) is relatively deficient. (c) Atherosclerotic tissues are low in chromium. These findings suggest that poor insulin regulation, chromium deficiency, and a high sugar intake may all be related in a way yet to be fully elucidated and that they may together comprise one of the significant factors in the development of atherosclerosis. It is interesting to note that the fiber found in whole foods (fruits, vegetables, whole grains, and legumes) that is effective in decreasing blood lipids and preventing atherosclerosis also has a modulating effect on blood glucose and insulin levels [97].

Other trace elements are being studied regarding their relationship to atherogenesis. The consistently negative correlations between hard water and cardiovascular disease have led to an increasing number of studies of the trace mineral content of such water. There is a growing consensus that calcium and magnesium are less important to the beneficial effects of hard water than are certain other trace elements. Those particularly thought to be of value are vanadium and lithium [98, 99].

A variety of studies have suggested that manganese deficiency might play a role in atherogenesis as well as zinc, cobalt, and perhaps copper (though excessively *high* levels of the latter are also though to predispose to myocardial infarction) [77]. Recent studies have also revealed a negative correlation between dietary selenium and coronary heart disease [100].

The diagnosis of trace mineral deficiencies may not be simple, however, since such elements as chromium cannot be well assessed through looking at the quite variable plasma levels [84]. Hair mineral analysis provides a promising possibility: chromium hair levels seem to be reliably correlated with general tissue levels [84]. Multiple trace element deficiencies are common in the American population [74] and these may be of some etiologic importance in patients with atherosclerosis. Lower dietary intakes seem to result from both the refinement of food and soil deficiencies [74]. Whole grain cereals, for example, are relatively rich in zinc, chromium, and selenium while refined grains are considerably lower. Lower-than-acceptable levels of soil manganese and zinc, for example, have been reported in a majority of states [101] and soil levels of selenium are low (as are dietary levels) in certain areas. Diets high in whole grains, leafy vegetables, and fruits seem to be especially high in trace minerals. This effect is magnified when the plants are grown on healthier soils [74]. Herbs and spices seem to owe their intensity of flavor to an ability to concentrate trace minerals that they contain in extraordinary quantities [74]. It is tempting to speculate that this may be responsible in part for their wide appeal.

Diets that, through various devices, manage to supply ample quantities of trace minerals would be expected to be correlated with a lower incidence of atherosclerosis and CHD. The corn meal milled from grain grown by the Hopi, for exam-

ple, supplied 2–3 times as much manganese as conventional corn meal furnished by the government, and the Hopi hominy grits four times as much manganese and 12 times as much zinc as the "enriched" grits available in the supermarket. The Hopi grains were high in trace elements and their traditional preparation of tortillas involves the use of mineral-rich ash from certain plants [102]. Coronary heart disease has been thought to be rare among these people [103].

General Nutrition in Atherogenesis

It is also important to consider the relationship between the general nutritional status and the development of atherosclerosis. Surveys show a gradual decrease in the intake of essential nutrients in the diet of the typical American. For example, the US Department of Agriculture Nationwide Food Consumption Survey in 1955 showed approximately 60% of all Americans receiving the RDA of the basic nutrients studied. A repeat of the study ten years later showed only 50% of Americans receiving the RDA in their diets: half the population was receiving a diet deficient in one or more nutrients [104]. The study was repeated in the late 1970s and the results (not completely tabulated) suggest a further deterioration in national dietary habits [105].

The American diet now contains 20%–25% of its calories as refined sugars and 40%–45% of the caloric intake as fats and oils. A diet high in such fuel-rich foods that contain almost no micronutrients (vitamins and trace minerals) can only gradually deplete the vitamin- and mineral-dependent metalloenzymes that are ultimately responsible for the integrity of the metabolic machinery.

The general nutritional status of a person depends on other factors, too (such as emotions), that can interact with nutrition. Emotional states can affect nutritional needs and nutritional deficiencies can affect one's emotional state [39]. Such an interaction might be: Mild, diet-induced nutritional deficiencies reduce one's capacity to respond comfortably to the demands of the environment. Uncertainty, apprehension, and anxiety result. This condition, with its autonomic and physiologic concomitants, places additional burdens on the body's metabolic machinery, thereby increasing the requirement for certain essential nutrients. The result is a shift toward a pattern of increased nutritional requirements with a greater tendency toward deficiency. This in turn further reduces the capacity of the organism to respond comfortably and so the situation worsens. Repeated turns of the screw eventually could lead to the development of a recognizable pathologic picture.

It is possible that a clearly causal role for specific nutritional factors in atherogenesis may not be proven by future research. Even so, one could conclude that a diet that leads to a general tendency toward cell death and tissue degeneration is suboptimal. Other, as yet unidentified, physiologic and/or psychological factors may operate during atherogenesis to localized the site of the degeneration to the arterial walls. Several dietary factors might serve to facilitate such a degenerative process in the arteries: a low-fiber diet interferes with the normal clearance of cholesterol from the body via the enterocolic excretion of bile acids while a diet high in fats and oils could further burden lipid metabolism. It may be necessary for psychological and emotional factors also to play a role in order to focus the process on the coronary arteries.

We have explored only the more compelling of the themes relating nutrition to atherogenesis. Evidence could be found to implicate any one of a large number of nutrients in the etiology of this disease, given a population sufficiently depleted of that nutrient possessing the predisposing genetic, emotional, and/or characterologic factors.

Certain general themes in the research literature are apparent: A broad range of studies have supported the beneficial effects of certain foods in preventing atherosclerosis: whole grains, especially in combination with legumes, fruits, and green and leafy vegetables. A marked increase in the proportion of such foods, to displace a significant portion of the caloric intake of fats, oils, and refined carbohydrates, would seem indicated. There is no indication that such measures can be harmful, and such dietary modifications might also play a preventive role for other diseases such as cancer and diabetes [106 – 110]. Many ethnic dishes from various parts of the world are com-

posed of just such basic components, demonstrating that these foods can be used as staples and need not be boring or unappealing.

This chapter has presented a clinical approach that involves the gradual transition from a typical American diet to one that incorporates increasing proportions of whole grains, legumes, vegetables, and fruits [39]. The major obstacle to such dietary modification seems to be the unfamiliarity of large segments of the population—both professional and lay—with the types of foods involved, how to prepare them, and the data supporting their beneficial use.

Nutrition in the Management of Acute Myocardial Infarction

In the care of the patient with acute myocardial infarction, the clinician is most concerned about minimizing demands in a compromised physiology to prevent recurrence and speed recovery. Several goals are important here:

1) Support the adrenals and other stress-response resources: B vitamins, especially pantothenic acid, can be helpful. Vitamin C is also important; 31 patients studied shortly after myocardial infarction were all found to have a fall in leucocyte ascorbic acid to scorbutic levels within 12 h [111]. To mollify the stress on the patient, vitamin-C therapy should be helpful. It seems possible that other nutrients may be needed in the same way to obviate the creation of internal stress.

2) Supply nutrients that will not increase (and, if possible, that will decrease) sludging and thrombogenesis: Formation of lipid peroxides increases during the platelet-release reaction. Tocopherol (vitamin E), an antioxidant known to inhibit such peroxidation reactions, has been found in vitro to exert a dose-dependent reduction in platelet aggregation. In vivo studies show increasing plasma and platelet levels up to doses of 1800 IU [112]. Further studies are needed to explore the therapeutic use of tocopherols as alternatives to more toxic anticoagulants.

3) Prevent coronary artery spasm: It has been shown in isolated coronary arteries from dogs that withdrawal of magnesium from a Krebs-Ringer incubation solution results in marked

vascular spasm. It is thought that magnesium functions to make calcium more available [113]. The use of magnesium salts in acute care is another area that deserves study.

4) Provide nutritional support for the tissue repair and restitution: All of the nutrition principles that apply to the primary prevention of atherosclerosis are important as acute care merges into convalescence. The most immediate concern is supplying adequate quantities of vitamins and minerals, especially trace minerals. A diet high in those foods mentioned earlier (whole grains, legumes, fresh fruits, and vegetables) should be implemented as soon as feasible to diminish the chances of further advancement of the atherosclerotic process. There are even data now emerging that suggest that the previously described careful dietary management might result in some degree of reversal of the atherosclerotic plaques [114]. Such reversal has been demonstrated in femoral arteries, though not, so far, in coronaries [115].

In contrast to the wealth of data available on nutrition and atherogenesis, relatively little work has been done on nutrition in the patient with an acute myocardial infarction. It is reasonable to think that the precise and timely furnishing of critical nutrients to the patient with myocardial damage could be of utmost importance to infarct healing and optimal scar formation.

References

1. Mann GV, Spoerry A, Gray M, Jarashow D: Atherosclerosis in the Masai. Am J Epidemiol 95:26–37, 1972.
2. Kannel WB, Gordon T: The Framingham diet study: diet and the regulations of serum cholesterol (sect 24). Washington DC: Dept HEW, 1970.
3. Nichols B, Ravenscroft C, Lamphiear DE, Ostrander LD: Independence of serum lipid levels and dietary habits. JAMA 236:1948–1953, 1976.
4. Hardinge MG, Crooks H, Stare F: Nutritional studies of vegetarians. IV. Dietary fatty acids and serum cholesterol levels. Am J Clin Nutr 10:516–524, 1962.
5. West RO, Hayes OB: Diet and serum choles-

terol levels: A comparison between vegetarians and non vegetarians in a Seventh Day Adventist group. Am J Clin Nutr 21:853–862, 1968.
6. Ruys J, Hickie JB: Serum cholesterol and triglyceride levels in Australian adolescent vegetarians. Br Med J 2:87, 1976.
7. Chen J: The effect of long-term vegetable diet on serum lipid and lipoprotein levels in man. Formosan Med Assoc J 65:65–77, 1966.
8. Hill P, Wynder E, Garbaczewski L, et al: Plasma hormones and lipids in men at different risk for coronary heart disease. Am J Clin Nutr 33:1010–1018, 1980.
9. Kirkeby K: Plasma lipids in a moderately low-fat, high-carbohydrate diet, rich in polyunsaturated fatty acids. Acta Med Scand 180:767–776, 1966.
10. Kritchevsky D: Fiber, lipids, and atherosclerosis. Am J Clin Nutr (Suppl 10) 31:565–574, 1978.
11. Taylor CB, Allen ES, Mikkelson B, Ho K: Serum cholesterol levels of Seventh-day Adventists. Paroi Arterielle 3:175–179, 1976.
12. Simons LA, Gibson JC, Paino C, Hosking M: The influence of a wide range of absorbed cholesterol in plasma cholesterol levels in man. Am J Clin Nutr 31:1334–1339, 1978.
13. Sachs F, Castelli WP, Donner A, Kass EH: Plasma lipids and lipoproteins in vegetarians and controls. N Engl J Med 292:1148–1151, 1975.
14. Barrow, JG, Quinlan CB, Cooper GR, et al: Studies in atherosclerosis. III. An epidemiologic study of atherosclerosis in Trappist and Benedictine monks: a preliminary report. Ann Intern Med 52:368–377, 1960.
15. Simons LA, Gibson JC, Paino C, et al: The influence of a wide range of absorbed cholesterol in plasma cholesterol levels in man. Am J Clin Nutr 31:1335, 1978.
16. Ophir O, Peer G, Gilad J, Blum M, Aviram A: Low blood pressure in vegetarians: the possible role of potassium. Am J Clin Nutr 37:755–762, 1983.
17. Phillips RL: Coronary heart disease mortality among Seventh Day Adventists with different dietary habits: a preliminary report. Am J Clin Nutr 31:191–198, 1978.
18. Liebman M, Bazzarre TL: Plasma lipids of vegetarian and non vegetarian males: effects of egg consumption. Am J Clin Nutr 38:612–619, 1983.
19. Keys AN, Kimura N, Kusukawa A, et al: Lessons from serum cholesterol studies in Japan,

Hawaii, and Los Angeles. Ann Intern Med 48: 83, 1958.

20. Stamler J: Lifestyles, major risk factors, proof and public policy. Circulation 58:1, 1976.

21. Malhotra SL: Epidemiology of ischemic heart disease in India, with special reference to causation. Br Heart J 29:895−905, 1967.

22. Williams R: Nutrition against disease. New York: Bantam, 1971.

23. Glueck CT: Dietary fat and atherosclerosis. Am J Clin Nutr 32:2703−2711, 1979.

24. Kritchevsky D, Tepper SA: Cholesterol vehicle in experimental atherosclerosis. J Atheroscler Res 7:647−651, 1967.

25. Speckman EW, Brink MF: Relationships between fat and mineral metabolism: a review. J Am Dietet Assoc 51:517, 1967.

26. Cohn PK: Serum lipid levels in angiographically defined coronary artery disease. Ann Intern Med 84:241−245, 1976.

27. Glueck GJ, Connor WE: Diet−coronary heart disease relationships reconnoitered. Am J Clin Nutr 31:727, 1978.

28. Becker N, Illingworth DR, Alaupovic P, et al: Effects of saturated, monounsaturated, and W-6 polyunsaturated fatty acids on plasma lipids, lipoproteins, and apoproteins in humans[1−3]. Am J Clin Nutr 37:355−360, 1983.

29. Dayton S, Pearce ML, Hashimoto S, Dixon WJ, Tomiyasu U: A controlled clinical trial of a diet high in unsaturated fat in preventing complications of atherosclerosis. Circulation (Suppl 2) 40:1969.

30. Miettinen M: Prevention of coronary heart disease by cholesterol lowering diet. Postgrad Med J (Suppl) 51:47−51, 1975.

31. Leren P: The effect of plasma cholesterol lowering diet in male survivors of myocardial infarction: a controlled trial. Acta Med Scand (Suppl) 466:1−92, 1966.

32. Glueck CJ: Dietary fat and atherosclerosis. Am J Clin Nutr 32:2703−2711, 1979.

33. Pearce ML, Dayton S: Incidence of cancer in men on a diet high in polyunsaturated fat. Lancet 1:464−467, 1971.

34. Ederer F: Cancer among men on cholesterol-lowering diets, experience from five clinical trials. Lancet 2:203−206, 1971.

35. Pinckney ER: The potential toxicity of excessive polyunsaturates. Am Heart J 85:723−726, 1973.

36. Bland J: Biochemical consequences of lipid peroxidation. J Chem Ed 55:151−155, 1978.

37. Mead JF: Dietary polyunsaturated fatty acids as potential toxic factors. Chemtech 2:70−71, 1972.

38. West EC, Redgrave TG: Reservations in the use of polyunsaturated fats in human nutrition. Am Lab: 23−30, 1975.

39. Ballentine RM: Diet and nutrition, a holistic approach. Honesdale PA: Himalayan, 1978.

40. Story JA: Dietary fiber and lipid metabolism: an update. In: Spiller GA, Kay RP (eds) Medical aspects of dietary fiber. New York: Plenum, 1980, pp. 137−152.

41. Varouny GV: Dietary fiber, lipid metabolism and atherosclerosis. Fed Proc 41:2801−2806, 1982.

42. Kay RP: Dietary fiber [review]. J Lipid Res 23:228 (tables 2 and 3), 1982.

43. Kay RP, Truswell AS: Effect of citrus pectin on blood lipids and fecal steroid excretion in man. Am J Clin Nutr 30:171−175, 1977.

44. Kelsay JL, Behall KM, Prather ES: Effect of fiber from fruits and vegetables on metabolic responses of human subjects. I. Bowel transit time, number of defecations, fecal weight, urinary excretions of energy and nitrogen and apparent digestibilities of energy, nitrogen and fat. Am J Clin Nutr 31:1149−1153, 1978.

45. Kay R Mcp, Truswell AS: Dietary fiber: effects on plasma and biliary lipids in man. In: Spiller GA, Kay Mcp (eds) Medical aspects of dietary fiber. New York: Plenum, 1980, pp. 153−173 (esp table 2, p. 158).

46. Liebman M, Smith MC, Iverson J, et al: Effects of coarse wheat bran fiber and exercise on plasma lipids and lipoproteins in moderately overweight men[1,2]. Am J Clin Nutr 37:71−81, 1983.

47. Chen WL, Anderson JW: Effect of plant fiber in descending plasma total cholesterol and increasing high-density lipoprotein cholesterol. Proc Soc Exp Biol Med 162:310−313, 1979.

48. Jenkins DJ, Leeds AR, Newton C, Cummings JH: Effect of pectin, guar gum, and wheat fiber on serum cholesterol. Lancet 2:1116−1117, 1975.

49. Wells AF, Ershoff BH: Beneficial effects of pectin in prevention of hypercholesterolemia and increase in liver cholesterol in cholesterol-fed rats. J Nutr: 87−92, 1961.

50. Sarathy R, Saraswathi G: Effect of tender cluster bean pods (Cyamopsis tetragonoloba) on cholesterol levels in rats[1−3]. Am J Clin Nutr 38: 295−299, 1983.

51. Schweizer T, Bekhechi AR, Koellreuter B, et al: Metabolic effects of dietary fiber from

dehulled soybeans in humans[1-2]. Am J Clin Nutr 38:1−11, 1983.

52. Ershoff BH: Antitoxic effects of plant fiber. Am J Clin Nutr 27:1395−1398, 1974.

53. Mendeloff AI: A critique of "fiber deficiency". Dig Dis 21:109−112, 1976.

54. Harrison VC, Peat G: Serum cholesterol and bowel flora in the newborn. Am J Clin Nutr 28:1351−1355, 1975.

55. Moore MC, Guzman MA, Schilling PE, Strong JP: Dietary atherosclerosis study on deceased persons. J Am Diet Assoc 68:216−223, 1976.

56. Trowell H: Dietary fiber and coronary heart disease. Rev Eur Etudes Clin Biol 17:345−349, 1972.

57. Kritchevsky D: Fiber, lipids and atherosclerosis. Am J Clin Nutr 31:S65−74, 1978.

58. Kritchevsky D: Nutrition and heart disease. Food Technol 33:39−42, 1979.

59. Connor WE, Connor SL: The alternative American diet. Adv Exp Med Biol 82:843−849, 1977.

60. Burslem D, Schonfeld G, Howald MA, Weidman SW, Miller JP: Plasma apoprotein & lipoprotein lipid levels in vegetarians. Metabolism 27:711−719, 1978.

61. Ginter E: Cholesterol: vitamin C controls its transformation to bile acids. Science 179:702−704, 1973.

62. Mathur K, Khan MA, Sharma RD: Hypocholesterolaemic effect of Bengal gram: a long term study in man. Br Med J 1:30−31, 1968.

63. Luyken R, Pikaar NA, Polman H, Schippers FA: The influence of legumes on the serum cholesterol level. Voeding 23:447−479, 1962.

64. Jenkins D, Wong GS, Patten R, et al: Leguminous seeds in the dietary management of hyperlipidemia[1-3]. Am J Clin Nutr 38:567−573, 1983.

65. Grande F, Anderson JT, Keys A: Effect of carbohydrates of leguminous seeds, wheat and potatoes on serum cholesterol concentration in man. J Nutr 86:313−317, 1965.

66. Portman OW, Mann GV, Wysocki AP: Bile acid excretion by the rat: nutritional effects. Arch Bioch Biophys 59:224, 1955.

67. Portman OW, Lawry EY, Bruno D: Effect of dietary carbohydrate on experimentally induced hypercholesterolemia and hyperbetalipoproteinemia in rats. Proc Soc Exp Biol Med 91:321, 1956.

68. Hodges RE, Krehl WA, Stone DB, Lopez A: Dietary carbohydrates and low cholesterol diets: effects on serum lipids of man. Am J Clin Nutr 20:198−208, 1967.

69. Kritchevsky D: Vegetable protein and atherosclerosis. J Am Oil Chem Soc 56:135−146, 1979.

70. Malinow MR, McLaughlin P, Naito HK, et al: Effect of alfalfa meal on shrinkage (regression) of atherosclerotic plaques during cholesterol feeding in monkeys. Atherosclerosis 30:27, 1978.

71. Sirtori CR, Agradi E, Conti F, Mantero O, Gatti E: Soybean-protein diet in the treatment of type II hyperlipoproteinemia. Lancet 1:275−277, 1977.

72. Grundy S, Abrams JJ: Comparison of actions of soy protein and casein on metabolism of plasma lipoproteins and cholesterol in humans[1-3]. Am J Clin Nutr 38:245−252, 1983.

73. Moore MC, Guzman MA, Schilling PE, Strong JP: Dietary−atherosclerosis study on deceased persons. J Am Diet Assoc 79:668−672, 1981.

74. Underwood EJ: Trace elements in human and animal nutrition. New York: Academic, 1977.

75. Chesters JK: Trace elements: adventitious yet essential dietary ingredients. Proc. Nutr Soc 35:15−22, 1976.

76. Perry HM: Minerals in cardiovascular disease. J Am Diet Assoc 62:631−637, 1973.

77. Masironi R: Trace elements and cardiovascular diseases. Bull WHO 40:305−312, 1969.

78. Schroeder HA: Chromium deficiency as a factor in atherosclerosis. J Chronic Dis 23:123−142, 1970.

79. Mertz W, Roginski EE: Effects of chromium (III) supplementation on growth and survival under stress in rats fed low-protein diets. J Nutr 97:531, 1969.

80. Tiptin IH, Schroeder HA, Perry HM, Cook MJ: Trace elements in human tissue. III. Subjects from Africa, the Near and Far East and Europe. Health Phys 2:403, 1965.

81. Tiptin IH, Cook MJ: Trace elements in human tissue. II. Adult subjects from the US. Health Phys 9:103, 1963.

82. Schroeder HA, Balassa JJ, Tipton IH: Abnormal trace metals in man. J Chronic Dis 15:941, 1962.

83. Schroeder HA: The role of chromium in mammalian nutrition. Am J Clin Nutr 21:230, 1968.

84. Hambridge KM: Chromium nutrition in man. Am J Clin Nutr 27:505−514, 1974.

85. Uusitupa M, Kumpulainen JT, Voutilainen E, et al: Effect of inorganic chromium supplementation on glucose tolerance, insulin response, and serum lipids in noninsulin-dependent diabetics[1-3]. Am J Clin Nutr 38:404−410, 1983.

86. Sowton E: Cardiac infarction and the glucose tolerance test. Br Med J 1:84−85, 1962.

87. Cohen AM, Shafrir E: Carbohydrate metabolism in myocardial infarction: behavior of blood glucose and free fatty acids after glucose loading. Diabetes 14:84−87, 1965.

88. Epstein FH: Hyperglycemia, risk factor in coronary heart disease. Circulation 36:609−619, 1967.

89. Yudkin J, Szanto S: Hyperinsulinism and atherogenesis. Br Med J 1:349, 1971.

90. Hallfrisch J, Reiser S, Prather ES: Blood lipid distribution of hyperinsulinemic men consuming three levels of fructose[1−5]. Am J Clin Nutr 37:740−748, 1983.

91. Cohen AM: Fats and carbohydrates as factors in atherosclerosis and diabetes in Yemenite Jews. Am Heart J 65:291−293, 1963.

92. Yudkin J: Diet and coronary thrombosis: hypothesis and facts. Lancet 2:152−162, 1957.

93. Yudkin J: Dietary fat and dietary sugar in relation to ischemic heart disease and diabetes. Lancet 2:4−5, 1964.

94. Yudkin J: Evolutionary and historical changes in dietary carbohydrates. Am J Clin Nutr 20:108−115, 1967.

95. Walker ARP: Sugar intake and coronary heart disease. Atherosclerosis 14:137−152, 1971.

96. Grande F: Sugar and cardiovascular disease. World Rev Nutr Diet 22:248−269, 1975:

97. Jenkins DJ: Dietary fiber and carbohydrate metabolism. In: Spiller GA, Kay RM (eds) Medical aspects of dietary fiber. New York: Plenum, 1980, pp 175−192.

98. Sharrett AR, Feinleib M: Water constituents and trace elements in relation to cardiovascular diseases. Prev Med 4:20−36, 1975.

99. Voors AW: Minerals in the municipal water and atherosclerotic heart death. Am J Epidemiol 93:259−266, 1971.

100. Salonen JT, Alfthan G, Huttunen JK, et al: Association between cardiovascular death and myocardial infarction and serum selenium in a match pair longitudinal study. Lancet 2:175−179, 1982.

101. Sauchelli V: Trace elements in agriculture. New York: Van Nostrand Reinhold, 1969.

102. Calloway DH, Giauque RD, Costa FM: The superior mineral content of some American Indian foods in comparison to federally donated counterpart commodities. Ecol Food Nutr 3:203−211, 1974.

103. Cohen LC, PHS physician Arizona, personal communication.

104. Labuza T, Sloan E: Food for thought. Westport CT: AVI, 1977.

105. Food and nutrient intakes of individuals in 1 day in the United States. Spring 1977, Nationwide Food Consumption Survey 1977−78, Preliminary Report no. 2, US Dept Agric, Science and Education Adm, 1980.

106. Anderson JW: Dietary fiber and diabetes. In: Spiller GA, Kay RM (eds) Medical aspects of dietary fiber. New York: Plenum, 1980, pp. 193−282.

107. Burkitt DP: Colon cancer: the emergence of a concept. In: Spiller GA, Kay RM (eds) Medical aspects of dietary fiber. New York: Plenum, 1980, pp. 75−82.

108. Armstrong B, Doll R: Environmental factors and cancer incidence and mortality in different countries, with special reference to dietary practices. Int J Cancer 15:617−631, 1975.

109. Reddy BS, Sharma C, Darby L, Laakso K, Wynder EL: Metabolic epidemiology of large bowel cancer: fecal mutagens in high-risk and low-risk populations for colon cancer. Mutat Res 72:511−522, 1980.

110. Trowell H: Diabetes mellitus and dietary fiber of starchy foods. Am J Clin Nutr (Suppl) 31:53−57, 1978.

111. Hume R, Weyers E, Rowan T, Reid DS, Hillis, WS: Leucocyte ascorbic acid levels after acute myocardial infarction. Br Heart J 34:238−243, 1972.

112. Steiner M, Anastasi J: Vitamin E, an inhibitor of the platelet release reaction. J Clin Invest 57:732−737, 1976.

113. Prasad DM, Altura BM: Magnesium deficiency produces spasms of coronary arteries. Science 208:198−200, 1980.

114. Blankenhorn DH: Reversibility of latent atherosclerosis. Mod Concepts Cardiovasc Dis 47:79−84, 1978.

115. Barndt R, Blankenhorn D, Crawford DW, Brooks SH: Regression and progression of early femoral atherosclerosis treated hyperlipidemic patients. Ann Intern Med 86:139−146, 1977.

16. THE ROLE OF ANTITHROMBOTIC THERAPY IN THE ACUTE ISCHEMIC SYNDROMES

Shaun Coughlin

Lewis T. Williams

The acute ischemic syndromes include unstable angina (with its subsets of new exertional angina, crescendo exertional angina, new rest angina, and crescendo rest angina), subendocardial myocardial infarction, and transmural myocardial infarction. Causes of myocardial ischemia in these syndromes include fixed coronary stenosis with myocardial oxygen demand exceeding supply, coronary vasospasm, and thrombosis of a coronary segment narrowed by atheroma or vasospasm [1–4] (see chapters 4–6). The extent to which each mechanism is operating in a particular patient or syndrome will obviously influence the efficacy of a particular therapeutic modality. The importance of thrombosis in the acute ischemic syndromes has been increasingly appreciated in recent years, with recent occlusive thrombus documented pathologically in 10% of cases of unstable angina, 35% of subendocardial infarcts, and 90% of transmural infarcts [5]. To best assess methods of intervention and the design of clinical trials, the process of arterial thrombosis is discussed below in the context of antithrombotic therapy.

Arterial Thrombosis

Arterial thrombosis is characterized by complex and incompletely understood interactions among hemodynamic forces, platelets, plasma-clotting factors, circulating factors, and the blood vessel wall. Platelets appear to play a central role in the process of arterial thrombosis [6–9]. Thrombosis does not occur in normal coronaries; rather, it typically occurs at sites of atherosclerotic narrowing. In experimentally stenosed vessels, cyclic alterations in flow attributable to platelet plugging have been reported [10, 11]. This phenomenon may occur in some patients with unstable angina. In instances of transmural infarction, endothelial defects are often found at the site of occlusive thrombi overlying atherosclerotic plaques [1, 12–14]. Thus, as discussed in chapter 6, the trigger for platelet aggregation and thrombus formation appears to involve abnormal hemodynamic forces and endothelial dysfunction at the site of stenosis. Platelet aggregation ex vivo is characterized by a two-step process, with a primary wave of aggregation occurring in response to stimuli such as ADP, thrombin, or epinephrine, and a secondary wave associated with platelet release of ADP and production of thromboxane A_2 [6, 15–17]. Platelets lacking ADP due to storage pool disease and platelets unable to synthesize thromboxane A_2 due to inhibition of cyclooxygenase by aspirin both exhibit defects in secondary aggregation [17–20, 21]. Since measures designed to trap extracellular ADP [22] or inhibit thromboxane production [21] prolong bleeding time, both ADP and

R.M. Califf and G.S. Wagner (eds.), ACUTE CORONARY CARE: Principles and Practice. Copyright © 1985. Martinus Nijhoff Publishing, Boston/Dordrecht/Lancaster.

thromboxane A_2 appear to play a role in promoting platelet aggregation in vivo. It is important to note, however, that despite inhibition of either mechanism in vivo, platelet aggregation and hemostatic plug formation still occur [21, 22]. In addition to promoting platelet aggregation, platelet-released thromboxane A_2 may cause local vasospasm, thereby further promoting stasis and thrombus formation [1, 23].

The membranes of activated platelets provide binding sites for the formation of active clotting factor complexes [24], thereby promoting local thrombin generation. Thrombin so produced may stimulate further platelet aggregation, independent of ADP release or thromboxane A_2 production [25, 26]. Thrombin also cleaves fibrinogen to fibrin, which polymerizes to form fibrin strands. Fibrin strands readily adhere to platelets [27], and fibrin deposition contributes to the stabilization of the loose primary hemostatic plug [8].

The vessel wall actively participates in the regulation of intravascular thrombosis through a variety of mechanisms. Vascular endothelial and smooth muscle cells produce prostacyclin, a labile arachidonic acid metabolite [28, 29] that is a potent vasodilator and inhibitor of platelet aggregation. Prostacyclin appears to act by stimulating adenylate cyclase activity; phosphodiesterase inhibitors have been reported to potentiate its action [30–32]. Production of prostacyclin can be experimentally increased by thrombin [33], angiotensin [34], bradykinin [34], platelet-produced prostaglandin endoperoxides [35], platelet-released serotonin, and platelet-derived growth factor [36]. Whether prostacyclin is a physiologically important local or circulating regulator of platelet function is unclear [37–42]. Its potential usefulness as a pharmacologic anticoagulant has been based on the observation that, in vivo, prostacyclin infusion decreases thrombus formation in response to vascular injury [43], and prevents thrombosis of partially stenosed coronary arteries [44, 45].

The endothelium exhibits ecto-ADPase activity [46], providing a mechanism for the degradation of extracellular ADP to adenosine, a vasodilator and platelet inhibitor [47, 48]. It has also been reported that endothelial cells can selectively release adenine nucleotides in response

to thrombin stimulation [49]. When endothelial prostacyclin synthesis was blocked with aspirin, stimulated cells were capable of inducing platelet aggregation. This effect was blocked by 2-azido-AMP, an antagonist of ADP [50]. Thus injured or stimulated endothelium may release enough ADP to activate platelets, while intact endothelium may degrade extracellular ADP, preventing excess platelet activation. A role for extracellular ADP in promoting thrombus formation in vivo has some experimental support [22]. ADP released from hemolyzed erythrocytes may also play a role in stimulating platelet aggregation [51].

Other endothelial cell properties relevant to the regulation of blood clotting include synthesis of plasminogen activator [52], uptake and degradation of biogenic amines [53], production of heparin sulfate [54], and binding of alpha 2-macroglobulin, a protease inhibitor [55].

Potential Sites of Pharmacologic Intervention

The above considerations and those presented in chapters 6 and 7 can be used to predict possible sites of intervention in the process of coronary thrombosis. Interventions can be arbitrarily classified as outlined in table 16-2 directed at prevention of thrombosis or at lysis of an established thrombus. Strategies for thrombus prevention can be divided into those directed at correction of conditions predisposing to or initiating thrombus formation, and those directed at factors mediating or modulating the thrombotic response to initiator (table 16-1).

The classification of the interventions into functional groups emphasizes the complexity and redundancy of the thrombotic process. Many stimuli are capable of activating platelets, and at least three mediators—ADP, thromboxane A_2, and thrombin [6, 15–17, 25, 26]—are capable of aggregating platelets by independent mechanisms. Thus, one might speculate that antiplatelet therapies directed against a single mediator such as thromboxane might be inadequate. In addition, platelet activation and activation of the plasma-clotting cascade are closely interrelated; thrombin is capable of activating platelets and causing fibrin deposition, and activated platelets promote thrombin generation. Thus, interven-

TABLE 16-1. Interventions that prevent or reverse thrombosis

1. Increase blood flow at the site of thrombosis
   a. Angioplasty
   b. Endarterectomy
   c. Vasodilators
      Nitrates (55)
      Calcium-channel blockers [56]
   d. Thrombolytic therapy
      Exogenous plasminogen activators (see chapter 6)
      Stimulation of endogenous plasminogen activator-production [63]
2. Reduce the thrombotic potential of the blood vessel wall
   a. Stimulation of endothelial prostacyclin synthesis
      Nitroglycerin [60]
      Captopril [61]
   b. Heparin
   c. Dextran sulfate [62]
   d. Stimulation of endothelial regeneration [57]
3. Inhibit thrombin production or action
   a. Heparin
   b. Vitamin-K antagonists
      Coumadin
   c. Hirudin-like compounds [85]
4. Inhibit platelet function
   a. Stimulation of platelet adenylate cyclase
      Prostacyclin [30−32, 66]
      PGE_1 [66]
      Adenosine [65]
   b. Inhibition of platelet cyclic AMP phosphodiesterase
      Dipyridamole [32]
   c. Blockade of platelet ADP receptors [50, 64]
   d. Reduction of extracellular ADP [21]
   e. Blockade of platelet serotonin receptors
      Methysergide
      Cyproheptadine [67, 68]
   f. Blockade of platelet alpha$_2$ receptors
      Yohimbine [69, 70]
   g. Inhibition of thromboxane A_2 production [71, 72]
      Inhibit acyl hydrolase activity
      Glucocorticoids [73]
      Quinacrine [74]
      Local anesthetics [75]
      Phenothiazines [76]
      Inhibit cyclooxygenase
      Aspirin [22, 77]
      Ibuprofen [78, 79]
      Inhibit thromboxane synthetase [80−82]
   h. Blockade of calcium influx [83, 84, 86, 87]

tions aimed at preventing the action of thrombin might be expected to prove useful in the prevention of arterial thrombosis, and use of combined antiplatelet and "antithrombin" therapy (e.g., prostacyclin and heparin) may be required to significantly inhibit thrombosis in some ischemic syndromes. Whether the risks of combined therapy are acceptable remains to be determined.

Clinical Trials

ACUTE MYOCARDIAL INFARCTION

Recent clinicopathologic and angiographic studies have demonstrated a high incidence of recent coronary thrombosis in association with transmural myocardial infarctions (see chapter 6). Thrombolytic studies utilizing intracoronary

TABLE 16-2. Clinical trials of anticoagulant drugs in acute myocardial infarction

Trial	Follow-up period	Deaths (% total pts)	
		Control	Intervention
Carleton et al. [107]	29 days	20.0	30
Medical Research Council [108]	28 days	18.0	16.2
Drapkin and Merskey [106]	21 days	19.5	13.5
Veterans Administration Coop. [109]	28 days	11.3	9.6

streptokinase suggest that myocardium can be salvaged with clot lysis, but only if reperfusion is achieved within 4−6 h after the onset of symptoms (see chapter 22). These observations suggest a causal role for coronary thrombosis in transmural infarction, but also suggest that thrombosis has generally occurred prior to patient presentation. Thus it would be too late for therapies designed to prevent thrombus formation to be useful. Data from numerous studies (table 16-2) have failed to show a consistent beneficial effect of anticoagulants (heparin followed by phenindione or warfarin) administered to patients early in the acute clinical phase of myocardial infarction (table 16-2, reviewed by May et al. [56]). Only one of these trials [57] reported a statistically significant difference for overall mortality between the intervention and control groups and this difference was mainly in women. "Antiplatelet" therapy (oral aspirin or persantine) was similarly ineffective when administered during the early hours of infarction (table 16-3, reviewed by May et al. [56]).

ANGINA PECTORIS

The finding that cyclic platelet aggregation occurs at sites of coronary stenosis [10, 11] has supported the proposal that platelet aggregates play a role in unstable angina. The transient and recurrent nature of these aggregates may provide a setting in which antithrombotic therapy is likely to have a significant clinical effect. A recent randomized, double-blind, placebo-controlled study conducted by Telford and Wilson [1, 12] evaluated the ability of heparin and/or atenolol to decrease the incidence of transmural infarction in patients presenting with "intermediate coronary syndrome." Patients included were those with recent onset of increasingly severe angina, deterioration of stable angina, and subendocardial ischemia with or without infarction. Heparin-

ization was begun (10000 U q6) immediately following recruitment. During the seven-day treatment period, three of 100 heparin-treated patients developed transmural infarctions, compared with 17 of the 114 who did not receive heparin. During the following seven weeks, four additional transmural infarctions occurred in the group that had received heparin, compared with three in the nonheparin-treated group. If confirmed, these results suggest that heparin treatment may reduce the incidence of transmural infarction in some subset of patients presenting with unstable angina or subendocardial infarction.

A recent multicenter, double-blind, placebo-controlled randomized trial examined the protective effects of aspirin against acute myocardial infarction and death in men with unstable angina [58]. The dose of aspirin utilized was 324 mg immediately upon randomization and daily thereafter for 12 weeks. Of 641 patients receiving placebo, 65 had acute myocardial infarcts during the trial period, compared with 31 of 625 patients receiving aspirin, a 51% reduction ($P = 0.0005$). The reduction in mortality in the aspirin group was also 51%—ten patients compared with 21 ($P=0.054$). If confirmed, these data suggest a protective effect of aspirin against acute myocardial infarction in men with unstable angina.

Several recent studies have evaluated the potential of prostacyclin in angina. Bergman and co-workers have reported that prostacyclin infusion prolonged the time to angina induced by rapid atrial pacing in ten patients with stable angina and angiographically proven coronary artery disease [59]. This effect probably relates mainly to the systemic hemodynamic effects of prostacyclin, as coronary sinus blood flow during atrial pacing was unaltered by prostacyclin infusion. Chierchia and co-workers evaluated the ef-

TABLE 16-3. Clinical trials of aspirin or dipyridamole in acute myocardial infarction

| | | | Deaths (% total pts) | |
Trial	Drug	Follow-up period	Control	Intervention
Gent et al. [110]	dipyridamole (400 mg/day)	28 days	5.8	15.7
Elwood and Williams [111]	Aspirin (300 mg/stat)	28 days	13.4	12.7

fects of prostacyclin infusion in nine patients with variant angina [60]. Despite producing antiplatelet and vasodilatory effects, prostacyclin infusion clearly benefited only one patient, with consistent reduction in the number of ischemic episodes during four consecutive periods of prostacyclin infusion alternated with placebo. Szczeklik and associates describe infusion of prostacyclin at $5-10$ ng/kg/min $\times$ 72 h in seven patients with rest angina who apparently had not responded to oral nitrates [61]. Symptoms disappeared in five patients and improved in two. These results are difficult to evaluate because the occurrence of myocardial ischemia was not assessed objectively, and the effects of PGI_2 were not compared with those of placebo. Uchida and co-workers have reported that intracoronary prostacyclin infusion resulted in dissolution of thrombus and coronary recanalization in three patients presenting with acute myocardial infarction [62]. These observations suggest that prostacyclin or its stable analogues may be useful in instances of myocardial ischemia due to a fixed stenoses with supply–demand imbalance [59], some cases of coronary vasospasm [60], and platelet activation initiating coronary thrombosis [61, 62]. The role of prostaglandins and prostaglandin inhibitors in ischemic heart disease has been the subject of a recent review [63].

POSTINFARCTION

Patients who have sustained a documented myocardial infarction are at high risk for a subsequent infarction [64]. Prophylactic antithrombotic therapy has thus been evaluated in this population. There have been six controlled randomized trials using aspirin in patients who have had myocardial infarction (table 16-4, reviewed by Mustard et al. [9]) [65–70]. The results of these trials have been extensively reviewed [9, 56, 71] (see chapter 17).

The dose of aspirin used in these studies varied from 300 to 1500 mg/day. The entry period for the trials varied from days to five years. In none of the studies involving aspirin or aspirin plus dipyridamole was there a significant reduction in death for patients receiving drug therapy compared with placebo. In five of the six studies the mortality rate in the aspirin-treated group was less than that in the placebo group and the aspirin tended to reduce the incidence of nonfatal myocardial infarction although this reduction was not statistically significant. Peto has combined the data from the six trials [72] and concluded that aspirin produced a 21% reduction in reinfarction ($P<0.001$), and a 16% reduction in cardiovascular mortality ($P<0.01$). However, the problems associated with data pooling have been extensively reviewed [73].

It can be argued that the dose of aspirin utilized in these trials did not favorably alter the balance between the vessel wall prostacyclin production and platelet thromboxane production in favor of the former [74]. Aspirin inhibits prostaglandin production by the irreversible acetylation of cyclooxygenase. Platelets lack the ability to resynthesize cyclooxygenase and thus a single dose of aspirin will inhibit platelet function for the platelet's seven- to ten-day circulating lifetime. In contrast, the vascular endothelium can synthesize new cyclooxygenase, restoring prostacyclin production within $6-48$ h. Aspirin, therefore (in theory), selectively inhibits platelet cyclooxygenase, altering the balance in favor of platelet inactivation. High doses of aspirin, however, do indeed inhibit vascular prostacyclin synthesis [74]. In addition, prostacyclin production is already compromised in atherosclerotic vessels [75]. Trials utilizing low doses of aspirin are currently underway. Because of the likelihood that there is both patient-to-patient variability in the overall response to aspirin and local variabil-

TABLE 16-4. Clinical trials of aspirin, aspirin plus dipyridamole, or sulfinpyrazone in long-term treatment of postmyocardial infarction patients

Trial	Drug	Follow-up period	Deaths (% total pts)	
			Control	Intervention
MRC I [96]	Aspirin (300 qd)	2.5 yrs	10.9	8.3
MRC II [94]	Aspirin (300 tid)	1 yr	14.8	12.3
Coronary drug project aspirin study [97]	Aspirin (324 tid)	10−28 mo	8.3	5.8
German−Austrian [95]	Aspirin (1500 qd)	2 yrs	10.6	8.5
AMIS [98]	Aspirin (500 bid)	3 yrs	9.7	10.8
Paris [99]	Aspirin (324 tid), dipyridamole (75 tid)	3−4 yrs	12.8	10.7
ART [113]	sulfinpyrazone (200 qid)	1−2 yrs	7.9	5.7
ARIS [114]	sulfinpyrazone (400 bid)	1−2 yrs	5.8	5.7

From Mustard et al. [9], with permission.

ity in normal and diseased vessels, aspirin's dual effect on both thromboxane and prostacyclin production is potentially a great disadvantage. Selective inhibition of thromboxane production by thromboxane synthetase inhibitors may overcome this problem.

There have been two clinical trials utilizing sulfinpyrazone for the prevention of reinfarction (table 16-4). Analysis of the anturane reinfarction trial suggests that sulfinpyrazone caused a reduction in sudden death during the first six months of therapy, but had no effect on the overall mortality rate or on the rate of reinfarction. This result is in contrast to that of the recent Italian study that reported a significant reduction in reinfarction in the sulfinpyrazone-treated group when compared with placebo. Total mortality, however, did not differ between the two groups. No effect was noted regarding sudden death (table 16-4, reviewed by May et al. [56]).

Five randomized clinical trials evaluated coumadinlike anticoagulants in the prevention of reinfarction and death in patients with previous myocardial infarcts. Three of the five studies showed a trend in favor of the anticoagulant group, but statistical significance was not achieved. One study reported a significant reduction in recurrent myocardial infarction. Review of these five randomized trials, which included

over 2300 patients, does not show conclusively that long-term anticoagulants lower the mortality in patients who have suffered a myocardial infarction [56].

Conclusion

The complexity of the phenomenon of intravascular thrombosis provides a number of potential sites of intervention in ischemic syndromes. There is considerable evidence to support a role for thrombosis in myocardial infarction and in unstable angina. Patients with acute infarctions are unlikely to respond to antithrombotic (as opposed to thrombolytic) therapy, whereas subsets of patients with unstable angina may respond to aggressive antiplatelet or anticoagulant therapy. Whether antiplatelet therapy is effective in the long-term prophylaxis against reinfarction is controversial. In retrospect, the therapeutic approaches used in recent clinical studies may not have provided an optimal antithrombotic effect. It is likely that further understanding of the physiology and pharmacology of platelets, the clotting cascade, and the blood vessel wall will greatly facilitate the development of more rational therapeutic strategies for preventing thrombotic phenomena that may play a role in myocardial ischemia.

TABLE 16-5. Anticoagulant drugs and long-term mortality after myocardial infarction

Trial	Intervention	Follow-up period	Deaths (% total pts)	
			Control	
Medical Research Council [115]	Phenindione	25 mo	21.3	14.9
Wasserman et al. [116]	Warfarin	36 mo	21.4	15.6
Seaman et al. [117]	Phenindione	72 mo	35.6	40.9
German–Austrian multicenter prospective clinical trial [95]	Phenprocoumon	24 mo	7.1	8.1
Sixty plus reinfarction trial [118]	Acenocoumarin/ Phenprocoumon	24 mo	15.4	11.6

References

1. Oliva PB: Pathophysiology of acute myocardial infarction, 1981. Ann Intern Med 94:236–250, 1981.
2. Oliva PB, Breckinridge JC: Arteriographic evidence of coronary arterial spasm in acute myocardial infarction. Circulation 56:366–374, 1977.
3. Maseri A, Labatte A, Baroldi G, Chierchia S, Marzilli M, Ballestra AM, Severi S, Parodi O, Biagini A, Distante A, Pesola A: Coronary vasospasm as a possible cause of myocardial infarction: a conclusion derived from the study of "preinfarction" angina. N Engl J Med 299:1271–1277, 1978.
4. De Wood MA, Spores J, Notske R, Mouser LT, Burroughs R, Golden MS, Lang HT: Prevalence of total coronary occlusion during the early hours of transmural myocardial infarction. N Engl J Med 303:897–902, 1980.
5. Buja LM, Willerson JT: Clinicopathologic correlates of acute ischemic heart syndromes. Am J Cardiol 47:343–356, 1981.
6. Henry RL: Platelet function. Semin Thromb Hemost 4:93–122, 1977.
7. Haft JI: Role of blood platelets in coronary artery disease. Am J Cardiol 43:1197–1206, 1979.
8. Packham MA, Mustard JF: Pharmacology of platelet-affecting drugs. Circulation 62:V-26–41, 1980.
9. Mustard JF, Kinlough Rathbone RL, Packham MA: Aspirin in the treatment of cardiovascular disease: a review. Am J Med 74:43–49, 1983.
10. Folts JD, Lalich JJ, Crowell EB, Rowe GG: Platelet aggregation produced by stenosis in dog coronary arteries [abstr]. Clin Res 23:183A, 1975.
11. Folts JD, Crowell EB Jr, Rowe GG: Platelet aggregation in partially obstructed vessels and its elimination with aspirin. Circulation 54:365–370, 1976.
12. Chapman I: Morphogenesis of occluding coronary artery thrombosis. Arch Pathol 80:256–261, 1965.
13. Horie T, Sekiguchi M, Hirosawa K: Coronary thrombosis in pathogenesis of acute myocardial infarction: histopathological study of coronary arteries on 108 necropsied cases using serial section. Br Heart J 40:153–161, 1978.
14. Ridolfi RL, Hutchins GM: The relationship between coronary artery lesions and myocardial infarcts: ulceration of atherosclerotic plaques precipitating coronary thrombosis. Am Heart J 93:468–486, 1977.
15. Holmsen H, Day HJ, Setkowsky CA: Secretory mechanisms: behaviour of adenine nucleotides during the platelet release reaction induced by adenosine diphosphate and adrenaline. Biochem J 129:67–82, 1972.
16. Smith JB, Ingerman C, Kocsis JJ, Silver MJ: Formation of prostaglandins during the aggregation of human blood platelets. J Clin Invest 52:965–969, 1973.
17. Samuelson B: Neurosci Res Bull 4:1017–1025, 1979.
18. Meyers K, Holmsen H, Seachord CI, Gorham J, Prieur D: Characterization of platelets from mink and cats with the Chediak-Higashi syndrome: 7th international congress on thrombosis and haemostasis, London, England, 15–20 July 1979. Thromb Haemost 42:218, 1979.
19. Meyers KM, Seachord CL, Holmsen H, Smith JB, Prieur DJ: A dominant role of thromboxane formation in secondary aggregation of platelets. Nature 282:331–333, 1979.

20. Smith JB, Willis AL: Aspirin selectively inhibits prostaglandin production in human platelets. Nature 231:235–237, 1971.

21. Schwartz BS, Leis LA, Johnson GJ: In vivo platelet retention in human bleeding-time wounds. II. Effect of aspirin ingestion. J Lab Clin Med 94:574–584, 1979.

22. Zawilska KM, Born GV, Begent NA: Effect of ADP-utilizing enzymes on the arterial bleeding time in rats and rabbits. Br J Haematol 50:317–325, 1982.

23. Hamberg M, Svensson J, Samuelsson B: Thromboxanes: a new group of biologically active compounds derived from prostaglandin endoperoxides. Proc Natl Acad Sci USA 72:2994–2998, 1975.

24. Shattil SJ, Bennett JS: Platelets and their membranes in hemostasis: physiology and pathophysiology. Ann Intern Med 94:108–118, 1980.

25. Kimlough-Rathbone RL, Packham MA, Reimers HJ, Casenave JP, Mustard JF: Mechanisms of platelet shape change, aggregation, and release induced by collagen, thrombin, or A23187. J Lab Clin Med 90:707, 1977.

26. Charo IF, Feinman RD, Detwiler TC: Interrelations of platelet aggregation and secretion. J Clin Invest 60:866, 1977.

27. Niewiarowski S, Regoeczi E, Stewart GJ, Senyl AF, Mustard JF: Platelet interaction with polymerizing fibrin. J Clin Invest 51:685–700, 1972.

28. Moncada S, Vane JR: Unstable metabolites of arachidonic acid and their role in haemostasis and thrombosis. Br Med Bull 34:129–135, 1978.

29. Moncada S, Gryglewski R, Bunting S, Vane J: An enzyme isolated from arteries transforms prostaglandin endoperoxides to an unstable substance that inhibits platelet aggregation. Nature 263:663–665, 1976.

30. Best LC, Martin TJ, Russell RG, Preston FE: Prostacyclin increases cyclic AMP levels and adenylate cyclase activity in platelets. Nature 267:850–851, 1977.

31. Gorman RR, Bunting S, Miller OV: Modulation of human platelet adenylate cyclase by prostacyclin (PGX). Prostaglandins 13:377–388, 1977.

32. Moncada S, Korbut R: Dipyridamole and other phosphodiesterase inhibitors act as antithrombotic agents by potentiating endogenous prostacyclin. Lancet 1:1286–1289, 1977.

33. Weksler BB, Ley CW, Jaffe EA: Stimulation of endothelial cell prostacyclin production by thrombin, trypsin, and the ionophore A 23187. J Clin Invest 62:923–930, 1978.

34. Gryglewski R, Korbut R, Splawinski J: Endogenous mechanisms which regulate prostacyclin release. Haemostasis 8:294–299, 1979.

35. Marcus A, Weksler BB, Jaffe EA, Broekman MJ: Synthesis of prostacyclin from platelet-derived endoperoxides by cultured human endothelial cells. J Clin Invest 66:979–986, 1980.

36. Coughlin SR, Moskowitz MA, Antoniades HN, Levine L: Serotonin receptor-mediated stimulation of bovine smooth muscle cell prostacyclin synthesis and its modulation by platelet-derived growth factor. Proc Natl Acad Sci USA.

37. Gryglewski RJ, Korbut R, Ocetkiewicz A: Generation of prostacyclin by lungs in vivo and its release into the arterial circulation. Nature 273:765–767, 1978.

38. Moncada S, Korbut R, Bunting S, Vane JR: Prostacyclin is a circulating hormone. Nature 273:767–768, 1978.

39. Bunting S, Moncada S, Reed P, Salmon JA, Vane JR: An antiserum to 5,6-dihydro prostacyclin (PGI$_1$) which also binds prostacyclin. Prostaglandins 15:565–563, 1978.

40. Amezcua JL, Parsons M, Oncada S: Unstable metabolites or arachidonic acid aspirin and the formation of the haemostatic plug. Thromb Res 13:477–488, 1978.

41. O'Grady J, Moncada S: Aspirin: a paradoxical effect on bleeding-time. Lancet 2:780, 1978.

42. Kelter JG, Hirsh J, Carter CJ, Buchanan MR: Thrombogenic effect of high-dose aspirin in rabbits: relationship to inhibition of vessel wall synthesis of prostaglandin I2-like activity. J Clin Invest 62:892–895, 1978.

43. Ubatuba FB, Moncada S, Vane JR: The effect of prostacyclin (PGT2) on platelet behaviour: thrombus formation in vivo and bleeding time. Thromb Haemost 41:425–435, 1979.

44. Aiken JW, Gorman RR, Shebuski RJ: Prevention of blockage of partially obstructed coronary arteries with prostacyclin correlates with inhibition of platelet aggregation. Prostaglandins 17:483–495, 1979.

45. Romson JL, Haack DW, Abrams GD, Lucchesi BR: Prevention of occlusive coronary artery thrombosis by prostacyclin infusion in the dog. Circulation 64:906–914, 1981.

46. Habliston DL, Ryan US, Ryan JW: Endothelial cells degrade ADP. J Cell Biol (Suppl) 79:206A, 1978.

47. Drury AN, Szent-Györgyi A: The physiological activity of adenine compounds with especial

reference to their action upon the mammalian heart. J Physiol (Lond) 68:213−237, 1929.

48. Haslom R, Rosson G: Effects of adenosine on levels of adenosine cyclic 3′,5′-monophosphate in human blood platelets in relation to adenosine incorporation and platelet aggregation. Mol Pharmacol 11:528−544, 1975.

49. Pearson J, Gordon J: Vascular endothelial and smooth muscle cells in culture selectively release adenine nucleotides. Nature 281:384−386, 1979.

50. Cusack NJ, Born GV: Effects of photolysable 2-azido analogues of adenosine, AMP and ADP on human platelets. Proc R Soc 197:515−520, 1977.

51. Rorvik TO, Holmsen I, Stormorken H: The release of ADP from red blood cells. Thromb Diath Haemorrh 19:77−83, 1968.

52. Lockutoff DJ, Edgington TE: Synthesis of a fibrinolytic activator and inhibitor by endothelial cells. Proc Natl Acad Sci USA 74:3903−3907, 1977.

53. Shepro D, D'Amore PA: Endothelial cell metabolism. In: Altura BM (ed) Vascular endothelium and basement membranes. Advances in microcirculation 9. Basel: S Karger, 1980, pp 161−205.

54. Buonassisi V, Root M: Enzymatic degradation of mucopolysaccharides from the surface of endothelial cell cultures. Biochim Biophys Acta 385:1−10, 1975.

55. Becker CG, Harpel PC: Alpha 2-macroglubulin on human vascular endothelium. J Exp Med 144:1−9, 1976.

56. May GS, Eberlein KA, Furberg CD, Passamani ER, De Mets DL: Secondary prevention after myocardial infarction: a review of long-term trials. Prog Cardiovasc Dis 24:331−352, 1982.

57. Drapkin A, Merskey C: Anticoagulant therapy after acute myocardial infarction: relation of therapeutic benefit of patient's age, sex, severity of infarction. JAMA 222:541, 1972.

58. Lewis HD Jr, Davis JW, Archibald DG, Steinke WE, Smitherman TC, Doherty JE III, Schnaper HW, Le Winter MM, Linares E, Pouget JM, Sabharwal SC, Chesler E, De Mots H: Protective effects of aspirin against acute myocardial infarction and death in men with unstable angina: results of a Veterans Administration cooperative study. N Engl J Med 309:396−403, 1983.

59. Bergman G, Daly K, Atkinson L, Rothman M, Richardson PJ, Jackson G, Jewitt DE: Prostacyclin: haemodynamic and metabolic effects in patients with coronary artery disease. Lancet 1:(8220), 569−572, 1981.

60. Chierchia S, Patrono C, Crea F, Ciabattoni G, De Caterina R, Cinotti GA, Distante A, Maseri A: Effects of intravenous prostacyclin in variant angina. Circulation 65:470−477, 1982.

61. Szczeklik A, Szczeklik J, Nizankowski R, Guszko P: Prostacyclin for acute coronary insufficiency. Artery 8:7, 1980.

62. Uchida Y, et al: In program and abstracts of the 5th international conference on prostaglandins, Milan. Fondazone Giovanni Lorenzini, 1982.

63. Pitt B, Shea MJ, Romson JL, Luccesi BR: Prostaglandins and prostaglandin inhibitors in ischemic heart disease. Ann Intern Med 99:83−92, 1983.

64. Weinblatt E, Shapiro S, Frank C, Sager RV: Prognosis of men after first myocardial infarction: mortality and first recurrence in relation to selected parameters. Am J Public Health 58:1329, 1968.

65. Elwood, P.C., Cochrane AL, Burr ML, Sweetnam PM, Williams G, Welsby E, Hughes SJ, Renton R: A randomized controlled trial of acetyl salicylic acid in the secondary prevention of mortality from myocardial infarction. Br Med J 1:436−440, 1974.

66. Breddin K, Loew D, Lechner K, Uberla K, Walter E: Secondary prevention of myocardial infarction: comparison of acetylsalicylic acid, phenprocoumon and placebo—a multicenter two-year prospective study. Thromb Haemost 41:225−236, 1979.

67. Elwood PC, Cochrane AL, Burr ML, Sweetnam PM, Williams G, Welsby E, Hughes SJ, Renton R: A randomized controlled trial of acetyl salicylic acid in the secondary prevention of mortality from myocardial infarction. Br Med J 1:436−440, 1974.

68. Coronary Drug Project Research Group: Aspirin in coronary heart disease. J Chronic Dis 29:625−642, 1976.

69. Aspirin Myocardial Infarction Study Research Group: A randomized, controlled trial of aspirin in persons recovered from myocardial infarction. JAMA 243:661−669, 1980.

70. Anturane Reinfarction Trial Research Group: Sulfinpyrazone in the prevention of sudden death after myocardial infarction. N Engl J Med 302:250−256, 1980.

71. Goldman L, Feinstein AR: Anticoagulants and myocardial infarction: the problems of pooling, drowning, and floating. Ann Intern Med 90:92−94, 1979.

72. Peto R: Biomedicine 28:24–36, 1975.
73. Chalmers TC, Matta RJ, Smith J Jr, Kunzler AM: Evidence favoring the use of anticoagulants in the hospital phase of acute myocardial infarction. N Engl J Med 297:1091–1096, 1977.
74. Weksler BB, Pett SB, Alonso D, Richter RC, Stelzer P, Subramanian V, Tack-Goldman K, Gay WA Jr: Differential inhibition by aspirin of vascular and platelet prostaglandin synthesis in atherosclerotic patients. N Engl J Med 308: 800–805, 1983.
75. Sinziger H, Silberbauer K, Feigl W, Wagner O, Winter M, Auerswald W: Prostacyclin activity is diminished in different types of morphologically controlled human atherosclerotic lesions. Thromb Haemost 42:803–804, 1979.

17. CLINICAL TRIALS OF MODIFICATION OF MORTALITY DURING ACUTE MYOCARDIAL INFARCTION

William T. Friedewald

Curt D. Furberg

Approximately 675,000 patients are admitted annually with a diagnosis of myocardial infarction (MI) to hospitals in the United States. Of these patients, 12%−15% will die during the hospitalization if this is their first MI; for recurrent MIs the percentage is even higher. To lessen this mortality, numerous interventions have been proposed and many have been critically evaluated in randomized controlled clinical trials.

This review addresses only pharmacologic interventions and only those started within minutes to three days after hospitalization with an MI and, in all but a few instances, completed while the patients were still hospitalized. General health care measures or surgical procedures are not evaluated, nor is long-term survival, i.e., greater than 90 days, considered.

Materials and Methods

This review considers controlled trials in MI patients reported prior to July 1983 and updates an earlier report [1]. Trials are included only if they had a total sample size of at least 100 patients with random assignment to intervention or control groups within a few hours to three days after admission. The period of follow-up in these trials was generally 3−4 weeks, but extended to as long as 90 days. The sample size criterion limits the eligible trials to those which might possibly

have had sufficient statistical power to detect a clinically important effect; a more restrictive requirement would have drastically limited the scope of this review. The requirement for randomization is a safeguard against bias in the allocation of patients to treatment. Finally, the criteria requirements of time from onset of infarct and length of follow-up limit this review to trials of acute intervention.

As "total mortality" is an end point reported in all the reviewed trials, it is an appropriate yardstick for comparing their results. This variable has the advantage that no element of judgment is required in its assessment and, as a result, the potential bias inherent in cause-specific end-point determination is avoided. Most of the trials considered in this review, however, were not primarily designed to assess "total mortality," and thus evaluation of such trials by this end point may well lead to conclusions different from those of the original reports. This end point is the most critical in determining overall efficacy of the intervention.

In many of the studies, the intervention was started as soon as possible after the patient was admitted to a hospital, often before the diagnosis of MI could be confirmed by characteristic electrocardiogram (ECG) changes and/or elevation of enzymes. Consequently, some patients were enrolled who later appeared not to have had an infarction. Despite this, wherever the data were presented in the report, all patients initially randomized are included in our mortality estimates, regardless of their ultimate diagnosis. It may be argued that this is needlessly stringent, but only by adopting such a conservative approach can the bias that can result form the differential withdrawal of randomized patients be reduced. In addition, this method removes the potentially serious problem of the use of differential diagnostic criteria for removing patients among the trials. Finally, this approach avoids the problem of excluding patients who would have potentially evolved to a completed infarction, but in whom therapy was effective in aborting such an event, which would lead to differential exclusion between the actively treated and control groups. The majority of the 59 reviewed trials reported their results based on all initially randomized patients.

The clinical trials reviewed are grouped into five major classes of intervention: (a) antiarrhythmics, (b) anticoagulants, (c) platelet-active drugs, (d) beta-blockers, and (e) thrombolytics. Agents in each of the last four classes theoretically have the additional advantage of potentially reducing the extent of myocardial injury or preventing reinfarction. Overlap exists between intervention class and the supposed mechanism of action, as any particular agent may have more than one effect. Three other interventions—glucose − insulin − potassium hyaluronidase, and vasodilators—are also briefly reviewed.

For each study the observed effect of the intervention has been standardized to the relative difference (i.e., the control group mortality minus the treatment group mortality divided by the control group mortality) to allow for variation in control group mortality rates. In addition the approximate 95% confidence limits have been determined [2] for this difference and plotted in figure 17-1. The numerical value of the relative difference in mortality (point estimate), which is given as a percentage in the figure, may seem to suggest that an intervention is "beneficial." When the confidence interval includes zero, however, the study results for total mortality are not statistically significant ($P>0.05$) and are, therefore, also consistent with either no benefit or even a negative effect from the intervention. A narrow

confidence interval is preferable since it expresses more certainty about the true effect of the intervention. Two related factors, large sample size and high mortality rate, narrow the width of this interval. Due to space limitations, individual trial treatment and control group mortality proportions are not presented; only the relative difference between the two groups.

Antiarrhythmic Drugs

During the evolution of an MI, the conditions predisposing to any particular arrhythmia change and, therefore, the time when an antiarrhythmic drug is first given is an important consideration. It is unrealistic to hope that any one agent will prove effective in suppressing all severe arrhythmias in all patients. Adverse effects are common and, consequently, for every patient the risk/benefit ratio must be carefully weighed. Fifteen trials of either quinidine, procainamide, disopyramide, lidocaine, or mexiletine qualify according to the criteria for inclusion in this review (table 17-1). (Beta-blockers are regarded as a separate category in this review.) Many of the newer agents that are being investigated (e.g., amiodarone, aprindine, encainide, ethmozine, flecainide, imipramine, and tocainide), as well as some of the more established (e.g., phenytoin and verapamil) are not included here because no trials meeting our review criteria have been reported.

The 15 trials that satisfy the review criteria ranged in size from 104 to 610 patients, and 11 of the trials were performed with a double-blind design. Each of the five drugs has been reported to suppress ventricular arrhythmias in the acute phase of an MI. As is evident in figure 17-1, however, not one of the trials has demonstrated a statistically significant reduction ($P<0.05$) in overall mortality. In fact, in eight of the 15 trials, there was a higher mortality in the treatment group.

Anticoagulants

Enthusiasm for a causal relationship between coronary thrombosis and MI has varied over the last 15 years, but such a relationship is currently widely accepted based on coronary angiographic

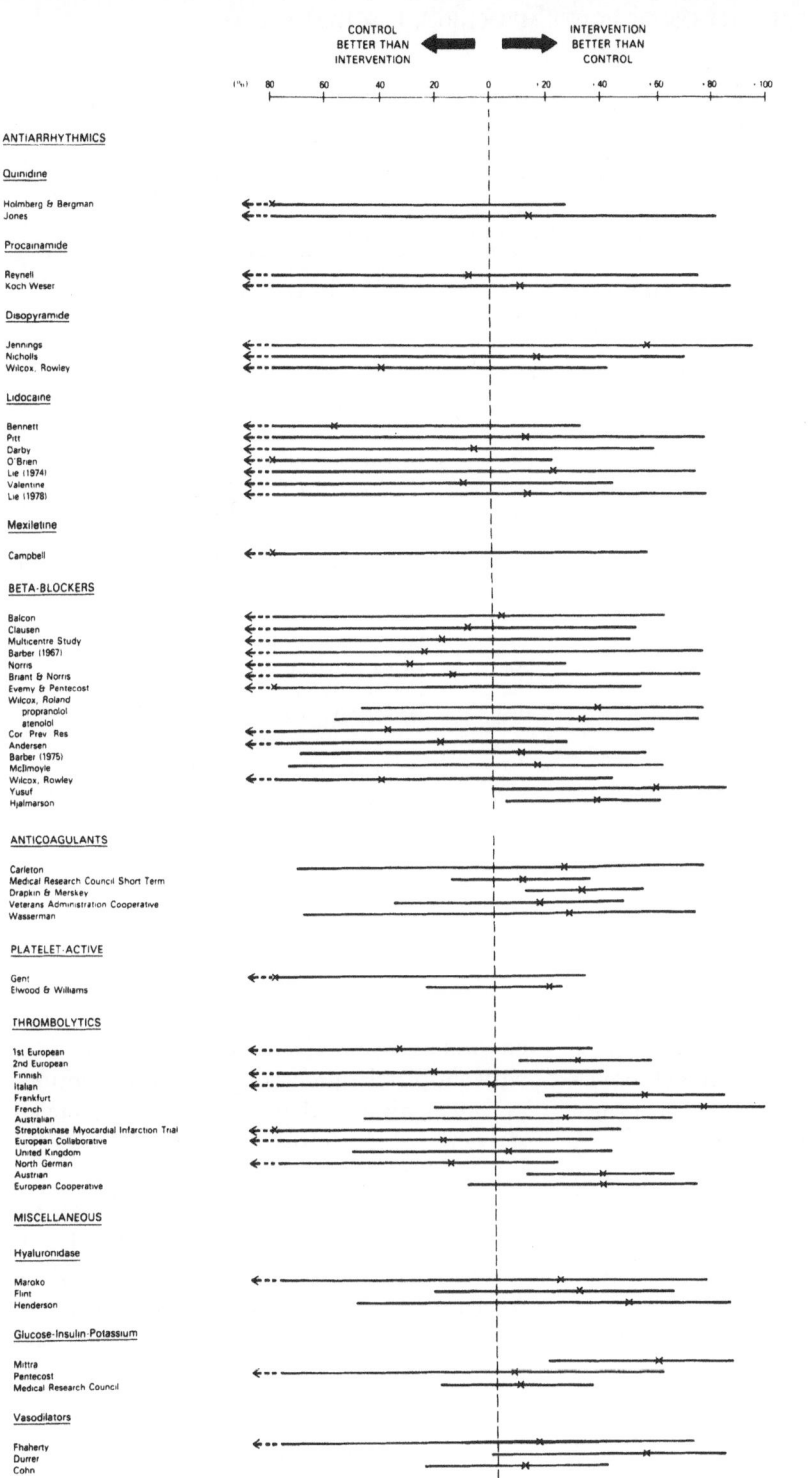

FIGURE 17-1. Estimates (x) as a percentage with approximate 95% confidence limits of the relative difference in total mortality between control and intervention in 59 short-term trials in the acute phase of myocardial infarction.

TABLE 17-1. Antiarrhythmic trials: design features

Trial	Type control	Number randomized	Length of follow-up (days)	Interventions
Quinidine				
Holmberg and Bergman [3]	Placebo	104	14	Quinidine 1.2 g/day × 14
Jones et al. [4]	Placebo	246	14	Quinidine 1.2 g/day × 3
Procainamide				
Reynell [5]	Usual Rx[a]	106	Hosp[b]	Procainamide 2−4 g/day × 14−21
Koch-Weser et al. [6]	Placebo	110	7	Procainamide 1 g stat + 2−4 g/day × 7
Disopyramide				
Jennings et al. [7]	Placebo	180	Hosp	Disopyramide 100 mg stat + 400 mg/day in CCU
Nicholls et al. [8]	Placebo	199	Hosp	Disopyramide 100 mg stat + 600 mg/day in hosp
Wilcox et al. [9]	Placebo	316	42	Disopyramide 450 mg/day × 42
Lidocaine				
Bennett et al. [10]	Usual Rx	610	Hosp	Lidocaine 60 mg stat IV + 0.5−1.0 mg/min/48 h
Pitt et al. [11]	5% Dextrose	222	Hosp	Lidocaine 75−100 mg stat IV + 2.5 mg/min/48 h
Darby et al. [12]	Usual Rx	322	Hosp	Lidocaine 200 mg stat IV + 2 mg/min/48 h
O'Brien et al. [13]	5% Dextrose	300	2	Lidocaine 75 mg stat IV + 2.5 mg/min/48 h
Lie et al. [14]	5% Glucose	225	CCU[c]	Lidocaine 100 mg stat IV + 3 mg/min/48 h
Valentine et al. [15]	Saline	364	30	Lidocaine 300 mg stat IM
Lie et al. [16]	Saline	321	Hosp	Lidocaine 300 mg stat IM
Mexiletine				
Campbell et al. [17]	Placebo	165	2	Mexiletine 600 mg stat + 750 mg/day × 2

[a]Rx, therapy.
[b]Hosp, length of follow-up is judged to be the period of hospitalization.
[c]CCU, length of follow-up is the period while in the coronary care unit.

and intraoperative demonstrations of thrombolytically resolvable occlusions. Administering anticoagulants as soon as possible after the first symptoms of acute ischemia might limit damage to the myocardium by reducing the risk of thrombus extension and recurrence. Also, the incidence of deep-vein thrombosis is reported to approach 40% in MI patients [18]. Early studies with historical controls [19] indicated that anticoagulants might have some additional impact on mortality in the acute phase of infarction. This possibility has been evaluated in five short-term controlled studies that meet our review criteria (table 17-2).

The five trials, which range in size from 125 to 1427 patients, incorporating an impressive total of 4010, have failed to clearly demonstrate that the use of anticoagulants in the acute phase of an MI reduces total mortality. Only one trial achieved results that attained statistical significance (figure 17-1). Four trials were single blind and the other unblinded.

Platelet-active Agents

The initial clinical impression that aspirin (acetylsalicylic acid) might prevent myocardial infarction was given additional credence when it was found that the drug inhibits platelet adhesion and aggregation, mediated through an effect on thromboxane A_2 [27]. Many other drugs [27] with antiplatelet properties have been identified as well. Only two short-term trials of platelet-active drugs satisfy the criteria for this review. One trial used a single 300-mg dose of aspirin and the other dipyridamole for 28 days. Each was double blind and placebo controlled (table 17-2).

One trial involved 120 and the other 2530 participants. Neither offered evidence to support the hypothesis that platelet-active agents prolong life in the acute phase of an MI (figure 17-1).

Beta-blocking Drugs

Approximately 20 beta-blockers are now available worldwide and each has differing potency, cardioselectivity, partial agonist activity, and local anesthetic and metabolic properties [28]. Despite these potentially important differences in the pharmacokinetic profiles of the individual drugs, there are no conclusive data establishing that their therapeutic benefit is the result of any of these specific properties rather than their beta-adrenergic blockade.

TABLE 17-2. Anticoagulant and platelet-active agent trials: design features

Trial	Type control	Number randomized	Length of follow-up (days)	Intervention(s)
Anticoagulants				
Carleton et al. [20]	Sham catheter	125	29	IV heparin
Med Research Council [21]	Low-dose phenindione	1427	28	IV heparin then phenindione
Drapkin and Merskey [22]	Placebo	1274	21	IV and SC heparin then phenindione
Vet Adm Cooperative [23]	Placebo	1037	28	SC heparin then warfarin
Wasserman et al. [24]	No anticoag	147	Hosp[a]	Warfarin
Platelet active				
Gent et al. [25]	Placebo	120	28	Dipyridamole 400 mg/day
Elwood and Williams [26]	Placebo	2530	28	Aspirin 300 mg stat

[a]Hosp, length of follow-up is judged to be the period of hospitalization.

Many patients with an acute MI have high plasma levels of free catecholamines. This may be counterproductive because, by enhancing oxygen consumption secondary to the increase in heart rate and contractility, there may be a fall in the threshold for cardiac arrhythmias. Beta-blockers have potent sympatholytic activity; hence, the rationale for their initial evaluation as an antiarrhythmic preventive measure after MI. It has also been theorized that by reducing myocardial oxygen demand they may also limit the size of a developing infarct.

Fifteen trials evaluating the effect of short-term administration of beta-blockers given early after an MI are included in this review. Of these, 13 used a double-blind design (table 17-3 and figure 17-1). In ten trials the beta-blocker was given orally throughout the study; in five an initial loading dose was given intravenously in the acute phase of the MI, followed by oral medication for the remainder of the trial.

Of these 15 trials ranging in size from 107 to 1395 patients, only that of Hjalmarson et al. [38] has demonstrated a significant reduction in mortality. In this trial, however, patients were followed for 90 days, which was substantially longer than any of the other trials and the sample size and number of deaths were the largest.

Thrombolytic Agents

Platelet aggregation combined with the deposition of a fibrin network is the basis for thrombus formation. The relative importance of the two

TABLE 17-3. Beta-blocker trials: design features

Trial	Type control	Number randomized	Length of follow-up (days)	Intervention(s)
Balcon et al. [29]	Placebo	155	28	Propranolol 80 mg/day
Clausen et al. [30]	No B-blocker	130	22	Propranolol 40 mg/day
Multicentre Study [31]	Placebo	226	28	Propranolol 80 mg/day
Barber et al. [32]	Placebo	107	28	Propranolol 160 mg/day
Norris et al. [33]	Placebo	536	21	Propranolol 80 mg/day
Briant and Norris [34]	Placebo	172	3	Alprenolol 400 mg/day
Evemy and Pentecost [35]	No B-blocker	128	28	Practolol 15 mg IV stat + 400 mg/day
Wilcox et al. [36]	Placebo	388	42	Propranolol 120 mg/day or atenolol 100 mg/day
Wilcox et al. [9]	Placebo	315	42	Oxprenolol 120 mg/day
Yusuf et al. [37]	No B-blocker	477	10	Atenolol 5 mg IV + 50 mg p.o. stat and 12 h + 100 mg/day
Hjalmarson et al. [38]	Placebo	1395	90	Metoprolol 15 mg IV stat + 200 mg/day p.o.
Cor Prev Res Group [39]	Placebo	313	56	Oxprenolol 80 mg/day
Andersen et al. [40]	Placebo	480	28	Alprenolol 5 mg IV stat + 400 mg/day
Barber et al. [41]	Placebo	500	90	Practolol 400 mg/day
McIlmoyle et al. [42]	Placebo	391	90	Metoprolol 15 mg IV stat + 200 mg/day

may differ in venous and arterial thrombi, but for both it has been assumed that antiplatelet agents and anticoagulants might prevent thrombus formation, and that fibrinolysis will cause thrombus dissolution. On this premise, thrombolytic agents have been given systemically to treat a wide variety of clinical conditions—pulmonary embolism, retinal vein or artery occlusions, deep-vein thrombosis, acute and chronic arterial thrombosis, and thrombosis in hemodialysis shunts. Their possible intracoronary thrombolytic effect for preserving ischemic myocardium when given within hours of onset of an MI has provoked the most recent clinical interest.

Two thrombolytic agents have been evaluated in large-scale clinical trials—urokinase, an enzyme produced by the kidneys that can be isolated from tissue culture or urine, and streptokinase, prepared from the streptococcus bacterium. Both act on the endogenous fibrinolytic system by promoting conversion of inactive plasminogen to the proteolytic enzyme plasmin [43].

After 13 trials involving 5197 patients (range 107−764), the question of whether or not systemic thrombolytic agents given in the acute phase of an MI prolong life is still unanswered (table 17-4 and figure 17-1). Three of the trials used a double-blind design, one was single blind, and the other nine were unblinded. The trend of the results in seven trials suggests benefit from intervention and, in three, the reduction in mortality is statistically significant ($P<0.05$). However, the high death rates in the control groups (over 26% during the hospital stay) in two of these trial raises some question as to whether the results can be generalized. In six trials there were more deaths in the intervention group than in the control group.

Recent reports in relatively small numbers of patients suggest that intracoronary administration of streptokinase may be effective, especially in patients with a transmural MI. If the agent is given by this route as soon as possible after the onset of MI symptoms, there is evidence from angiography and serum enzyme determinations that an occluded coronary artery may recanalize with associated relief of ischemic chest pain. This therapy offers hope for the future, but it requires proper evaluation by clinical trials before being generally advocated [57]. Several trials are either in progress or in preparation to evaluate intracoronary and/or intravenous thrombolytic therapy.

Miscellaneous

There are a number of interventions that do not fit into the five major drug classes considered, but are of interest and have been studied in the

TABLE 17-4. Thrombolytic agent trials: design features

Trial	Type control	Number randomized	Length of follow-up (days)	Intervention Initial[b]	Maintenance
Amery et al. [44]	Heparin	192	Hosp[a]	SK 1250	104/h × 12
European Working Party [45]	Heparin	764	Hosp	SK 250	100/h × 24
Heikinheimo et al. [46]	Glucose	426	42	SK 600	var × 48 h
Dioguardi et al. [47]	Heparin	321	40	SK 250	150/h × 3
Breddin et al. [48]	Laevulose	206	Hosp	SK 250	500/3 h
Brochier et al. [49]	Heparin	120	30	UK —	2700
Bett et al. [50]	Heparin	534	Hosp	SK 250	100/h × 18
Ness et al. [51]	Heparin or glucose	107	21	SK 250	100/h × 24
European Collaborative [52]	Glucose	341	21	UK var	var × 18
Aber et al. [53]	None	660	42	SK 250	100/h × 24
Poliwodo et al. [54]	Heparin	483	40	SK 250	100/h × 16
Benda et al. [55]	None	728	40	SK 500	750/4 h 1500/16 h
European Cooperative [56]	Glucose	315	21	SK 250	100/h × 24

[a]Hosp, length of follow-up is judged to be the period of hospitalization.
[b]SK, streptokinase; UK, urokinase; var, variable dosage; units are in thousands.

post-acute MI patient. These are glucose–insulin–potassium (GIK), hyaluronidase, and vasodilators.

Three clinical trials of GIK, all non-double-blind, qualify for consideration. Mittra [58] randomized 170 patients within 48 h of the onset of MI symptoms, and after 14 days of intervention there were ten deaths in the 85 GIK patients and 24 in the 85 control patients ($P<0.05$). Regrettably, two subsequent trials could not confirm these results. Pentecost et al. [59] randomized 200 patients within 48 h of their MI, and at the time of discharge from hospital, usually a period of four weeks, mortality in the 100 intervention patients was almost identical to that in 100 control patients who received usual care (15 vs 16 deaths, respectively). The Medical Research Council [60] in the United Kingdom randomized 986 patients and, at the end of 28 days of follow-up, no significant difference in total mortality was evident between the study groups (103 deaths in the 480 GIK group; 115 deaths in the 488 controls). The results of these three trials are presented graphically in figure 17-1.

After a preliminary nonrandomized study demonstrating that hyaluronidase accelerated the fall of ST-segment elevation in MI patients, Maroko and colleagues [61] conducted a trial in 111 patients with presumed MI and randomized them to either hyaluronidase, given as an intravenous bolus every 6 h for 48 h, or to the control group. Based on a 33-lead precordial unipolar ECG, they presented evidence of reduced ECG signs of myocardial necrosis in the hyaluronidase group, but by the time of hospital discharge, mortality in the hyaluronidase group was not significantly different from that of control patients (eight deaths out of 54 hyaluronidase patients and 11 deaths out of 57 controls). Flint et al. [62] assessed in a randomized double-blind clinical trial the benefit of intravenous GL enzyme (hyaluronidase) in 483 patients enrolled within 6 h of the onset of MI symptoms. A single injection of 200,000 IU GL enzyme or an indistinguishable placebo was given in the emergency department. At 30 days or hospital discharge there were 22 deaths in 240 of the enzyme-treated group and 32 in 243 of the placebo group (a large but not statistically significant difference). Henderson et al. [63] in their trial of the same preparation randomized 192 patients within 12 h of symptom onset. Among the 165 patients who were diagnosed as having definite or possible MI, one of the 84 in the GL group died within two weeks as compared with seven of the 81 in the placebo group. At 120 days the mortality rates were not significantly different: 7.2% (six out of 83 patients on GL, one lost to follow-up) versus 13.9% (11 out of 79 controls, two lost to follow-up). The findings from these recent trials of hyaluronidase (figure 17-1) are encouraging and further evaluation of its efficacy is underway.

Finally a few trials of vasodilators have been published. A trial of intravenous nitroglycerin by Flaherty et al. [64] was initiated in patients within 18 h of onset of pain and continued for 48 h. A preliminary report revealed that 11 (20.8%) of 53 patients in the nitroglycerin group died during the three-month follow-up period as compared to 11 (24.4%) of 45 in the placebo group. Durrer et al. [65] stopped their trial of nitroprusside in 328 patients when the difference in one-week mortality between the intervention and control groups reached nominal statistical significance ($P<0.05$). At four weeks of follow-up there were nine (5.5%) deaths in the 163 patients given nitroprusside compared with 20 (12.1%) among the 165 controls ($P<0.05$). Intervention was initiated within 12 h of onset of symptoms of an MI and continued for 24 h. In contrast in the trial by Cohn et al. [66] 812 MI patients with left ventricular filling pressure of 12 mmHg or higher were randomized within 24 h of an MI. In the 407 patients given a nitroprusside infusion over 48 h, 47 died during a three-week period, as compared with 42 in the 405 patients given placebo. After 13 weeks, the number of deaths was 69 in the nitroprusside group and 77 in the placebo group. Neither of these differences was statistically significant (figure 17-1).

Discussion

The value of 22 different short-term interventions administered in the period shortly after the onset of symptoms of an MI has been examined in 59 randomized, controlled clinical trials ranging in size from 104 to 2530 patients and involving a total of over 24,000. Total mortality has been chosen as the response variable for this review. As stated, most of the trials were not designed to assess mortality and, consequently, were often too small to test the hypothesis that an intervention prolongs life. Of the 59 trials, 27 randomized fewer than 250 patients, only 14 randomized more than 500 patients, and only six randomized more than 1000 patients. More importantly from a design aspect, 27 of the 59 trials reported a total of 25 or fewer deaths. For the results of such small trials to achieve statistical significance ($P<0.05$) with a two-sided test, the intervention would need to reduce mortality by over 50%. Even with 50 total deaths a true benefit from intervention that exceeds 40% would be necessary to reach statistical significance. It is not surprising, therefore, that the majority of the trial findings are inconclusive with regard to total mortality. If there were a true, reasonably large effect, however, one would expect a preponderance (the actual number dependent on the sample sizes of each trial and the true effect) of the trials to have a lower mortality in the treated compared with control groups.

Eight classes of intervention have been considered in this review and the composite results for each class are equivocal. Eight of the 15 antiarrhythmic studies show a trend favoring intervention, seven favoring control. In no instance are the results statistically significant. Nine of the trials had fewer than 250 participants and not one recorded a total of more than 50 deaths. Quinidine, procainamide, disopyramide, lidocaine, and mexiletine have all been reported to suppress ventricular arrhythmias in the critical period after MI, but none of the trials adequately document that this effect is accompanied by a prolongation of life. Several large-scale, multicenter studies are now being mounted to address this question.

Support for the use of beta-blockers in the long term after MI has developed with a reduction in total mortality by about 22% in the first $1-2$ years after MI [67], but the effect on mortality of beta-blockade during the acute phase of an infarction is uncertain. Of the 15 short-term trials reviewed, eight reported a high mortality in the beta-blocker group, but there were fewer than 25 deaths in six of the trials and fewer than 50 in 12. The negative results of some of these smaller studies must be weighed against the favorable outcome in a recently published large study of metoprolol [38]. Nevertheless, further trials of sufficient scope are underway to help resolve the issue of whether beta-blockers prescribed within hours of an acute MI reduce mortality during the acute period.

All five short-term anticoagulant trials found a lower mortality in the treated compared with the control group. Three of the five enrolled more than 1000 subjects and each of these recorded over 100 fatal events, but only one attained statistical significance ($P<0.05$). This one trial by Drapkin and Merskey [22] reported only a modest relative difference of 9% (nonsignificant) for men, who comprised 66% of the study, but for women the relative difference was 52% with a control group mortality of 31%. With these somewhat unusual results reported from this trial, there remains no clear evidence to support the use of anticoagulants acutely after MI although the data are suggestive.

In contrast to any arguable benefit that platelet-active agents might confer in the long term, especially during the first several months after the infarct, neither of the two trials reviewed here indicate any benefit from using them in the short term during the early stages of an MI.

Thrombolytic agents given intravenously have been studied in 13 randomized, controlled trials involving more than 100 patients. In three studies, including the two largest, the reduction in mortality in the intervention group at the time of hospital discharge, or shortly afterward, was statistically significant. Hemorrhagic complications with the high doses of streptokinase and urokinase used in the past are not uncommon. Intracoronary application appears promising, but the technique is specialized and is unlikely to be available to the majority of patients. Active investigation of the role of intravenous and intracoronary administration of these agents as well as a new agent, tissue plasminogen activator, is underway.

One of the three trials of GIK, none of three trials of hyaluronidase, and one of the three trials of vasodilators reached statistical significance for the total mortality end point.

After a considerable commitment of time and resources, it is disappointing to conclude that the effect of available short-term interventions in the acute phase of an MI has not been more definitively determined. The striking feature in each of the interventions is the inconsistency of the results among individual trials. Benefit in a particular subgroup, however, might be masked by the lack of an effect in the majority of patients. It can be argued that in acute-phase trials a proportion of subjects with massive myocardial damage are inevitably going to die as a result of their MI, regardless of intervention. A negative outcome in these individuals might well dilute a small, but nevertheless important, effect in patients with less severe infarcts.

At this time no single form of intervention has been conclusively shown to reduce mortality in the acute phase of an MI. Two interventions (beta-blockers and thrombolytic agents) in the acute inhospital phase of MI have shown promising, though not conclusive, results. Three other interventions (anticoagulants, hyaluronidase, and vasodilators) have shown somewhat less promising, though still encouraging, overall results. The efficacy and safety of all these interventions and others need to be further assessed in trials of sufficient scope before their ultimate usefulness can be decided.

References

1. May GS, Chir B, Furberg CD, Eberlein KA, Geraci BJ: Secondary prevention after myocardial infarction: a review of short-term acute phase trials. Prog Cardiovasc Dis 25:335−359, 1983.
2. Cornfield J: A statistical problem arising from retrospective studies: proceedings of the 3rd Berkeley symposium on mathematical statistics and probability. Berkeley: University of California Press, 1956.
3. Holmberg S, Bergman H: Prophylactic quinidine treatment in myocardial infarction: a double-blind study. Acta Med Scand 181:297−304, 1967.
4. Jones DT, Kostuk WJ, Gunton RW: Prophylactic quinidine for the prevention of arrhythmias after acute myocardial infarction. Am J Cardiol 33:655−660, 1974.
5. Reynell PC: Prophylactic procaine amide in myocardial infarction. Br Heart J 23:421−424, 1961.
6. Koch-Weser J, Klein SW, Foo-Canto LL, Kastor JA, De Sanctis RW: Antiarrhythmic prophylaxis with procainamide in acute myocardial infarction. N Engl J Med 281:1253−1260, 1969.
7. Jennings G, Model DG, Jones MBS, Turner PP, Besterman EMM, Kidner PH: Oral disopyramide in prophylaxis of arrhythmias following myocardial infarction. Lancet 1:51−54, 1976.
8. Nicholls DP, Haybyrne T, Barnes PC: Intravenous and oral disopyramide after myocardial infarction. Lancet 2:936−938, 1980.
9. Wilcox RG, Rowley JM, Hampton JR, Mitchell JRA, Roland JM, Banks DC: Randomized placebo-controlled trial comparing oxprenolol with disopyramide phosphate in immediate treatment of suspected myocardial infarction. Lancet 2:765−769, 1980.
10. Bennett MA, Wilner JM, Pentecost BL: Controlled trial of lignocaine in prophylaxis of ventricular arrhythmias complicating myocardial infarction. Lancet 2:909−911, 1970.
11. Pitt A, Lipp H, Anderson ST: Lignocaine given prophylactically to patients with acute myocardial infarction. Lancet 1:612−616, 1971.
12. Darby S, Bennett MA, Cruickshank JC, Pentecost BL: Trial of combined intramuscular and intravenous lignocaine in prophylaxis of ventricular tachyarrhythmias. Lancet 1:817−819, 1972.
13. O'Brien KP, Taylor PM, Croxson RS: Prophylactic lidocaine in hospitalized patients with acute myocardial infarction. Med J Aust (Suppl) 2:36−37, 1973.
14. Lie KI, Wellens HJ, Van Capelle FJ, Durrer D: Lidocaine in the prevention of primary ventricular fibrillation: a double-blind, randomized study of 212 consecutive patients. N Engl J Med 291:1324−1326, 1974.
15. Valentine PA, Frew JL, Mashford ML, Sloman JG: Lidocaine in the prevention of sudden death in the prehospital phase of acute infarction: a double-blind study. N Engl J Med 291:1327−1331, 1974.
16. Lie KI, Liem KL, Louridtz WJ, Janse MJ, Willebrands AF, Durrer D: Efficacy of lidocaine in preventing primary ventricular fibrillation within 1 hour after a 300 mg intramuscular injection: a double-blind, randomized study of 300 hospitalized patients with acute myocardial infarction. Am J Cardiol 42:486−488, 1978.
17. Campbell RWF, Achuff SC, Pottage AP, Murray A, Prescott LF, Julian DG: Mexiletine in the prophylaxis of ventricular arrhythmias during acute myocardial infarction. J Cardiovasc Pharmacol 1:43−52, 1979.
18. Gazes PC, Gaddy JE: Bedside management of acute myocardial infarction. Am Heart J 97:782−796, 1979.

19. Manson DI, Fullerton HW: Anticoagulant therapy in cardiac infarction. Br Med J 1:6–8, 1956.

20. Carleton RA, Sanders CA, Burack WR: Heparin administration after acute myocardial infarction. N Engl J Med 263:1002–1005, 1960.

21. Assessment of short-term anticoagulant administration after cardiac infarction: report of working party on anticoagulant therapy in coronary thrombosis to the Medical Research Council. Br Med J 1:335–342, 1969.

22. Drapkin A, Merskey C: Anticoagulant therapy after acute myocardial infarction: relation of therapeutic benefit of patient's age, sex, and severity of infarction. JAMA 222:541–548, 1972.

23. Results of a cooperative clinical trial: anticoagulants in acute myocardial infarction. JAMA 225:724–729, 1973.

24. Wasserman A, Gutterman LA, Yoe KB, Kemp VE Jr, Richardson DW: Anticoagulants in acute myocardial infarction. Am Heart J 71:43–49, 1966.

25. Gent AE, Brook CGD, Foley TH, Miller TN: Dipyridamole: a controlled trial of its effect in acute myocardial infarction. Br Med J 4:366–368, 1968.

26. Elwood PC, Williams WO: A randomized controlled trial of aspirin in the prevention of early mortality in myocardial infarction. J R Coll Gen Pract 29:413–416, 1979.

27. Packham MA, Mustard JF: Pharmacology of platelet-affecting drugs. Circulation (Suppl 5) 62:V26–40, 1980.

28. Frishman WH: Multifactor actions of beta-adrenergic blocking drugs in ischemic heart disease: current concepts. Circulation (Suppl 1) 67: I-11–18, 1983.

29. Balcon R, Jewitt DE, Davies JPH, Oram S: A controlled trial of propranolol in acute myocardial infarction. Lancet 2:917–919, 1966.

30. Clausen J, Felsby M, Jorgensen FS, Nielsen BL, Roin J, Strange B: Absence of prophylactic effect of propranolol in myocardial infarction. Lancet 2:920–924, 1966.

31. A multicentre trial: propranolol in acute myocardial infarction. Lancet 2:1435–1437, 1965.

32. Barber JM, Murphy FM, Merrett JD: Clinical trial of propranolol in acute myocardial infarction. Ulster Med J 36:127–130, 1967.

33. Norris RM, Caughey DE, Scott PJ: Trial of propranolol in acute myocardial infarction. Br Med J 2:398–400, 1968.

34. Briant RB, Norris RM: Alprenolol in acute myocardial infarction: double-blind trial. N Z Med J 71:135–138, 1970.

35. Evemy KL, Pentecost BL: Intravenous and oral practolol in the acute stages of myocardial infarction. Eur J Cardiol 7:391–398, 1978.

36. Wilcox RG, Roland JM, Banks DC, Hampton JR, Mitchell JRA: Randomised trial comparing propranolol with atenolol in immediate treatment of suspected myocardial infarction. Br Med J 1:885–888, 1980.

37. Yusuf S, Sleight P, Rossi P, Ramsdale D, Peto R, Furze L, Sterry H, Pearson M, Motwani R, Parish S, Gray R, Bennett D, Bray C: Reduction in infarct size, arrhythmias and chest pain by early intravenous beta blockade in suspected acute myocardial infarction. Circulation (Suppl 1) 67: I-32-41, 1983.

38. Hjalmarson A, Elmfeldt D, Herlitz J, Holmberg S, Malek I, Nyberg G, Ryden L, Swedberg K, Vedin A, Waagstein F, Waldenstrom A, Waldenstrom J, Wedel H, Wilhelmsen L, Wilhelmsson C: Effect on mortality of metoprolol in acute myocardial infarction: a double-blind randomised trial. Lancet 2:823–827, 1981.

39. Coronary Prevention Research Group: An early intervention secondary prevention study with oxprenolol following myocardial infarction. Eur Heart J 2:389–393, 1981.

40. Andersen MP, Bechsgaard P, Frederiksen J, Hansen DA, Jurgensen HJ, Nielsen B, Pedersen F, Pedersen-Bjergaard O, Rasmussen SL: Effect of alprenolol on mortality among patients with definite or suspected acute myocardial infarction. Lancet 2:865–868, 1979.

41. Barber JM, Boyle McC, Chaturvedi NC, Singh N, Walsh MJ: Practolol in acute myocardial infarction. Acta Med Scand (Suppl) 587:213–219, 1975.

42. McIlmoyle, Evans A, McBoyles D, Cran G, Barber JM, Elwood H, Salathia K, Shanks R: Early intervention in myocardial ischemia: proceedings of the British Cardiac Society. Br Heart J 47:188, 1982.

43. Brogden RN, Speight TM, Avery GS: Streptokinase: a review of its clinical pharmacology, mechanism of action and therapeutic uses. Drugs 5: 357–445, 1973.

44. Amery A, Roeber G, Vermeulen HJ, Verstraete M: Single-blind randomised multicentre trial comparing heparin and streptokinase treatment in recent myocardial infarction. Acta Med Scand (Suppl) 505:3–33, 1969.

45. European Working Party: Streptokinase in recent myocardial infarction: a controlled multicentre trial. Br Med J 3:325–331, 1971.

46. Heikinheimo R, Ahrenberg P, Honkapohja H,

Iisalo E, Kallio V, Konttinen Y, Leskinen O, Mustaniemi H, Reinikainene M, Siitonen L: Fibrinolytic treatment in acute myocardial infarction. Acta Med Scand 189:7−13, 1971.

47. Dioguardi N, Mannucci PM, Lotto A, Rossi P, Levi GF, Lomanto B, Rota M, Mattei G, Proto C, Fiorelli G, Agostoni A: Controlled trial of streptokinase and heparin in acute myocardial infarction. Lancet 2:891−895, 1971.

48. Breddin K, Ehrly AM, Fechler L, Frick D, Koenig H, Kraft H, Krause H, Krzywanek HJ, Kutschera J. Loesch HW, Ludwig O, Mikat B, Rausch F, Rosenthal P, Sartory S, Voigt G, Wylicil P: Die Kurzzeitfibrinolyse beim akuten Myokardinfarkt. Dtsch Med Wochenschr 98:861−873, 1973.

49. Brochier M, Raynaud R, Planiol T, Fauchier JP, Griguer P, Archambaud D, Pellios A, Clisson M: Le traitement par l'urokinase des infarctus du myocarde et syndromes de menace. Arch Mal Coeur 68:563−569, 1975.

50. Bett HN, Biggs JC, Castaldi A, Chesterman CN, Hale GS, Hirsch J, Isbister JP, McDonald IG, McLean KH, Morgan JJ, O'Sullivan EF, Rosenbaum M: Australian multicentre trial of streptokinase in acute myocardial infarction. Lancet 1:57−60, 1973.

51. Ness PM, Simon TL, Cole C, Walston A: A pilot study of streptokinase therapy in acute myocardial infarction: observations on complications and relation to trial design. Am Heart J 88:705−712, 1974.

52. A European Collaborative Study: Controlled trial of urokinase in myocardial infarction. Lancet 2:624−626, 1975.

53. Aber CP, Bass NM, Berry CL, Carson PHM, Dobbs RJ, Fox KM, Hamblin JJ, Haydu SP, Howitt G, MacIver JE, Portal RW, Raftery EB, Rousell RH, Stock JPP: Streptokinase in acute myocardial infarction: a controlled multcentre study in the United Kingdom. Br Med J 2:1100−1104, 1976.

54. Poliwoda H, Schneider B, Avenarius HJ: Untersuchungen zum klinischen Verlauf des akuten Myokardinfarktes. Gemeinschaftsstudie an 26 krankenhaeusern in Norddeutschland. Teil 1: Die fibrinolytische Therapie des Myodarkinfarktes mit Streptokinase. Med Klin 72:451−458, 1977.

55. Benda L, Haider M, Ambrosch F: Ergebnisse der oesterreichischen Herzinfarktstudie mit Streptokinase. Wiener Klin Wochenshr 89:779−783, 1977.

56. European Cooperative Study Group: Streptokinase in acute myocardial infarction. N Engl J Med 301:797−802, 1979.

57. Furberg CD: Clinical value of intracoronary streptokinase. Am J Cardiol 53:626−627, 1984.

58. Mittra B: Potassium, glucose, and insulin in treatment of myocardial infarction. Lancet 2:607−609, 1965.

59. Pentecost BL, Mayne NMC, Lamb P: Controlled trial of intravenous glucose, potassium, and insulin in acute myocardial infarction. Lancet 1:946−948, 1968.

60. Medical Research Council Working-Party on the Treatment of Myocardial Infarction: Potassium, glucose, and insulin treatment for acute myocardial infarction. Lancet 2:1355−1360, 1968.

61. Maroko PR, Hillis LD, Muller JE, Tavazzi L, Heyndrickx GR, Ray M, Chiariello M, Distante A, Askenazi J, Salerno J, Carpentier J, Reshetnaya NI, Radvany P, Libby P, Raabe DS: Favorable effects of hyaluronidase on electrocardiographic evidence of necrosis in patients with acute myocardial infarction. N Engl J Med 296:898−903, 1977.

62. Flint EJ, Cadigan PJ, DeGiovanni J, et al: Effect of GL enzyme (a highly purified form of hyaluronidase) on mortality after myocardial infarction. Lancet 1:871−874, 1982.

63. Henderson A, Campbell RWF, Julian DG: Effect of a highly purified hyaluronidase preparation (GL enzyme) on electrocardiographic changes in acute myocardial infarction. Lancet 1:874−876, 1982.

64. Flaherty JT, Becker LC, Weisfeldt ML, Weiss JL, Gerstenblith G, Kallman CH, Bulkley BH: Results of a prospective randomized clinical trial of intravenous nitroglycerin in acute myocardial infarction. Circulation 62:III-82, 1980.

65. Durrer JD, Lie KI, Van Capelle FJL, et al: Effect of sodium nitroprusside on mortality in acute myocardial infarction. N Engl J Med 306:1121−1128, 1982.

66. Cohn JN, Franciosa JA, Francis GS, et al: Effect of short-term infusion of sodium nitroprusside on mortality rate in acute myocardial infarction complicated by left ventricular failure. N Engl J Med 306:1129−1135, 1982.

67. Frishman WH, Furberg CD, Friedewald WT: B-adrenergic blockade for survivors of acute myocardial infarction. N Engl J Med 310:830−837, 1984.

III. METHODS FOR DIAGNOSING AND SIZING MYOCARDIAL INFARCTIONS

18. SERUM CK-MB IN DIAGNOSIS AND ASSESSMENT OF ACUTE MYOCARDIAL INFARCTION

Richard D. White

Peer Grande

Galen S. Wagner

When coronary care units were first developed in the early 1960s, it became important to make a prompt diagnosis regarding presence or absence of an acute myocardial infarct (AMI) to optimize the use of these specialized facilities. This diagnosis was extremely difficult when no new Q waves appeared on the electrocardiogram (ECG) during the first $24-48$ h following CCU admission. Total "cardiac" enzyme determinations were an alternative, and when glutamic oxaloacetic transaminase (SGOT), lactic dehydrogenase (LDH), and creatine kinase (CK) all remained within normal limits, the diagnosis of an acute infarct was excluded. However, a variety of other body tissues could be the source of transient elevations of each of these enzymes. The first attempt to specifically identify the tissue of origin of an enzyme was the electrophoretic method for separating the isoenzymes of LDH [1]. This improvement over the use of total LDH was still suboptimal, because (a) an elevation in LDH_1 could result from hemolysis as well as from myocardial necrosis, and (b) the results were expressed as ratios of one isoenzyme (LDH_1) to another (LDH_2) rather than the absolute level of a particular isoenzyme.

It was important to determine whether an isoenzyme of other than LDH could be identified, which would be a more sensitive and specific marker of an AMI. The goal was the identification of an isoenzyme that was normally not detectable in the serum and was specific for myocardium. Thus, one would only need to document the presence or absence of the specific myocardial isoenzyme to identify or exclude the diagnosis of a myocardial infarction.

Serum CK-MB for Diagnosis of Myocardial Infarction

Reliable quantitative methods for separation of CK isoenzymes were developed in the 1970s. When the three CK isoenzymes were measured in human tissue extracts, most authors found myocardium to be the only source of CK isoenzyme MB. Although traces of CK-MB were found in skeletal muscle in some studies, the concentration of CK-MB was very low compared with the concentration in myocardium [2–7]. Therefore, serum CK-MB was judged to be a potentially reliable diagnostic test for AMI.

The first methods for separation of the CK isoenzymes were qualitative electrophoretic assays [2, 3, 8]. These methods were not highly sensitive and therefore serum levels of $25-30$ U/l of CK-MB were required for its identification. Now serum CK-MB can be analyzed accurately by several techniques, such as quantitative elec-

R.M. Califf and G.S. Wagner (eds.), ACUTE CORONARY CARE: Principles and Practice. Copyright © 1985. Martinus Nijhoff Publishing, Boston/Dordrecht/Lancaster.

trophoresis [9, 10], batch adsorption—desorption chromatography [11], column chromatography [9], antibody inhibition [12], and radioimmunoassay [13]. With more sensitive analytical techniques the presence of small amounts of CK-MB in normal sera has been documented, but this increased sensitivity may not necessarily be a clinical advantage. As shown by Wagner et al. [14], high levels of both specificity and sensitivity for the diagnosis of AMI had been achieved using the original less-sensitive technique.

The clinical evaluation of the more-sensitive assays of CK-MB has been difficult, mainly because of the absence of a "gold standard" for acute infarct diagnosis. Figure 18-1 shows the theoretical distribution of results of any quantitative diagnostic test. The figure illustrates the influence of the "discriminative level" on the rates of false and true negative and positive results. Increasing the discriminative level results in more false negative tests, lowering it results in more false positive tests. To identify the optimally accurate discriminative level of a quantitative test, it is necessary to make a descriptive study of patients suspected for the disease. As demonstrated in figure 18-1, the optimal discriminative level of a quantitative diagnostic test (i.e., serum CK-MB) cannot be determined from studying normal persons. It is a well-known experience that patients suspected for a disease, but in whom the diagnosis is disproven, may have results of biochemical tests different from normals. Serum CK-MB is below 5 U/l in normals, whereas the optimal discriminative level for diagnosis of AMI is 25—30 U/l [15—17].

Some patients in whom AMI was suspected clinically, but not proven by other tests, have peak CK-MB above the upper limit in normals, but below that of patients with proven MI. In a group of 401 patients with suspected AMI, 23% showed presence of minimally elevated CK-MB [10]. These might indeed be patients with "preinfarction" states. Having not completely infarcted, they might then be at risk for acute infarction with its attendant complications after discharge from the hospital.

A cooperative prospective study was performed to confirm the optimal discriminative peak CK-MB value for AMI diagnosis, to identify the clinical characteristics of patients with peak lev-

els less than that value, and to follow these patients after discharge to determine whether there was a high incidence of subsequent AMI [21] and/or death. All of the patients with appearance of new Q waves on serial ECGs and all with conclusively positive multiple other enzyme results had peak levels of serum CK-MB (on at least twice-daily determinations) >25 U/l.

The group of 115 patients with peak CK-MB from 5 to 24 U/l were followed for one year. Among 76 patients with accompanying severe medical problems, such as cardiac or respiratory failure, 25 (33%) died from a cardiac event. However, none of the 39 patients without coexisting serious medical problems died during one year of follow-up. Thus, "minimally elevated" CK-MB (5—24 U/l) occurs most often in association with severe acute medical problems and, in patients without such problems, does not indicate a poor prognosis. Patients with peak CK-MB values in this diagnostic "grey zone" may or may not have had small acute infarcts, but should not be considered to be in a "preinfarction" state.

Several studies have shown serum CK-MB to be more reliable than other individual tests for AMI. In table 18-1 the predictive values of the diagnostic tests for AMI are shown. The predictive value of a negative test was significantly highest for CK-MB. Therefore, CK-MB was most reliable for disproving the AMI diagnosis. The predictive values of a positive test were highest for ECG and CK-MB: the reliable methods for confirming the suspected diagnosis AMI. Several studies have shown similar high diagnostic effectiveness of CK-MB [8, 10, 16, 18—20].

It is important to consider the time course of CK-MB appearance in the serum during an AMI. Irvin et al. [22] have performed every 1—2 hour CK-MB serum sampling in 21 consecutive patients. A range of 3—15 hours after acute onset of symptoms is required before CK-MB is abnormally elevated. A negative test prior to 15 h, therefore, would have no diagnostic value. The peak CK-MB occurred between 11 and 38 h. Therefore sampling at 8 hourly intervals during the initial 36 h would be required to identify the approximately peak value. CK-MB remained in the abnormal range between 18 and 85 h. Therefore, sampling 12 and 24 h after onset of symp-

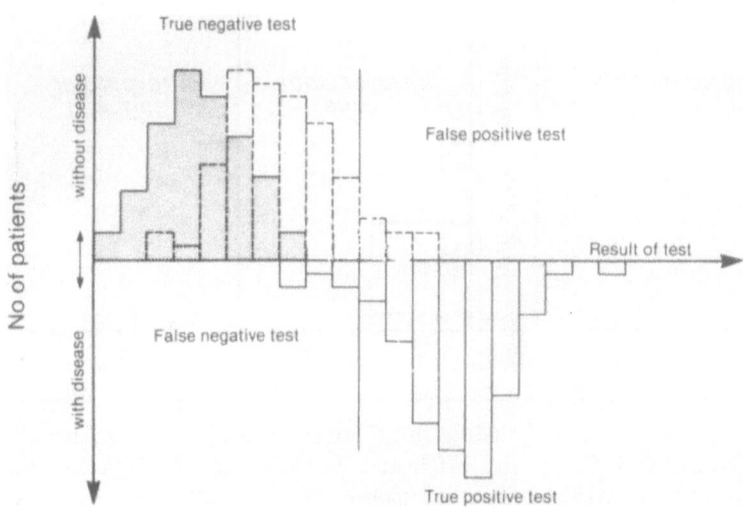

FIGURE 18-1. Diagnostic frequency distribution. A diagnostic test result is indicated for three populations. Above the horizontal line are (a) one group of healthy controls (shaded), and (b) one group of patients suspected of the disease in whom the diagnosis finally was disproven. Below the horizontal line are (c) those in whom the diagnosis was proven. The vertical line indicates the chosen discriminative limit.

TABLE 18-1. Predictive value of single tests and ECG in diagnosis of acute myocardial infarction ($n = 401$)

Predictive value of	CK-MB	SGOT	CK	LDH	ECG
Positive test	0.98	0.87	0.74	0.77	1.00
Negative test	1.00	0.97	0.98	0.98	0.77

toms would be likely to detect an abnormal value if it were present.

Serum CK-MB for Estimation of Acute Myocardial Infarct Size

The reason for developing methods to assess the extent of AMI size arises from the hypothesis that infarct size is a major determinant of prognosis and that limitation of infarct size can influence the prognosis favorably.

In the earliest studies, depletion of CK from myocardium in experimental animals correlated well with morphologic criteria of infarction, ST changes and microsphere-measured blood flow [23, 24]. Several assumptions must be fulfilled,

however, for serum CK-MB to be considered a reliable marker for estimation of infarct size. Figure 18-2 demonstrates the compartments, distribution, and elimination pathways for CK-MB. Since the kinetics of CK-MB are complicated and incompletely described—and the available methods for estimation of tissue damage from biochemical markers is limited—most studies have used simple one-compartment models. Although such models are simplifications of complex biologic systems, several studies have confirmed their clinical usefulness. The total appearance of CK-MB in plasma estimated by these models correlates well with several other indirect measures of infarct size: angiographic estimates of left ventricular asynergy and ejection fraction

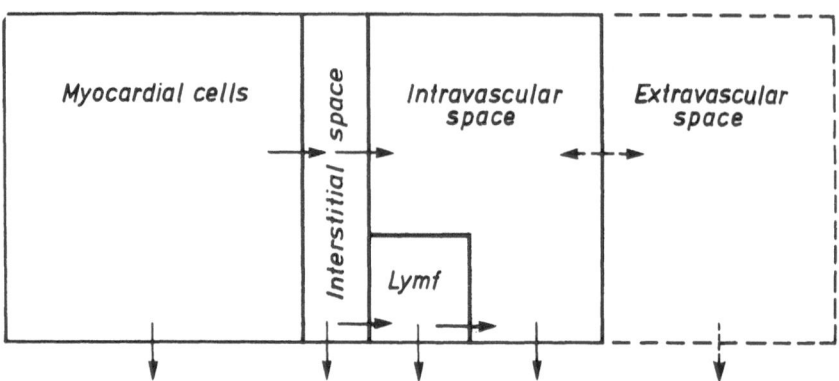

FIGURE 18-2. Theoretical distribution compartments and elimination pathways for CK-MB molecules. (Lymf is lymph.)

[25], precordial mapping of Q-wave and ST-segment changes [26], thallium-201 scintigraphy [27], ventricular dyssynergy estimated by echocardiography [28], and myocardial positron-emission tomography with ^{11}C-labeled palmitate [29]. Both infarct size estimated from serum CK [30], and serum CK-MB [31, 32], have shown highly significant correlation to extent of myocardial necrosis determined at autopsy. Although the coefficients of correlation between serum CK-MB-estimated infarct size and all the other indices of infarct size achieved r values of 0.75−0.95, the standard error of the estimate showed the relationship to be only semiquantitative. Usually the standard error of the estimate was 25%, which gives (at the 95% confidence limit) a range of ±50%. However, since the range of possible infarct sizes among patients is very large, i.e., in one study between 4 and 160 g, the enzymatic estimates may be clinically useful.

Of particular clinical interest are the studies demonstrating a significant relationship between enzymatically estimated infarct size and prognosis. Using CK in frequent blood sampling, Sobel and co-workers have demonstrated a close relationship between estimated infarct size, heart failure, ventricular dysrhythmia, and mortality [33, 34]. A practical approach, using serum CK-MB sampled three times a day, also showed a close relationship between the estimated infarct size and one-year mortality [35]. Table 18-2 shows the result of a multivariate analysis of the prognostic variables related to one-year survival after AMI [36]. This analysis was based on in-

formation available at day 7 after the acute event. Of the 12 variables tested, heart failure and serum CK-MB-estimated infarct size were most closely related to one-year survival.

Estimations of infarct size by serum CK-MB are useful as end points in clinical trials designed to evaluate infarct-limiting therapy. Methods for predicting infarct extent from only the early portion of the CK release curve have been reported, and applied to study interventions that might alter the magnitude of infarction [37, 38]. By predicting the infarct size, the treated patients are used as their own controls. However, accurate prediction of the "enzymatic infarct size" requires that blood sampling be continued beyond the length of time when any size-limiting intervention would be likely to be effective. Ryan et al. showed that only if values 2 h or more beyond the peak CK were included did predicted and actual CK-estimated infarct size agree [39]. Therefore, enzymatic evaluation of infarct size limitation must be performed in classically designed studies with control groups.

During recent years, studies have been performed to elucidate the weakness of serum CK-MB estimates of infarct size. Although the quantity of serum CK-MB has correlated well with left ventricular ejection fraction in most studies, others have found a poor correlation in patients with inferior infarcts. It has been hypothesized that this is due to the concomitant presence of right ventricular infarction in some patients with

TABLE 18-2. Prognostic variables associated with one-year survival (Cox model multvariate analysis, $n = 274$)

Prognostic variable	Significance
Sex	—
Hypertension	—
Infarct localization	—
Pulmonary edema	—
Cardiogenic shock	—
Cardiac dysrhythmias	—
Cardiac arrest	—
Age	0.02
Previous infarct	0.02
NYHA class	0.015
CK-MB-estimated infarct size	0.01
Heart failure	0.001

inferior infarcts, but not in patients with anterior infarcts. The right ventricular free wall is quite thin, however, and one wonders whether infarction of even a large extent of this wall could be capable of releasing a significant amount of CK-MB into the blood. Roberts and associates [40, 41] diagnosed right ventricular infarction by right heart hemodynamics, and found similar serum CK-estimated infarct sizes in patients with inferior and anterior infarcts. The left ventricular ejection fraction was significantly more decreased among patients with anterior, and the right ventricular ejection fraction with inferior, infarct locations. Prognosis was much better for patients with inferior infarction than for those with anterior infarcts and similar CK-MB values. In a recent study comparing serum CK-MB-estimated infarct size and infarct size estimated by QRS score [42] a much higher coefficient of correlation was found for anterior than inferior infarcts ($r = 0.75$ vs $r = 0.35$) (see chapter 19). These findings indicate that right ventricular infarction, in some patients with inferior infarcts, may contribute significantly to the enzymatically estimated infarct size.

One important determinant of the serum level of any enzyme released by infarcted myocardium is the level of perfusion of the tissue. The value of reperfusion therapy (intravenous or intracoronary streptokinase) in limiting the extent of an acute

MI, as determined by most indirect measurements of MI size [43, 44], has been well demonstrated, but infarct sizing via CK-MB has not yielded similar results. It has been demonstrated that reperfusion alters both CK [45—47] and CK-MB [48—50] kinetics by reducing the time until the appearance of serum peak values. Peak CK values have been shown to increase markedly after reperfusion (2—3 times higher [45, 46, 51, 52]), while changes in peak CK-MB values have not always been significant [48, 49].

Evaluations of the effect of reperfusion on the enzymatic evaluation of acute MI size have yielded conflicting results. Some experimental studies have found that alterations in kinetics of total CK due to reperfusion did not significantly change the estimation of MI size [46, 47], but others have demonstrated that reperfusion led to significant overestimation of the extent of necrosis [45]. Whether or not the alterations in CK-MB kinetics invalidate the use of the time—activity curves for sizing acute MIs has not yet been determined, but it seems reasonable to expect that the differences in the time course of appearance of serum CK-MB would obviate its use in patients receiving reperfusion therapy.

Conclusion

Serum CK-MB can now be analyzed accurately by several techniques: quantitative electrophoresis, batch adsorption—desorption chromatography, column chromatography, and immunoinhibition. In the early diagnosis of AMI, serum CK-MB is the most reliable diagnostic enzyme, and the only diagnostic test with both a high diagnostic sensitivity and specificity. Estimation of infarct size can be performed fairly reliably by serum CK-MB but, like other methods, certain limitations are present. Therefore it is necessary to evaluate infarct size by multiple methods.

References

1. Moller CE, Raabo E: Diagnostic use of fractionated lactate dehydrogenase activity (LD) in myocardial infarction. Acta Med Scand 175:31—42, 1964.
2. Roe CR, Limbird LE, Wagner GS, Nerenberg

ST: Combined isoenzyme analysis in the diagnosis of myocardial injury: application of electrophoretic methods for the detection and quantitation of the creatine phosphokinase MB isoenyzme. J Lab Clin Med 80:577−590, 1972.

3. Konttinen A, Somer H: Determination of serum creatine-kinase isoenzymes in myocardial infarction. Am J Cardiol 29:817−820, 1972.

4. Smith AF: Separation of tissue and serum creatine kinase isoenzymes on polyacryl-amide gel slabs. Clin Chim Acta 39:351−359, 1972.

5. Somer H, Dirbowitz V, Donner M: Creatine kinase isoenzyme in neuromuscular disease. J Neurol Sci 29:129−136, 1976.

6. Goto I, Nagamine M, Katsuki S: Creatine phosphokinase isoenzymes in muscle. Arch Neurol 20:422−429, 1969.

7. Roberts R, Sobel B: Creatine kinase isoenzymes in the assessment of heart disease. Am Heart J 95:521−528, 1978.

8. Roberts R, Henry PD, Witteveen SAGJ, Sobel BE: Quantification of serum creatine phosphokinase isoenzyme activity. Am J Cardiol 33:650−654, 1974.

9. Wong PC-P, Smith AF: Comparison of 3 methods of analysis of the MB isoenzyme of creatine kinase in serum. Clin Chim Acta 65:99−107, 1975.

10. Grande P, Christiansen C, Naestoft J: Creatine kinase isoenzyme MB assay by electrophoresis. Scand J Clin Lab Invest 39:207−212, 1979.

11. Henry PD, Roberts R, Sobel BE: Rapid separation of plasma creatine kinase isoenzymes by batch adsorption on glass beads. Clin Chem 21:844−849, 1975.

12. Gerhardt W, Ljungdahl L, Börjesson J, Hofvendahl S, Hedenäs B: Creatine kinase B-subunit activity in human serum. I. Development of an immunoinhibition method for routine determination of S-creatine kinase B-subunit activity. Clin Chim Acta 78:29−41, 1977.

13. Roberts R, Parker CW, Sobel BE: Detection of acute myocardial infarction by radioimmunoassay for creatine kinase MB. Lancet 2:319−322, 1977.

14. Wagner GS, Roe CR, Limbird LE, Rosati RA, Wallace AG: The importance of identification of the myocardial-specific isoenzyme of creatine phosphokinase (MB form) in the diagnosis of acute myocardial infarction. CIrculation 47:263−269, 1973.

15. Grande P, Christiansen C, Pedersen A, Christiansen MS: Optimal diagnosis in acute myocardial infarction: a cost-effectiveness study. Circulation 61:723−728, 1980.

16. Ljungdahl L, Gerhardt W, Hofvendahl S: Serum creatine kinase B subunit activity in diagnosis of acute myocardial infarction. Br Heart J 43:514−522, 1980.

17. Scandinavian Committee on Enzymes: Creatine kinase (EC 2.7.3.2) and creatine kinase B-subunit activity in serum in suspect myocardial infarction: The Nordic Clinical Chemistry Project (NORDKEM), Helsinki, Finland, 1981.

18. Blomberg DJ, Kimber WD, Burde MD: Creatine kinase isoenzymes: predictive value in the early diagnosis of acute myocardial infarction. Am J Med 59:464−469, 1975.

19. Roark SF, Wagner GS, Izlar HL Jr, Roe CR: Diagnosis of acute myocardial infarction in a community hospital. Circulation 53:965−969, 1976.

20. Kraft J, Aastrup H, Schrøder P: Diagnostic value for acute myocardial infarction of creatine kinase and lactate dehydrogenase isoenzymes compared with total enzymes: creatine kinase isoenzyme specificity for myocardial damage. Acta Med Scand 203:167−174, 1978.

21. White RD, Grande P, Califf L, Palmeri ST, Califf RM, Wagner GS: Diagnostic and prognostic significance of minimally elevated creatine kinase MB in suspected acute myocardial infarction. Am J Cardiol (in press).

22. Irvin R, Cobb F, Roe C: Acute myocardial infarction and MB creatine phosphokinase. Arch Intern Med 140:329−334, 1980.

23. Shell WE, Kjekshus JK, Sobel BE: Quantitative assessment of the extent of myocardial infarction in the conscious dog by means of analysis of serial changes in serum creatine phosphokinase activity. J Clin Invest 50:2614−2625, 1971.

24. Maroko PR, Kjekshus JK, Sobel BE, Watanabe T, Covell JW, Ross J Jr, Braunwald E: Factors influencing infarct size following experimental coronary artery occlusions. Circulation 43:67−81, 1971.

25. Rogers WJ, McDaniel HG, Smith LR, Mantle JA, Russel RO, Rackley CE: Correlation of angiographic estimates of myocardial infarct size and accumulated release of creatine kinase MB isoenzyme in man. Circulation 56:199−205, 1977.

26. Yusuf S, Lopez R, Maddison A, Maw P, Ray N, McMillan S, Sleight P: Value of electrocardiogram in predicting and estimating infarct size in man. Br Heart J 42:283−293, 1979.

27. Henning H, Schelberg HR, Righetti A, Ashburn WL, O'Rourke RA: Dual myocardial imaging with technetium-99m pyrophosphate and thallium-201 for detecting, localizing and sizing

acute myocardial infarction. Am J Cardiol 40: 147−155, 1977.

28. Visser CA, Lie KI, Kan G, Meltzer R, Durrer D: Detection and quantification of acute, isolated myocardial infarction by two dimensional echocardiography. Am J Cardiol 47:1020−1025, 1981.

29. Ter-Pogossian MM, Klein MS, Markham J, Roberts R, Sobel BE: Regional assessment of myocardial metabolic integrity in vivo by positron-emission tomography with ^{11}C-labeled palmitate. Circulation 61:242−255, 1980.

30. Bleifeld W, Mathey D, Hanrath P, Buss H, Effert S: Infarct size estimated from serial serum phosphokinase in relation to left ventricular hemodynamics. Circulation 55:303−311, 1977.

31. Grande P, Hansen BF, Christiansen C, Naestoft J: Estimation of acute myocardial infarct size in man by serum CK-MB measurements. Circulation 65:756−764, 1982.

32. The MILIS Study Group (personal communication).

33. Sobel BE, Brenahan GF, Shell WE, Yoder RD: Estimation of infarct size in man and its relation to prognosis. Circulation 46:640−648, 1972.

34. Geltman EM, Ehsani AA, Campbell MK, Schechtman K, Roberts R, Sobel BE: The influence of location and extent of myocardial infarction on long-term ventricular dysrhythmia and mortality. Circulation 60:805−814, 1979.

35. Grande P, Christiansen C, Pedersen A: Influence of acute myocardial infarct size on acute and one-year mortality. Eur Heart J 4:20−25, 1982.

36. Grande P, Nielsen AA, Wagner GS, Christiansen C: Quantitative influence of serum CK-MB estimated infarct size and other prognostic variables on one year mortality after acute myocardial infarction. Br Heart J (in press).

37. Shell WE, Lavelle JF, Covell FW: Early estimation of myocardial damage in conscious dogs and patients with evolving acute myocardial infarction. J Clin Invest 52:2579−2590, 1973.

38. Shell WE, Sobel BE: Protection of jeopardized ischemic myocardium by reductions of ventricular afterload. N Engl J Med 291:481−486, 1974.

39. Ryan W, Karliner JS, Gilpin EA, Covell JW, De Luca M, Ross J: The creatine kinase curve area and peak creatine kinase after acute myocardial infarction: usefulness and limitations. Am Heart J 101:162−168, 1981.

40. Strauss HD, Sobel BE, Roberts R: The influence of occult right ventricular infarction on enzymatically estimated infarct size, hemodynamics and prognosis. Circulation 62:503−508, 1980.

41. Marmor A, Geltman EM, Biello DR, Sobel BE, Siegel BA, Roberts R: Functional response of right ventricle to myocardial infarction: defence on the site of left ventricular infarction. Circulation 62:1005−1011, 1981.

42. Grande P, Hindman N, Saunamäki K, Wagner GS: Comparison of noninvasive techniques for estimation of myocardial infarct size. (In preparation.)

43. Rentrop P, Blanke H, Karsch KR, et al: Changes in left ventricular function after intracoronary streptokinase infusion in clinically evolving myocardial infarction. Am Heart J 102:1188−1193, 1981.

44. Markis JE, Malagold M, Parker JA, et al: Myocardial salvage after intracoronary thrombolysis with streptokinase in acute myocardial infarction: assessment by intracoronary thallium-201. N Engl J Med 305:777−782, 1981.

45. Vatner SF, Baig H, Manders WT, et al: Effect of coronary artery reperfusion on myocardial infarct size calculated from creatine kinase. J Clin Invest 61:1048, 1978.

46. Jarmakani JM, Limbird L, Graham TC, et al: Effects of reperfusion on myocardial infarct, and the accuracy of estimating infarct size from serum creatine phosphokinase in the dog. Cardiovasc Res 10:245, 1976.

47. Ganz W, Geft I: What is the role of thrombolytic therapy in acute myocardial infarction? Cardiovasc Clin 13:163−172, 1983.

48. Anderson JL, Marshall HW, Bray BE, et al: A randomized trial of intracoronary streptokinase in the treatment of acute myocardial infarction. N Engl J Med 308:1312−1318, 1983.

49. Schröder R, Biamino G, Leitner E-Rv, et al: Intravenous short-term infusion of streptokinase in acute myocardial infarction. Circulation 67: 536−643, 1983.

50. Blanke H, Von Hardenberg D, Cohen M, Kaiser H, Karsch KR, Holt J, Smith H, Rentrop P: Patterns of creatine kinase release during acute myocardial infarction after nonsurgical reperfusion: comparison with conventional treatment and correlation with infarct size. JACC 3:675−680, 1984.

51. Bresnahan GF, Roberts R, Shell WE, Ross J, Sobel BE: Deleterious effects due to hemorrhage after myocardial reperfusion. Am J Cardiol 33: 82−86, 1974.

52. Sharma GP, Hornay G: Serum CPK enzymes in myocardial ischemia followed by reperfusion. In: Fajaddin M, Bhata B, Siddiqui HH, et al (eds) Advances in myocardiology, vol 2. Baltimore: University Park Press, 1980, pp 383−396.

19. THE ABILITY OF THE QRS COMPLEX TO DETERMINE THE LOCATION AND SIZE OF MYOCARDIAL INFARCTS

Robert A. Warner

Galen S. Wagner

Raymond E. Ideker

The standard 12-lead electrocardiogram (ECG) remains the principal clinical method for evaluating patients with suspected acute ischemic syndromes and for establishing the diagnosis of "transmural" myocardial infarction. QRS complex changes are the most specific of the electrocardiographic indicators of myocardial infarction (MI). ST-segment and T-wave changes of all descriptions can be caused by reversible myocardial ischemia. Even many of the QRS changes of infarction can be mimicked by bundle branch block or ventricular hypertrophy. This chapter considers the relationships between specific QRS changes and both the location and the extent of myocardial infarcts.

Infarct Location

Specific changes in the QRS complex are indicative of infarcts in various locations in the heart, as indicated in chapter 9, in which Roberts and Gardin present terminology derived from anatomic observations and apply these to the changes in the QRS complex of the ECG. They consider "parallelism" in terminology to be very important and therefore consider the primary infarct locations within the left ventricle to be either "anterior" or "posterior." However, the interventricular septum in the living human is not parallel to the median sagittal plane of the body with the right ventricle to the right and the left ventricle to the left of that plane (figure 19-1). Rather, the septum is rotated so that the right ventricle is anterior and rightward and the left ventricle is posterior and leftward. Also, the conically shaped heart is tilted so that the "posterior" wall is inferior and posterior, and the "anterior" wall is superior and anterior.

It is also important to consider (see chapter 9) the common location of myocardial infarcts within both the "anterior" (or superior) and the "posterior" (or inferior) walls. As these authors note, "anterior" infarcts are primarily apical rather than basal (figure 19-2A) [1], and therefore do not occupy the more superior aspect of the anterior wall. Therefore, the changes in QRS complex produced by such infarcts do not tend to appear in leads directed superiorly and inferiorly (II, III, and aVF), but rather appear in those directed anteriorly and posteriorly (V_1 and V_2). Infarcts in this location cause the summation of early QRS forces to be directed away from leads V_1 and V_2 and are therefore termed "anterior" (AMI).

"Posterior" infarcts primarily involve the basal aspect of the left ventricle (figure 19-2B) because the vessel involved (the posterior descending branch of either the right or the left circumflex)

R.M. Califf and G.S. Wagner (eds.), ACUTE CORONARY CARE: Principles and Practice. Copyright © 1985. Martinus Nijhoff Publishing, Boston/Dordrecht/Lancaster.

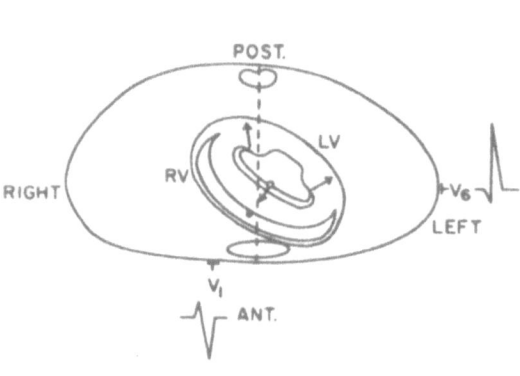

FIGURE 19-1. This is a schematic diagram of a cross-sectional view of the human thorax at the level of the ventricles. Most of the right ventricle but also a significant amount of the left ventricle lies to the right of the midline. Therefore, lead V_1 rather than lead V_6 is oriented perpendicularly in relationship to the interventricular septum. The right bundle is indicated as a dot on the right side of the septum and the left bundle as a dot on the left side. The direction of electrical activation via the three aspects of the left bundle is indicated. Infarction of the anteroseptal region would cause the summation of electrical forces to be directed away from lead V_1. Conversely, infarction of the "posterolateral" free wall would cause the summation of forces to be directed toward lead V_1.

does not extend to the apex in most patients [2]. These infarcts commonly cause QRS changes in leads directed superiorly and inferiorly (II, III, and aVF), rather than in those directed anteriorly and posteriorly (V_1 and V_2) [3]. Because the initial aspect of the QRS complex is directed away from leads II, III, and aVF, these infarcts are best termed "inferior" (IMI).

"Anterior" infarcts involve as much as three-fourths of the ventricular septum because of the length of the septal perforating branches of the left anterior descending artery. "Inferior" infarcts also may involve the septum, but only in its posterior fourth to third because of the short length of the septal perforating branches of the posterior descending artery [2].

"Anterior" infarcts may involve the anterior aspect of the free wall of the left ventricle and cause QRS forces to be directed away from the laterally oriented leads such as I and aVL [1]. "Inferior" infarcts may involve the posterior aspect of the free wall of the left ventricle and cause

forces to be directed toward the anteriorly oriented leads such as V_1 and V_2. Thus, the "true posterior" infarct location (which causes an increase in R-wave size in leads V_1 and V_2) lies lateral to, rather than basal to, the typical "inferior" infarct location [3].

Infarction in the distribution of a "nondominant" circumflex artery (does not supply the posterior descending branch) is much less common than in the other two locations [4]. When this does occur, however, it causes either increase in R-wave size in leads V_1 and V_2 ("true posterior") or increase in Q-wave size in leads I and aVL ("lateral").

Because the apex of the left ventricle lies nearest leads V_5 and V_6, infarction causes the initial aspect of the QRS complex to be directed away from these leads. Infarction of the apex rarely occurs alone, but rather as a part of extensive anterior infarction [5]. Less commonly, infarction of the posterior aspect of the apex is a part of extensive inferior infarction [3].

ECG versus VCG for Infarct Diagnosis

The ECG is one of the most widely used tests in clinical medicine and is generally considered to be an excellent means of diagnosing either acute or previous myocardial infarcts. When traditional methods of interpretation are used, however, the ECG often fails to perform optimally. A Q-wave duration of at least 40 ms (0.04 s) has commonly been considered as the QRS abnormality diagnostic of a myocardial infarction (see chapter 9). However, computer simulation of human heart activation by Selvester et al. [6] has indicated that a 30-ms Q wave in some leads (I, II, aVL, aVF, V_5, and V_6), a 20-ms Q wave in others (V_4), and, indeed, any Q wave in others (V_1, V_2, and V_3) are diagnostic of infarction. Conversely, even a 40-ms Q wave normally occurs in lead III. Therefore, nontraditional definitions of "abnormal Q waves" are required for optimal ECG diagnosis of infarcts.

A 30-ms Q wave in lead aVF has been found to have between 60% [7, 8] and 90% [3] sensitivity for the diagnosis of an isolated inferior myocardial infarction. Though lead III should be more sensitive, as noted above, its use is limited by inadequate specificity. Alternatively, lead II

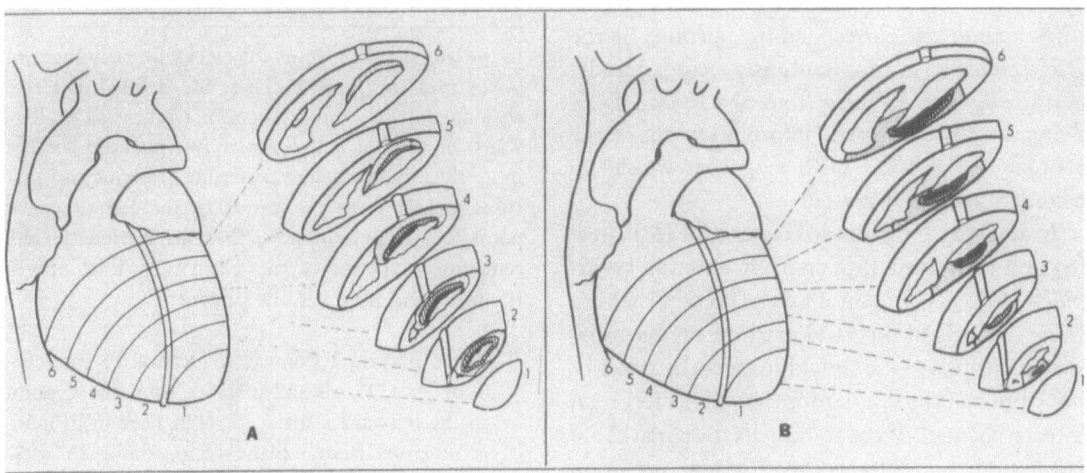

FIGURE 19-2. Typical anterior infarcts of various sizes are indicated in the distribution of the left anterior descending coronary artery in panel A, and inferior infarcts in the distribution of the posterior descending coronary artery are similarly indicated in panel B. Locations of small (solid), medium (solid + hatched), and large (solid + hatched + stippled) lesions are indicated in the six cross-sectioned slices in both areas. Small anterior infarcts are in the anterior aspect of the apex and they spread to involve the middle and basal aspects of the anterior wall as well as the apex circumferentially. Small inferior infarcts occur at the junction between the middle and basal aspects of the wall.

would be even more specific for diagnosis of IMI, but its sensitivity would be even less than that of aVF.

Standard ECG criteria have been shown to be insensitive for diagnosis of anterior MI [9], but new criteria proposed from computer simulation by Selvester et al. [6] identified 90% of isolated autopsy-proven anterior infarcts [1], and similar criteria were found to have 83% sensitivity by Warner et al. [10] for AMI identified at catheterization.

Various investigators have found that the vectorcardiogram (VCG) is superior to the traditional ECG for diagnosing myocardial infarcts [7, 9–12]. A recent study that compared the performances of three sets of traditional ECG to three sets of VCG criteria for IMI [12] showed that, although each of the ECG criteria sets were highly specific, their sensitivities ranged from only 4% to 34%. Thus, when applied to a population with IMI proven at catheterization, the traditional ECG criteria missed between 66% and 96% of all the infarcts. In contrast, each of the VCG criteria sets exhibited at least 90% specificity and at least 82% sensitivity.

However, the VCG is used much less commonly than is the ECG. Even the best diagnostic test will make no more than a minor impact on the management of patients with a particular disease if that test is applied to only a small portion of the population at risk for that disease. Therefore, it has been necessary to develop a new method of interpreting ECGs that permits derivation from the ECG, information that previously has been thought to be contained only in the VCG [8, 13, 14]. This method combines the diagnostic capabilities of the VCG with the ubiquity of the ECG, and has resulted in improved ability to diagnose MI, even under circumstances in which the VCG is not available.

Application of this method of interpretation requires that the ECGs be obtained using three-channel machines. These machines, which have been in widespread clinical use for several years, simultaneously record leads I, II, and III, then leads AVF, aVL, and aVF, then leads V_1, V_2, and V_3, and finally leads V_4, V_5, and V_6. Three-channel recorders were developed to facilitate the display of the entire ECG on a single $8\frac{1}{2} \times 11''$ sheet of paper. In addition to being more convenient, ECGs obtained using such devices contain significantly more diagnostic information than do those recorded with single-channel machines. The three-channel machines make it possible to analyze the temporal relationships among the corresponding portions of the QRS complexes of simultaneously recorded leads, permitting one to infer from a standard ECG diagnostically important information about the contour of the VCG QRS loop that would be recorded from that patient.

In applying the proposed criteria for IMI alone [8] and combined IMI and left anterior hemiblock [13], it is important to be certain that the three channels of the ECG machine are recorded simultaneously. One should inspect the times of inscription of the standardization marks recorded by each channel. If the standardization marks are not recorded simultaneously, then a correction for the discrepancy should be made. For example, if the standardization mark in channel 2 is inscribed 20 ms later than the marks in channels 1 and 3, then the QRS complexes in leads II and aVL are considered to have actually begun 20 ms earlier than is apparent on the write-out.

New ECG Criteria for Diagnosis of IMI

The VCG criteria upon which the new ECG criteria for diagnosing IMI are based are those of Starr et al. (table 19-1) [7]. These VCG criteria were chosen because they were shown by Hurd et al. to have the best overall diagnostic performance of three different sets of VCG criteria for IMI [12]. Several components of the VCG criteria should be emphasized: (a) at least the initial portion of the QRS loop in the frontal plane must be clockwise. (b) The very initial portion of the QRS loop may be directed inferiorly. Since this means that the first part of the loop is represented on the positive half of the axis of one or more of the inferior leads, it follows that the ECG of a patient with an IMI need not have Q waves in each of leads II, III, and aVF. (c) If the initial portion of the loop does proceed inferiorly from the origin, IMI can be diagnosed only if this part of the loop is entirely to the right of the origin. These three considerations led to the proposed ECG criteria for diagnosing IMI indicated in table 19-2.

Figure 19-3 demonstrates the method by which the direction of rotation of the QRS loop in the frontal plane can be inferred from the ECG. Figure 19-4 illustrates the importance of noting

TABLE 19-1. VCG criteria for IMI of Starr et al. [7]

In the frontal plane, generally clockwise early superior forces must be present. These are defined as forces that are initially either superior (rightward or leftward) or inferior and completely rightward for not more than 10 ms before becoming superior and that subsequently cross the x-axis to the left of the E point (or, less commonly, the entire efferent limb remaining superior to the x-axis). At least one of the following must also be present:

1. Time from the E point to the leftward x intercept of at least 25 ms and distance from the E point to the leftward x intercept of at least 0.30 mV.
2. A maximal frontal plane vector above 15° (less than 15°).
3. A maximal superior deviation of at least 0.10 mV and a ratio of maximal superior deviation to maximal inferior deviation of at least 1:5.

TABLE 19-2. ECG criteria for IMI

In the absence of counterclockwise rotation in the frontal plane:

1. Q waves of 30 ms or longer in lead II,

   and/or

2. Regression of initial inferior forces from lead III to lead II.

whether "regression of initial inferior forces from lead III to lead II" is present. "Regression of initial inferior forces from lead III to lead II" means that, at the instant that the QRS begins, the electrical forces recorded by lead II are less positive than those being recorded by lead III. This phenomenon may be manifested in any of the following ways: (a) an initial R wave in lead III associated with a lower R wave, an isoelectric segment, or a Q wave in lead II; (b) an isoelectric segment in lead III associated with a Q wave in lead II; or (c) a Q wave in lead III associated with a deeper Q wave in lead II. Regression of initial inferior forces from lead III to lead II occurs on the ECG because the QRS loop (as indicated by the VCG) begins to move in the frontal plane, rightward from the origin. A 30-ms or longer Q wave in lead II is approximately equivalent to the 25-ms initial superior time included in the VCG criteria of Starr et al. [7].

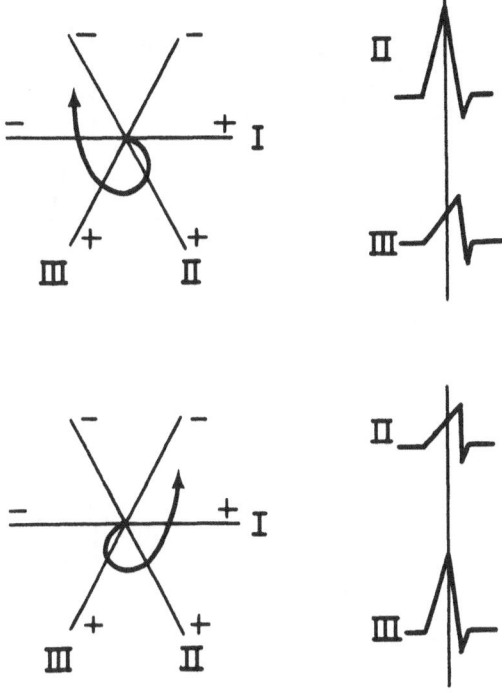

FIGURE 19-3. Two VCG loops in the frontal plane superimposed upon diagrams of the triaxial reference system. To the right of each loop are diagrams of the QRS complexes in scalar leads II and III that correspond to that loop. In the upper panel, the direction of rotation of the loop is clockwise. Since the initial portion of the loop is maximally represented on the positive half of the axis of lead II before it is maximally represented on the positive half of the axis of lead III, the peak of the R wave in lead II precedes the peak of the R wave in lead III. In the lower panel, the direction of rotation of the loop is counterclockwise. Since the initial portion of the loop is maximally represented on the positive half of the axis of lead III before it is maximally represented on the positive half of the axis of lead II, the peak of the R wave in lead III precedes the peak of the R wave in lead II.

Evaluation of the New Criteria

The diagnostic performance of the proposed criteria was tested using two series of patients [8]. The first series consisted of 333 patients studied in an ad hoc manner using an unblinded experimental design. The criteria were then applied to a confirmatory series of 94 patients using a blinded design (i.e., the electrocardiographer did not know the anatomic findings of each patient at the time the ECGs were read). For both the initial and confirmatory series, patients with and without IMI were identified using data obtained at cardiac catheterization. Patients with IMI were defined by >75% narrowing of the dominant coronary artery and asyneresis, akinesia, or dyskinesia of the inferior wall of the left ventricle as shown on contrast ventriculography in the right anterior oblique (RAO) projection. Patients without IMI were those without significant obstruction of the dominant coronary artery

and without abnormal motion of the inferior left ventricular wall. The sensitivities and specificities of the proposed ECG criteria in the initial and confirmatory series were, respectively: 91% and 92%, and 94% and 100%. The diagnostic performance of the proposed ECG criteria was statistically superior to the performances of two sets of more-traditional ECG criteria and equivalent to the performance of the VCG criteria from which the proposed criteria were derived.

Thus, either more optimally defined criteria based simply on scalar Q-wave dimensions or, more complexly, on vector initial force directions, can improve the accuracy of the standard 12-lead ECG for diagnosis of IMI. Such criteria have been developed, however, using ECGs that do not contain the potentially confounding factors such as bundle branch block or ventricular hypertrophy. It is also important to optimize the ability to use the ECG for infarct diagnosis in the presence of such factors.

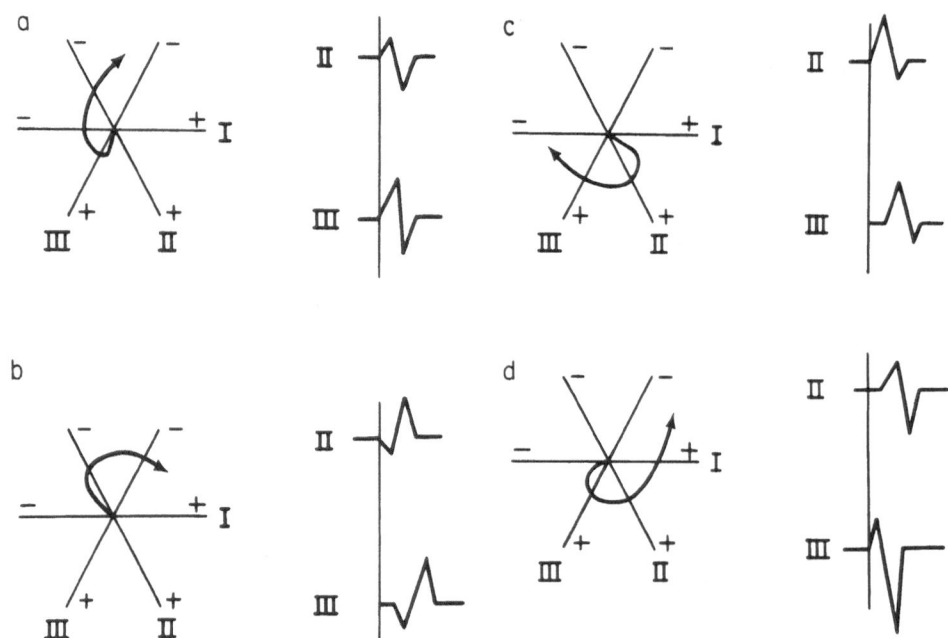

FIGURE 19-4. VCG QRS loops in the frontal plane superimposed upon diagrams of the triaxial reference system. To the right of each loop are diagrams of the QRS complexes in scalar leads II and III that correspond to that loop. When a segment of loop is represented on the positive half of a given lead axis (the left half in lead I and the inferior halves in leads II and III), the portion of the scalar QRS complex that corresponds to this segment is inscribed above the isoelectric line in that lead. Conversely, when a segment of the loop is represented on the negative half of a lead axis, the corresponding part of the QRS complex in this lead is inscribed below the isoelectric line. The magnitude of the deflection of a given portion of a QRS complex in a lead axis is related to the extent to which the corresponding segment of the VCG loop parallels the axis of that lead. For example, if the initial 10 ms of the loop is perpendicular to the axis of lead II, but not to leads I and III, then the QRS complexes recorded by lead II will appear to begin 10 msec later than those recorded by leads I and III.

The QRS complexes in panels A and B meet the proposed criteria for inferior infarction and the QRS complexes in panels C and D do not. (A) Clockwise loop that initially travels to the right of the E point and remains inferior for only a short time. Because the initial portion of the loop is more nearly parallel to the positive half of the axis of lead III than it is to the positive half of lead III, the R wave in lead III is taller than the R wave in lead II. (B) Clockwise loop that initially travels superiorly and to the right of the E point. Because the initial portion of the loop is perpendicular to the axis of lead III, the first portion of the Q wave in lead II coincides with an isoelectric segment in lead III. (C) Clockwise loop that initially travels inferiorly and to the left of the E point (thereby failing to conform to the VCG criteria of Starr et al. [7]). Since the initial portion of the loop is perpendicular to the axis of lead III and is more nearly parallel to the positive half of the axis of lead II, the initial part of the R wave in lead II coincides with an isoelectric segment in lead III. Thus, there is progression, rather than regression, of the initial inferior forces from lead III to lead II. (D) Counterclockwise loop that initially is perpendicular to the axis of lead II and is more nearly parallel to the positive half of the axis of lead III. Although this results in regression of initial inferior forces from lead III to II, because the peak of the R wave in lead III precedes the peak of the R wave in lead II, counterclockwise rotation in the frontal plane can be inferred. Therefore, the proposed criteria for inferior infarction are not met.

IMI in the Presence of Left Anterior Hemiblock

The traditional ECG diagnosis of IMI is more difficult when left anterior hemiblock (LAHB) coexists. One reason this combination presents a special diagnostic problem is that both IMI and LAHB tend to shift the QRS axis leftward in the frontal plane. Another reason is that in LAHB the ventricular activation occurring via the inferiorly directed posterior fascicle of the left bundle branch [15, 16] predominates. This decreases the ability of IMI to produce Q waves in leads II, III, and aVF. The diagnosis of combined IMI and LAHB is easier using the VCG than the traditional ECG because each of the abnormalities is associated with a characteristic change in contour of the QRS loop in the frontal plane. Since IMI causes clockwise rotation of the initial forces and LAHB causes counterclockwise rotation (most importantly of the terminal forces), combined IMI and LAHB exhibits clockwise rotation of the initial portion and counterclockwise rotation of the terminal portion of the QRS loop in the frontal plane [17−20]. This contour can be inferred from the ECG using the principles illustrated in figure 19-1. The proposed criteria for combined IMI and LAHB are shown in table 19-3.

The sensitivity and specificity of the proposed criteria were tested using ECGs obtained under clinical circumstances in which the presence and absence, respectively, of combined IMI and LAHB were highly likely [14]. Thirty-five patients with LAHB alone were identified: each had clinical, enzymatic and serial ECG evidence of isolated acute AMI and, in the course of these infarcts, developed left-axis deviation that was not previously present. Each of the 35 patients also manifested atrioventricular block as their infarcts continued to evolve. Patients [14] with clinical, enzymatic, and serial ECG evidence of isolated acute IMI were also identified. None of these patients had evidence of LAHB prior to their IMIs. Finally, 17 patients were identified with the combination of IMI and LAHB by: (a) clinical, enzymatic, and serial ECG evidence of acute IMI; and (b) ECGs obtained prior to the changes of acute IMI in which the QRS complexes in leads aVR and aVL both ended in R waves, with the peak of the terminal R wave in lead aVL preceding the peak of the terminal R wave in lead aVR. In a previous study, the above findings in leads aVR and aVL were identified as reliable markers of the presence of LAHB [13]. The ECG findings listed in table 19-4 were present only in the last and not in the first two groups of patients. The sensitivity and specificity of the proposed ECG criteria were each 100% and were statistically superior to each of ten combinations of traditional ECG criteria for combined IMI and LAHB.

New ECG Criteria for Diagnosis of AMI

Anterior myocardial infarction (AMI) would be expected to diminish the magnitude of the anteriorly directed electrical forces of depolarization. Therefore, the traditional ECG criteria for AMI require that Q waves and/or R waves of reduced amplitude be present in some combination of the right precordial leads. Warner et al. [10] evaluated the diagnostic performances of six different sets of such traditional ECG criteria on 116 patients in whom previous AMI was shown to be

TABLE 19-3. Performances[a] of criteria for the diagnosis of IMI

Series	Group	n	Proposed %	VCG[b] %	aVF[c] %	2, 3, aVF[d] %
Initial	Cases	139	91	81	59	29
	Noncases	194	92	98	92	96
Confirmatory	Cases	47	94	—	64	28
	Noncases	47	100	—	94	98

[a]The tabulated percentages are the observed sensitivities and specificities for the observed cases and noncases, respectively.
[b]VCG data are based on 67 cases and 86 noncases from the initial series. There were no VCGs in the confirmatory series.
[c]30-ms or longer Q wave in lead aVF (without regard to leads II or III).
[d]30-ms or longer Q wave in each of leads II, III, and aVF.

TABLE 19-4. EKG criteria for combined IMI and
LAHB

1. Leads aVR and aVL both end in R waves, with the
   peak of the terminal R wave in lead aVR occurring later than the peak of the terminal R wave
   in lead aVL.

and

2. A Q wave of any magnitude is present in lead II.

TABLE 19-5. Performances of the traditional ECG
criteria for AMI in groups A and B

Set of criteria	Sensitivity (%)	Specificity (%)	Relative odds
Lipman and Massie	64	99	176:1
McConahay			
Possible	53	100	113:1
Definite	42	100	72:1
Horan and Flowers	78	95	67:1
Chung	36	100	56:1
Friedman	61	93	21:1

either present or absent by cardiac catheterization. Patients with AMI (36) were defined as
those with a 75% or greater narrowing of the left
anterior descending coronary artery and either
akinesia or dyskinesia of the anterior left ventricular wall on contrast ventriculography in the
right anterior oblique projection. Patients without AMI (80) were defined as those with normal
coronary arteries and normal left ventriculograms.
Patients with left bundle branch block, left ventricular or type-C [21] right ventricular enlargement, and left anterior hemiblock were excluded
from both groups. The results of this evaluation
are shown in table 19-5.

In various sets of VCG criteria for AMI, the
duration of time that the initial QRS forces are
anterior to the point of origin is an important
diagnostic parameter [9, 22, 23]. This amount of
time can be estimated from the ECG (recorded at
the standard paper speed of 25 mm/s) as follows:
the widths of the initial R waves in each of leads
V_1-V_4 are compared with the widths of the
spaces between the 40-ms time lines of the ECG
paper. Therefore, measurement of the duration of
anteriorly directed forces of depolarization can be
obtained from the ECG as well as the VCG. The
abilities of a total of 28 different ECG parameters
of the magnitude of anterior forces (table 19-6) to
discriminate between patients with and without
AMI were determined [10]. The various combinations of the 28 parameters were also tested to
determine whether any combinations were superior to the individual parameters for diagnosing
AMI. The ten best parameters and combinations
of parameters for identifying AMI are listed in
table 19-7: nine utilize a measurement of the
duration of initial anterior forces. The diagnostic
performance of the best of the ECG criteria for
AMI (Q wave of any magnitude or an initial R

wave <20 ms in lead V_2) was compared with
that of the best of the traditional ECG criteria
for AMI (table 19-5—Lipman and Massie). The
former was superior to the latter (P <0.25).

Since abnormalities other than AMI can reduce
the magnitude of the anteriorly directed electrical forces of depolarization, it was also important
to evaluate the effects of several of these other
abnormalities upon the specificities of the various
criteria for AMI. Warner et al. [10] studied an
additional 83 patients who met angiographic
criteria for "no AMI" as follows: 32 patients with
left ventricular enlargement [24], 29 patients
with type-C right ventricular enlargement [25],
and 22 patients with left anterior hemiblock
[13]. Both left ventricular and type-C right ventricular enlargement reduced the specificity of
the criterion of "a Q wave or an R wave 20 ms in
duration in V_2" to only 81% and 83%, respectively. Left anterior hemiblock did not affect the
specificity of this criterion. However, the specificities for AMI of the more stringent criterion of
"a Q wave (of any magnitude) in lead V_2" were
97% in patients with either left ventricular or
type-C right ventricular enlargement and 100%
in left anterior hemiblock. As a result of the
analysis of all 199 patients, the comprehensive
criteria for diagnosing AMI listed in table 19-8
are recommended.

Infarct Size

Since the standard 12-lead ECG has proven valuable for infarct diagnosis, it is important to determine its value and limitations for infarct
sizing. The QRS complex that indicates presence
of infarction is also altered by ventricular hypertrophy and intraventricular conduction delays,

TABLE 19-6. Parameters used to evaluate initial anterior forces

Amplitudes of the initial R waves in leads V_1, V_2, V_3, and V_4

Durations of the initial R waves in leads V_1, V_2, V_3, and V_4

Ratios of the amplitudes of the R and S waves in leads V_1, V_2, V_3, and V_4

Sums of amplitudes of initial R waves in leads $V_1 + V_2$, $V_2 + V_3$, $V_1 + V_3$, and $V_1 + V_2 + V_3$

Sums of durations of initial R waves in leads $V_1 + V_2$, $V_2 + V_3$, $V_1 + V_3$, and $V_1 + V_2 + V_3$

Presence of poor progression or of regression of the amplitude of initial R waves in leads V_1 to V_4

Presence of poor progression or of regression of the duration of initial R waves in leads V_1 to V_4

Presence of Q waves in leads V_1, V_2, V_3, and/or V_4.

TABLE 19-7. Performances of the ten best criteria for AMI

Parameter	Sensitivity (%)	Specificity (%)	Relative odds
QinV2 or			
DRV2<20ms	83	99	483:1
QinV2	64	100	178:1
DRV3<30ms	86	96	147:1
ARV123<4.5mm	86	96	147:1
DRV2<20ms or			
DRV3<20ms	86	96	147:1
QinV2 or			
ARV3<1mm or			
DRV2<20ms or			
DRV3<20ms	86	96	147:1
QinV2 or			
DRV3<20ms	81	97	138:1
DRV123<55ms	83	96	117:1
DRV23<70ms	86	95	117:1
DRV3<30ms	78	97	115:1

QinV2 = Q wave of any magnitude in lead V_2; DRV2 = duration of initial R wave in lead V_2; DRV3 = duration of initial R wave in lead V_3; ARV123 = sum of amplitudes of initial R waves in leads V_1, V_2, and V_3; ARV3 = amplitude of initial R wave in lead V_3; DRV123 = sum of durations of initial R waves in leads V_1, V_2, and V_3; DRV23 = sum of durations of initial R waves in leads V_2 and V_3.

TABLE 19-8. Proposed ECG criteria for the diagnosis of AMI

In the absence of both LVE and type-C RVE:
A Q wave (of any magnitude) or an initial R wave less than 20 ms in duration is present in lead V_2.
In the presence of either LVE or type-C RVE:
A Q wave (of any magnitude) is present in lead V_2.

and infarcts on opposing myocardial walls tend to "cancel" QRS changes. These factors might diminish the usefulness of the ECG for infarct sizing. Evaluation of the capabilities of the ECG requires knowledge of the sequence of human heart activation, development of hypothetical criteria for the effects of alteration in this sequence by infarcts of various sizes and, finally, testing of these hypotheses using the standard of anatomically sized infarcts.

Following the documentation of the sequence of electrical activation of the myocardium in both experimental animals [26] and man [27], Solomon and Selvester simulated this sequence in a computerized model [28]. By sequentially eliminating areas of myocardium of various sizes in the distributions of the major coronary arteries, they were able to simulate the effect of infarctions of varying sizes in the different anatomic locations upon the electrical activity recorded from the body surface [29]. Results from these processes permitted the formulation of a scoring system using both qualitative and quantitative observations of the QRS complex [6]. This 32-point scoring system was designed so that each point would indicate infarction of approximately 3% of the left ventricle.

At the time of these observations, it had not yet been proven that there was a close relationship between specific QRS changes on ECG and anatomic infarct location. Therefore, studies were designed to determine whether there were specific and sensitive quantitative QRS criteria for both inferior [7] and anterior [9] infarct locations. These studies demonstrated both high sensitivity and specificity for criteria obtained from the Frank lead vectorcardiogram and, thereby, established the relationship between QRS changes and infarct location. A subsequent study demonstrated the limitations of these criteria [30] in patients with left ventricular hypertrophy.

An initial series of studies evaluated the ability of a simplified version of this scoring system that considered only Q- and R-wave durations and R/Q- or R/S-wave amplitude ratios for estimating the extent of single infarcts in patients without the confounding factors of ventricular hypertrophy or bundle branch block on ECG and for whom postmortem measurement of anatomic infarct size had been obtained. A preliminary evaluation of both intra- and interobserver variability and a determination of the specificity of the scoring system in normal controls were performed [31]. Each of the 37 criteria included in this simplified 29-point version (table 19-9) of the scoring system was required to achieve at least 95% specificity in a control population proven to be free of both coronary atherosclerosis and ventricular wall motion abnormality by cardiac catheterization. Hearts obtained from postmortem examinations evaluated by a common protocol were studied. Only those patients with a single infarction present at postmortem examination were included. A previously described method for estimating the anatomic extent of myocardial infarcts from postmortem hearts [32] was used as the standard for infarct size. A system was devised for dividing each of the transverse heart

TABLE 19-9. Scoring system for estimating the size of myocardial infarction

Lead	criteria (no. of points)		Maximum points
I	Q$\geq$30ms(1)	R/Q$\leq$1(1)	2
II	Q$\geq$40ms(2)		2
	Q$\geq$30ms(1)		
aVL	Q$\geq$30ms(1)	R/Q$\leq$1(1)	2
aVF	Q$\geq$50ms(3)	R/Q$\leq$1(2)	5
	Q$\geq$40ms(2)	R/Q$\leq$2(1)	
	Q$\geq$30ms(1)		
V$_1$	Any Q(1)		4
	R$\geq$50ms(2)		
	R$\geq$40ms(1)	R/S$\geq$1(1)	
V$_2$	Any Q or R $\leq$20ms(1)		4
	R$\geq$60 ms(2)		
	R$\geq$50 ms(1)	R/S$\geq$1.5(1)	
V$_3$	Any Q or R $\leq$30ms(1)		1
V$_4$	Q$\geq$20ms(1)	R/Q or R/S$\leq$0.5(2)	3
		R/Q or R/S$\leq$1(1)	
V$_5$	Q$\geq$30ms(1)	R/Q or R/S$\leq$1(2)	3
		R/Q or R/S$\leq$2(1)	
V$_6$	Q$\geq$30ms(1)	R/Q or R/S$\leq$1(2)	3
		R/Q or R/S$\leq$3(1)	

slices into octants for precise localization of the infarcts. In 21 patients with anterior infarcts the correlation between the QRS score obtained from the final ECG prior to death and the measured infarct size was $r = 0.80$ [1], in 31 patients with inferior infarcts the correlation was $r = 0.74$ [3], and in 20 patients with posterolateral infarcts the correlation was $r = 0.72$ [4].

The left ventricular ejection fraction has been shown to have important prognostic ability in patients with recent acute myocardial infarction [33, 34]. Palmeri et al. [35] documented a good correlation between the QRS score and the left ventricular ejection fraction at three weeks, eight weeks, and one year following an acute myocardial infarction and this was confirmed by other investigators [36, 37]. In an additional study of all patients undergoing cardiac catheterization and subsequently receiving only medical management, the prognostic capability of the QRS scoring system was documented [38].

Summary

Many technologic advances have been required to facilitate the studies presented in this chapter to evaluate the ability of the common 12-lead ECG for locating and sizing myocardial infarcts. This improved understanding has become particularly important since sophisticated, but potentially dangerous, medical (see chapter 6) and surgical (see chapter 35) therapies have been developed. Their success requires immediate implementation when the patient first presents with symptoms of acute myocardial ischemia or infarction. A standard 12-lead ECG may be the only method sufficiently cost and time effective to determine which patients should receive aggressive medical or surgical therapy versus rest on the CCU. Comparison of the relationship between the quantitative changes on the initial and subsequent ECGs may also prove useful for clinical determination of the outcome of the various forms of therapy for these patients.

References

1. Ideker RE, Wagner, GS, Ruth WK, Alonso DR, Bishop SP, Bloor CM, Fallon JT, Gottlieb GJ, Hackel DB, Phillips HR, Reimer KA, Roark SF, Rogers WJ, Savage RM, White RD, Selvester RH: Evaluation of a QRS scoring system for estimating myocardial infarct size. II. Correlation with quantitative anatomic findings for anterior infarcts. Am J Cardiol 49:1604–1614, 1982.

2. James TN: Anatomy of the coronary arteries. New York: Paul Hoeber, 1961.

3. Roark SF, Ideker RE, Wagner GS, Alonso DR, Bishop SP, Bloor CM, Fallon JT, Gottlieb GJ, Hackel DB, Phillips HR, Reimer KA, Rogers WJ, Ruth WK, Savage RM, White RD, Selvester RH: Evaluation of a QRS scoring system for estimating myocardial infarct size. III. Correlation with quantitative anatomic findings for inferior infarcts. Am J Cardiol 51:382–389, 1983.

4. Ward RM, White RD, Ideker RE, Hindman NB, Alonso DR, Bishop SP, Bloor CM, Fallon JT, Gottlieb GJ, Hackel DB, Hutchins GM, Phillips HR, Reimer KA, Roark SF, Rochlani SP, Rogers WJ, Ruth WK, Savage RM, Weiss JL, Selvester RH, Wagner GS: Evaluation of a QRS scoring system for estimating myocardial infarct size. IV. Correlation with quantitative anatomic findings for posterolateral infarcts. Am J Cardiol 53:706–714, 1984.

5. Savage RM, Wagner GS, Ideker RE, Podolsky SA, Hackel DB: Correlation of postmortem anatomic findings with electrocardiographic changes in patients with myocardial infarction: retrospec-

6. Selvester RH, Sanmarco ME, Solomon JC, Wagner GS: The ECG: QRS change. In: Wagner GS (ed) Myocardial infarction: measurement and intervention. The Hague: Martinus Nijhoff, 1982, pp 23–50.

7. Starr JW, Wagner GS, Behar VS, Walston A II, Greenfield JC Jr: Vectorcardiographic criteria for the diagnosis of inferior myocardial infarction. Circulation 49:829–836, 1974.

8. Warner R, Hill NE, Sheehe PR, Mookherjee S, Fruehan CT, Smulyan H: Improved electrocardiographic criteria for the diagnosis of inferior myocardial infarction. Circulation 66:422, 1982.

9. Starr JW, Wagner GS, Draffin RM, Reed JB, Walston A II, Behar VS: Vectorcardiographic criteria for the diagnosis of anterior myocardial infarction. Circulation 53:229–234, 1976.

10. Warner RA, Reger M, Hill NE, Mookherjee S, Smulyan H: Electrocardiographic criteria for the diagnosis of anterior myocardial infarction: importance of the duration of precordial R waves. Am J Cardiol 52:690–692.

11. Lee GB, Wilson WJ, Amplatz K, Tuna N: Correlation of the vectorcardiogram and electrocardiogram with the coronary arteriogram. Circulation 38:189, 1968.

12. Hurd HP, Starling MR, Crawford MH, Diabal PW, O'Rourke RA: Comparative accuracy of electrocardiographic and vectorcardiographic criteria for inferior myocardial infarction. Circulation 63:1025, 1981.

13. Warner RA, Hill NE, Mookherjee S, Smulyan H: Improved electrocardiographic criteria for the diagnosis of left anterior hemiblock. Am J Cardiol 51:723, 1983.

14. Warner RA, Hill NE, Mookherjee S, Smulyan H: Electrocardiographic criteria for the diagnosis of combined inferior myocardial infarction and left anterior hemiblock. Am J Cardiol 51:716, 1983.

15. Catellanos A, Chahine RA, Chapunoff E, Gomez J, Portillo B: Diagnosis of left anterior hemiblock in the presence of inferior wall myocardial infarction. Chest 60:543, 1971.

16. Rosenbaum MB, Elizari MV, Lazzari JO: The hemiblocks. Oldsmar: Tampa Tracings, 1970, pp 227, 223 and 273.

17. Benchimol A, Desser KB, Schumacher J: Value of the vectorcardiogram for distinguishing left anterior hemiblock from inferior infarction with left axis deviation. Chest 61:74, 1972.

18. Kulbertus HE, Collignon P, Humblet L, Deleval-Rutten F: Left axis deviation in inferior infarction: vectorcardiographic recognition of concomitant left anterior hemiblock. Chest 60:362, 1971.

19. Kohn PM, Harris AH: Vectorcardiographic analysis of left axis deviation in the differentiation of diaphragmatic infarction and parietal block. Dis Chest 47:492, 1965.

20. Castellanos A, Chahine RA, Chapunoff E, Gomez J, Portillo B: Diagnosis of left anterior hemiblock in the presence of inferior wall myocardial infarction. Chest 60:543, 1971.

21. Chou T-C, Helm RA, Kaplan S: Clinical vectorcardiography, 2nd edn. New York: Grune and Stratton, 1974, pp 103−113.

22. Hugenholtz PG, Forkner CE Jr, Levine HD: A clinical appraisal of the vectorcardiogram in myocardial infarction. II. The Frank system. Circulation 24:825, 1961.

23. Hoffman I: Clinical vectorcardiography in adults: part 1. Am Heart J 100:329, 1980.

24. Romhilt DW, Estes EH: A point-score system for ECG diagnosis of left ventricular hypertrophy. Am Heart J 75:752, 1968.

25. Selvester RH, Rubin HB: New criteria for the electrocardiographic diagnosis of emphysema and cor pulmonale. Am Heart J 69:437, 1965.

26. Scher AM, Young AC: The pathway of ventricular depolarization in the dog. Circ Res 4:461−469, 1956.

27. Durrer D, Van Dam RT, Freud GE, Janse MJ, Meijler FL, Arzbaecher RC: Total excitation of the isolated human heart. Circulation 41:899−912, 1970.

28. Solomon JC, Selvester RH: Simulation of measured activation sequence in the human heart. Am Heart J 85:518−524, 1973.

29. Selvester RH, Wagner JO, Rubin HB: Quantitation of myocardial infarct size and location by electrocardiogram and vectorcardiogram. In: Snellen HA, et al (eds) Quantitation in cardiology. The Hague: Leiden University Press, 1972, pp 31−44.

30. Phillips HR, Starr JW, Behar VS, Walston A II, Greenfield JC Jr, Wagner GS: Evaluation of vectorcardiographic criteria for the diagnosis of myocardial infarction in the presence of left ventricular hypertrophy. Circulation 53:235−240, 1976.

31. Wagner GS, Freye CJ, Palmeri ST, Roark SF, Stack NC, Ideker RE, Harrell FE, Selvester RH: Evaluation of a QRS scoring system for estimating myocardial infarct size. I. Specificity and observer agreement. Circulation 65:342−347, 1982.

32. Ideker RE, Behar VS, Wagner GS, Starr JW, Starmer CF, Lee KL, Hackel DB: Evaluation of asynergy as an indicator of myocardial fibrosis. Circulation 57:715−725, 1978.

33. Borer JS, Rosing DR, Miller RH, Stark RM, Kent KM, Bacharach SL, Green MV, Lake CR, Cohen H, Holmes D, Donohue D, Baker W, Epstein SE: Natural history of left ventricular function during the year after acute myocardial infarction: comparison with clinical, electrocardiographic and biochemical determinations. Am J Cardiol 46:1−12, 1980.

34. Shah PK, Pichler M, Berman DS, Singh BN, Swan HJC: Left ventricular ejection fraction determined by radionuclide ventriculography in early stages of first transmural myocardial infarction: relation to short term prognosis. Am J Cardiol 45:542−546, 1980.

35. Palmeri ST, Harrison DG, Cobb FR, Morris KG, Harrell FE, Ideker RE, Selvester RH, Wagner GS: A QRS scoring system for assessing left ventricular function after myocardial infarction. N Engl J Med 306:4−9, 1982.

36. Seino Y, Staniloff HM, Shell WE, Mickle D, Shah PK, Vyden JK: Evaluation of a QRS scoring system in acute myocardial infarction: relation to infarct size, early stage left ventricular ejection fraction, and exercise performance. Am J Cardiol 52:37−42, 1983.

37. Roubin GS, Shen WF, Kelly DT, Harris PJ: The QRS scoring system for estimating myocardial infarct size: clinical, angiographic and prognostic correlations. JACC 2:38−44, 1983.

38. Bounous EP, Hinohara T, Califf RM, Harrell FE, Ideker RE, Selvester RH, Wagner GS: The prognostic significance of a QRS scoring system for estimation of left ventricular infarct size in patients with coronary artery disease.

20. RADIONUCLIDE TECHNIQUES FOR DIAGNOSING AND SIZING OF MYOCARDIAL INFARCTION

Frans J. Th. Wackers

Radionuclide techniques have acquired an important place in the evaluation of patients with acute ischemic heart disease. Because of the noninvasive nature of the techniques and the capability to perform studies at the patient's bedside, these studies can be obtained in critically ill patients with little discomfort to the patient. Two techniques are employed: (a) myocardial imaging, and (b) assessment of right and left ventricular function. The field of nuclear cardiology and its applications is still evolving as new and sophisticated computer software is becoming widely available and new radiotracers are being introduced.

Radionuclide Techniques

THALLIUM-201 MYOCARDIAL SCINTIGRAPHY (see chapter 51)

Thallium-201 accumulates in the body in proportion to the distribution of cardiac output. In the myocardium the distribution of thallium-201 reflects coronary blood flow. In normal subjects, the accumulation in the left ventricle is more or less homogeneous. In patients with acute myocardial infarction, the area of infarction is visualized as an area deficient of radiotracer uptake [1]. Thallium-201 myocardial imaging preferably is performed in multiple views in order to visualize all myocardial segments as completely as pos-

sible: anterior view, 45° left anterior oblique view, and left lateral view. For the latter view, the patient is turned on the right side, so that accurate visualization of the posterior wall can be achieved. For static imaging of myocardial infarction, computer acquisition is not necessary. When quantitation of defect size is performed, acquisition in 128 × 128 matrix and generation of circumferential count profiles is the preferred technique. Visual analysis of thallium-201 images preferably is performed using a continuous gray scale.

TECHNETIUM-99m-PYROPHOSPHATE MYOCARDIAL IMAGING

Technetium-99m-labeled Sn-pyrophosphate is a bone-imaging agent, which has been found to accumulate in acutely infarcted myocardium. The uptake occurs in the peripheral zones of an area of necrosis on depositions of calcium−apatite crystals. Intense myocardial accumulation of technetium-99m-pyrophosphate is specific for acute myocardial infarction [2]. As for thallium imaging, pyrophosphate imaging is performed in three standard views. Myocardial imaging is performed $1\frac{1}{2}-2$ h after injection of the radiopharmaceutical when the blood pool is cleared of radiotracer. An important aspect of imaging with this radiopharmaceutical is quality control of labeling efficiency.

R.M. Califf and G.S. Wagner (eds.), ACUTE CORONARY CARE: Principles and Practice. Copyright © 1985. Martinus Nijhoff Publishing, Boston/Dordrecht/Lancaster.

MULTIGATED CARDIAC BLOOD POOL IMAGING

For multigated cardiac blood pool imaging, the patient's red blood cells are labeled with technetium-99m. To achieve this, the red cells are "pretreated" with cold stannous—pyrophosphate, followed 15 min later by an injection of 20 mCi of technetium-99m. Imaging is performed with a single crystal gamma camera that is interfaced with a dedicated minicomputer. Data acquisition is performed in frame mode, using the electrocardiographic R wave as a synchronizing signal. Each RR interval is divided in 16—32 equal segments. The summed serial data acquired for each segment from 200 to 300 heartbeats are stored in computer memory. For data analysis, the summed images of each frame are displayed as an endless loop movie. Usually three standard views are obtained: anterior view, left anterior oblique view, and left lateral view. Left ventricular ejection fraction is calculated after background correction from the left anterior oblique image: end-diastolic counts minus end-systolic counts, divided by end-diastolic counts [3]. The studies further allow for evaluation of the size of the various chambers, great vessels, and regional wall motion.

FIRST-PASS RADIONUCLIDE ANGIOGRAPHY

For reliable first-pass angiocardiography, high count rate capability of the detection system is a necessity. The conventional single-crystal cameras are presently not capable of acquiring sufficiently high count rates. Therefore, these studies are preferably performed employing a multicrystal gamma camera. It is to be expected that further development of digital gamma cameras will allow adequate count rate first-pass studies in the near future. After a rapid bolus injection of the radioactive tracer, the first transit of the radioactive tracer through the central circulation is monitored. Right and left ventricular ejection fraction can be calculated by generating a time—activity curve over regions of interest over the ventricles and counts in end-diastole and end-systole.

GATED FIRST-PASS ANGIOCARDIOGRAPHY

The gated first-pass technique is a modification and combination of the multigated technique and first-pass technique. The injection technique is the same as for first-pass studies. However, the acquisition is performed using the R wave of the electrocardiogram as a synchronizing signal. The data acquisition is discontinued as soon as the bolus enters the main pulmonary artery. These studies are preferably performed in the right anterior oblique position and, since no background activity is present, the right ventricular ejection fraction can be calculated in the usual manner without need for background subtraction.

The Diagnosis of Myocardial Infarction

THALLIUM-201 MYOCARDIAL SCINTIGRAPHY

Thallium-201 myocardial imaging is a reliable sensitive technique for detecting acute myocardial infarction. During the first 6 h after onset of chest pain, > 90% of patients with myocardial infarction have abnormal thallium-201 images [1]. Figure 20-1 shows an example of acute myocardial infarctions at different anatomic locations as visualized by thallium-201. With increasing time interval after onset of chest pain, the sensitivity of thallium-201 scintigraphy to detect infarction decreases. This is particularly true in patients with nontransmural or small myocardial infarction (figure 20-2). Large myocardial infarctions are indefinitely visible on thallium-201 scans. Serial myocardial scintigraphy demonstrated that frequently perfusion defects present in patients with acute myocardial infarction during the acute phase decrease in size when the time interval between onset of chest pain and imaging increases. A possible explanation for this phenomenon is that during the *acute* phase of myocardial infarction both ischemic and necrotic myocardium is demonstrated, whereas on later scans only infarcted myocardium is visualized. It seems likely that this difference in defect size represents an area of jeopardized myocardium. We observed that, in patients who demonstrated such a decrease in size of defect, a postmyocardial infarction thallium-201 exercise test was able to "reproduce" the acute image on the immediately postexercise images. The location of myocardial infarction as assessed from multiple-view scans correlates well with electrocardiographic location

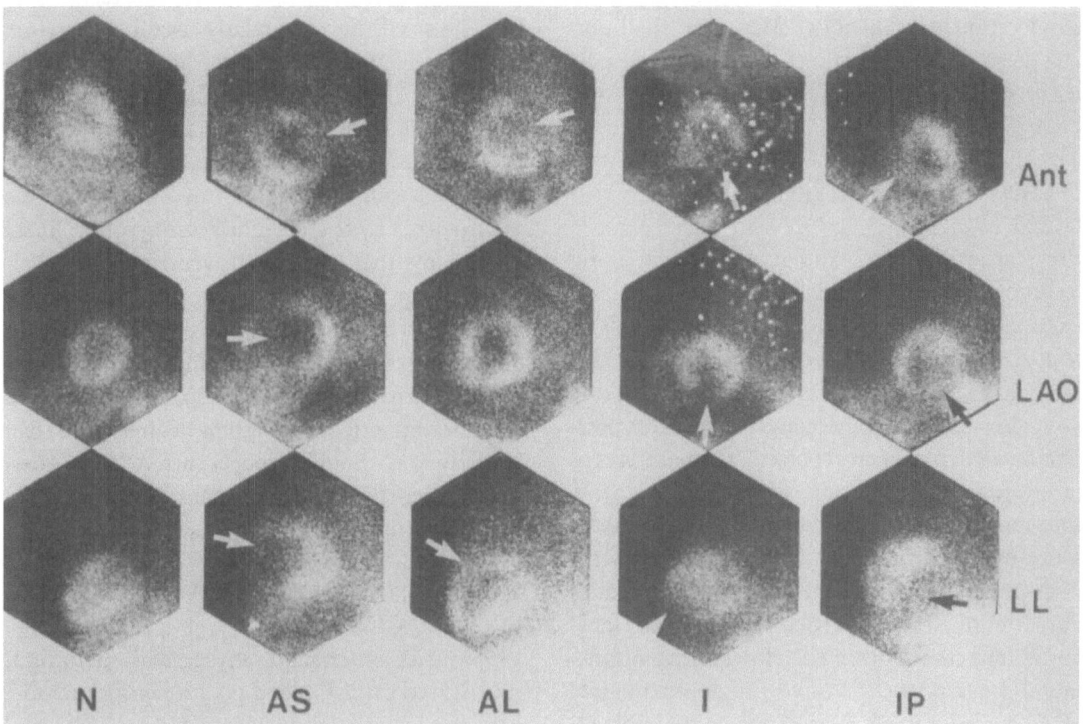

FIGURE 20-1. Typical examples of acute myocardial infarction visualized with thallium-201 myocardial scintigraphy in anterior (ANT), 45° anterior oblique (LAO), and left lateral (LL) projections.
The first column shows a normal (N) thallium-201
scan. The second to fourth columns show defects
(arrows) caused by acute myocardial infarction involving the anteroseptal (AS), anterolateral (AL), inferior
(I), and inferoposterior (IP) walls. From Wackers et al.
[1], with permission.

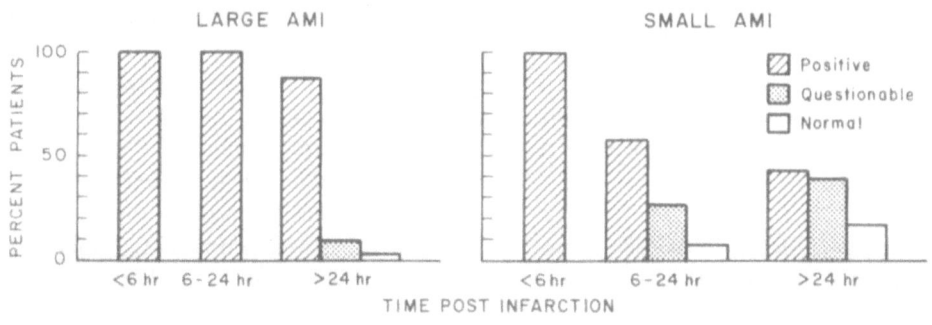

FIGURE 20-2. Results of thallium-201 scintigraphy in
patients with biochemically large and biochemically
small acute myocardial infarction in relation to time
interval after onset of chest pain.

of infarction. Also, the correlation with postmortem location is excellent [4]. Moreover, thallium-201 scans are more accurate in recognizing posterior wall involvement than the electrocardiogram.

TECHNETIUM-99m-PHYROPHOSPHATE IMAGING

The enthusiasm for employing this imaging technique for diagnosing acute myocardial infarction has declined in recent years. This is related to the fact that the sensitivity of this imaging method is the highest between 24 and 48 h after infarction. Although some early positive results have been reported, they are exceptions rather than the rule. Nevertheless, in the appropriate time frame the sensitivity to detect acute myocardial infarction with technetium-99m-pyrophosphate imaging is high, exceeding 90% (figure 20-3). In particular, almost all transmural infarcts are detected. However, nontransmural infarcts are detected in approximately 60%. If repeat imaging is performed, almost all myocardial infarcts can be detected [5]. The intensity and configuration of technetium-99m-pyrophosphate uptake in the myocardium have been reported to be of prognostic significance. Massive uptake or a "donut" appearance indicates large myocardial infarction and poor prognosis. The intensity of accumulation of technetium-99m-pyrophosphate in an infarct usually tapers approximately $5-7$ days after onset of acute chest pain. In most patients the imagines are negative at discharge. However, 10% of the patients may have a persistent positive technetium-99m-pyrophosphate scan after myocardial infarction. It has been suggested that this finding is of prognostic significance. Patients demonstrating this pattern appear to have more recurrent infarction, recurrent angina, and a greater incidence of congestive heart failure.

DUAL-ISOTOPE MYOCARDIAL IMAGING

Combined imaging of thallium-201 and technetium-99m-pyrophosphate can be useful in two clinical situations. First, in small and nontransmural myocardial infarction, both thallium-201 and technetium-99m-pyrophosphate imaging are less sensitive. When the two techniques are combined, however, almost all myocardial infarcts will be detected by either of the two techniques [6]. This will be particularly useful in patients with nondiagnostic electrocardiograms who are admitted to rule out myocardial infarction. Second, when right ventricular infarction is suspected, dual myocardial imaging is useful for precise anatomic location of myocardial necrosis as visualized by technetium-99m-pyrophosphate uptake in either left or right ventricle. The thallium image provides an anatomic marker for localizing the septum of the left ventricle. In employing dual-isotope imaging, we have demonstrated that right ventricular involvement in inferior infarction was far more frequent than initially was thought and occurred in approximately one-third of the patients with acute inferior infarction [7].

MULTIGATED CARDIAC BLOOD POOL IMAGING

In patients with acute myocardial infarction, multigated cardiac blood pool imaging provides particularly useful clinical information. Regional wall motion abnormalities can be detected by multiple-view imaging indicating the site and extent of myocardial infarction. Calculation of right and left ventricular ejection fraction provides an objective measure of the degree of impairment to cardiac function. Patients with anterior wall myocardial infarction as a rule have lower left ventricular ejection fraction than patients with inferior myocardial infarction, reflecting that anterior myocardial infarcts usually are large. Many patients with inferior wall myocardial infarction may have well-preserved global left ventricular function. However, a subgroup can be identified with a lower left ventricular ejection fraction. The latter patients often have on the electrocardiogram, in addition to inferior ST-segment elevation, anterior ST-segment depression. This most likely reflects reciprocal changes from extensive posterior infarction.

In patients with acute myocardial infarction, marked spontaneous changes of left ventricular ejection fraction may occur during the first 24 h after infarction [9]. Although overall mean left ventricular ejection fraction in a group of patients is unchanged, one-third demonstrate improvment, one-third demonstrate deterioration, and one-third demonstrate no change of left ventricu-

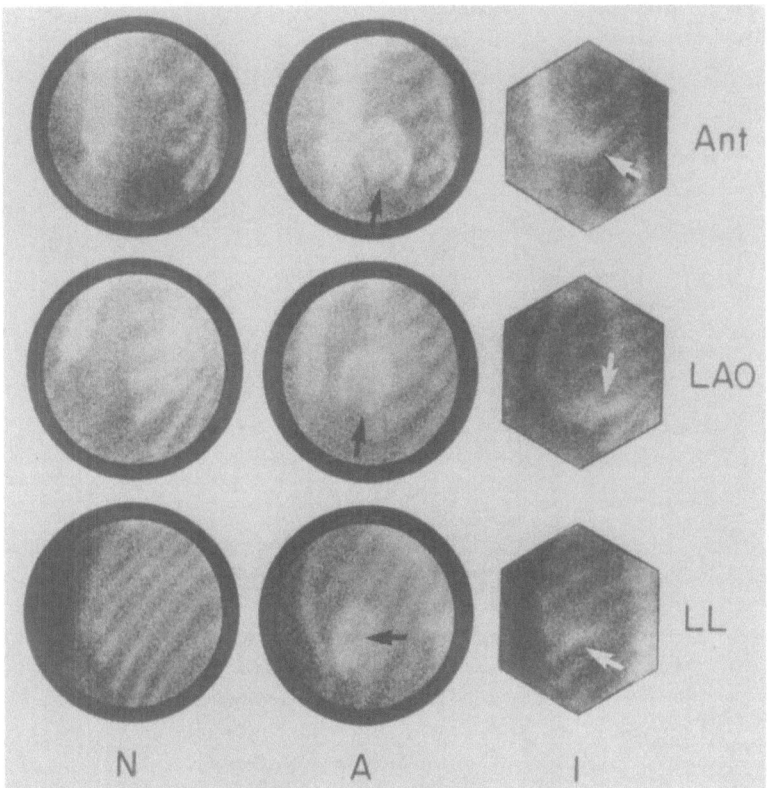

FIGURE 20-3. Typical examples of acute myocardial infarction visualized with technetium-99m-pyrophosphate in anterior (ANT), 45° left anterior oblique (LAO), and left lateral (LL) projections. The first column shows a normal scan. The bony skeleton is visualized. The second and third columns show abnormal accumulation (arrows) of technetium-99m-pyrophosphate in acute myocardial infarction involving the anterior (A) and inferior (I) walls.

lar ejection fraction. These spontaneous changes in left ventricular function have no apparent correlation to infarct extension or changes in loading conditions. They probably represent intrinsic changes in myocardial contractility. This finding has important practical consequences for analysis of results of acute interventions, such as intercoronary streptokinase infusion in patients with acute myocardial infarction. In order to assess the effect of such modalities, large numbers of patients need to be studied to achieve statistical significance. As mentioned above, right ventricular involvement in the setting of inferior infarction is a common phenomenon occurring in ap-

proximately one-third of patients with acute inferior wall infarction. Consistent with findings by technetium-99m-pyrophosphate imaging is that approximately one-third of the patients with inferior infarction have depressed right ventricular ejection fraction.

For a rapid, bedside diagnosis of right ventricular infarction, multigated blood pool images are extremely useful. A typical patient shows a markedly dilated, hypokinetic right ventricle with often preserved left ventricular function (figure 20-4). The degree of right ventricular and left ventricular involvement is variable and represents a continuum. At one end there is predominant right ventricular infarction, inbetween biventricular infarction, and at the opposite end of the spectrum there is predominant left ventricular infarction with either minimal or no right ventricular involvement. In view of the importance of recognizing the syndrome of right ventricular infarction, and the relative ease with which these data can be obtained by multigated blood pool imaging, we feel that in each patient

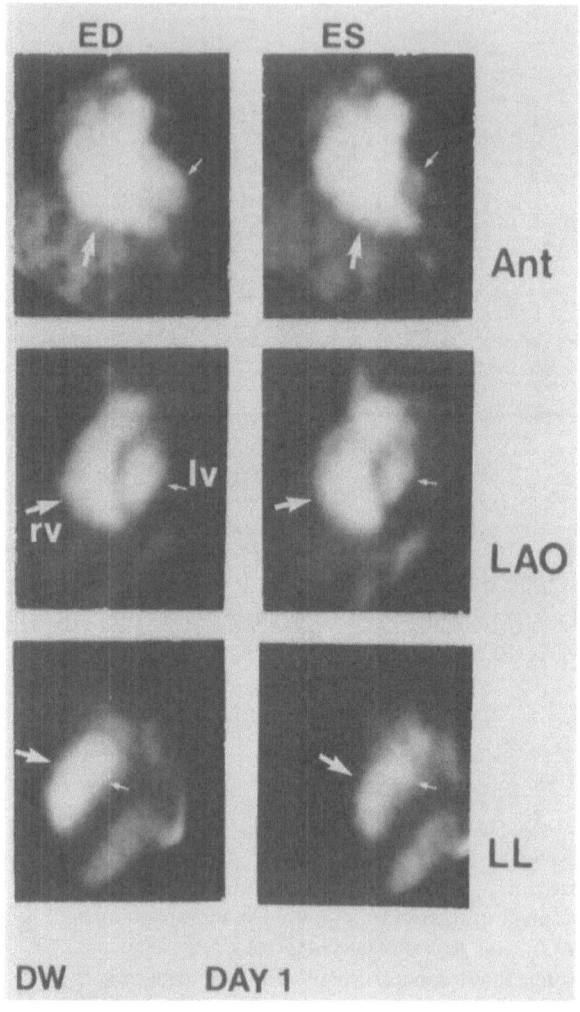

FIGURE 20-4. Typical example of multigated cardiac blood pool imaging in a patient with predominant right ventricular (RV) infarction and normal left ventricular (LV) function. On the three views: anterior (ANT), 45° left anterior oblique (LAO), and left lateral (LL), it can be appreciated that the RV is markedly dilated and diffusely hypokinetic. These images are typical for right ventricular infarction. ED, end-diastole; ES, end-systole.

with inferior wall infarction and hypotensive episodes this particular radionuclide study is indicated—the more so since hemodynamic parameters are not always unequivocally diagnostic. Right ventricular ejection fraction in these patients should be quantitated by the gated first-pass technique. A remarkable finding is that, in many of these patients who initially have severely depressed right ventricular ejection fraction, spontaneous improvement may occur during the subsequent days. As with global left ventricular and right ventricular ejection fraction, also regional wall motion may demonstrate spontaneous changes over the course of time.

Size of Myocardial Infarction

THALLIUM-201 MYOCARDIAL SCINTIGRAPHY

The extent of myocardial perfusion defects on thallium-201 scans correlates well with the extent of necrosis or scar tissue found at postmortem [4] (figure 20-5). However, planar thallium-

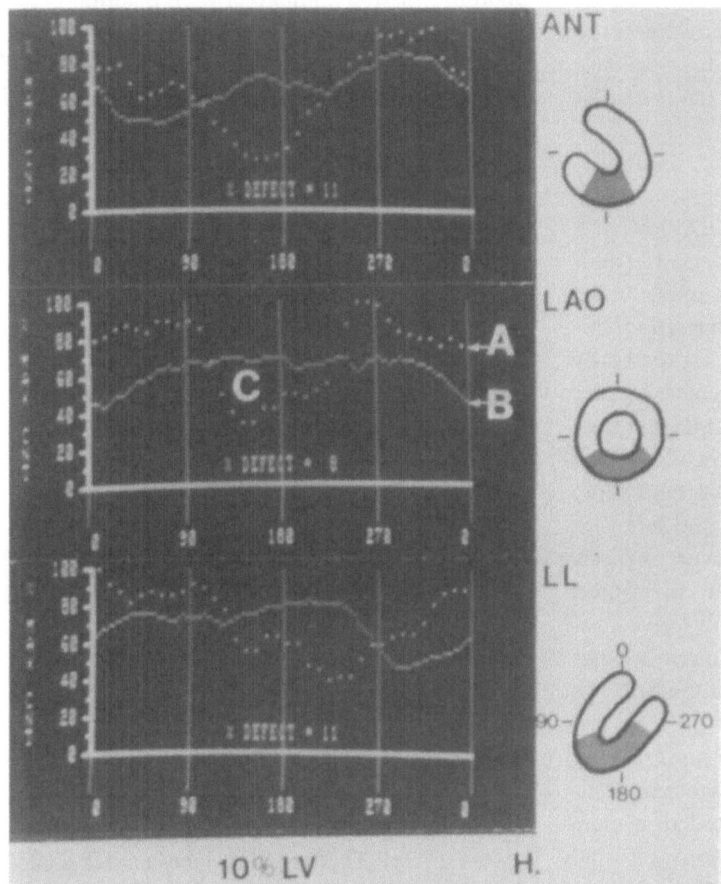

FIGURE 20-5. Example of quantitation of thallium-201 perfusion defect by circumferential profile analysis. The patient's thallium-201 scan indicated an inferoapical perfusion defect on three views, schematically shown as shaded areas. The circumferential profiles (dotted lines, A) for each view display the distribution of thallium-201 throughout the ventricle from 0° to 360°. The lower limit of normal thallium-201 distribution is displayed as continuous lines (B). The area of the perfusion defect (dotted line below the continuous line, (C) is expressed as "percent of whole left ventricle." In the example shown, the size of the myocardial perfusion defect, on three views, averages 10% of the left ventricle.

201 imaging is intrinsically limited in totally visualizing all myocardial segments. More recently, single-photon emission tomography with thallium-201 in patients with recent myocardial infarction demonstrated a close correlation ($r = 0.89$) between infarct volume as calculated from tomographic images and CK-MB release curves.

It is of clinical relevance that the size of thallium-201 defects in patients with acute myocardial infarction is of prognostic significance. Recent studies strongly suggest that, in patients with acute myocardial infarction, the size of resting thallium-201 perfusion defects effectively discriminates between high- and low-risk groups for late cardiac events [11, 12].

TECHNETIUM-99m-PYROPHOSPHATE IMAGING

Infarct sizing on the basis of abnormal accumulation of technetium-99m-pyrophosphate in the myocardium has been attempted initially by three-dimensional reconstruction from planar images. In experimental animals, a good correlation could be demonstrated only for anterior infarctions. More recently, good results have been reported employing single-photon emission tomography for estimating size of infarction [13].

In addition, also the pattern of uptake is of significance: the intensity and area of technetium-99m-pyrophosphate accumulation has been correlated with occurrence of postdischarge cardiac events.

MULTIGATED BLOOD POOL EQUILIBRIUM OR FIRST-PASS ANGIOCARDIOGRAPHY

Although there exists a general inverse relationship between infarct size and calculated value for left ventricular ejection fraction, in any individual patient, infarct size cannot be estimated by this measured value. This is understandable since, in normal subjects, left ventricular ejection fraction may vary over a wide range, dependent upon the patient's state of activity or sympathetic tone. Nevertheless, assessment of right and left ventricular function in patients with acute myocardial infarction is extremely useful in clinical management, since it provides an objective measure of residual myocardial function. Left ventricular ejection fraction is of prognostic significance. An ejection fraction of 30% or less predicts a high risk for death from pump failure early after myocardial infarction, whereas well-preserved cardiac function is related to a more favorable outcome [14]. It is conceivable that quantitative analysis of regional wall motion abnormalities would also provide an index of infarct size, but no reliable and validated methods are as yet available. Thus, although assessment of left ventricular and right ventricular function does not allow direct sizing of myocardial infarction, it is nevertheless the single most useful clinical parameter in patients with acute myocardial infarction.

Summary

In patients with acute myocardial infarction, radionuclide techniques are extremely useful. The procedures are noninvasive and serial studies can be performed at the bedside. For the diagnosis of myocardial infarction, thallium-201 myocardial imaging during the acute hours of infarction is the most sensitive. During the subacute phase of infarction, technetium-99m pyrophosphate myocardial imaging is very specific, but less sensitive. Sizing of myocardial infarction probably best is performed using thallium-201 single-photon emission tomography or planimetry of planar images. For clinical management of patients, the assessment of the right and left ventricular function by gated cardiac blood pool imaging is of invaluable significance in management of patients and permits categorization of patients according to their risk for future complications. In patients with acute myocardial infarction, two questions are to be answered: First, to what degree is left and right ventricular function impaired? And, second, how much myocardium is at risk for future myocardial infarction? Radionuclide techniques provide answers to these important questions.

References

1. Wackers FJTh, Busemann Sokole E, Samson G, Van der Schoot JB, Lie KI, Liem KL, Wellens JJ: Value and limitations of thallium-201 scintigraphy in the acute phase of myocardial infarction. N Engl J Med 295:1−5, 1976.
2. Parkey RW, Bonte FJ, Meyer SL, Atkins JM, Curry GL, Stokely EM, Willerson JT: A new method for radionuclide imaging of acute myocardial infarction in humans. Circulation 50:540−546, 1974.
3. Wackers FJTh, Berger HJ, Johnstone DE, Goldman L, Reduto LA, Langou RA, Gottschalk A, Zaret BL: Multiple gated cardiac blood pool imaging for left ventricular ejection fraction: validation of the technique and assessment of variability. Am J Cardiol 43:1159−1166, 1979.
4. Wackers FJTh, Becker AE, Samson G, Busemann Sokole E, Van der Schoot JB, Vet AJTM, Lie KI, Durrer D, Wellens HJJ: Location and size of acute transmural myocardial infarction estimated from thallium-201 scintiscans: a clinicopathological study. Circulation 56:72−78, 1977.
5. Falkoff M, Parkey RW, Bonte FJ, Lewis JS, Buja LM, Dehmer G, Willerson JT: Technetium-99m stannous pyrophosphate myocardial scintigraphy: serial imaging to detect myocardial infarcts in patients. Clin Cardiol 1:163−168, 1978.
6. Berger HJ, Gottschalk A, Zaret BL: Dual radionuclide study of acute myocardial infarction: comparison of thallium-201 and technetium-99m stannous pyrophosphate imaging in man. Ann Intern Med 88:145−154, 1978.
7. Wackers FJTh, Lie KI, Busemann Sokole E, Res J, Van der Schoot, Durrer D: Prevalence of right ventricular involvement in inferior wall infarc-

tion assessed with myocardial imaging with thallium-201 and technetium-99m-pyrophosphate. Am J Cardiol 42:358−362, 1983.

8. Kelly MJ, Giles RW, Simon TR, Berger HJ, Langou RA, Zaret BL, Wackers FJTh: Multigated equilibrium radionuclide angiocardiography: improved detection of left ventricular wall motion abnormalities and aneurysms by the addition of the left lateral view. Radiology 139:167−173, 1981.

9. Wackers FJTh, Berger HJ, Weinberg MA, Zaret BL: Spontaneous changes in left ventricular function over the first 24 hours of acute myocardial infarction: implications for evaluating early therapeutic interventions. Circulation 66:748−754, 1982.

10. Tamaki S, Nakajima H, Murakami T, Yui Y, Kambara H, Kadota K, Yoshida A, Kawaai C, Tamaki N, Mukai T, Ishii Y, Torizuka K: Estimation of infarct size by myocardial emission computed tomography with thallium-201 and its relation to creatine kinase−MB release after myocardial infarction in man. Circulation 66: 994−1001, 1982.

11. Silverman KJ, Becker LC, Bulkley BM, Burow RD, Mellits ED, Kallman CH, Weisfeldt ML: Value of early thallium-201 scintigraphy for predicting mortality in patients with acute myocardial infarction. Circulation 61:996−1003, 1980.

12. Perez-Gonzales J, Botvinick EH, Dunn R, Rahimtoola S, Ports T, Chatterjee K, Parmley WW: The late prognostic value of acute scintigraphic measurement of myocardial infarction size. Circulation 66:960, 1982.

13. Holman BL, Goldhaber SZ, Kirsch C-M, Polak JF, Friedman BJ, English RJ, Wynne J: Measurement of infarct size using single photon emission computed tomography and technetium-99m-pyrophosphate: a description of the method and comparison with patient prognosis. Am J Cardiology 50:503−511, 1982.

14. Shah PK, Pichler M, Berman DS, Singh BN, Swan HJ: Left ventricular ejection fraction determined by radionuclide ventriculography in early stages of first transmural myocardial infarction: relation to short-term prognosis. Am J Cardiol 45:542−546, 1980.

21. THE CLINICAL DIAGNOSIS OF RIGHT VENTRICULAR INFARCTION

David G. Harrison

Melvin L. Marcus

The diagnosis of right ventricular infarction is often overlooked for at least three reasons: (a) Infarction of the right ventricle is, with rare exception, associated with left ventricular infarction. Thus, clinical events caused by right ventricular infarction are often erroneously attributed to left ventricular infarction. (b) The routine 12-lead electrocardiogram, heavily relied upon to assist in the diagnosis of left ventricular infarction, is of limited value in the diagnosis of right ventricular infarction. (c) While anatomic evidence of right ventricular infarction has been recognized for many decades, only recently has the clinical presentation of this entity been described.

Importance of Making the Right Diagnosis of Right Ventricular Infarction

Autopsy series [1—3] and clinical studies using several independent noninvasive techniques [4—6] have found that approximately one-third of all patients with inferior infarction have associated right ventricular infarction (see table 21-1). Since inferior infarction occurs frequently, this suggests that a sizable minority of patients admitted to the coronary care unit have right ventricular infarction. *It is useful for the clinician to realize that approximately one in three patients with inferior infarction will likely have associated necrosis of the right ventricle.* Fortunately, only a small number of these (approximately 3%—4% of all

patients with infarction of either ventricle) have compromised hemodynamics because of right ventricular infarction. For this reason, one might question the need to establish the diagnosis of right ventricular infarction in a hemodynamically stable patient with minimal likelihood of having necrosis of the right ventricle. While clinically such an effort may seem unnecessary, accurate diagnosis of right ventricular infarction may be warranted for investigational purposes and may identify those few patients at risk for subsequent untoward events early in the course of their myocardial infarction.

Anatomy and Physiology

The majority of the right ventricle in man is perfused by the right coronary artery, although a small region of the anterior free wall is supplied by small branches of the left anterior descending artery [7]. In older autopsy studies, and more recently in studies using positron emission tomography [8], occasional patients have been identified with right ventricular infarction associated with anterior myocardial infarction. However, the great majority of patients with right ventricular infarction have necrosis of the inferior left ventricle.

Pathophysiology

Following infarction of a sufficient quantity of the right ventricle, this chamber's ability to pump

R.M. Califf and G.S. Wagner (eds.), ACUTE CORONARY CARE: Principles and Practice. Copyright © 1985. Martinus Nijhoff Publishing, Boston/Dordrecht/Lancaster.

TABLE 21-1. Incidence of right ventricular infarction: literature reviewed

Author	Techniques used	Incidence of RVI	
		All patients	Inferior MI
Klein et al. [6]	Radionuclide ventriculogram ^{99m}Tc-Pyp scintigraphy Right heart catheterization Autopsy Echocardiography Right precordial ECG	b	58/110 (52.7%)
Sharpe et al. [4]	^{99m}Tc-Pyp scintigraphy Radionuclide ventricle Echocardiography Right heart catheterization	6/26 (0.23)	6/15 (0.40)
Candell-Riera et al. [39]	^{99m}Tc-Pyp scintigraphy Electrocardiography Echocardiography Right heart catheterization Right precordial ECG	b	18/42[a] (0.42)
Erhardt et al. [37]	Right precordial ECG and/or autopsy	b	25/92 (0.27)
Cintron et al. [12]	Bedside exam	16/96 (0.17)	16/44 (0.36)
Wartman and Hellerstein [1]	Autopsy	13.8%	
Croft et al. [34]	Right precordial ECG Clinical findings Radionuclide ventriculography ^{99m}Tc-Pyp scintigraphy	10/33 (0.30)	b
Isner and Roberts [3]	Autopsy	33/236 (0.14)	33/139 (0.24)
		Average = 37±10% (SD)	

[a] Diagnosis based on positive right ventricular ^{99m}Tc-Pyp uptake.
[b] Data not presented in the manuscript.

blood through the pulmonary circulation to the left atrium and ventricle is reduced. This reduction in right ventricular forward output and many of the clinical features of this disorder are due to two major factors: (a) decreased pumping ability of the right ventricle, i.e., reduced systolic function, and (b) abnormal diastolic function. The abnormal diastolic function is in part due to an inability of the right ventricle to appropriately dilate after infarction due to restraining effects of the pericardium [9, 10]. This diminution in right ventricular compliance accounts for the frequently observed Kussmaul's sign and elevation of the jugular venous pressure [10−12]. Reduction of systolic function is manifested by a decrease in right ventricular ejection fraction, which, together with the alteration in diastolic

function, reduces cardiac output. These factors may result in a life-threatening reduction of cardiac output.

Clinical Features of Right Ventricular Infarction

The clinical features of right ventricular infarction have been the subject of several reports [10−12]. These have been somewhat difficult to interpret because there has been no "gold standard" to assure that all patients included in these reports truly had right ventricular infarction and that patients excluded did not have right ventricular infarction. Despite these unavoidable flaws, these studies have clearly shown that right ventricular infarction may present as a spectrum ranging from no clinical manifestations to shock associated with evidence of right ventricular failure.

The "typical" patient with extensive right ventricular infarction may present with electrocardiographic evidence of inferior wall myocardial infarction, hypotension, and evidence of right ventricular failure. Findings compatible with this failure include elevated venous pressure, Kussmaul's sign [10-12] and, less commonly, evidence of tricuspid regurgitation [13]. These findings are most often not associated with evidence of left ventricular failure.

The absence of left ventricular failure, i.e., the absence of pulmonary edema on chest x-ray, or the lack of evidence on physical examination of pulmonary congestion is very important but is often difficult to establish clinically. Among older patients, particularly those with superimposed lung disease, pulmonary rales are a common finding. Rotman et al. have examined the incidence of rales in the absence of elevated pulmonary artery diastolic pressures [14]. Among 15 patients with rales, one-third had a pulmonary artery diastolic pressure less than 15 mmHg. In their series, the combination of an S_3 gallop and pulmonary rales, however, was always associated with an elevated pulmonary artery diastolic pressure. Riley et al. have shown that a ventricular gallop sound was more common in patients with elevated left ventricular or pulmonary artery end-diastolic pressures than in those with normal left ventricular or pulmonary artery diastolic pressures. Substantial overlap existed between groups, however, so that the presence of a ventricular gallop alone could not be used to predict left ventricular filling pressures [15].

Several investigators have examined the accuracy of the chest x-ray in detecting left heart failure early in the course of myocardial infarction [16-18]. While this clinical tool is quite helpful in caring for patients with chronic cardiac disease, it seems to be of limited use early in the course of acute myocardial infarction. These limitations relate to inability to obtain an upright PA film, the occasional presence of interstitial fibrosis masquerading as interstitial edema and most importantly, a significant time lag (often as great as 6 h) between the development of hemodynamic alterations characteristic of left ventricular failure and the typical x-ray manifestations of pulmonary congestion [16, 18].

Hemodynamic Features of Right Ventricular Infarction

Because the clinical findings of right ventricular infarction may be misleading, placement of a Swan-Ganz catheter in the severely ill patient is often helpful in establishing the diagnosis of right ventricular infarction and indispensable in their subsequent management.

The hemodynamic findings in patients with right ventricular infarction have been reported on several occasions [10, 11, 19]. It should be stressed that patients included have been seriously ill and that minor degrees of right ventricular necrosis may not be associated with notable hemodynamic alterations.

Cohn et al. [11] first reported the clinical findings in six patients with probable right ventricular infarction. These investigators pointed out that the ratio of right ventricular end-diastolic pressure to left ventricular end-diastolic pressure was significantly greater than 1 among patients with right ventricular infarction whereas, among patients with left ventricular infarction alone, this ratio was significantly less than 1.

More recent studies have confirmed the findings of Cohn et al. Lorell and co-workers [10] reported the hemodynamic findings in 12 patients with right ventricular infarction. These patients all had elevations of right atrial pressure with normal or near-normal pulmonary capillary wedge pressure. Further, several features present suggested pericardial tamponade or constriction. These included equalization of right atrial, right ventricular, and pulmonary capillary wedge pressures, Kussmaul's sign, and a characteristic "dip and plateau" or "square root" appearance of the right ventricular diastolic pressure trace (see figure 21-1). The later findings were postulated to be secondary to the combined effects of right ventricular dysfunction and the restraining effects of the pericardium.

Management of the acutely ill patient with right ventricular infarction is greatly enhanced by monitoring pulmonary artery, right atrial,

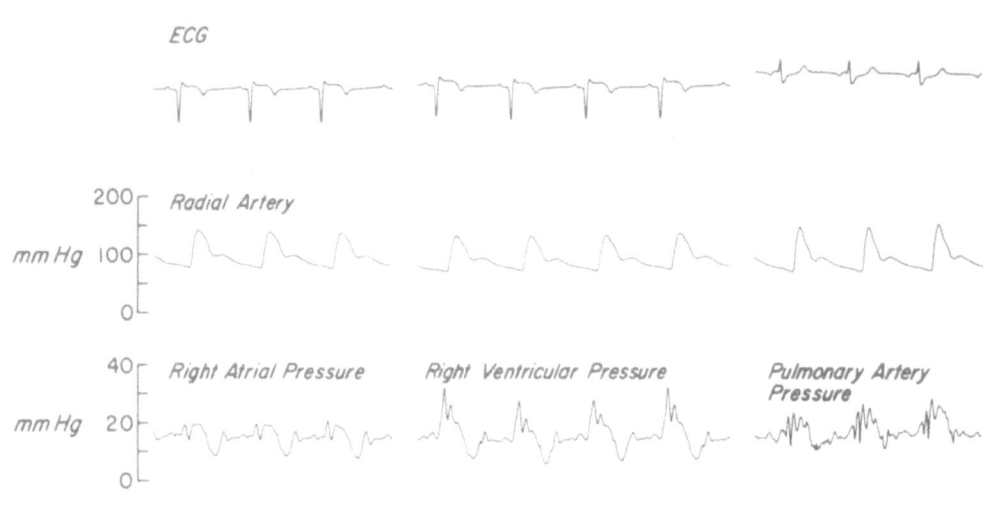

FIGURE 21-1. ECG, arterial pressure, and right heart pressures in a patient with right ventricular infarction. There is elevation of right atrial and right ventricular end-diastolic pressures. The right atrial pressure trace demonstrates a prominent Y descent. During diastole, both the right atrial and right ventricular pressure tracings demonstrate a characteristic dip and plateau configuration. The pulmonary artery pressure is not elevated. From Lorell et al. [10], with permission.

and pulmonary capillary wedge pressures. The hemodynamic consequences of right ventricular infarction are primarily related to underfilling of the left ventricle. While the ability of the infarcted right ventricle to increase its output by increasing right ventricular diastolic volume is undoubtedly diminished in right ventricular infarction, it is not abolished. Thus three of 12 patients in one series [10] and three of six in another [11] improved with volume expansion. Because the goal of such therapy is to increase pulmonary capillary wedge pressure to an optimum level (approximately 14−18 mmHg), direct monitoring of this pressure is invaluable.

Thus, invasive monitoring is an important therapeutic tool and is helpful in establishing the diagnosis of right ventricular infarction. It should be stressed that other processes, including chronic lung disease, acute pulmonary emboli, and pericardial constriction, may produce similar hemodynamic alterations and thus should be considered when the results of right heart catheterization suggest right ventricular infarction. For these reasons, it is clear that no hemodynamic alterations are entirely specific for right ventricular infarction. Also because small amounts of right ventricular necrosis may not produce hemodynamic changes, normal hemodynamic findings do not exclude right ventricular infarction.

Scintigraphic Studies Used in the Diagnosis of Right Ventricular Infarction

In the clinical setting, three scintigraphic techniques have gained widespread acceptance and are commonly used in the diagnosis and treatment of cardiovascular diseases. These include thallium-201 scintigraphy for identification of both ischemic [20, 21] and infarcted [22, 23] myocardium, radionuclide angiography, and the use of the infarct-avid agent technetium-99m pyrophosphate (^{99m}Tc-Pyp). The usefulness of each of these in the diagnosis of right ventricular infarction will be considered.

THALLIUM-201 SCINTIGRAPHY (see chapter 51) Thallium-201 scintigraphy identifies infarcted left ventricular myocardium by the absence of regional uptake and lack of redistribution to that area on subsequent examinations [22, 23]. Unfortunately the nonhypertrophied right ventricle is inconsistently visualized with current methodology. Thus the detection of a thallium-201 uptake deficit is not a reliable marker of right ventricular infarction.

RADIONUCLIDE ANGIOGRAPHY
(see chapters 25 and 52)

Recently, it has become possible to estimate left ventricular ejection fraction, to determine the presence or absence of wall motion abnormalities, and to assess left ventricular volumes by using radionuclide angiography. Two different technologies have evolved. The most widely used approach requires that technetium-99m pyrophosphate (^{99m}Tc-Pyp) be tagged to red blood cells (earlier techniques used albumin) and thus remain in the "blood pool." A gamma camera, linked to specialized computer equipment, is used to collect counts from a variety of positions over the precordium. By "gating" these counts with the patient's electrocardiogram, estimations of left ventricular ejection fraction and left ventricular volumes can be obtained.

The second approach, commonly referred to as the "first pass" technique, involves collecting emitted counts from the various cardiac chambers as the isotope, initially injected into the circulation by a peripheral vein, passes through these chambers.

This method is best performed using specially designed equipment not suited for gated studies, but can be performed fairly adequately using equipment designed for gated studies. Newer-generation computer software may further improve on the ability of single-crystal detection system to estimate accurately ejection fraction by using this "first pass" technique.

Early work by Steele et al. [24] examined the accuracy of the first-pass approach in determining the right ventricular ejection fraction. These investigators found that this technique correlated well with values obtained from right ventricular cineangiograms. Steele et al. [24] showed that the right ventricular ejection fraction is normally approximately 10% lower than the left ventricular ejection fraction. Others have confirmed this finding [25, 26].

Unfortunately the gated blood pool scintigraphic approach visualizing the right ventricle is complicated by the fact that no one view completely separates the right ventricle from other cardiac structures. Attempts have been made to solve this problem by using multiple regions of interest around the right ventricle and averaging the ejection fractions obtained from each. Experience at the University of Iowa has shown this approach to be frought with error and largely unreliable.

Fortunately, in the process of performing a multigated radionuclide angiogram, a first-pass study can be performed as the technetium-99m is initially bolused into the circulation. Thus, an accurate estimate of right ventricular ejection fraction and wall motion can be obtained by the first-pass technique. Subsequently, assessment of left ventricular wall motion and ejection fraction is possible using the gated approach.

Despite the fact that a number of studies have shown that the mean right ventricular ejection fraction is reduced in patients with right ventricular infarction [4, 6, 25], several potential pitfalls exist in using this technique to diagnose right ventricular infarction. A number of disease processes including chronic pulmonary hypertension due to lung disease, left ventricular failure, or congenital heart disease may reduce right ventricular ejection fraction independent of right ventricular infarction. Second, it is likely that small amounts of right ventricular necrosis produce little or no alteration in right ventricular ejection fraction. Lastly, several investigators have shown that the right ventricular ejection fraction following right ventricular infarction is only transiently diminished. Reduto et al. [25] found that, after left ventricular infarction, the left ventricular ejection fraction remained consistently depressed. In contrast, after right ventricular infarction, the initially depressed right ventricular ejection fraction improved in 50% of patients during a 13-day period. Klein et al. [6] showed that the right ventricular ejection fraction increased from a mean of $21\pm8\%$ after right ventricular infarction to a mean of $43\pm9\%$ approximately two months later. This latter value is similar to that found in normal patients. Thus, a normal right ventricular ejection fraction several weeks after suspected right ventricular infarction does not exclude the presence of previous right ventricular infarction.

Detection of Right Ventricular Infarction Using Infarct-Avid Agents

A variety of agents have been shown to localize preferentially to infarcted myocardium. These include iodine-133, [97]Hg-fluoroscein, and [203]Hg-fluoroscine, [99m]Tc-(Sn)-tetracycline, and ^{99m}Tc-Pyp [27]. Of these, ^{99m}Tc-Pyp has gained widespread popularity as a useful clinical tool in diagnosing myocardial infarction. This popularity is in part due to the excellent quality of images obtained with ^{99m}Tc-Pyp. Furthermore, numerous experimental studies [28−30] and several clinical studies have clearly shown that ^{99m}Tc-Pyp scanning can discriminate between infarcted and ischemic myocardium [31]. It is thought that technetium pyrophosphate complexes to tissue calcium that is released from infarcted myocardium. The time of removal of tissue calcium from infarcted myocardium is highly variable. In the experimental animal, ^{99m}Tc-Pyp can be shown to accumulate in infarcted tissue within 6 h of coronary occlusion [32], but sufficient quantities of ^{99m}Tc-Pyp are not present in the infarct to allow images of diagnostic quality for 12−24 h after coronary occlusion [12]. The intensity of uptake into infarcted myocardium likely increases thereafter and reaches a peak at approximately 24−72 h after the onset of infarction. Scintigrams suitable for diagnosis may be obtained from 12 h to six days after acute myocardial infarction [27].

ACCURACY OF [99m]TC-PYP SCINTIGRAPHY IN ESTABLISHING THE DIAGNOSIS OF RIGHT VENTRICULAR INFARCTION

If certain precautions are taken, ^{99m}Tc-Pyp scintigrams are extremely sensitive and specific in detecting myocardial necrosis of either the right or left ventricles. While certain processes not primarily involving the myocardium are occasionally responsible for a falsely positive scan (fractured ribs, calcified aortic valves, muscle contusions), these entities are relatively uncommon and usually easily recognized. Processes other than acute coronary occlusion occasionally cause myocardial uptake of ^{99m}Tc-Pyp, but these have been shown to generally involve myocardial necrosis [33]. Even some patients with persistently positive scintigrams after myocardial infarction have been shown to have histologic evidence of ongoing tissue necrosis [33].

The ^{99m}Tc-scintigram is of particular use in diagnosing right ventricular infarction. It is the only currently widely available procedure that can definitely localize the area of infarction to the right ventricle.

SEPARATION OF RIGHT VENTRICULAR FROM LEFT VENTRICULAR [99m]TC-PYP UPTAKE

In the $30°−60°$ left anterior oblique view, the septum is positioned left of the image and the left and right ventricles are clearly separated by the interventricular septum. The exact angulation necessary to obtain this result varies from patient to patient. This variability is easily recognized and appropriate alterations of camera angle may be readily made.

Wackers et al. [5] initially reported an effective method of discriminating between left and right ventricular technetium uptake. These investigators used dual scanning with thallium-201 and ^{99m}Tc-Pyp. Using this approach the thallium-201 scan obtained in the $45°$ LAO view was used to identify the left ventricular outline, and a subsequent ^{99m}Tc-Pyp scan performed with the patient in an identical position. Because the energy spectra of these isotopes are different, it was possible (by appropriately setting the energy windows) to visualize the image produced by each isotope independent of the other (differential imaging). The chest wall was marked so that the two views could be superimposed. Recognition of right ventricular uptake could thus be separated from left ventricular uptake by identifying a region of technetium uptake anterior to the left ventricular image obtained with thallium-201.

Sharpe et al. [4] have identified the respective positions of the right and left ventricular chambers by using a radionuclide angiogram performed in the same projection as the ^{99m}Tc-Pyp scintigram. Right ventricular infarction was deemed present if technetium uptake was visualized anterior to the position of the left ventricle in the $45°$ LAO view. These investigators found a good correlation between this evidence of right ventricular infarction and a variety of other noninvasive techniques.

While the above "combined" approaches may help clearly discriminate right ventricular from left ventricular ^{99m}Tc-Pyp uptake, it is usually quite easy to separate left and right ventricular uptake by using only a ^{99m}Tc-Pyp scintigram. This is because right ventricular infarction is almost always associated with inferior left ventricular infarction. When the 45° LAO view is used, uptake in the inferior left ventricle, the septum, and the right ventricular free wall produces a classic "W" sign (see figure 21-2). The right ventricular free wall extends toward the sternum and can usually be readily separated from the septum and left ventricular inferior wall. One of the above "combined" approaches would be required to identify clearly the position of the left ventricle when right ventricular infarction without left ventricular infarction is suspected and/or if either cardiac position or chest wall configuration is strikingly abnormal. Thus, Klein et al. [6], Croft et al. [34], and D'Arcy and Nanda [35] have utilized ^{99m}Tc-Pyp scintigraphy alone to identify right ventricular infarc-

tion with success and have reported results similar to those reported by Wackers et al. [5] and Sharpe et al. [4].

Electrocardiographic Identification of Right Ventricular Infarction

Traditionally the nonhypertrophied right ventricle, in the absence of conduction disturbances, has been considered to be electrocardiographically silent and this technique has been dismissed as being of little use in the diagnosis of right ventricular infarction [2]. Several recent reports, however, have contradicted this dogma. Erhardt and coworkers, in a series of interesting clinical reports, have shown that lead CR_4R (a lead placed at the fifth intercostal space in the right midclavicular line) is quite useful in identifying patients with right ventricular infarction. In this initial report [36], he studied 12 patients who died and were subsequently found to have infarction of the right ventricle at autopsy. In ten of these 12, ST-segment elevation was noted in lead

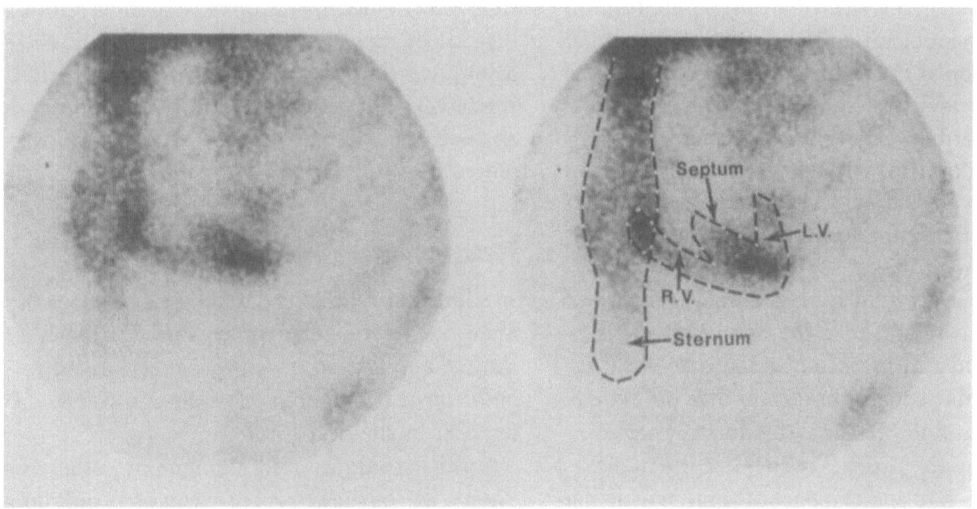

FIGURE 21-2. Left anterior oblique ^{99m}Tc-Pyp scintigram showing uptake in a large portion of the right ventricular free wall indicating extensive right ventricular infarction. In this view, the right ventricle (RV) is usually easily separated from the left ventricle (LV) by the interventricular septum. The detector position needed to separate those structures is generally 30°–45° left anterior oblique.

CR_4R. In contrast, only one of nine patients with inferior wall myocardial infarction without right ventricular infarction had this finding. In a subsequent report [37], Erhardt and co-workers reconfirmed these results and in addition examined 74 patients with acute inferior wall myocardial infarction who survived. Among these patients, hemodynamic complications suggesting the presence of right ventricular infarction were more common when ST-segment elevation was present in lead CR_4R than when this finding was absent. Finally these workers showed that CR_4R may show ST-segment elevation in the absence of inferior wall myocardial infarction when right ventricular infarction resulted from extension of anterior wall left ventricular infarction.

Chou et al. [38] examined 11 patients with inferior wall myocardial infarction. In five cases, right ventricular infarction was established at subsequent autopsy and, in six cases, the diagnosis was based on hemodynamic data. Among these 11 patients, eight manifested ST-segment elevation of 1 mm or greater in lead V_1. Unfortunately these investigators did not include a control group in their study. Candell-Riera et al. [39] compared the electrocardiographic finding of ST-segment elevation in lead V_4R (a precordial lead position at the right fourth intercostal space at the midclavicular line) to multiple other findings compatible with right ventricular infarction. Among 22 patients with elevated ST segments in lead V_4R, 15 had evidence of right ventricular infarction by technetium pyrophosphate scintigraphy. Only three of 20 patients without ST-segment elevation in lead V_4R had technetium pyrophosphate uptake in the right ventricle. Elevation of the right ventricular end-diastolic pressure to a value equal to or greater than pulmonary capillary wedge pressure was much more common among the patients with ST-segment elevation in this lead and evidence of right ventricular dilatation on echocardiography was more common among patients with ST-segment elevations in V_4R.

More recently, Croft et al. [34] examined the frequency of ST-segment elevations in at least one right precordial lead ($V_4R - V_6R$) and compared this finding with right ventricular ejection fraction by radionuclide ventriculography and technetium pyrophosphate scintigraphy. Figure 21-3 provides a comparison of ECG findings in one of their patients with and one without right ventricular infarction. Right ventricular ejection fraction estimated by radionuclide ventriculogram was significantly lower in patients with ST-segment elevation in at least one of the examined right precordial leads than in those without this finding. The finding of ST-segment elevation in at least one of the three right precordial leads examined was 91% specific and 90% sensitive for the diagnosis of right ventricular infarction as established by ^{99m}Tc-Pyp scintigraphy. Klein et al. [6] examined a larger number of patients with acute inferior wall myocardial infarction and compared the accuracy of lead V_4R in detecting right ventricular infarction with ^{99m}Tc-Pyp scintigraphy, echocardiography, hemodynamic monitoring, and radionuclide ventriculography. The sensitivity of this finding was 82.7%, specificity 76.9%, positive predictive value 70%, and negative predictive value 87.7%.

Thus, there exists a substantial amount of data to suggest that right precordial electrocardiography may be valuable in the early recognition of right ventricular infarction. It should be stressed that all of these studies have shown that these techniques do not detect all patients with right ventricular infarction and, if the diagnosis is clinically suspected, further studies are warranted.

Future Diagnostic Tools of Potential Use

In addition to the several diagnostic tools already mentioned, two other procedures, currently of limited application, may prove useful in the recognition and diagnosis of right ventricular infarction in the near future.

Cardiac computerized tomography, otherwise known as "fast CT," is currently used only in a few centers in the United States [40]. This procedure, coupled with intravenous injection of small quantities of iodinated contrast material, allows visualization of both the left and the right ventricle throughout the cardiac cycle. Because infarcted and normal myocardium have different uptake of contrast material, infarcted tissue is readily differentiated from noninfarcted tissue.

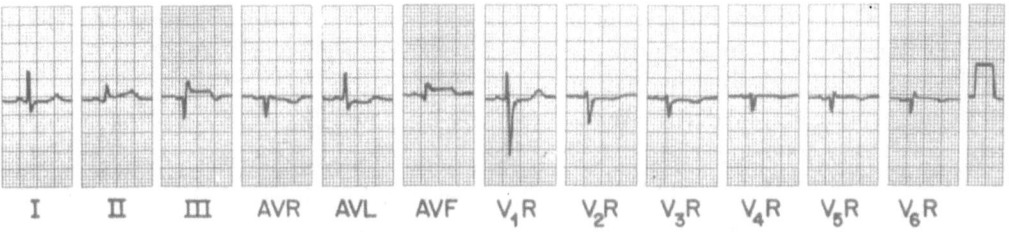

I   II   III   AVR   AVL   AVF   V₁R   V₂R   V₃R   V₄R   V₅R   V₆R

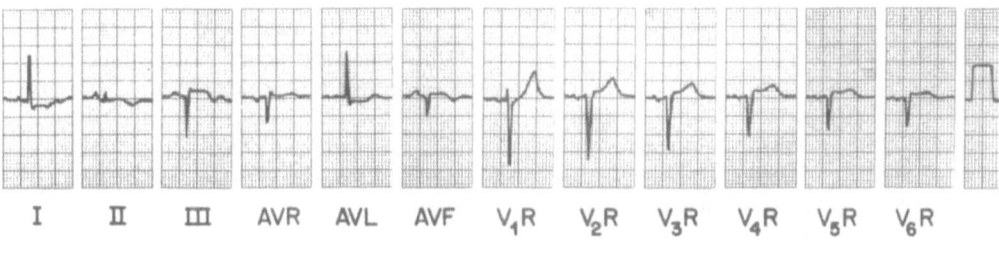

I   II   III   AVR   AVL   AVF   V₁R   V₂R   V₃R   V₄R   V₅R   V₆R

FIGURE 21-3. Electrocardiographic findings in a patient without (above) and a patient with (below) right ventricular infarction associated with inferior infarction. Notice in both electrocardiograms the presence of ST-segment elevation and Q waves in the inferior leads. The right precordial leads in the lower electrocardiogram demonstrate diffuse ST-segment elevation. From Croft et al. [34], with permission.

Positron emission tomography (PET) has been used in several centers to visualize perfusion of the left ventricle. Unfortunately, until recently it was difficult to consistently visualize the right ventricle and therefore PET has not been used extensively to diagnose right ventricular infarction. Newer-generation PET scanning devices have the capability of more consistently visualizing the right ventricle and it is conceivable that right ventricular infarction may be readily identified using this technology (E.M. Geltman, personal communication).

The utility of cardiac imaging using nuclear magnetic resonance (NMR) has recently been reviewed [41]. Theoretically, NMR should be quite useful in identifying the edema associated with infarction of either the left or right ventricle. The sensitivity and specificity of this methodology in accurately identifying right ventricular infarction have not been determined.

Summary

The major obstacle to diagnosis of right ventricular infarction is that the physician caring for a patient may not consider its presence. A rule of thumb is that the diagnosis of right ventricular infarction should be considered in any patient with hemodynamic compromise following inferior wall myocardial infarction. The diagnostic procedures used to establish this diagnosis will largely depend on what technology is most commonly performed at that particular institution. In the acute phase, right precordial chest leads, and in particular leads $V_4R - V_6R$, may be useful in detecting the presence of right ventricular infarction. However, the absence of findings in these electrocardiographic leads does not rule out the presence of right ventricular infarction. When dealing with a critically ill patient, right heart catheterization and monitoring of pulmonary artery and pulmonary capillary wedge pressure are invaluable, though other disease entities may mimic the hemodynamic findings of right ventricular infarction. The diagnosis and treatment of the critically ill patient with right ventricular infarction are greatly aided by knowledge of right heart and pulmonary capillary wedge pressures. During the several days following the onset of infarction, either ^{99m}Tc-Pyp scintigraphy or radionuclide ventriculography may be helpful in further confirming the diagnosis. At present, technetium-99m pyrophosphate scintigraphy, if performed correctly, is as close to being a "gold standard" as any widely available technology for diagnosing right ventricular infarction.

References

1. Wartman WB, Hellerstein HK: The incidence of heart disease in 2,000 consecutive autopsies. Ann Intern Med 28:41−65, 1948.
2. Wade WG: The pathogenesis of infarction of the right ventricle. Br Heart J 21:545−554, 1959.
3. Isner JM, Roberts WC: Right ventricular infarction complicating left ventricular infarction secondary to coronary heart disease: frequency, location, associated findings and significance from analysis of 236 necropsy patients with acute or healed myocardial infarction. Am J Cardiol 42:885−894, 1978.
4. Sharpe DN, Botvinick EH, Shames DM, Schiller NB, Massie BM, Chatterjee K, Parmley WW: The noninvasive diagnosis of right ventricular infarction. Circulation 57:483−490, 1978.
5. Wackers JT, Lie KI, Sokole EB, Res J, Van der Schoot JB, Durrer D: Prevalence of right ventricular involvement in inferior wall infarction assessed with myocardial imaging with thallium-201 and technetium-99m pyrophosphate. Am J Cardiol 42:358−362, 1978.
6. Klein HO, Tordjman T, Ninio R, Sareli P, Oren V, Lang R, Gefen J, Pauzner C, Di Segni E, David D, Kaplinsky E: The early recognition of right ventricular infarction: diagnostic accuracy of the electrocardiographic V$_4$R lead. Circulation 67:558−565, 1983.
7. James TH: Anatomy of the coronary arteries. New York: Harper and Row, 1961.
8. Geltman EM, Biello D, Galie E, Baird T, Roberts R, Sobel BE: Right ventricular injury with anterior as well as inferior infarction documented by positron tomography [abstr]. Circulation (Suppl 4) 64:235, 1981.
9. Goldstein JA, Vlahakes GJ, Verrier ED, Schiller NB, Tyberg JV, Ports TA, Parmley WW, Chatterjee K: The role of right ventricular systolic dysfunction and elevated intrapericardial pressure in the genesis of low output in experimental right ventricular infarction. Circulation 65:513−522, 1982.
10. Lorell B, Leinbach RC, Pohost GM, Gold HK, Dinsmore RE, Hutter AM Jr, Pastore JO, Desanctis RW: Right ventricular infarction: clinical diagnosis and differentiation from cardiac tamponade and pericardial constriction. Am J Cardiol 43:465−471, 1979.
11. Cohn JN, Guiha NH, Broder MI, Limas CJ: Right ventricular infarction: clinical and hemodynamic features. Am J Cardiol 33:209−214, 1974.
12. Cintron GB, Hernandez E, Linares E, Aranda JM: Bedside recognition, incidence and clinical course of right ventricular infarction. Am J Cardiol 47:224−227, 1981.
13. Wells DE, Befeler B: Dysfunction of the right ventricle in coronary artery disease. Chest 66:230−235, 1974.
14. Rotman M, Chen JTT, Seningen RP, Hawley J, Wagner JS, Davidson RM, Gilbert MR: Pulmonary arterial diastolic pressure in acute myocardial infarction. Am J Cardiol 33:357−362, 1974.
15. Riley CP, Russell RO, Rackley CE: Left ventricular gallop sound and acute myocardial infarction. Am Heart J 86:598−602, 1973.
16. Kostuk W, Barr JW, Simon AL, Ross J Jr: Correlations between the chest film and hemodynamics in acute myocardial infarction. Circulation 48:624−632, 1973.
17. Harrison MO, Conte PJ, Heitzman ER: Radiological detection of clinically occult cardiac failure following myocardial infarction. Br J Radiol 44:265, 1971.
18. Fluck DC, Valentine PA, Treister B, Higgs B, Reid DN, Steiner RE, Mounsey JPD: Right heart pressures in acute myocardial infarction. Br Heart J 29:748, 1967.
19. Rotman M, Ratliff NB, Hawley J: Right ventricular infarction: a haemodynamic diagnosis. Br Heart J 36:941−944, 1974.
20. Pohost GM, Zir LM, Moore RH, McKusick KA, Guiney T, Beller GA: Differentiation of transiently ischemic from infarcted myocardium by serial imaging after a single dose of thallium-201. Circulation 55:294, 1977.
21. Hamilton GW, Trobaugh BG, Ritchie JL, Williams DL, Weaver WD, Gould KL: Myocardial imaging with intravenously injected thallium-

201 in patients with suspected coronary artery disease: analysis of technique and correlation with electrocardiographic, coronary anatomic and ventriculographic findings. Am J Cardiol 39:347, 1977.

22. Wackers FJ, Sokole EB, Samson G, Van der Schoot JB, Lie KI, Leim KL, Wellens HJJ: Value and limitations of thallium-201 scintigraphy in the acute phase of myocardial infarction. N Engl J Med 295:1–5, 1976.

23. DiCola VC, Downing SE, Donabedian RK, Zaret BL: Pathophysiological correlates of thallium-201 myocardial uptake in experimental infarction. Cardiovasc Res 11:141, 1977.

24. Steele P, Kirch D, Le Free M, Battock D: Measurement of right and left ventricular ejection fractions by radionuclide angiocardiography in coronary artery disease. Chest 70:51–61, 1976.

25. Reduto LA, Berger HJ, Cohen LS, Gottschalk A, Zaret BL: Sequential radionuclide assessment of left and right ventricular performance after acute transmural myocardial infarction. Ann Intern Med 89:441, 1978.

26. Maddahi J, Berman DS, Matsuoka DT, Waxman AD, Stankus KE, Forrester JS, Swan HJC: A new technique for assessing right ventricular ejection fraction using rapid multiple-gated equilibrium cardiac blood pool scintigraphy: description, validation and findings in chronic coronary artery disease. Circulation 60:581, 1979.

27. Marcus ML, Go RT, Ehrhardt JC: Infarct avid imaging techniques. In: Myocardial infarction: measurement and intervention. The Hague: Martinus Nijhoff, 1982, pp. 325–346.

28. Buja LM, Parkey RW, Dees JH, Stokely EM, Harris RA Jr, Bonte JF, Willerson JT: Morphologic correlates of technetium-99m stannous pyrophosphate imaging of acute myocardial infarcts in dogs. Circulation 52:596, 1975.

29. Buja LM, Parkey RW, Stokely EM, Bronte FJ, Willerson JT: Pathophysiology of technetium-99m stannous pyrophosphate and thallium-201 scintigraphy of acute anterior myocardial infarcts in dogs. J Clin Invest 57:1508, 1976.

30. Marcus ML, Tomanek RJ, Ehrhardt JC, Kerber RE, Brown DD, Abboud FM: Relationships between myocardial perfusion, myocardial necrosis and coronary occlusion. Circulation 54:647, 1976.

31. Shen AC, Jennings RB: Myocardial calcium and magnesium in acute ischemic injury. Am J Pathol 67:417, 1972.

32. Doherty PW, McLaughlin PR, Billingham M, Kernoff R, Goris ML, Harrison DC: Cardiac damage produced by direct current countershock applied to the heart. Am J Cardiol 43:225, 1979.

33. Poliner LR, Buja LM, Parkey RW, Bonte FJ, Willerson JT: Clinicopathologic findings in 52 patients studied by technetium-99m stannous pyrophosphate myocardial scintigraphy. Circulation 59:257, 1979.

34. Croft CH, Nicod P, Corbett JR, Lewis SE, Huxley R, Mukharji J, Willerson JT, Rude RE: Detection of acute right ventricular infarction by right precordial electrocardiography. Am J Cardiol 50:421–427, 1982.

35. D'Arcy B, Nanda NC: Two-dimensional echocardiographic features of right ventricular infarction. Circulation 65:167–173, 1982.

36. Erhardt LR: Clinical and pathological observations in different types of acute myocardial infarction. Acta Med Scand Suppl 560, 1974.

37. Erhardt LR, Sjogren A, Wahlberg I: Single right-sided precordial lead in the diagnosis of right ventricular involvement in inferior myocardial infarction. Am Heart J 91:571–576, 1976.

38. Chou T, Van der Bel-Kahn J, Allen J, Brockmeier L, Fowler NO: Electrocardiographic diagnosis of right ventricular infarction. Am J Med 70:1175–1180, 1981.

39. Candell-Riera J, Figueras J, Valle V, Alvarez A, Gutierrez L, Cortadellas J, Cinca J, Salas A, Rius J: Am Heart J 101:281–287, 1981.

40. Higgins CB (ed): CT of the heart and great vessels: experimental evaluation and clinical application. Mt Kisco NY: Futura, 1983.

41. Kaufman L, Crooks L, Sheldon P, Hricak H, Herfkens R, Bank W: The potential impact of nuclear magnetic resonance imaging on cardiovascular diagnosis. Circulation 67:251–257, 1983.

IV. METHODS FOR MONITORING THE PATIENT WITH ACUTE MYOCARDIAL ISCHEMIA

22. HEMODYNAMIC MONITORING IN ACUTE MYOCARDIAL INFARCTION

Robert K. Stack

Richard S. Stack

Since the advent of the coronary care unit and continuous electrocardiographic monitoring, pump failure has replaced dysrhythmia as the leading cause of inhospital death due to acute myocardial infarction (MI) [1−3]. The flow-directed pulmonary artery catheter (Swan-Ganz catheter) offers the ability to precisely monitor therapeutic interventions that may lead to a reduction in short-term mortality and morbidity resulting from pump failure and other mechanical complications of acute myocardial infarction [4−6].

Indications

Swan-Ganz catheterization, because of potential complications and cost, is not indicated in many cases of uncomplicated acute MI [7]. In some instances, however, the hemodynamic data may provide the key to rational management. Forrester et al. found that elevated pulmonary capillary wedge pressure (greater than 18 mmHg) and low cardiac index (less than 2.2 l/min/m^2) could be predicted clinically 83% of the time [8]. However, in certain unstable patients this degree of accuracy is not acceptable. In addition, hemodynamic parameters may change rapidly in acutely ill patients and the noninvasive clinical evaluation may lag behind the actual hemodynamic alterations. Indications for hemodynamic monitoring include, but are not limited to, the presence of pulmonary edema and/or cardiogenic

shock, pulmonary congestion that does not respond to conventional therapy, and the onset of signs or symptoms of peripheral hypoperfusion in the presence of an apparently adequate left ventricular filling pressure [4−12]. The data obtained from right heart catheterization have also been shown to predict prognosis [9, 13] and aid in the diagnosis of other complications of acute MI such as acute mitral regurgitation [14], ventricular septal defect [15], pericardial tamponade [16], pulmonary embolism [17], and infarction of the right ventricle [18].

Static Accuracy: Balancing and Calibrating Pressure-Monitoring Equipment

To avoid potentially disastrous errors in the analysis of hemodynamic data, it is essential that all physicians who perform Swan-Ganz catheterization be familiar with their pressure-monitoring equipment. The accuracy of zero determinations and gain settings must be confirmed *by the physician* responsible for the procedure.

Although various manufacturers differ in the degree of sophistication and labeling of amplifier controls, they each have some form of position control and a gain (sensitivity) control. In addition, many employ a separate zero or "R balance" device for balancing transducers. The following is a description of a typical pressure-monitoring system.

R.M. Califf and G.S. Wagner (eds.), ACUTE CORONARY CARE: Principles and Practice. Copyright © 1985. Martinus Nijhoff Publishing, Boston/Dordrecht/Lancaster.

Prior to calibration, each transducer should be flushed and cleared of all evidence of trapped air. With the transducer electrically isolated from the amplifier, the position control is adjusted to the baseline of the strip chart recorder and/or monitoring screen. The transducer is then activated and is opened to room air at the midchest level of the supine patient. The zero control is adjusted until the tracing is inscribed exactly on the baseline throughout the entire range of gain settings. The transducer is then connected to an external manometer and the pressure resulting in a desired full-scale deflection is applied to the transducer. The gain control is then employed to adjust the tracing to a full-scale deflection on the strip chart recorder and/or monitoring screen.

Dynamic Accuracy: Adjusting the Frequency Response and Damping Coefficient

Although careful attention to static accuracy is essential for accurate pressure determinations, the dynamic accuracy of pressure waveforms must also be considered. The two major determinants of dynamic accuracy are the natural frequency and the damping coefficient [19]. If the pressure-monitoring system has a low natural frequency (< 20 Hz), in the range of the physiologic waveforms being recorded, significant overshoot may occur secondary to the phenomenon of resonance. If the damping coefficient of the system is also low ("underdamped") the degree of error will be further exaggerated.

Most modern catheter−manifold-tubing systems have both a low natural frequency and a low damping coefficient. The low natural frequency is usually due to small amounts of inapparent trapped air at the site of various tubing connections. Other major factors that result in a low natural frequency include: long tubing, narrow tubing, compliant tubing, and higher viscosity of the fluid in the tubing (e.g., presence of contrast material). The low damping coefficient generally observed in pressure-monitoring systems can be corrected with the use of newly available mechanical damping needles introduced into the tubing system (e.g., Correc Torr, Norton Company). The importance of dynamic accuracy

for faithful reproduction of physiologic waveforms is shown in figure 22-1.

Technique of Catheter Insertion

Insertion requires central venous access, which may be gained percutaneously via the internal or external jugular, femoral, right, or left subclavian or antecubital approaches. Antecubital cutdowns may also be performed. Following local anesthesia, cannulation of the vein is accomplished using an introducer sheath. After the transducers are balanced and calibrated, the integrity of the balloon is tested in a basin of saline. The Swan-Ganz catheter is advanced through the introducer to the right atrium, where the pressure waveforms are recorded. Samples of blood from the superior and inferior vena cavae and right atrium should also be obtained at this time if a possible intracardiac shunt is suspected. The balloon is inflated and the catheter is advanced into the right ventricle, where the pressure waveforms are recorded. The catheter is then introduced into the pulmonary artery and should be allowed to advance until a pulmonary wedge pressure is obtained. The balloon is deflated and the pulmonary artery pressure is recorded. Cardiac output may be determined using the thermodilution technique [20, 21]. After all pressure measurements, cardiac output, and oxygen samples are obtained, the catheter should be anchored at the insertion site with a suture and a sterile dressing applied. A chest x-ray should be obtained to confirm the position of the catheter and to exclude the presence of a pneumothorax. Normal pressures, cardiac index, and AVO_2 difference are shown in table 22-1 [22]. Normal pressure waveforms obtained with an optimally damped Swan-Ganz catheter are shown in figure 22-2.

Complications

Complications may develop during the use of Swan-Ganz catheterization. Although most of these are minor, serious complications and fatalities can occur [23−29]. Complications associated with venous access include pneumothorax, hemothorax, arterial puncture and hematoma, and infection at the puncture site. Ventricular arrhythmias are associated with passage through

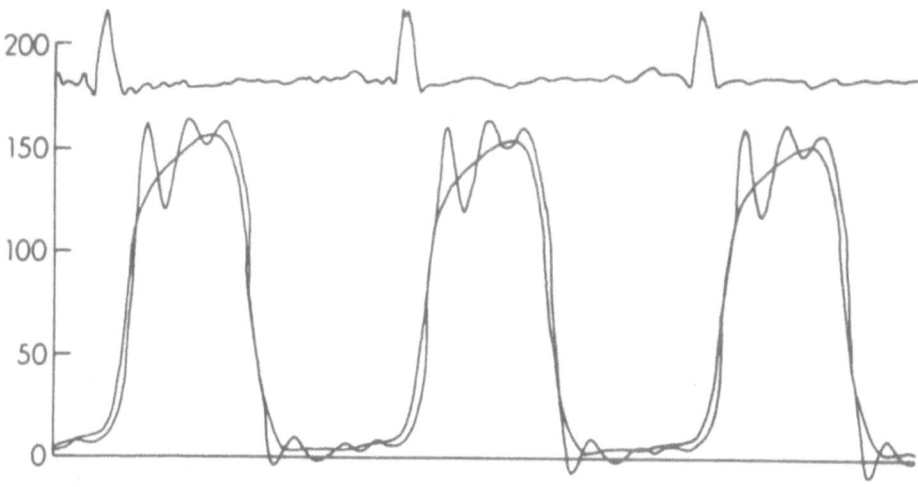

FIGURE 22-1. An underdamped left ventricular fluid-filled catheter tracing (with multiple peaks and overshoot) is compared with a simultaneous micromanometer pressure recording.

TABLE 22-1. Normal hemodynamic values

		Range	Mean
C_1		$2.8-4.2$ l/min/m^2	3.4
AVO$_2$ difference		$30-48$ ml/l blood	38
Art pressure	Systolic	$90-140$ mmHg	130
	Diastolic	$6-90$	70
	Mean	$70-105$	85
RA	Max.	$2-14$	7
	Min.	$-2-6$	2
	Mean	$-1-8$	4
RV	Systolic	$15-28$	24
	End-diastolic	$0-8$	4
PA	Systolic	$15-28$	24
	Diastolic	$5-16$	10
	Mean	$10-22$	16
PCWP	Max.	$9-23$	16
	Min.	$1-12$	6
	Mean	$6-15$	9
Systolic vascular resistance		$900-1400$ dyn$-$s/cm^5	1150 dyn$-$s/cm^5
Pulmonary vascular resistance		$150-250$	200

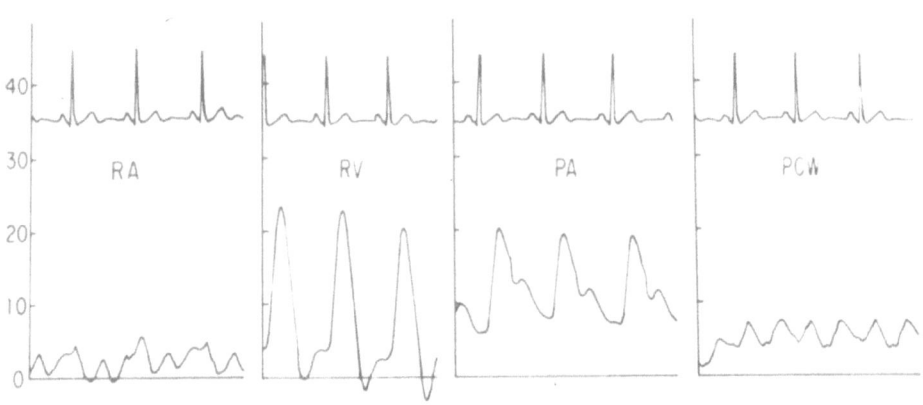

FIGURE 22-2. Optimally damped Swan-Ganz pressure tracings.

the right ventricle [23—26]. The incidence of ectopy is increased in the presence of hypoxia, shock, electrolyte abnormalities, acidosis, or when the time required to cannulate the pulmonary artery is prolonged greater than 20 min [23], and is decreased by the use of prophylactic lidocaine [30].

Transient right bundle branch block with or without left anterior fascicular block has been reported to occur in as many as 5% of right heart catheterizations [31, 32]. Complete heart block has been reported with preexisting left bundle branch block [33, 34] and, therefore, a prophylactic temporary pacemaker may be indicated in this setting.

Pulmonary complications include hemoptysis, infarction, and pulmonary artery rupture [27—29]. Most fatalities attributed to pulmonary complications of Swan-Ganz catheterization have been secondary to the rare occurrence of pulmonary artery rupture and hemorrhage. Most fatalities have occurred in elderly patients with pulmonary hypertension, associated with prolonged inflation of the balloon or migration and impaction of the deflated catheter tip. Nonfatal pulmonary embolus and infarction are more common occurrences [24, 25, 26]. Deep-vein thrombosis including superior vena cava syndrome has also been reported [35, 36]. Other unusual complications include catheter-related sepsis [24, 37], catheter knotting, damage to pulmonary or tricuspid valve leaflets, and the

development of a clinically insignificant thrombocytopenia [38—41].

Use of Hemodynamic Data

Patients with acute myocardial infarction may be divided into clinical subsets on the basis of hemodynamic data [12] (see chapter 11). Hemodynamic classification can provide both therapeutic and prognostic information [9, 11, 12, 42]. In table 22-2, patients are categorized on the basis of cardiac index, arterial pressure, and pulmonary capillary wedge pressure. Patients in subset IB generally have a good prognosis requiring no hemodynamic intervention and may be candidates for early hospital discharge. The systemic and wedge pressures in patients in subset IC will respond to fluid infusion, but treatment may not be necessary since the cardiac index is in the normal range. Hypertension (subset IA) should be treated if it persists after relief of chest pain, and a beta-blocking agent may reduce the discrepancy between myocardial oxygen supply and demand [43, 44].

Patients with elevated pulmonary capillary wedge pressure and normal cardiac index (subset II) may benefit from diuretic therapy, thereby reducing preload, left ventricular size, wall tension, and oxygen demand. In the presence of systolic hypertension the addition of vasodilator agents may be necessary. The rare circumstance of high output failure with hypotension (subset

TABLE 22-2. Therapeutic subsets

Cardiac index	BP		pcw < 18	pcw ≥ 18
			Subset I	*Subset II*
	A ↑		Treat pain, vasodilator, propranolol	Diuretics, vasodilator
≥ 2.2 l/min/m²	B N1		No Rx	Diuretics
	C ↓		Fluids or no Rx	Inotropic agent
			Subset III	*Subset IV*
	A ↑		Fluids → vasodilator	Vasodilator
< 2.2 l/min/m²	B N1		Fluids	Vasodilator, inotropic agent
	C ↓		Fluids	Inotropic agent balloon pump, vasodilator

IIC) should stimulate a search for an underlying mechanical or metabolic cause.

In the presence of pulmonary capillary wedge pressure less than 18 mmHg and decreased cardiac index less than 2.2 l/min/m² (subset III), volume expansion to a pulmonary capillary wedge pressure of 18−20 mm can optimize cardiac output by the Frank-Starling mechanism [45, 46]. If a bradydysrhythmia is present, either an increase in parasympathetic tone or sinus node dysfunction is present. Such patients may require atropine or temporary cardiac pacing, but volume infusion and/or a decrease in or discontinuation of nitrate therapy may suffice.

Patients with a depressed cardiac index and pulmonary capillary wedge pressure greater than 18 mmHg (subset IV) have a poor prognosis [8, 9, 13]. It is in these patients that vasodilator therapy may be of considerable benefit. A decrease in afterload affects the left ventricular function curve in the same direction as an increased inotropic state without the associated increase in oxygen demand [47, 49]. The size of the left ventricle may also be reduced, further reducing the left ventricular work. Nitrates and nitroprusside also have a direct effect on venous capacitance, resulting in a decreased preload. Cardiac output is increased, preload is decreased, and heart rate and blood pressure may remain unchanged due to the augmentation of stroke volume in the presence of a diminished peripheral vascular resistance. Inotropic agents and/or an intraaortic balloon pump may be required to maintain an adequate perfusion pressure in these patients if vasodilators fail.

In addition to the determination of hemody-namic subsets, data obtained from Swan-Ganz catheterization can also provide critical diagnostic information regarding complications of acute myocardial infarction. Acute mitral regurgitation or ventricular septal defect may occur in the setting of acute infarction with potentially fatal consequences (see chapter 45). Diagnosis using noninvasive methods may be difficult or impossible. Although new systolic murmurs are frequently present, they occasionally may be absent [50].

The differential diagnosis of these two major complications is possible with a Swan-Ganz catheter. Oximetry will show an abnormal stepup in PO_2 in the right ventricle in the presence of a ventricular septal defect. This disorder may also be suspected when the thermodilution cardiac output curve loses its normally smooth exponential downslope and develops a second recirculation peak. Acute mitral regurgitation may be suspected by the presence of a large V wave in the pulmonary capillary wedge tracing (see figure 22-3). However, limitations of this sign in chronic mitral regurgitation have recently been documented in a study by Fuchs et al. where large V waves were also seen in patients with ventricular septal defect, prosthetic mitral valve, mitral stenosis, and congestive heart failure [51]. One-third of their patients with documented severe mitral regurgitation had trivial V waves (less than 5 mmHg), but none of the patients in their study had mitral regurgitation of acute onset and thus the sensitivity of this sign to diagnose the presence of acute mitral regurgitation during infarction remains uncertain. Both acute mitral regurgitation and ventricular septal rupture may

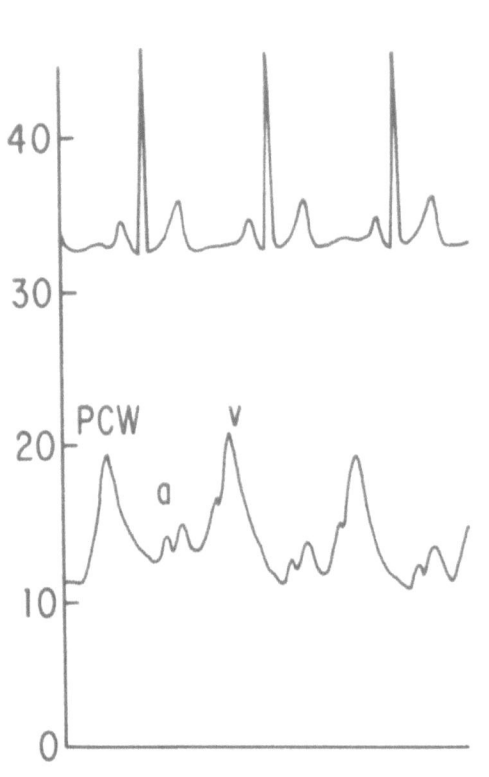

FIGURE 22-3. Prominent V waves are recorded in a pulmonary capillary wedge tracing obtained from a patient with severe mitral regurgitation.

myocardial infarction [60]. If diagnosed and managed early (see chapter 45), however, surgical cure has been reported [61]. Pulmonary embolus is not an uncommon occurrence in the preinfarction period and differentiation from extension of infarction may be clinically difficult. When ventilation–perfusion scans are indeterminant, the finding of a pulmonary artery diastolic pressure markedly elevated over the pulmonary capillary wedge pressure can corroborate the preliminary diagnosis of pulmonary embolus and indicate the need for a pulmonary arteriogram [17].

Summary

Swan-Ganz catheterization is often a very useful adjunct to the management of selected patients with acute myocardial infarction. The rate of serious complications is low and the therapeutic and prognostic information obtained may be essential for adequate patient management. As further research elucidates the value of various methods of coronary reperfusion aimed at acute myocardial salvage, Swan-Ganz catheterization will likely play a key role in optimizing hemodynamics and thus minimizing myocardial oxygen requirements during the early stages of acute myocardial infarction.

respond initially to vasodilator therapy or intraaortic counterpulsation balloon pumping [52–56]. Surgical correction is almost always the treatment of choice following stabilization [14, 15].

Right ventricular infarction (see chapter 21) may occur in as many as 40% of cases of acute inferior myocardial infarction [57, 58]. Hemodynamic data are often very helpful in establishing this diagnosis. Sendon et al. found that right atrial pressure that was approximately equal to pulmonary capillary wedge pressure suggested right ventricular infarction [59]. The finding of a y descent, equal or deeper than the x descent, was also highly suggestive. The sensitivity and specificity of these criteria, however, depend on the clinical situation, and similar findings may be seen in constrictive pericarditis and restrictive cardiomyopathy. Pericardial tamponade associated with myocardial rupture is an underdiagnosed and generally fatal complication of acute

References

1. Killip T III, Kimball JT: Treatment of myocardial infarction in a coronary care unit. Am J Cardiol 20:457–464, 1967.
2. Friedberg CK: General treatment of acute myocardial infarction. Circulation 39:IV-252–260, 1969.
3. Norris RM, Brandt PWT, Lee AJ: Mortality in a coronary-care unit analysed by a new coronary prognostic index. Lancet x: 278–281, 1969.
4. Durrer JD, Lie KI, Van Capelle FJL, Durrer D: Effect of sodium nitroprusside on mortality in acute myocardial infarction. N Engl J Med 306: 1121–1128, 1982.
5. Shell WE, Sobel BE: Protection of jeopardized ischemic myocardium by reduction of ventricular afterload. N Engl J Med 291:481–486, 1974.
6. Chatterjee K, Swan HJC, Kaushik VS, Jobin G, Magnusson P, Forrester JS: Effects of vasodilator therapy for severe pump failure in acute myocardial infarction on short-term and late prognosis. Circulation 53:797–802, 1976.

7. Dalen JE: Bedside hemodynamic monitoring. N Engl J Med 301:1176–1178, 1979.

8. Forrester JS, Diamond GA, Swan HJC: Correlative classification of clinical and hemodynamic function after acute myocardial infarction. Am J Cardiol 39:137–145, 1977.

9. Weber KT, Janicki JS, Russell RO, Rackley CE: Identification of high risk subsets of acute myocardial infarction: derived from the myocardial infarction research units cooperative study data bank. Am J Cardiol 41:197–203, 1978.

10. McHugh TJ, Forrester JS, Adler L, Zion D, Swan HJC: Pulmonary vascular congestion in acute myocardial infarction: hemodynamic and radiologic correlations. Ann Intern Med 76:29–33, 1972.

11. Russell RO Jr, Mantle JA, Rogers WJ, Rackley CE: Current status of hemodynamic monitoring: indications, diagnoses, complications. Crit Care Cardiol x:1–13, 1981.

12. Forrester JS, Diamond G, Chatterjee K, Swan HJC: Medical therapy of acute myocardial infarction by application of hemodynamic subsets (first of two parts). N Engl J Med 295:1356–1413, 1976.

13. Ratshin RA, Rackley CE, Russell RO Jr: Hemodynamic evaluation of left ventricular function in shock complicating myocardial infarction. Circulation 45:127–139, 1972.

14. Nishimura RA, Schaff HV, Shobb C, et al: Papillary muscle rupture complicating acute myocardial infarction: analysis of 17 patients. Am J Cardiol 51:373, 1983.

15. Radford MJ, Johnson RA, Daggot WM, et al: Ventricular septal rupture: a review of clinical and physiologic features and an analysis of survival. Circulation 64:545, 1981.

16. Shabetai R, Fowler NO, Guntheroth WG: The hemodynamics of cardiac tamponade and constrictive pericarditis. Am J Cardiol 26:480–489, 1970.

17. Sasahara AA, Cannilla JE, Morse RL, Sidd JJ, Tremblay GM: Clinical and physiologic studies in pulmonary thromboembolism. Am J Cardiol 20:10–20, 1967.

18. Lopez-Sendon J, Coma-Canella I, Gamallo C: Sensitivity and specificity of hemodynamic criteria in the diagnosis of acute right ventricular infarction. Circulation 64:515–525, 1981.

19. Grossman W: Pressure measurement. In: Grossman W (ed) Cardiac catheterization and angiography. Philadelphia: Lea and Febiger, 1980, pp 103–115.

20. Ganz W, Donoso R, Marcus HS, Forrester JS, Swan HJC: A new technique for measurement of cardiac output by thermodilution in man. Am J Cardiol 27:392–396, 1971.

21. Swan HJC, Ganz W: Measurement of right atrial and pulmonary arterial pressures and cardiac output: clinical application of hemodynamic monitoring. Chicago: Year Book Medical, 1982, pp 453–473.

22. Schlant RL, Sonnenblick EH, Gorlin R: Normal physiology of the cardiovascular system. In: Hurst JW (ed) The Heart. 1982, pp 75–114.

23. Sprung CL, Jacobs LJ, Caralis PV, Karpf M: Ventricular arrhythmias during Swan-Ganz catheterization of the critically ill. Chest 79:413–415, 1981.

24. Boyd KD, Thomas SJ, Gold J, Boyd AD: A prospective study of complications of pulmonary artery catheterizations in 500 consecutive patients. Chest 84:245–249, 1983.

25. Elliott CG, Zimmerman GA, Clemmer TP: Complications of pulmonary artery catheterization in the care of critically ill patients: a prospective study. Chest 76:647–652, 1979.

26. Cairns JA, Holder D: Ventricular fibrillation due to passage of a Swan-Ganz catheter. American Journal of Cardiology 35:589, 1975.

27. Foote GA, Schabel SI, Hodges M: Pulmonary complications of the flow-directed balloon-tipped catheter. N Engl J Med 290:927–931, 1974.

28. Pape LA, Haffajee CI, Markis JE, Ockene IS, Paraskos JA, Dalen JE, Alpert JS: Fatal pulmonary hemorrhage after use of the flow-directed balloon-tipped catheter. Ann Intern Med 90:344–347, 1979.

29. Hart U, Ward DR, Gillilian R, Brawley RK: Fatal pulmonary hemorrhage complicating Swan-Ganz catheterization. Surgery 91:24–27, 1982.

30. Shaw TJI: The Swan-Ganz pulmonary artery catheter: incidence of complications, with particular reference to ventricular dysrhythmias, and their prevention. Anaesthesia 34:651–656, 1979.

31. Luck JC, Engel TR: Transient right bundle branch block with 'Swan-Ganz" catheterization. Am Heart J 92:263–264, 1976.

32. Castellanos A, Ramirez AV, Mayorga-Cortes A, Pefkaros K, Rozanski JJ, Sprung C, Myerburg RJ: Left fascicular blocks during right-heart catheterization using the Swan-Ganz catheter. Circulation 64:1271–1276, 1981.

33. Thomson IR, Dalton BC, Lappas DG, Lowenstein E: Right bundle-branch block and complete heart block caused by the Swan-Ganz catheter. Anesthesiology 51:359–362, 1979.

34. Abernathy WS: Complete heart block caused by the Swan-Ganz catheter. Chest 65:349, 1974.

35. Dye LE, Segall PH, Russell RO Jr, Mantle JA, Rogers WJ, Rackley CE: Deep venous thrombosis of the upper extremity associated with use of the Swan-Ganz catheter. Chest 73:673−675, 1978.

36. Snow P: Swan-Ganz catheter and superior vena cava syndrome [letter to editor]. JAMA 243: 1525, 1980.

37. Hunter D, Moran JF, Venezio FR: Osteomyelitis of the clavicle after Swan-Ganz catheterization. Arch Intern Med 143:153−154, 1983.

38. Lipp H, O'Donoghue K, Resnekow L: Intracardiac knotting of a flow-directed balloon catheter [letter to editor]. N Engl J Med 284:220, 1971.

39. Ettinghausen SE, Pearlman SH, Brandstetter RD: Tricuspid valve erosion from Swan-Ganz catheters. Chest 80:509−510, 1981.

40. Ford SE, Manley PN: Indwelling cardiac catheters: an autopsy study of associated endocardial lesions. Arch Pathol Lab Med 106:314−317, 1982.

41. Kim YL, Richman KA, Marshall BE: Thrombocytopenia associated with Swan-Ganz catheterization in patients. Anesthesiology 53:261−262, 1980.

42. Bleifeld W, Hanrath P, Mathey D, Merx W: Acute myocardial infarction. V. Left and right ventricular haemodynamics in cardiogenic shock. Br Heart J 36:822−834, 1974.

43. Mueller HS, Ayers SM, Religa A, Evans RG: Propranolol in the treatment of acute myocardial infarction: effect on myocardial oxygenation and hemodynamics. Circulation 49:1078−1087, 1974.

44. Vatner SF, Baig H, Manders WT, Ochs H, Pagani M: Effects of propranolol on regional myocardial function, electrograms, and blood flow in conscious dogs with myocardial ischemia. J Clin Invest 60:353−360, 1977.

45. Russell RO Jr, Rackley CE, Pombo J, Hunt D, Potanin C, Dodge HT: Effects of increasing left ventricular filling pressure in patients with acute myocardial infarction. J Clin Invest 49:1539−1550, 1970.

46. Crexells C, Chatterjee K, Forrester JS, Dikshit K, Swan HJC: Optimal level of filling pressure in the left side of the heart in acute myocardial infarction. N Engl J Med 289:1263−1266, 1973.

47. Massie BM, Chatterjee K: Vasodilator therapy of pump failure complicating acute myocardial infarction. Med Clin North Am 63:25−51, 1979.

48. Sonnenblick EH, Downing SE: Afterload as a primary determinant of ventricular performance. Am J Physiol 204:604−610, 1963.

49. Chatterjee K, Parmley WW, Ganz W, Forrester J, Walkinsky P, Crexells C, Swan HJC: Hemodynamic and metabolic responses to vasodilator therapy in acute myocardial infarction. Circulation 48:1183−1193, 1973.

50. Forrester JS, Diamond G, Freedman S, Allen HN, Parmley WW, Matloff J, Swan HJC: Silent mitral insufficiency in acute myocardial infarction. Circulation 44:877−883, 1971.

51. Fuchs RM, Heuser RR, Yin FCP, Brinker JA: Limitations of pulmonary wedge V waves in diagnosing mitral regurgitation. Am J Cardiol 49: 849−854, 1982.

52. Chatterjee K, Parmley WW, Swan HJC, Berman G, Forrester J, Marcus HS: Beneficial effects of vasodilator agents in severe mitral regurgitation due to dysfunction of subvalvular apparatus. Circulation 48:684−690, 1973.

53. Goodman DJ, Rossen RM, Holloway EL, Alderman EL, Harrison DC: Effect of nitroprusside on left ventricular dynamics in mitral regurgitation. Circulation 50:1025−1032, 1974.

54. Harshaw CW, Grossman W, Munro AB, McLaurin LP: Reduced systemic vascular resistance as therapy for severe mitral regurgitation of valvular origin. Ann Intern Med 83:312−316, 1975.

55. Tecklenberg PL, Fitzgerald J, Allaire BI, Alderman EL, Harrison DC: Afterload reduction in the management of postinfarction ventricular septal defect. Am J Cardiol 38:956−958, 1976.

56. Gold H, Lunbach R, Sanders C, et al: Intraaortic balloon pumping for ventricular septal defect or mitral regurgitation complicating acute myocardial infarction. Circulation 47:1191−1196, 1973.

57. Cohn JN, Guiha NH, Broder MI, Limas CH: Right ventricular infarction: clinical and hemodynamic features. Am J Cardiol 33:209−214, 1974.

58. Roberts R, Marmor AT: Right ventricular infarction. Annu Rev Med 34:377−390, 1983.

59. Lopez-Sendon J, Coma-Canella I, Gamallo C: Sensitivity and specificity of hemodynamic criteria in the diagnosis of acute right ventricular infarction. Circulation 64:515−525, 1981.

60. Bates RJ, Beutler S, Resnekov L, Anagnostopoulos CE: Cardiac rupture: challenge in diagnosis and management. Am J Cardiol 40:429−437, 1977.

61. Cobbs BW, Hatche CR, Roberson PH: Cardiac rupture: three operations with two long term survivors. JAMA 223:232, 1973.

23. THE USE OF ECHOCARDIOGRAPHIC TECHNIQUES FOR DETERMINING CARDIAC FUNCTION DURING ACUTE MYOCARDIAL INFARCTION

Randolph P. Martin

Two-dimensional echocardiography (2DE) has proven to be a clinically useful diagnostic and prognostic noninvasive modality. Advances in instrumentation have led to the widespread use of this technique, not only in standard noninvasive laboratories, but also in such critical care areas as the coronary care unit and surgical−medical intensive care units. 2DE is a truly portable, totally noninvasive technique with no known biologic hazards. It can be performed serially and provides high-resolution (2−4 mm) rapid tomographic information about cardiac chambers, valves, pericardial structures, and great vessels. The ability to image the heart rapidly through multiple tomographic planes allows the clinician to use this noninvasive test to determine quickly the differential diagnoses in patients who come to hospitals with chest-pain syndromes (table 23−1).

This technique allows the echocardiographer quickly to visualize total cardiac anatomy, and this noninvasive modality is the only widely applied noninvasive test that allows for visualization of segmental and subsegmental wall motion and thickening analysis of both the left and right ventricles. 2DE, therefore, allows for the rapid assessment of the location and extent of segmental wall motion abnormalities in the patient with suspected or proven coronary ischemia/acute

myocardial infarction (MI). This information provided by 2DE about the extent of segmental wall motion abnormalities and viable residual myocardium offers diagnostic and prognostic information when the patient is imaged in the early hours after an acute myocardial ischemic event. Additionally, this technique has great use in rapidly assessing the complications of an acute myocardial infarction (MI) (table 23-2).

Nuclear techniques have been useful in the evaluation of patients with known or suspected coronary artery disease. 2DE, however, has the unique advantage, noted above, that allows the physician to visualize the heart in multiple tomographic planes, providing clear and definite anatomic visualization of great vessels, valves, papillary muscles, and segmental−global ventricular function. By imaging the heart from multiple transducer positions, the echocardiographer is able actually to visualize cardiac size, shape, and function in a three-dimensional sense. However, 2DE (even when coupled with Doppler ultrasound) is a very useful diagnostic tool only when applied in the appropriate clinical setting. Technology never replaces conventional clinical diagnoses, but technology can be extremely cost effective and aid greatly in diagnosis and prognosis when judicially applied in the proper clinical setting. 2DE (especially when coupled with

R.M. Califf and G.S. Wagner (eds.), ACUTE CORONARY CARE: Principles and Practice. Copyright © 1985. Martinus Nijhoff Publishing, Boston/Dordrecht/Lancaster.

TABLE 23-1.

Advantages of 2DE for CCU
    Noninvasive—no biological hazard
    Portable—rapid bedside use
    Serial studies
    M-mode—Doppler
    Rapid tomographic assessment of total cardiac
        anatomy
        Chamber size
        Valvular integrity
        LV−RV global—segmental function
        Great vessels (proximal)
        Pericardial abnormalities
    Aids in differential diagnosis of chest pain
        Pericardial abnormalities
        Mitral valve prolapse
        Myopathies (IHSS, congestive)
        Type-I aortic dissection

TABLE 23-2.

Role of 2DE in suspected AMI−CAD
    Diagnostic—Rapid assessment of
                Segmental−Global LV−RV
                function
    Prognostic—Clinical course
                Wall motion index
                Ejection fraction
                Multivessel disease
                Remote asynergy
                Lack of hyperkinesis
    Detect complication of AMI
        Free-wall rupture—hemopericardium
        VSD
        Papillary muscle dysfunction
        Aneurysm
        Myopathy
        LV thrombi

Doppler) has tremendous diagnostic and prognostic value in the patient with known or suspected acute MI. The ability to aid in the differential diagnoses of patients with chest-pain syndromes, and to detect the consequences of MI, as well as the extent of left ventricular wall motion abnormalities, makes this technique extremely valuable in these patients. It is again emphasized that this is a portable, rapidly available technique that can go to the patient's bedside and provide information in the early hours after the onset of a severe ischemic process.

Acute Myocardial Infarction Diagnosis

Experimental animal studies utilizing the 2DE technique have shown that acute ligation of a coronary artery quickly leads to a rapid decrease in segmental systolic wall thickening that shortly proceeds to dyskinesis and thinning of the ischemic segment. These changes can be visualized as soon as 30 s after acute ligation and precede the onset of ECG changes [1, 2]. Such animal work has shown further a very good correlation between the localization of experimental infarction by 2DE and the postmortem anatomic extent of MI. It is important to note that, if total ligation is continued for greater than 20 min, the striking segmental wall motion abnormalities observed in the animal model do not return to normal even

though blood flow is reestablished. Therefore, acute severe ischemic events that do not progress to complete transmural myocardial infarcts will produce very characteristic segmental wall motion abnormalities if visualized by 2DE within 4−6 h after the onset of the event.

Several authors have shown that 2DE, like both radionuclide and contrast angiography, allows the accurate grading of segmental wall motion abnormalities. Unlike these techniques, 2DE is unique in its ability to allow actual visualization of systolic wall thickening [3]. Parisi et al. [4] found a 95% sensitivity and 84% specificity of 2DE in the detection of wall motion abnormalities when compared with angiography. 2DE, with its unique ability to visualize segmental and subsegmental wall thickening as well as endocardial wall motion, is sensitive for diagnosing high-grade segmental wall motion abnormalities of the left ventricular inferior wall, the right ventricle, and basal ventricular septum—areas not easily or well visualized by nuclear techniques.

Several studies have confirmed the ability of 2DE clearly to diagnose high-grade segmental wall motion abnormalities in patients with transmural and subendocardial myocardial infarcts. The ability of this technique accurately to diagnose acute segmental wall motion abnormalities in patients soon after admission to coronary care units was first noted by Heger et al. [5]. They performed 2DEs on 44 patients within 4 h of admission for known or suspected MI, and were able to obtain adequate left ventricular (LV) examinations in over 84% of these. There was an excellent correlation between ECG localization of the MI and 2DE asynergy in the infarct zone. These authors subsequently [6] demonstrated that the degree of overall LV dysfunction, as determined by the early-acute 2DEs, correlated well with the patient's prognosis. The fewer the number of LV segments showing high-grade segmental wall motion abnormalities on the acute early 2DE images, the better was the overall functional status of the patient.

Work from the author's laboratory [7] has shown that 2DE is not only an extremely accurate diagnostic tool in patients with acute MI, but offers valuable prognostic information. 2DE, early after the onset of chest pain, provides very accurate diagnostic information about the location and extent of segmental wall motion abnormalities. Additionally, 2DE provides prognostic information about the patient's clinical course and the number of coronary artery vessels involved with high-grade stenotic lesions. This study [7] and that by Horowitz et al. [8] have shown the high sensitivity of 2DE to diagnose accurately "transmural" MI. Patients within 12 h of admission for the initial episode of severe chest pain that was suspected to represent an acute MI were studied [8]. High-grade segmental wall motion abnormalities were seen in 94% of the 33 patients who eventually evolved a "transmural" MI. Of these 33, 18 had nondiagnostic changes on their admission ECGs. The two patients who were missed by 2DE, and had normal wall motion, had uncomplicated clinical courses. Of their 32 patients without clinical evidence of MI, 84% (27) had normal segmental and regional wall motion on their admission-initial 2DE, and all had uncomplicated hospital courses. Patients with totally normal left and right ventricular size, shape, and function, when imaged soon after a chest-pain event, will seldom have clinical confirmation of a "transmural" MI.

Patients with transmural MI commonly have high-grade (akinetic and dyskinetic) segments that can be clearly visualized. There is a very characteristic location for anterior (figure 23-1) versus inferior or posterior locations of MI (fig-

ures 23-2 and 23-3) that the echocardiographer comes to recognize easily. Furthermore, patients with nontransmural MI generally have severe hypokinesis or akinesis, but not necessarily dyskinesis or marked thinning of the involved segment. Loh et al. [9] have demonstrated the usefulness of 2DE in diagnosing "nontransmural" MI. These authors investigated 30 patients with acute chest-pain syndromes and nondiagnostic ECG findings. Ten (83%) of 12 patients who eventually evolved a nontransmural MI had 2DE evidence of significant segmental wall motion abnormalities, while all 18 patients without MI had normal wall motion.

Thus, many studies have clearly shown that 2DE is a sensitive technique for detecting high-grade segmental wall motion abnormalities in patients who have significant chest pain due to acute MI—either transmural or nontransmural [5–10]. 2DE can be easily applied to approximately 90% of patients admitted with chest-pain syndrome (84%–95% of patients can be successfully imaged). It is important to recognize that the speed with which the 2DE is performed is critical. 2DE performed days after a severe chest-pain episode does not offer the same diagnostic and prognostic information as that applied within hours (table 23-3).

Differential Diagnostic Role

Many patients are admitted to coronary care units (CCUs) for "rule-out MI." 2DE is extremely useful for detecting true cardiac conditions (other than acute MI) that produce significant chest pain. Foremost among these would be type-1 aortic dissections, pericardial abnormalities, mitral valve prolapse, and IHSS. All of these conditions can be easily recognized by 2DE, which aids in accurately triaging the "rule-out MI" patient. These capabilities enhance the cost effectiveness of 2DE.

Prognostic Role of Two-Dimensional Echocardiogram in the CCU

Since 2DE offers complete tomographic visualization of multiple segments of left and right ventricular free walls, it allows the echocardiographer to determine not only the location of

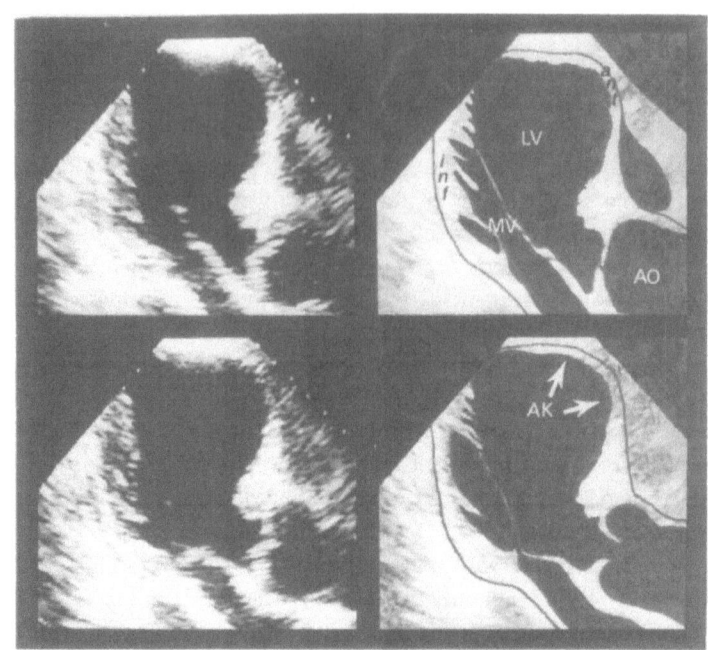

FIGURE 23-1. A four-panel illustrative example of an anterior septal myocardial infarction. The panels on the left show actual stop-frame images, with the panel on the right showing diagrammatic drawings. The top frames are labeled "diastole"; the bottom frames, "systole." This apical two-chamber view clearly shows the akinetic (AK) segment involving the apical anterior septal wall.

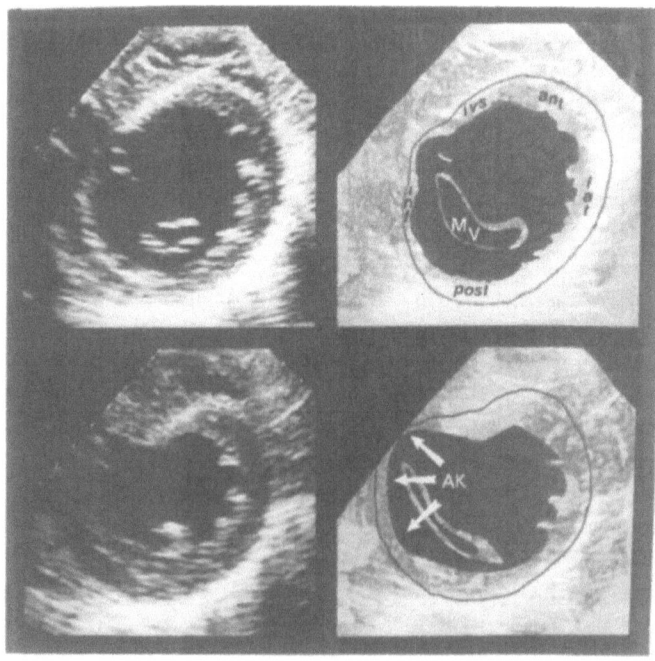

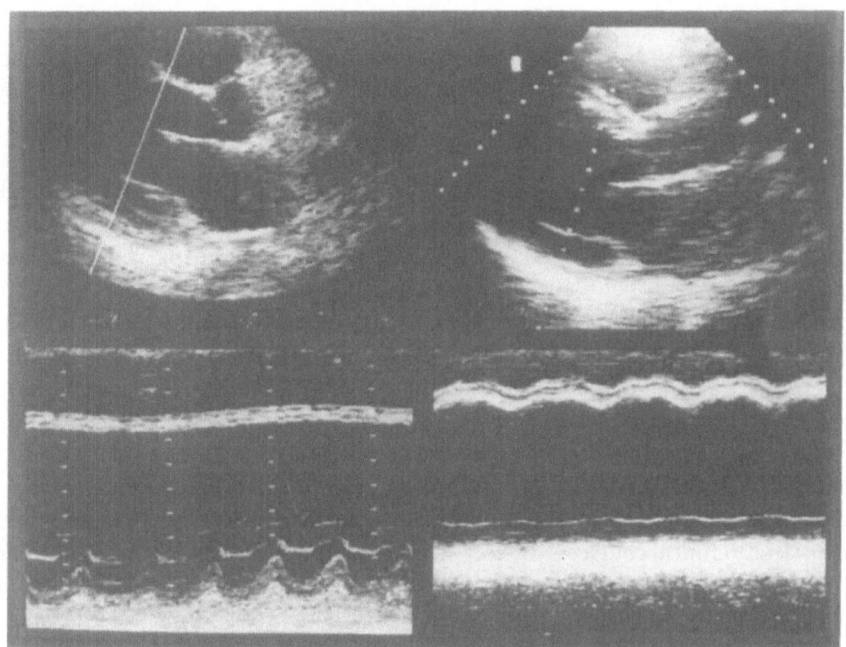

FIGURE 23-3. Illustrative two-dimensional (top panels) and M-mode (bottom panel) echoes on patients with anterior myocardial infarction (left panel) and inferior myocardial infarction (right panel). Patients with extensive anterior septal MIs will often show a thin nonmoving interventricular septum on both the 2D and M-mode. Those patients with characteristic inferior MIs on the parasternal long-axis view will often show a thinned area underlying the chordal and posterior mitral leaflet structures on the 2DE, and a thin if not hard to recognize posterior wall on the M-mode echo.

FIGURE 23-2. Stop-frame images with schematic drawings taken during diastole (top panel) and systole (bottom panel) of a patient with an inferior myocardial infarction. These views are obtained from a parasternal short-axis view. The akinetic (AK) inferior wall can clearly be seen to have the outward characteristic motion during systole.

TABLE 23-3. Summary of use of 2DE in acute MI

Feasibility—84%–95% of patients can be
    successfully imaged
Diagnostic—Sensitivity 93%–94% (SWMA = MI)
    Specificity 84% (no SWMA = no MI)
Prognostic—Clinical course
    Normal echo—good prognosis
    Extent of SWMA—prognosis worsens
  Multivessel disease
  Remote asynergy
  Lack of hyperkinesis

SWMA, high-grade segmental wall motion abnormalities

segmental wall motion abnormalities but their extent. 2DE performed soon after admission to the CCU for acute MI offers prognostic information concerning (a) the patient's clinical course—even earlier than conventional clinical parameters, and (b) the presence of severe multivessel coronary artery stenosis. 2DE is able to detect ischemic and/or jeopardized (but not infarcted) myocardium, and may be an excellent technique for following interventions that aid in its salvage.

Many authors have shown that the extent of an MI can be determined from a "wall motion index" [6, 7, 11]. The wall motion index is based upon the ability of the 2DE accurately to visualize segmental and subsegmental left and right ventricular free wall motion and thickening. Each segment can be given a score (with normal, hypokinesis, akinesis, and dyskinesis each having an assigned numerical value). Adding all the scores for each segment and dividing by the number of segments analyzed gives a wall motion index. The wall motion index is an accurate and early discriminator between those patients who are going to be survivors of their acute MI and those who will be nonsurvivors or who will develop major complications such as cardiogenic shock [7, 12]. This author's laboratory has shown that many clinical and laboratory parameters, especially those available soon after the patient's admission, do not accurately discriminate between those patients who will or will not have major complications and/or die. The wall motion index, which shows the extent of segmental wall motion abnormalities and indicates ischemia remote from the area of infarction, provides an

early prognostic role of 2DE in patients with acute MI. This index would be extremely useful if intervention is aimed at preserving ischemic, but not infarcted, myocardium. This author's group has shown that the wall motion index alone (not age, sex, previous MI or angina NYHA classification, location of MI, admission blood pressure, chest x-ray, or Killip class) accurately predicted those patients who developed cardiogenic shock and/or died during the acute hospitalization.

Our group has also shown that early acute 2DE provides the ability to detected significant multivessel coronary artery disease. In the vast majority of patients, a very good agreement exists between the ECG localization of infarction and 2DE localization of high-grade segmental wall motion abnormalities. However, 2DE may detect high-grade segmental wall motion abnormalities in a zone remote from the ECG infarction zone. Previous work in nuclear cardiology has shown that there can clearly be remote zones of asynergy that do not correspond to a single infarct vascular region. This has been termed "remote asynergy" or "ischemia at a distance." Remote asynergy is associated with a higher incidence of death, cardiogenic shock, reinfarction, or angina during the acute hospital course [7]. The presence of remote asynergy on 2DE correctly identified 77% of patients with severe multivessel disease. These results suggest that critical multivessel disease can be detected in patients imaged soon after the onset of an acute MI by the presence of remote asynergy and/or the lack of a hyperkinetic remote zone.

Many studies have shown that predischarge 2DE, like predischarge exercise testing, offers significanct information concerning the patient's short-term and one-year prognosis. It is important to recognize that the segmental wall motion abnormalities obtained on 2DE often overestimate the eventual pathologic size of the acute MI. The 2DE, in its ability to show ischemia as well as infarction, shows the ramifications of reversible hypoperfusion as well as infarction. The 2DE extent of asynergy closely correlates with the thallium defect. The various interventions aimed at salvaging the ischemic myocardium should be effectively evaluated by 2DE techniques.

Right Ventricular Infarction

Right ventricular (RV) infarction may frequently complicate inferior−posterior LV infarction, and is an important clinical syndrome whose early recognition has major therapeutic implications (see chapter 21). While RV infarction was thought initially to be a fairly rare occurrence, as many as 25−45% of patients with inferior MIs may have RV infarction [13, 14]. Certain characteristics of 2DE findings are seen in patients with RV infarction [15]. These patients often have akinetic or dyskinetic motion of the RV free wall, and will often have RV dilatation as well as possible paradoxical interventricular septal motion. Since the rapid diagnosis of RV involvement with inferior MI can lead to the proper invasive and hemodynamic management of the patient, 2DE seems to be an extremely valuable technique in patients with inferior MI in whom the question of RV involvement is either unsuspected or not clinically recognized.

Detection of the Mechanical Complications of Myocardial Infarction

Just as 2DE has proven to be useful in the rapid confirmation or diagnosis of the presence and extent of segmental wall motion abnormalities in patients with acute MI, it is also a very useful technique for detecting infarct complications (LV free-wall rupture, ventricular septal defect, papillary or chordal ruptures, ventricular aneurysms, LV thrombi). Since the majority of mechanical complications may be surgically correctable if diagnosed early, 2DE can be a valuable triage tool in any patient with suspected or known complications of MI. Not only does 2DE determine the presence of the presumed complications, but important prognostic information about residual LV or RV function can be noninvasively obtained in these critically ill patients. As such, 2DE often allows for the judicious use of invasive and surgical procedures and determines those patients in whom aggressive management is warranted.

Ventricular Free-Wall Rupture

Rupture of the free wall of the left ventricle occurs in up to 10% of hospital infarct deaths (see chapter 45). It is four times more frequent in women with an acute MI, especially those over the age of 60 who are hypertensive. It often occurs within the first week (3rd−5th day) and primarily occurs in anterior transmural infarctions involving at least 20% of the LV circumference. Often the free-wall rupture occurs near the junction of normal and infarct tissue. When imaging the patient with acute MI, 2DE often shows an area of demarcation between akinetic or dyskinetic infarct segments and normal segments. These areas may be those at which potential free-wall rupture might occur. When a patient presents, 3−5 days after admission, with recurrent chest pain, sudden hemodynamic collapse, and electromechanical dissociation, the diagnosis of presumed free-wall rupture is suggested. In this clinical setting, the final maneuver in a resuscitation is a pericardiocentesis attempting to diagnose and relieve tamponade secondary to hemopericardium. If, soon after CPR is instituted, 2DE visualization of the heart is obtained (often from the subcostal view), the presence or absence of a hemopericardium can be quickly diagnosed. This author has utilized a portable 2DE technique during multiple resuscitations in the CCU to determine the presence or absence of hemopericardium. The actual free-wall rupture of the ventricle can be visualized in selected cases. Since blood in the pericardial space will organize quite quickly, this organizing pericardial effusion can often be seen by 2DE within minutes of its occurrence. If a hemopericardium is present and responsible for the patient's hemodynamic collapse, the early detection may allow for possible intervention and potential salvage of the patient.

Rupture of the Ventricular Septum

Ventricular septal defects (VSDs) that occur after acute MI are less frequent than free-wall rupture (see chapter 45). The incidence is less than 1%. The majority of VSDs occur the first week after the MI: 60% of the VSDs occur with anterior MI and primarily involve the apical portion of the interventricular septum; the remaining 40% occur with inferior MI and involve the inferior basal portion of the interventricular septum. The size of the VSD and the presence or absence of a septal aneurysm often determine the hemodynamic consequences and likelihood for surgical survival. There is a very high mortality with acute VSD, with 25% of patients dying within three days, 65% within two weeks, and 90% within two months. 2DE has been widely applied to the detection and localization of acute and suspected postmyocardial infarction VSDs [16, 17] (figure 23-4). By determining residual and global LV and RV function, 2DE has been useful for determining prognosis in patients with suspected postmyocardial infarction VSD [7].

While the patient with an acute VSD often has a very loud holosystolic murmur and a sternal to left parasternal systolic thrill, the differentiation between a VSD and acute mitral regurgitation-type murmur may be difficult. 2DE, especially when coupled with Doppler echocardiography, allows for the rapid visualization of sizable VSDs. The Doppler is quickly able to distinguish between predominant mitral regurgitation and VSDs that are too small to be accurately visualized by 2DE. While Swan-Ganz catheterization has been the classic bedside hemodynamic method to determine shunt size, 2DE offers visualization of the site and size of the VSD, and the presence of accompanying septal aneurysm, and gives segmental analysis of LV function that can be used in determining those patients who may be good surgical candidates [18].

Mitral Regurgitation: Postmyocardial Infarction

2DE can be a useful diagnostic test in those patients with acute or chronic mitral regurgitation (MR) status-post-MI who have acute or late congestive heart failure. Papillary muscle dysfunction due to infarction of the papillary muscle head can lead to MR. 2DE can be used to visualize scarring and fibrosis of the papillary head adjacent to an infarct zone. These patients often present with late congestive heart failure and chronic MR. Acute papillary muscle rupture or chordal rupture can lead to severe acute MR, which may occur in up to as many as 1% of patients status-post-MI. Since total rupture of the papillary head is associated with a high degree of mortality, the immediate recognition of partial or complete papillary muscle rupture by 2DE may aid in improved survival rates for these patients. Since the median survival for patients with partial papillary muscle rupture is three days, immediate diagnosis is needed if surgical correction is going to be undertaken. 2DE allows for determination, even in the difficult subject,

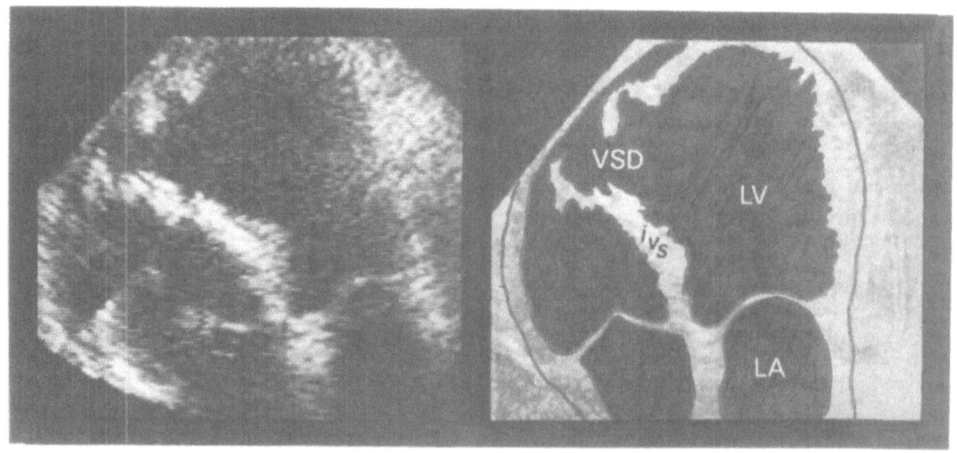

FIGURE 23-4. A stop-frame apical four-chamber view on a patient who developed a ventricular septal defect status-postanterior septal MI. The large VSD is clearly visualized.

of a flail mitral leaflet. Additionally, MR secondary to either papillary muscle ischemia or anatomic distortion of the mitral papillary apparatus in the setting of a large inferior aneurysm can be quickly determined by 2DE (figure 23-5).

There are many cases in which the classic physical findings that allow one to differentiate between acute MR and acute VSD status-post-MI are not present. 2DE has been very useful in quickly determining whether a VSD or MR is present. With the widespread advent of accurate continuous-wave/pulsed-wave Doppler coupled to 2DE, the ability to sample quickly for regurgitant blood flow in left and right atria and to sample along the ventricular septum will aid in further differentiation between VSD and MR acutely after MI. Some patients have very small VSDs that cannot be visualized but are easily detected by the simultaneous 2DE—Doppler technique. If no VSD is visualized by 2DE and no turbulent flow is found in the region of the ventricular system, the etiology of the murmur (and symptoms) is often acute MR. This is quickly confirmed by the Doppler technique. Additionally, 2DE can give the differential diagnosis for acute MR, namely, papillary—chordal rupture, papillary infarction fibrosis without rupture, and inferior aneurysm with distortion of the mitral apparatus.

Left Ventricular Aneurysms

LV aneurysms occur in 5%—15% of survivors of acute MI. Since the five-year survival for a patient with a proven LV aneurysm may be less than 20%, accurate early diagnosis is important as it may determine potential surgical candidates. Surgical results or repair of ventricular aneurysms really depend upon the associated extent of coronary artery disease, the extent and location of the LV aneurysm, the residual LV function, associated VSDs or papillary muscle rupture, and the timing after acute MI. Most ventricular aneurysms develop 6—12 weeks after acute MI. They are four times more common at the apex and anterior segments of the ventricle than in the posterior—inferior areas. Patients often show signs and symptoms of increasing congestive heart failure, recurrent angina pectoris, ventricular ar-

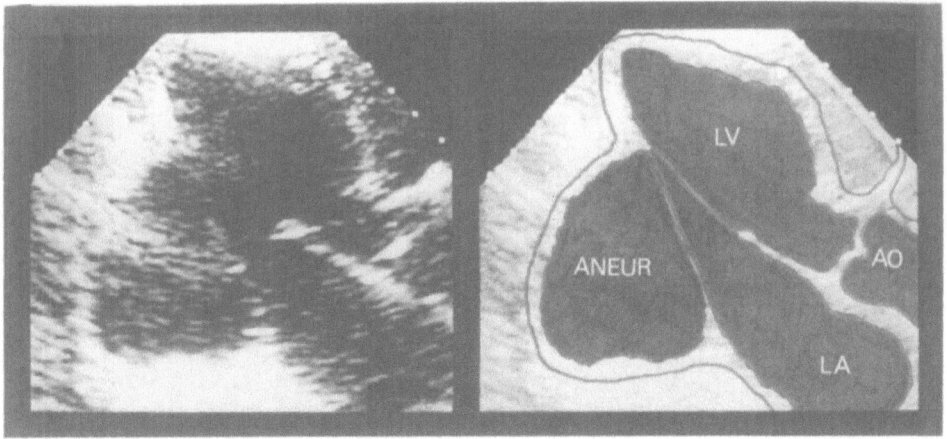

FIGURE 23-5. A low parasternal view on a patient with an inferior MI who was suspected of having a VSD. The 2DE clearly showed a sizable inferior aneurysm (ANEUR), but with intact ventricular septum and papillary muscle apparatus. The harsh murmur was therefore secondary to mitral regurgitation due to the extreme distortion of the papillary muscle apparatus from the sizable aneurysm.

rhythmias, or systemic embolization. The clinical diagnosis of ventricular aneurysms, based upon physical diagnosis, anterior ST-segment elevation, and LV bulge on chest X-ray, is of limited sensitivity.

The M-mode technique has not been extremely useful for detecting and localizing ventricular aneurysms. 2DE has been shown to be a very accurate and reliable tool not only for determining the presence and location of ventricular aneurysms, but for assessing residual LV function. Most 2D echocardiographers refer to ventricular aneurysms as being systolic segmental dyskinetic areas that exhibit marked thinning (both in systole and diastole) and lead to an abnormal segmental contour of the ventricle in both diastole and systole. 2DE is the only currently available imaging technique that allows for direct visualization of wall thickness, segmental and subsegmental wall motion, and the presence of mural thrombi.

Many authors have shown 2DE to be very accurate in confirming, when compared with standard angiographic techniques, the presence and location of ventricular aneurysms after MI [18, 19] (figures 23-5 and 23-6). Lengyel et al. [18] defined an aneurysm on 2DE as being a segmental, well-demarcated bulge in the left ventricle in diastole and systole that had thin dyskinetic walls. These authors found a 93% sensitivity and an 84% specificity of the 2DE technique when compared with angiography in diagnosing true ventricular aneurysms in 76 patients suspected of having LV aneurysms.

2DE has also proven extremely useful in diagnosing false or pseudo-aneurysms [20]. Pseudo-aneurysms are perforations of the LV free wall that lead to a localized hemopericardium limited from further expansion by the pericardium. In contradistinction to true aneurysms of the left ventricle, pseudo-aneurysms are prone to rupture and therefore their accurate diagnosis is of extreme clinical importance. 2DE has been an accurate noninvasive technique for determining the presence and location of pseudo-aneurysms and may, in fact, be superior to angiography where overlap of segments may lead to a missed diagnosis [11]. The 2DE features of pseudo-aneurysms are a sharp discontinuity of the LV endocardium at the neck or mouth of the pseudo-aneurysm. The mouth or neck of the pseudo-aneurysm is very narrow when compared with the enlarged and somewhat globular body of the pseudo-aneurysm. Since 2DE also gives an accurate qualification–quantification assessment of LV function, this technique is useful in determining those patients who represent good surgical candidates and should undergo invasive tests.

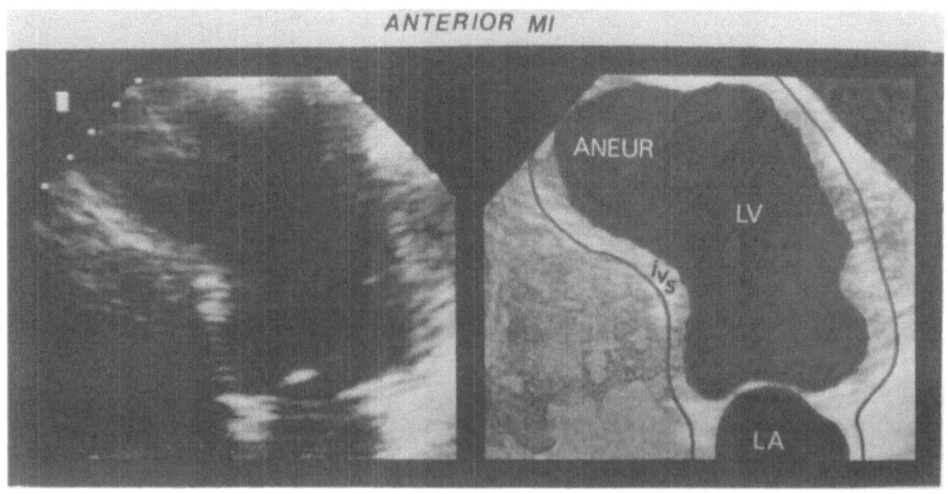

FIGURE 23-6. An apical four-chamber view of a large apical septal aneurysm (ANEUR) after an anterior septal MI.

Left Ventricular Thrombi

2DE detection of LV thrombi is often dramatic and raises many therapeutic questions (figure 23-7). Autopsy studies have shown that 20%—60% of patients with transmural MIs will have LV thrombi at the time of their postmortem examination, but systemic embolization only occurs in 3%—5% of patients with acute MI. The presence of LV thrombi is related to the size of the MI, as anterior wall infarctions generally have larger areas of necrosis and more commonly have associated LV thrombi. The ability of 2DE to detect LV thrombi is well known. Organized thrombi, which have a higher acoustic impe-

dence than the surrounding nonclotted blood, are easier to detect than those freshly formed thrombi that may appear as a homogeneous swirling group of echoes within the LV cavity. Technical considerations play a strong role in the 2DE detection of thrombi and differentiation from artifacts. The false-positive rate for erroneously concluding that an artifact (reverberation) or true anatomic feature (trabecular band) is an LV thrombi may be as high as 15%—20%. However, 2DE does allow for the accurate diagnosis of the presence, size, and location of LV thrombi in the setting of coronary artery disease.

Stratton et al. [21] found a higher incidence of thrombi in transmural anterior MIs than other MIs, and a higher incidence of LV aneurysm accompanying the thrombi. While De Maria et al. [22] have shown systemic embolization only in anterior MIs with thrombi confined to the apex, the question of visualization of thrombi and potential embolization is an important one. Stratton et al. [21] found that 35% of their patients with proven thrombi had clinical evidence of systemic embolizations. This is, however, a higher incidence of embolization than other studies have shown. Autopsy studies have shown that 33%—64% of patients with MI and cardiac thrombi have evidence of systemic embolization, but many of these are silent.

Since the ECG has excellent resolution, it should aid in the detection of ventricular thrombi. The question as to whether the thrombi that are detected have a morphologic pattern or a motion pattern that is predictive of embolization has not been well investigated. It is the author's opinion that very large mobile thrombi, especially those in the LV apex, or those that have dependent trailing edges that swirl around within the LV cavity, may be more likely to embolize. While anticoagulation carries well-known risks, it is the author's opinion that those patients with sizable, mobile thrombi, or thrombi with large swirling edges, should undergo oral anticoagulation. Follow-up studies should be performed on a six-month to yearly basis. Various studies have shown disappearance of thrombi with and without anticoagulation when follow-up echoes were obtained. If the thrombus disappears over time, the discontinuance of the anticoagulants could be considered.

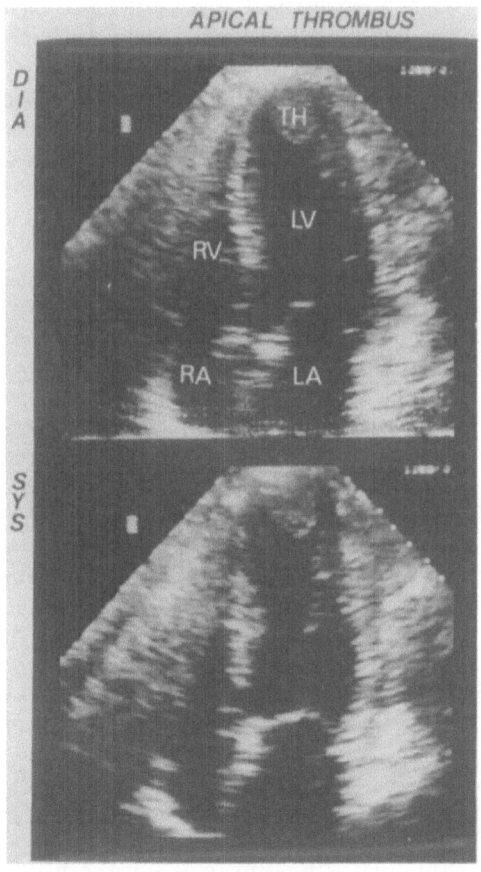

FIGURE 23-7. An apical four-chamber view taken at diastole (top panel) and systole (bottom panel) showing a discrete circular apical thrombus (TH) in a patient with an apical infarction.

Late Congestive Heart Failure after Myocardial Infarction

2DE allows for a prompt etiologic diagnosis in those patients who suffer congestive heart failure months or years after MI (table 23-4). Since the etiology centers around suspected ventricular aneurysm, MR secondary to papillary muscle dysfunction, or ischemic end-stage cardiomyopathies, 2DE can quickly be used to distinguish a cardiomyopathy from an actual aneurysm. As the proper diagnosis is obtained, proper therapeutic management can be entertained.

TABLE 23-4.

CHF after myocardial infarction (late)
Etiology: Aneurysm
      Mitral regurgitation-
          papillary muscle dysfunction
      Ischemic myopathy
2DE quickly distinguishes:
      Ischemic myopathy vs localized aneurysm
      Papillary muscle ischemia vs mitral valve
          abnormalities

References

1. Battler A, Foelicher VF, Gallagher KP, et al: Dissociation between regional myocardial dysfunction and ECG changes during ischemia in the conscious dog. Circulation 62:735, 1980.
2. Meltzer RS, Woythaler JN, Buda AJ, Griffin JC, Harrison WD, Martin RP, Harrison DC, Popp RL: Two-dimensional echocardiographic quantification of infarct size alteration by pharmacologic agents. Am J Cardiol 44:257–262, 1979.
3. Stamm RB, Carabello B, Watson D, Taylor G, Beller GA, Martin RP: Comparison of regional wall motion determined by two-dimensional echocardiography, radionuclide angiography, and left ventriculography. In: Rijsterborgh H (ed) Echocardiography. The Hague: Martinus Nijhoff, 1981, pp 103–107.
4. *Parisi AF, Moynihan PF, Folland ED, Feldman CL*: Quantitative detection of regional left ventricular contraction abnormalities by two-dimensional echocardiography. II. Accuracy in coronary artery disease. Circulation 63:761–767, 1981.
5. Heger JJ, Weyman AE, Wann LS, Dillon JC, Feigenbaum H: Cross-sectional echocardiography in acute myocardial infarction: detection and localization of regional left ventricular asynergy. Circulation 60:531–538, 1979.
6. Heger JJ, Weyman AE, Wann LS, Rogers EW, Dillon JC, Feigenbaum H: Cross-sectional echocardiographic analysis of the extent of left ventricular asynergy in acute myocardial infarction. Circulation 61:1113–1118, 1980.
7. Gibson RS, Bishop HL, Stamm RB, Crampton RS, Beller GA, Martin RP: Value of early two-dimensional echocardiography in patients with acute myocardial infarction. Am J Cardiol 49:1110–1119, 1982.
8. Horowitz RS, Morganroth J, Parrotto C, Chin CC, Soffer J, Pauletto FJ: Immediate diagnosis of acute myocardial infarction by two-dimensional echocardiography. Circulation 65:323–329, 1982.
9. Loh IK, Charuzi Y, Beeder C, et al: Early diagnosis of nontransmural myocardial infarction by two-dimensional echocardiography. Am Heart J 104:963, 1982.
10. Eaton LW, Weiss JL, Bukley BH, et al: Regional cardiac dilatation after acute myocardial infarction: recognition by two-dimensional echocardiography. N Engl J Med 300:57, 1979.
11. Nixon JV, Narahara A, Smitherman TC: Estimation of myocardial involvement in patients with acute myocardial infarction by two-dimensional echocardiography. Circulation 62:1248, 1980.
12. Stamm RB, Gibson RS, Bishop HL, Carabello B, Beller GA, Martin RP: Echocardiographic detection of infarct-localized asynergy and remote asynergy during acute myocardial infarction: Correlation with the extent of angiographic coronary disease. Circulation 67:233–244, 1983.
13. Wackers FJ, Lie KI, Sokole EB, et al: Prevalence of right ventricular involvement in inferior wall myocardial infarction assessed with myocardial imaging with thallium-201 and technetium-99m pyrophosphate. Am J Cardiol 42:358, 1978.
14. Sharpe DN, Botvinick EH, Shames DM, et al: The noninvasive diagnosis of right ventricular infarction. Circulation 57:483, 1978.
15. D'Arcy BD, Nanda NC: Two-dimensional echocardiographic features of right ventricular infarction. Circulation 65:167, 1982.
16. Bishop HL, Gibson RS, Stamm RB, Beller GA, Martin RP: Role of two-dimensional echocardiography in the evaluation of patients with ventricular septal rupture post-myocardial infarction. Am Heart J 102:965–971, 1981.

17. Drobac M, Gilbert B, Howard R, et al: Ventricular septal defect after myocardial infarction: diagnosis by two-dimensional echocardiography. Circulation 67:335, 1983.

18. Lengyel M, Tajik AJ, Seward JB, Hagler DJ, Smith HC: Sensitivity and specificity of two-dimensional echocardiography in the detection of left ventricular aneurysms [abstr]. Am J Cardiol 45:436, 1980.

19. Baur HR, Daniel JA, Nelson RR: Detection of left ventricular aneurysm on two-dimensional echocardiography. Am J Cardiol 50:191, 1982.

20. Gatewood RP Jr, Nanda NC: Differentiation of left ventricular pseudo-aneurysm from true aneurysm with two-dimensional echocardiography. Am J Cardiol 46:869−877, 1980.

21. Stratton JR, Leighty SW Jr, Pearlman AS, Ritchie JL: Detection of left ventricular thrombus by two-dimensional echocardiography: sensitivity, specificity, and causes of uncertainty. Circulation 66:156−166, 1982.

22. De Maria AN, Bommer W, Neuman NA, Grehl T, Weinart L, De Nardo S, Amsterdam EA, Mason DT: Left ventricular thrombi identified by cross-sectional echocardiography. Ann Intern Med 90:14−18, 1981.

24. THE POTENTIAL USEFULNESS OF DOPPLER ULTRASOUND IN MYOCARDIAL INFARCTION

Stephen M. Teague

In acute myocardial infarction, Doppler ultrasound examination offers noninvasive bedside evaluation of ventricular function and systolic murmurs. Areas of application include measurement of cardiac output, determination of ejection velocity, and differentiation of mitral regurgitation from ventricular septal defect. These functions may be accomplished with or without concomitant M-mode and two-dimensional echocardiographic examinations. Doppler flow information augments anatomic and motion analysis available in these imaging formats.

Satumora introduced clinical cardiac Doppler technology in 1957. Relatively recent technical advances in range resolution, signal processing, and velocity display led to current instrumentation that can be mastered by most clinicians familiar with M-mode ultrasonic techniques. Widespread appreciation and use of Doppler ultrasound has lagged behind that of the imaging modalities, however. M-mode and two-dimensional ultrasound images may be related directly to anatomy; Doppler examination produces flow profiles understood from a perspective of fluid dynamics. The abstract nature of Doppler information impairs an immediate understanding. This obstacle vanishes once the basic principles, limitations, and applications of the technique are understood.

The Doppler Principle

In Doppler ultrasonography, targets moving within the ultrasonic beam shift the frequency of the returning (backscatter) signal by an amount proportional to target velocity. Movement toward the transducer produces a backscatter frequency above the transmitted frequency, while movement away from the transducer shifts the backscatter frequency below the transmitted frequency. The Doppler instrument compares the frequency of the backscattered signal with that of the transmitted signal (f_c), and the difference (f_d) between the two reflects the velocity (v) and direction of the target within the ultrasonic beam. A critical factor governing the magnitude of the velocity signal is the angle ($\ominus$) subtended by the ultrasonic beam and velocity vector of the target. The relationship between these factors is described by the Doppler equation:

$$v = \frac{f_d C}{2 f_c \cos} \ominus$$

where C = 1560 m/s, the speed of ultrasound in blood.

One of the goals of the bedside Doppler examination is to align the beam with the target velocity vector, so that $\ominus$ = 0 or 180°. Subsequently, cos $\Theta = 1$, or -1 and only then will the observed Doppler shift relate directly to target velocity:

$$V = \frac{Cf_d}{2f_c}$$

For physiologic measurements, the Doppler shift frequency f_d fortuitously ranges across the audio spectrum. Doppler instruments have an acoustic output that conveys this information. The Doppler shift frequency is also available in a graphical display, where v or f_d is displayed on the y-axis versus time. The result is a record of target velocity variation over time. An electrocardiogram and phonocardiogram may be simultaneously displayed for identification of systole, diastole, and valve motion. These principles are illustrated in figure 24-1.

CONTINUOUS AND PULSED DOPPLER MODES
Currently, the clinician can choose between two modes of Doppler operation. In continuous-wave mode (CW), velocities are registered all along the ultrasonic beam; there is no practical limit to velocity detection, but the range of the moving target (s) cannot be determined. This mode is utilized in survey examinations looking for high-velocity jet phenomena resulting from stenotic/regurgitant valvular disease and ventricular septal defect. Only in this mode may the highest velocities be quantified. In a complementary fashion, pulsed mode (PM) discriminates the range (location) of moving targets, but sharp velocity detection limitations exist. After finding and quantifying high-velocity intracardiac phenomena with CW, PM is utilized to localize the lesion. In myocardial infarction, this is of chief importance in distinguishing ventricular septal defect from mitral regurgitation. It is desirable to have Doppler instrumentation capable of both PM and CW modes.

THE BEDSIDE DOPPLER EXAMINATION
The patient is examined in the supine or lateral decubitus position. To minimize the observation angle Θ, the aortic arch is examined from the suprasternal notch, while the mitral valve is studied from the ventricular apex. The ventricular septum is approached from the left sternal bor-

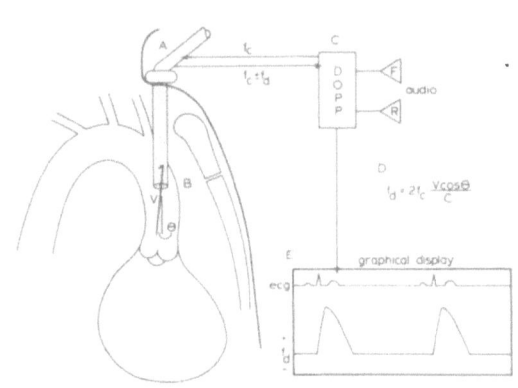

FIGURE 24-1. Ejected aortic root blood (B) encounters Doppler beam emitted by a transducer in the suprasternal notch (A). The transmitted frequency, f_c, is backscattered and shifted by interaction with the blood elements. The magnitude and direction of this shift is determined by the Doppler equation (D) and is electronically extracted by the Doppler instrument (C). Acoustic signals representing this shift appear in forward (F) and reverse (R) speakers. The shifts are also displayed graphically versus time (E), along with the electrocardiogram.

der. Often, acoustic windows from two or more costal interspaces must be utilized to examine the entire septum. These cardinal positions are shown in figure 24-2. From these positions, the Doppler beam is steered utilizing the acoustic and visual displays. In general, the transducer is aligned to obtain (a) maximum Doppler signal strength, (b) maximal displayed velocity, and (c) clear identification of systolic and diastolic events. If simultaneous M-mode or two-dimensional scanning is available, anatomic location of the Doppler beam may be ascertained. It must be emphasized that it is of far greater importance to obtain optimum Doppler signals than anatomic images in simultaneous examination.

Aortic Flow Profiles

Technically, the easiest Doppler examination is the assessment of ascending aortic velocity with the transducer in the suprasternal notch. The beam is directed slightly right or left of midline, to develop the highest systolic Doppler shift in the display and acoustic output of the instru-

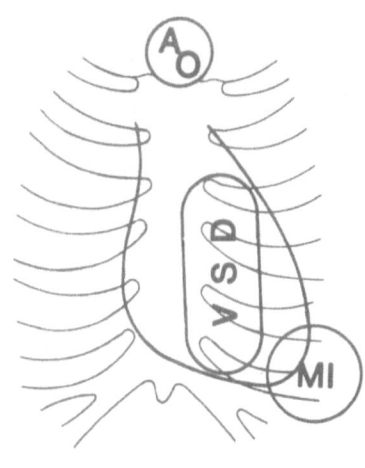

FIGURE 24-2. Transducer locations for examination of the aortic arch (A_0), interventricular septum (VSD), and mitral valve (MI).

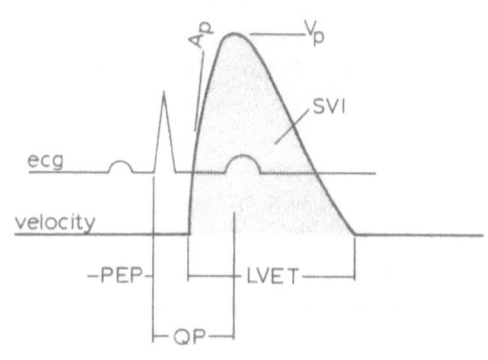

FIGURE 24-3. Information available from simultaneous electrocardiographic and Doppler aortic arch velocity measurement. A_p and V_p represent peak acceleration and velocity, respectively. Stroke volume is estimated by the area under the velocity profile (SVI). See text for details of systolic time intervals PEP, LVET, and QP.

ment. Clicks produced by aortic valve opening and closing may or may not be obtained. The simplicity of the examination belies the wealth of available information, as seen in figure 24-3. If a simultaneous electrocardiogram is recorded, the following parameters may be derived: preejection period (Q wave to earliest ejection), time to peak, velocity (Q wave to peak velocity), and left ventricular ejection time (time between valve clicks, or time of systolic ejection). Peak ejection velocity and peak acceleration (slope of the initial rise in systolic velocity) may be determined.

SYSTOLIC TIME INTERVALS

The systolic time relationship of preejection period divided by left ventricular ejection time (PEP/LVET) may be calculated from these measurements. Systolic time intervals measured by electrocardiography, phonocardiography, and carotid pulse tracings have been evaluated in the setting of acute infarction. Despite shortening of total electromechanical systole in response to increased adrenergic tone, abnormalities in PEP/LVET have correlated with left ventricular dysfunction. In a series of 30 patients with acute infarction, PEP/LVET has been shown to correlate with cardiac index ($r = -0.81$) [1]. In 127 patients with chronic significant coronary artery disease, PEP/LVET correlated with angiographic left ventricular ejection fraction ($r = -0.76$) [2]. The magnitude of PEP/LVET paralleled the short-term prognosis in patients with acute infarction [3].

PEAK VELOCITY AND ACCELERATION

Invasive studies using velocity-detecting catheters and electromagnetic flow meters have established the usefulness of aortic arch velocity and acceleration determinations in acute infarction. After characterizing the left ventricle as an impulse generator, Rushmer et al. demonstrated acute deterioration of ejection velocity and acceleration after occlusion of a major coronary artery in the dog [4]. Further observations in dogs subjected to inotropic stimulation and coronary ligation demonstrated the close relationship between inotropic state and ejection acceleration [5]. Limited changes in preload (by posture) minimally influenced acceleration.

Velocity and acceleration are not pure indices of left ventricular systolic performance, however. Manipulation of afterload with nitroprusside infusion in animal models strongly influenced peak acceleration as did profound reductions of preload by exsanguination [6–8].

Limited clinical studies have investigated peak acceleration and peak velocity in patients with coronary artery disease. In chronic coronary disease, catheter-tipped velocity transducers in the aorta revealed peak velocity and acceleration to be inversely related to the severity and extent of angiographically proven coronary disease [9]. Peak velocity and acceleration correlated with angiographic ejection fraction ($r = 0.88$) in 12 of these patients. A similar clinical study of 40 patients undergoing routine catheterization correlated peak velocity and acceleration with stroke volume. Both velocity and acceleration, however, failed to discriminate patients ranked by left ventricular end-diastolic pressure, cardiac index, and ejection fraction [10]. Electronic filtering of the velocity and acceleration signals may have biased these results, as lower values of acceleration and velocity were reported in this study than those previously published [9, 11, 12]. Jewitt and co-workers studied 24 patients with coronary artery disease, 14 during acute infarction complicated by congestive failure [13]. Peak velocity and acceleration were depressed in acute infarction, but there was measurement overlap in the two groups and a statistical analysis was not performed. Velocity and acceleration measurements successfully discriminated between survivors and nonsurvivors ($P < 0.001$) in this study.

Noninvasive Doppler aortic arch velocity determination was introduced in 1975 by Angelsen et al. [14], Huntsman et al. [15], and Light [16]. Buchtal et al. employed the technique in the study of 21 patients with recent infarction, six with hypovolemic shock, and seven with septic shock [17]. Reductions in ejection time and peak velocity correlated with deteriorating clinical status, while improvement was marked by increases in these parameters.

In summary, Doppler aortic velocity determinations should be of use in acute infarction through the determination of systolic time intervals, peak ejection velocity, and peak ejection acceleration. The usefulness of these parameters in the determination of left ventricular performance has been established independent on the noninvasive Doppler technique. It is anticipated that future investigations will reveal quantitative relationships between hemodynamic status in acute infarction and the Doppler aortic velocity profile.

CARDIAC OUTPUT

Stroke volume and cardiac output may be obtained noninvasively by determining the area under the aortic velocity profile and the diameter of the aortic root. The latter requires independent imaging of aortic diameter by M-mode or two-dimensional echo, while the former requires mathematical integration of Doppler aortic velocity. Recall that integration of velocity over a finite time yields distance. In like manner, integration of the aortic velocity profile over a systolic ejection period yields the distance traveled by the ejected blood during systole. Multiplication of this distance by the area of the aortic root yields stroke volume. Cardiac output is then obtained in the product of stroke volume and heart rate. It is of interest that cardiac output may be calculated at many points in the cardiac chambers by using this technique: in the aorta, pulmonary artery, and across the mitral valve. The required measurements are mean area in the region of flow, area under the velocity profile, and heart rate.

A number of assumptions and limitations of this methods are apparent. Aortic dimensions must be known with great precision, and the assumption that aortic diameter is constant during systole is not always valid [18]. Like all Doppler velocity measurements, the results are strongly influenced by the angle between the Doppler beam and the flow vector. Finally, the velocity profile is assumed to be uniform across the aorta during systole.

Despite these sources of measurement error, the Doppler technique has been validated in the accurate assessment of stroke volume and cardiac output. In six dogs, thermodilution stroke volume was found to be proportional to the area under the Doppler aortic velocity curve [19]. Despite wide swings in stroke volume by fluid infusion and exsanguination, a correlation coefficient of 0.95 was found between the two techniques. A subsequent animal study compared Doppler cardiac output with electromagnetic flow meter output in the ascending aorta [20]. A correlation coefficient of 0.96 was found, with all data lying close the line of identity despite manipulations of fluid infusion, exsanguination, and dopamine infusion.

Several studies have validated Doppler cardiac output determinations in man. Utilizing M-mode or two-dimensional echo assessment of the aortic root diameter and pulsed or continuous-wave Doppler evaluation of aortic root velocity, echo estimates of cardiac output agreed closely with Fick determinations [21, 22]. In neonates and children presenting a wide range of Fick cardiac output (403–3260 ml/min), Berman and associates observed a correlation coefficient of 0.96 against Doppler output estimates [23]. In a similar pediatric population, a correlation coefficient of 0.95 between Doppler cardiac output and indicator-dilution cardiac output was found [24]. Huntsman et al. studied 53 patients using continuous-wave Doppler and A-mode aortic root diameter determinations during measurement of thermodilution cardiac output [25]. Patients with acute infarction, respiratory failure, and recent or ongoing surgery were included. Adequate studies were obtained in 85% of the 53, with the regression between Doppler and thermodilution outputs described by a slope of 0.95 and an offset of 0.38 ($r = 0.94$, $n = 110$). Cardiac output ranged between 2 and 11 l/min in this group. These data are shown in figure 24-4.

QUANTITATIVE LIMITATIONS
Repeatability and interobserver variability do not seem to impede an accurate noninvasive assessment of the aortic arch velocity profile [26, 27]. Of more concern is the accurate echo assessment of arch diameters; error in this measurement is raised to the second power in the cardiac output determination. Echocardiographic technicians identify the aortic root by the presence of aortic leaflet motion. This is in the sinuses of Valsalva, however, and an erroneously large diameter may be measured here. It is important to scan up the arch above this level for diameter determination.

Doppler techniques are best in the detection of peak velocity. The aortic root velocity profile is almost flat so that peak velocity approximates mean velocity, and subsequently this measurement may be carried on for quantitative pur-

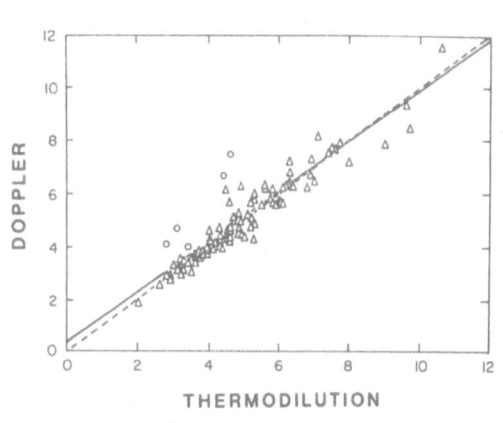

FIGURE 24-4. Comparison between Doppler and thermodilution estimates of cardiac output in 45 patients undergoing simultaneous measurement. From Huntsman et al. [25], with permission.

poses. Lesions producing nonlaminar flow disturbances in the root, such as aortic stenosis and high cardiac output states, invalidate this relationship between mean and peak velocities, and quantification is not reliable. High-velocity flow disturbances produce unique Doppler phenomena, however, and these phenomena allow identification and localization of jet lesions such as mitral regurgitation and ventricular septal defect.

Evaluation of Systolic Murmurs

New systolic murmurs may accompany myocardial infarction, acutely or in the convalescent phase. When the new murmur coexists with hemodynamic deterioration, an urgent need arises for the detection and quantification of ventricular septal defect and mitral regurgitation (see chapter 45). Bedside Doppler examination offers this capability.

In both mitral regurgitation and ventricular septal defect, blood flows between cardiac chambers under high pressure and across channels of small caliber. The pressure gradient produces high flow velocities (up to 6 m/s) distal to such orifices and disturbed flow profiles result. When the Doppler beam encounters these high-velocity jets, a characteristic pattern is produced consist-

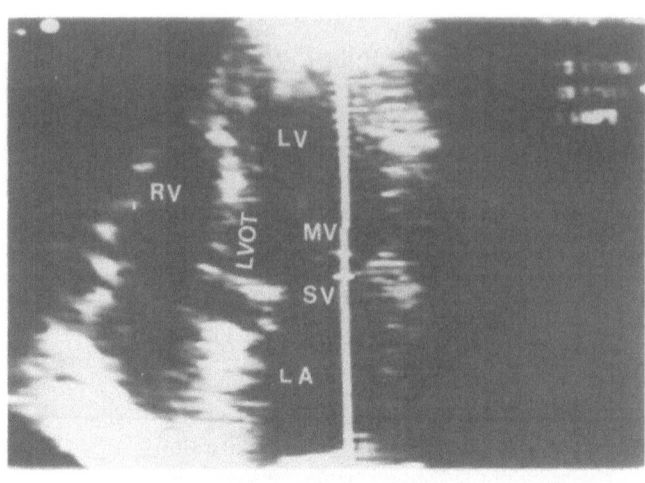

A

FIGURE 24-5. Apical ultrasonic examination of a patient hospitalized with acute inferior infarction, holosystolic murmur, and giant V waves on the wedge pressure tracing. (A) An apical four-chamber two-dimensional echocardiographic view localizes the pulsed mode Doppler sample volume (SV) in the left atrium (LA) posterior to the mitral valve (MV). (B) Pulsed mode Doppler recording of velocity information (f_d) versus time from the SV. Note systolic disturbed flow indicated by the disorganized spectral pattern at arrows. The twin velocity peaks of laminar mitral diastolic flow are seen. At surgery a flail posterior mitral valve leaflet was found.

ing of harsh, high-frequency acoustic output and spectral broadening in the graphical display [28]. Using pulsed Doppler techniques, the disturbed flow can be localized in the right ventricular outflow tract or along the ventricular septum in the presence of ventricular septal defect. In mitral regurgitation, the flow disturbance is found in the left atrium behind the mitral valve. The peak velocities present in these jets always exceed the limitations of the pulsed mode. In the continuous-wave mode, the beam may be aligned carefully along the jet axis, and the peak velocity may be transduced. Relating peak velocity to the driving pressure gradient through the Bernoulli equation, the pressure in the chamber receiving the jet may be deduced noninvasively if systolic ventricular (systemic) pressure is known [29]. It may be possible to grade the severity of the lesion by the systolic pressure in the receiving chamber.

MITRAL REGURGITATION

Clinical trials have assessed the sensitivity and specificity of pulsed mode Doppler ultrasound in the detection of mitral regurgitation. Of 47 patients with chest-pain syndromes undergoing cardiac catheterization and Doppler examination by Abbasi and associates, 21 had mitral regurgitation by Doppler examination [30]. By ventriculography, 23 had mitral regurgitation, for a sensitivity of 92%. Of the 24 patients with no mitral regurgitation by catheterization, one had mitral regurgitation by Doppler, for a specificity

of 96% (figure 24-5). Similar figures are reported by Gehring et al. in a study of 112 patients [31]. Both groups found that the severity of regurgitation could be estimated by mapping the extent of systolic flow disturbances in the left atrium, and a correlation with angiographic regurgitant grade was found.

VENTRICULAR SEPTAL DEFECT

Stevenson and associates studied the ability of pulsed Doppler ultrasound to differentiate ventricular septal defect from mitral regurgitation in 40 pediatric patients [32]. Of the 16 undergoing catheterization, ten had ventricular septal defect and six had mitral regurgitation. Pulsed Doppler ultrasound correctly identified these lesions. In one patient with Doppler systolic flow disturbance in both the right ventricle and left atrium, both ventricular septal defect and mitral regurgitation were found by catheterization.

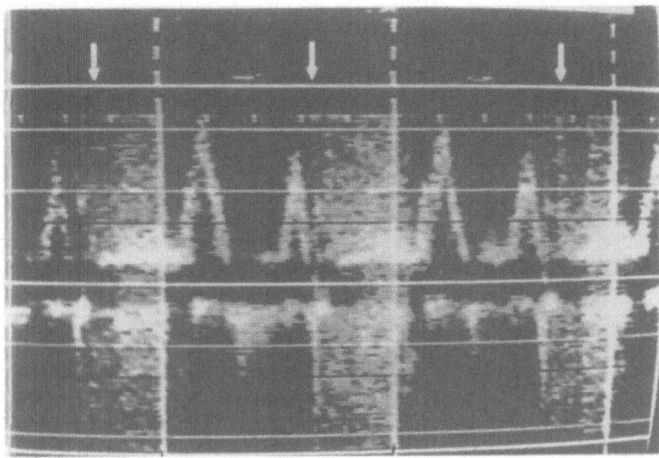

B

Limitations of Doppler Ultrasound

Doppler ultrasound shares many of the problems of two-dimensional and M-mode angiography. Adequate studies are often difficult or impossible to obtain in obese or emphysematous patients. Since the targets of the Doppler beam are the formed elements of blood, the backscatter signal is always of weaker amplitude than that of cardiac walls and valves. It may be difficult to distinguish flow information in this noisy background, particularly if the patient is anemic.

Technical skill is required to obtain valid Doppler quantitative results. It is always necessary to minimize the Doppler angle ($\ominus$) and maximize the peak recorded velocity. These requirements may necessitate observations from sites remote from standard echocardiographic views. In the pulsed mode, results may be invalidated if the actual velocities surpass the detection limits of the device.

Summary

Doppler ultrasound is a new technology that allows detection of the rate, direction, and contour of blood flow noninvasively. In patients with acute infarction, it is possible to determine stroke volume and cardiac output by using this technique. It may be possible to determine the location and significance of systolic murmurs complicating the course of infarction. This method has significant promise in the evaluation of systolic time intervals and in ejection-phase indices of acceleration and velocity.

Although the routine application of Doppler ultrasound in the coronary care unit is unclear at this time, these proven and potential benefits indicate an important role in the future.

References

1. Lewis RP, Rittgers S, Forester WF, Boudoulas H: A critical review of the systolic time intervals. Circulation 56:146–158, 1977.
2. Lewis RP, Boudoulas H, Welch TG, Forester WF: Usefulness of systolic time intervals in coronary artery disease. Am J Cardiol 37:787–796, 1976.
3. Northover BJ: Left ventricular systolic time intervals in patients with acute myocardial infarction. Br Heart J 43:506–513, 1980.
4. Rushmer RF, Watson N, Harding D, Baker D: Effects of acute coronary occlusion on performance of right and left ventricles in intact unanesthetized dogs. Am Heart J 66:522, 1963.
5. Noble MIM, Trenchard D, Guz A: Left ventricular ejection in conscious dogs. I. Measurement and significance of the maximum acceleration of blood from the left ventricle. Circ Res 19:139–147, 1966.
6. Van den Bos GS: Indices of contractility in the intact heart. Proc R Soc Med 65:545–547, 1972.
7. Van den Box GC, Elzinga G, Westerhof N, Noble MIM: Problems in the use of indices of

myocardial contractility. Cardiovasc Res 7: 834—848, 1973.

8. Hof RP, Hof A: Acceleration of blood in the aorta: a parameter useful for evaluating cardiotonic and afterload reducing substances. J Pharmacol Methods 6:67—95, 1981.

9. Bennett ED, Else W, Miller GAH, Sutton GC, Miller HC, Noble MIM: Maximum acceleration of blood from the left ventricle in patients with ischaemic heart disease. Clin Sci Mol Med 46: 49—59, 1974.

10. Kolettis M, Jenkins BS, Webb-Peploe MM: Assessment of left ventricular function by indices derived from aortic flow velocity. Br Heart J 38:18—31, 1976.

11. Rudewald B: Hemodynamics of the human ascending aorta as studied by means of a differential pressure technique. Acta Physiol Scand (Suppl 187) 54:1—64, 1962.

12. Gabe IT, Gault JH, Ross J, Mason DT, Mills CJ, Shillingford JP, Braunwald E: Measurement of instantaneous blood flow velocity and pressure in conscious man with a catheter tip velocity probe. Circulation 40:603—614, 1969.

13. Jewitt D, Gabe I, Mills C, Maurer B, Thomas M, Shillingford J: Aortic velocity and acceleration measurements in the assessment of coronary heart disease. Eur J Cardiol 1:299—305, 1974.

14. Angelsen BAJ, Aaslid R, Brubakk AO: Transcutaneous aortic blood velocity measurement by pulsed ultrasonic Doppler meter. In: Proceedings of the 3rd Nordic meeting on medical and biological engineering. Paper 49. Tampere: Finnish Society for Medical Engineering, 1975.

15. Huntsman LI, Gams E, Johnson CC, Fairbanks E: Transcutaneous determination of aortic blood flow velocities in man. Am Heart J 89:605—612, 1975.

16. Light H: Transcutaneous aortovelography: a new window on the circulation? Br Heart J 38:433—442, 1976.

17. Buchtal A, Hanson GC, Peisach AR: Transcutaneous aortovelography: potentially useful technique in management of critically ill patients. Br Heart J 38:451—456, 1976.

18. Greenfield JC, Patel DJ: Relation between pressure and diameter in the ascending aorta of man. Circ Res 10:778—781, 1962.

19. Colocousis JS, Huntsman LL, Curreri PW: Estimation of stroke volume changes by ultrasonic Doppler. Circulation 56:914—917, 1977.

20. Darsee JR, Mikolich JR, Walter PF, Schlant RC: Transcutaneous method of measuring Doppler cardiac output. I. Comparison of transcutaneous and juxta-aortic Doppler velocity signals with catheter and cuff electromagnetic flowmeter measurements in closed and open chest dogs. Am J Cardiol 46:697—612, 1980.

21. Hoekenga DE, Greene ER, Loeppky JA, Mathews EC, Richards KL, Luft UC: A comparison of noninvasive Doppler cardiographic and simultaneous Fick measurements of left ventricular stroke volume in man. Circulation 62:III-199, 1980.

22. Magnin PA, Stewart JA, Myers S, Von Ramm O, Kisslo JA: Combined Doppler and phased-array echocardiographic estimation of cardiac output. Circulation 63:388—392, 1981.

23. Berman W Jr, Eldridge M, Yabek S, Dillon T, Alverson D, Rupas D, Bouma K, Hendon L: Pulsed Doppler determination of cardiac output in neonates and children [abstr]. Circulation 64: IV-167, 1981.

24. Hoenecke HR, Goldberg SJ, Carnahan Y, Sahn DJ, Allen HD, Valdex-Cruz LM: Controlled quantitative assessment of pulmonary and aortic flow by range gated pulsed Doppler in children with cardiac disease. Circulation 64:IV-167, 1981.

25. Huntsman LL, Stewart DK, Barnes SR, Franklin BS, Colocousis JS, Hessel EA: Noninvasive Doppler determination of cardiac output in man: clinical validation. Circulation 67:593—602, 1983.

26. Gardin JM, Burn C, Hughes C, Henry WL: Are Doppler aortic flow velocity measurements reproducible [abstr]? Circulation 64:IV-205, 1981.

27. Gisvold SE, Brubakk AO: Measurements of instantaneous blood-velocity in the human aorta using pulsed Doppler ultrasound. Cardiovasc Res 16:26—33, 1982.

28. Lorch GS, Rubenstein S, Baker DW, Dooley T, Dodge HT: Doppler echocardiography: use of graphical display system. Circulation 56:576—585, 1977.

29. Hatte L, Angelsen B: Doppler ultrasound in cardiology: physical principles and clinical applications. Philadelphia: Lea and Febinger, 1982.

30. Abbasi AS, Allen M, De Cristofaro D, Ungar I: Detection and estimation of the degree of mitral regurgitation by range-gated pulsed Doppler echocardiography. Circulation 61:143—147, 1980.

31. Gehring J, Lindlbauer R, Borst K, Strobel M: Nichtinvasive Diagnostik der Mitralinsuffizienz mit der gepulsten Doppler-echokardiographie. Dtsch Med Wochenschr 104:1474—1477, 1979.

32. Stevenson JG, Kawabori J, Guntheroth WG: Differentiation of ventricular septal defect from mitral regurgitation by pulsed Doppler echocardiography. Circulation 56:14—18, 1977.

25. THE USE OF SERIAL RADIONUCLIDE ANGIOGRAPHY FOR MONITORING FUNCTION DURING ACUTE MYOCARDIAL INFARCTION

Sebastian T. Palmeri

In the past, the principal treatment goals of coronary care units were to reduce myocardial oxygen demands and to prevent the arrhythmic complications of the myocardial infarction. In the 1970s, several major therapeutic and technological breakthroughs appeared that have given the physician a better understanding of the pathophysiologic process of infarction, as well as the opportunity to alter its natural history significantly. The first of these innovations was the Swan-Ganz catheter, which provided the physician with continuous hemodynamic information. This, in turn, allowed him to provide superior supportive measures and the opportunity to intervene more aggressively in an attempt to limit infarct size. Coincident with these developments came refinements in catheterization equipment and techniques that permitted the safe performance of coronary arteriography during the early stages of an evolving myocardial infarction. This further increased our understanding of the infarct process and also permitted interventions directed not only at the ischemic or injured myocardium, but directly against the offending coronary artery obstructive lesion. While many of these treatment modalities remain investigational, they have nevertheless drastically changed the role of the physician in his approach to the infarct patient. The physician is no longer the passive observer, but, rather, is now faced with the dilemma of choosing the most appropriate management course. This chapter outlines the role of radionuclide angiography in monitoring left ventricular function in the acute infarct setting. The role of radionuclide perfusion scanning for diagnosing and sizing myocardial infarctions and the role of exercise radionuclide angiography for determining prognosis and long-term management are presented in chapters 20 and 52.

Radionuclide Angiography

Nuclear cardiology is a growing discipline with increasingly more sophisticated scintillation cameras, computers, programming, and biologically useful radioisotopes. Popular current techniques include myocardial perfusion imaging and cardiac blood pool imaging including both first-pass and multigated techniques.

First-pass radionuclide angiograms are generally obtained after the intravenous injection of 10 mC of technetium-99m pertecnetate. Precordial counts are recorded in a binary form using a multicrystal gamma camera linked to a dedicated computer. A high-frequency time—activity curve is obtained from a left ventricular region of interest.

Multigated radionuclide angiograms are obtained after the labeling of the cardiac blood pool either with radioactive human serum albumin or the in vivo red blood cell labeling with technetium-99m. Precordial counts are recorded using a standard Anger camera. The data are collected either in the list or histogram mode with the computer dividing the average RR interval into equal segments of time to create a series of frames. These frames construct an average cardiac cycle acquired over $1-2$ min. The frames are connected and displayed in a rapid-sequence endless-loop movie format. High-temporal-resolution left ventricular time−activity curves are also generated from left ventricular and background regions of interest.

First-pass methods require less acquisition time than multigated methods, which facilitate acquisitions performed during certain interventions such as exercise stress testing, but the resulting count rates are lower and thereby limit the analysis of regional function. Since the inferior wall is not obscured by the right ventricle in the RAO projection, geometric formulas can be used to estimate absolute left ventricular volumes and cardiac output. The first-pass technique also provides the advantages of providing information regarding pulmonary transit times and the presence or absence of intracardiac shunts. First-pass methods require highly sophisticated equipment, which is costly and cumbersome and rarely permits bedside examination.

Multigated angiograms require approximately 2 min of acquisition time, but the resultant images are generally of higher quality. Serial images can be obtained for $4-6$ h without re-administration of the radioisotope, which permit multiple views and scans assessing the acute and delayed effects of several interventions; this has obvious clinical advantages for coronary care unit imaging. In addition, commercially available multigated systems are easily portable. Finally, the multigated technique is better suited for imaging patients when extrasystoles or arrhythmias are present, which is often the case, in the acute postinfarction period.

Left Ventricular Function

The ideal noninvasive test would provide direct quantifiable information regarding myocardial cellular ischemia and necrosis. While thallium perfusion imaging (see chapter 51) and newer methods such as positron emission tomography and nuclear magnetic resonance attempt to provide such information, cardiac blood pool imaging is designed to assess the mechanical properties of the heart. It can therefore provide only indirect information regarding infarct size and ischemia. Although cardiac blood pool imaging can provide information regarding all phases of the cardiac cycle, the focus of this discussion will be on ejection fraction and segmental wall motion analyses, both of which are indices of cardiac systolic function.

EJECTION FRACTION

The left ventricular ejection fraction has been shown to be a useful mechanical expression of the inotropic or contractile state of the heart [1, 2]. For example, when the ejection fraction is low, the ejection volume is small relative to the end-diastolic volume. Therefore less work is being performed per given fiber length, that is, contractility is reduced. It is important to note that all mechanical measures of the inotropic state of the heart are sensitive to afterload (systemic arterial pressure) and preload (venous return) changes. With the preload stable, there is an almost linear inverse relationship between afterload and the ejection fraction [3]. Even under different loading conditions, however, changes in the left ventricular ejection fraction may still reflect changes in contractility if these changes are in directions opposite to the anticipated responses.

Heart rate is also a major determinant of cardiac performance. Increasing the frequency of contraction exerts a positive inotropic effect through the interval strength relationship [4]. Increasing the heart rate may also affect the loading conditions of the heart by reducing the duration of diastolic filling. Heart rate therefore significantly influences left ventricular ejection.

The interpretation of ejection phase indices (including the ejection fraction) can be even more complicated in the abnormal heart. For example, in the normal heart, stroke volume is maintained during periods of increased afterload by compensatory changes in the preload. When contractility is depressed in the basal state, however, the preload reserve may be maximally utilized even under resting conditions. Therefore, elevations in afterload that are well tolerated by the normal heart will result in an afterload mismatch and a fall in the cardiac output. In the special circumstances of mitral regurgitation or ventricular septal defects, there is a reduction in the left ventricular afterload. Therefore, a normal ejection fraction may be maintained in the face of a severely impaired left ventricle. Finally, in contrast to acutely produced alterations in preload and afterload, the heart adapts differently to chronic volume and/or pressure overload, namely, by dilatation or hypertrophy.

WALL MOTION ANALYSIS

Newer computer programs for quantitative measurements of regional function have enhanced the importance of wall motion analysis as a method of sizing myocardial infarcts, defining relative amounts of ischemic or jeopardized myocardium, and assessing the effects of therapeutic interventions. Histopathologic studies have demonstrated an almost linear relationship between the severity of the regional contraction abnormality and the percentage of muscle loss [5, 6]. While akinetic and dyskinetic segments contain significant amounts of fibrosis, hypokinetic segments appear to be comprised principally of viable myocardium. Therefore, interventions designed to limit infarct size might be assessed based on their effects on these regions of mild dysenergy. Such an approach should be cautious, however, since there are several pathophysiologic and practical factors complicating such an analysis [7]. Normalization of regional contraction abnormalities may not mean improved regional function if they merely reflect changes in the loading conditions of the heart or are secondary to enhanced contractility in the neighboring nonischemic myocardium. Furthermore, enhanced systolic function may be transient and might ultimately further compromise the ischemic zones. However, the time course of resolution of wall motion abnormalities after reinstitution of blood flow may be variable. It has generally been believed that, in the absence of necrosis, restoration of coronary blood flow would result in prompt and total return to normal function, but there is increasing evidence that transiently ischemic myocardium may remain depressed for several hours or days before normal metabolic and mechanical function is appreciated [8]. This was recently demonstrated by a reperfusion study using intracoronary streptokinase by Stack et al. [9] (see chapter 34). Therefore, an intervention may be beneficial in increasing regional blood flow and reducing ischemia, without causing immediate improvement in overt regional systolic function. It should also be noted that clinically apparent regional changes in systolic function are generally reflected in changes in the global left ventricular ejection fraction [10–12]. In some cases, however, compensatory changes in remote areas of normal myocardium may mask the global effect of regional dysfunction secondary to an acute infarction or transient ischemia [9]. Therefore, when assessing the efficacy of an intervention, both global and regional changes should be carefully considered, as well as the hemodynamic conditions in which they occur.

Natural History Studies

In 1982, Wackers and his colleagues at Yale obtained multigated radionuclide angiograms on 34 patients within 12 h of their first Q-wave infarctions [13]. Scans were performed on admission, and 2, 4, and 24 h later. Although the mean left ventricular ejection fraction did not change during this period, 56% of the individual patients demonstrated significant changes from an increase of 32% to a decrease of 14% in their left ventricular ejection fractions (table 25-1). The authors remarked that diminishing afterload, preload, and myocardial ischemia might have all contributed to the increase in the left ventricular ejection fraction during the acute phase observed in some patients, while withdrawal of enhanced sympathetic tone and infarct extension or expansion might have caused the decline in the ejection fraction seen in others.

Also in 1982, Nemerovski et al. reported the results of a similar group of 54 patients at UCLA who underwent serial radionuclide studies after their first Q-wave infarction [14]. Both left and right ventricular ejection fractions were recorded on days 1, 3, and 10 after the acute infarctions. Even over this slightly longer period of observation, no significant change in the mean ejection fractions was observed: 42%–46% and 42%–48% for the left and right ejection fractions, respectively. However, considerable individual variations were again noted. From the admission

TABLE 25-1. RNA results in the early postinfarction period

	Ejection fraction (%)[a]		Patients (%) with ΔEF		Number of patients
	Early	Follow-up	Increase	Decrease	
Wackers et al. [13]					
Left ventricle	44	47	32	24	34
Nemerovski et al. [14]					
Left ventricle	42	46	39	26	54
Right ventricle	42	48	48	14	
Schelbert et al. [15]					
Left ventricle	42	45	54	26	63
Steele et al. [16]					
Left ventricle	41	49	12[b]	NA	26
Right ventricle	52	57	46[b]	NA	

[a]Ejection fractions not corrected for technical laboratory differences.
[b]Patients (%) with initial abnormal ejection fractions that became normal.
NA, data not presented in the published report.

to the final radionuclide study, the left ventricular ejection fraction increased in 39% of the patients and decreased in 26%. The right ventricular ejection fraction increased in 48% and decreased in 14% of the patients.

Serial radionuclide cardiac blood pool scans were first obtained in a series of postinfarction patients by Schelbert et al. at the University of California in San Diego in 1976 [15]: 63 patients underwent first-pass radionuclide angiography within five days of their acute myocardial infarction; 13 patients (21%) had had previous myocardial infarctions. The mean left ventricular ejection fraction for the group was 44% with a range of 22%−60% (normal ⩾52%): 60% of the patients had left ventricular ejection fractions greater than 40; 10% of the patients had ejection fractions less than 30%. Within the first five days, 50 patients underwent repeat studies. A slight but statistically insignificant increase in the resting left ventricular ejection fraction was noted, 42%−45%. Of these patients, 54% improved, 26% deteriorated, and the left ventricular ejection fraction was unchanged in 20%. A total of 43 of these patients had early and late (mean 20 months) follow-up radionuclide studies. The left ventricular ejection fraction was again noted to increase from 45% to 49%, which was a statistically significant improvement ($P<0.01$): 61% of the patients improved, 23%

declined, and 16% were unchanged.

In 1977, Steele et al. performed serial radionuclide probe studies in 26 patients on days 1, 2, 3, and 12 after their first infarctions [16]. The mean left ventricular ejection fraction rose on successive days from an initial value of 41% to 46% and then to 48%, to the final recording of 49% on the 12th postinfarction day. The right ventricular ejection fraction also was noted to improve, especially in those patients with acute inferior wall myocardial infarctions whose initial ejection fraction was 50% (normal ⩾52%) and rose to a peak value of 58% by the third postinfarction day.

Although each of these studies is small and consequently generalization must be cautious, there appears to be a slight improvement in resting right and left ventricular function over time in the majority of patients surviving an acute myocardial infarction. Individual differences can be attributable to the presence or absence of prior myocardial infarctions or continued ischemia, hemodynamic differences, and differences in the patients' admission and subsequent drug treatment regimens. If the evolution of a patient's cardiac function after infarction could be assessed independently of these confounding factors, additional pathophysiologic, clinical, and prognostic information might be obtained as outlined in table 25-2.

TABLE 25-2. Interpretation of serial changes in left ventricular function after infarction

Ejection fraction		Interpretation
Early	Late	
Normal	Normal	Small infarct with well-preserved residual LV function
	Abnormal	Declining function reflects either reinfarction, continued ischemia, withdrawal of compensatory mechanisms, or changes in therapy
Abnormal	Normal	Small infarct with compensation by normal viable myocardium or early restoration of coronary blood flow with late recovery of "stunned" myocardium
	Abnormal	Significant percent of myocardium loss at the time of the acute or prior infarction

Clinical and Hemodynamic Classifications

In 1973, Kostuk et al. performed first-pass radionuclide angiography on 64 patients within one month of their acute myocardial infarctions [17]. The mean left ventricular ejection fraction was 38% with a wide range of ejection fractions, 8%–67%. Of the 64 patients, 58 (91%) had left ventricular ejection fractions depressed below normal (normal ⩾52%). The authors also noted a correlation between the radionuclide-derived ejection fractions and the National Institutes of Health Myocardial Infarct Research Units (MIRU) clinical classification scheme (table 25-3). The mean left ventricular ejection fraction for the 21 patients in class I (no clinical evidence of impaired left ventricular function) was approximately 49%, the ejection fraction was 35% for the 32 patients in class II (mild to moderate left ventricular failure) and 30% for the class-III patients (overt pulmonary edema), and the left ventricular ejection fraction was 10% for the five patients in cardiogenic shock, class IV. Schelbert et al. confirmed this correlation between the left ventricular ejection fraction and the MIRU clinical classification in their 63 patients studied within one week of an acute myocardial infarction [15]. Class-I patients had a mean left ventricular ejection fraction of 52%, class-II patients 40%, and the class-III patients had a left ventricular ejection fraction of 33%. The authors noted, however, that there was considerable variability

of individual left ventricular ejection fractions within each class. While the overall left ventricular ejection fraction was normal in class-I patients, 44% of these patients had depressed left ventricular ejection fractions (less than 52%) and 11% had ejection fractions less than 40%. While none of the patients in class II had normal ejection fractions, only half were below 40%. There was less variability in class-III patients, with none of the patients having normal ejection fractions, 84% of the patients having ejection fractions below 40%, and 42% having ejection fractions less than 30%.

Wynne et al. compared the left ventricular ejection fractions derived from their equilibrium radionuclide angiograms to the commonly used Killip classification [18]. All of their patients were studied within two days of their first Q-wave infarction. The mean left ventricular ejection fraction was 50% for the Killip class-I patients (no clinical evidence for left ventricular dysfunction), 40% for the class-II patients (mild to moderate left ventricular dysfunction as evidenced by either an S_3 gallop or pulmonary rales), and 20% for the patients combined into Killip classes III (overt pulmonary edema) and IV (cardiogenic shock). Sanford et al. confirmed the association between the Killip classess and the left ventricular ejection fractions in a group of 100 patients studied in an earlier phase of their acute infarctions (within 8 h of the onset of their chest pain) [19]. The left ventricular ejection fraction declined linearly from 50% to 42% to 27% in the

TABLE 25-3. Correlation between early postinfarction left ventricular ejection fraction and clinical classification

	LVEF (%) functional class			LVEF range/functional class		
	I	II	III—IV	I	II	III—IV
Kostuk et al. [17]	49	35	21	NA	NA	NA
Schelbert et al. [15]	52	40	33	37—60	24—52	23—42
Wynne et al. [18]	50	40	20	NA	NA	NA
Sanford et al. [19]	50	42	27	17—71	7—76	20—42
Rigo et al. [20]	42	35	19	31—53	26—45	14—23

Ejection fractions not corrected for technical laboratory differences.
NA, data not presented in the published report.

Killip classes I, II, and III, respectively. The authors also noted there was significant individual variability within each classification similar to that which had been previously reported by Schelbert et al. The range of left ventricular ejection fractions in the 41 class-I patients was approximately 17%—71%, with four patients (10%) having a left ventricular ejection fraction of less than 30%. The class-II patients had an even greater range, 7%—76%, with 15 patients (36%) having left ventricular ejection fractions of less than 30%.

Rigo et al. performed equilibrium radionuclide angiograms and right heart catheterizations in 38 patients within 48 h of acute myocardial infarction [20]. The patients were divided into three groups based on their hemodynamic studies. Group-I patients had normal hemodynamics with a left ventricular filling pressure of $\leqslant 15$ mm/Hg, cardiac index $\geqslant 2.5$ l/min/m^2, and a systolic arterial pressure greater than 90 mm/Hg. Group-II patients had either an increased left ventricular filling pressure or an abnormal cardiac index, or both, with a normal systolic arterial pressure. Group-III patients were in cardiogenic shock with a systolic arterial pressure of less than 80 mmHg. In spite of the fact that the patients in group I could be considered to be in a low-risk subgroup with uncomplicated myocardial infarctions, 12 of the 13 patients in this group had abnormal ventricular ejection fractions. The mean left ventricular ejection fraction for the entire group was 42%. The 22 patients in group II had a mean left ventricular ejection fraction of 35% and the three patients in cardiogenic shock had severely depressed left ventricular ejection fractions, mean 19%.

It can be concluded from these studies that the left ventricular ejection fraction is closely correlated with the commonly used clinical and hemodynamic classification schemes. Patients with no clinical or hemodynamic evidence for left ventricular failure will have left ventricular ejection fractions close to normal. Patients with clinical evidence for mild to moderate left ventricular dysfunction will have left ventricular ejection fractions reduced approximately 15 EF% units, and patients in pulmonary edema or cardiogenic shock will have severely depressed left ventricular ejection fractions. However, the great individual patient variability within each class should be emphasized. This, in part, reflects the small number of patients in each of the reported series. It also reflects important variables not being considered, such as the patient's history of prior myocardial infarction, the presence of continued ischemia, associated right ventricular dysfunction, and various hemodynamic and iatrogenic variables.

Prognostic Indices

The major determinants of the short-term prognosis of a patient suffering an acute myocardial infarction are the size of the infarct and the functional status of the residual myocardium. Postmortem studies have demonstrated that patients who have cardiogenic shock complicating their acute myocardial infarction generally have 40% or more of the left ventricular myocardium destroyed by the acute or prior infarcts [21, 22]. This association between increasing infarct size and increasing mortality has been confirmed by other clinical indices, including serial analysis of serum creatine phosphokinase changes [23]. The inverse relationship between infarct size and the functional status of the residual myocardium as reflected in the global left ventricular ejection fraction has also been demonstrated by ECG and CK isozyme analyses [11, 17, 24]. A Duke University study of patients three weeks after acute myocardial infarction demonstrated a significant inverse relationship between ECG-estimated infarct size and the radionuclide-derived left ventricular ejection fraction, $r = -0.88$ [11]. Previously, Kostuk et al. had reported a similar relationship between infarct size estimated by CK analysis and the global left ventricular ejection fraction, $r = -0.71$ [17]. In addition to demonstrating the relationship between CPK enzymes and left ventricular ejection fraction, the authors also reported that the mean left ventricular ejection fraction was significantly higher in the survivors of the acute infarction, 40%, compared with the nonsurvivors, 26% (table 25-4). In fact, in their series the left ventricular ejection fraction of 25% divided patients into relative high- and low-risk subgroups with an 8% one-month mortality for the patients with initial ejection fractions above 25%, and a 58% one-month mortality for those patients with ejection fractions below 25%. Rigo et al. found almost identical results with the mean left ventricular ejection fraction for their survivors being 38% compared with 27% for the nonsurvivors [20]. In the Rigo series, no one with an ejection fraction greater than 40% died within the three-month follow-up period.

The value of the initial left ventricular ejection fraction for predicting early mortality was also demonstrated by Schelbert et al., who divided their patients into two subgroups, those with normal left ventricular ejection fractions ($\geq 52\%$) and those with depressed ejection fractions [15]. None of the patients with normal ejection fractions died in the first two months after their infarctions, while the mortality rate was 19% for those patients with depressed ejection fractions. The predictive value of this simple classification of high- and low-risk patients based on the left ventricular ejection fraction was confirmed in the UCLA series reported by Nemerovski et al. [14]. None of their patients with initial normal left ventricular ejection fractions died, but those patients with severely depressed ejection fractions (less than 30%) had a 23% mortality rate. The authors also noted that an intermediate group of patients with ejection fractions between 31% and 53% had an inhospital mortality of 3%.

In addition to classification schemes that are based on single values for any given indices of cardiac function, it is likely that prognostic information is contained in the directional changes and the magnitude of the changes that these indices make during the immediate postinfarction period. The focus of the analysis in table 25-2 is on the resting left ventricular ejection fraction, which primarily reflects infarct size. Treating the ejection fraction as a continuous function would permit a more sophisticated analysis than merely dichotomizing patients into normal versus abnormal subgroups. In addition, the importance of identifying the presence and extent of postinfarction residual ischemia cannot be overemphasized [25].

Clinical Trials

Dunn and his associates used radionuclide angiography to assess the role of sublingual nitroglycerin on global and regional left and right ventricular function following an acute myocardial

TABLE 25-4. Early postinfarction left ventricular ejection fraction and short-term prognosis

	Overall mortality (%)	Follow-up Period	Ejection fraction (%)		Mortality (%)		Mortality (%)	
			Survivors	Non-survivors	Normal EF	Abnormal EF	EF>30%	EF<30%
Kostuk et al. [17]	17	1 mo	40	26	NA	NA	8	58
Rigo et al. [20]	16	3 mo	38	27	0	16	7	44
Schelbert et al. [15]	12	2 mo	NA	NA	0	19	NA	NA
Nemerovski et al. [14]	7	Inhospital	NA	NA	0	10	2	23

NA, data not presented in published reports.

infarction [26]. At the time of their initial post-infarction radionuclide angiogram (mean 36 h), the global left ventricular ejection fraction was 51% and was abnormal in nine of 18 patients. The global right ventricular ejection fraction was 42%, and was abnormal in eight of 18 patients, which included eight of the ten patients with inferior wall myocardial infarction. From the early to the predischarge radionuclide angiograms, the global left ventricular ejection fraction rose significantly in seven of 18 patients, but the mean left ventricular ejection fraction was unchanged. On the other hand, the mean right ventricular ejection fraction did rise significantly from 42% to 52% ($P<0.02$) with ten of 18 patients appreciating an increase in the right ventricular ejection fraction.

At the time of the early study, 16 patients had abnormal regional ejection fractions in the ECG-identified site of the myocardial infarction. Following nitroglycerin, the mean global left and right ventricular ejection fractions rose significantly, 51%−55% ($P<0.02$) and 42%−47% ($P<0.05$), respectively. The global left ventricular ejection fraction increased in six patients while the regional left ventricular ejection fraction increased in 12 of the 18 patients. Five patients increased their ejection fraction in the infarct zone, four patients in the noninfarct zone, and three patients increased their ejection fraction in both zones following nitroglycerin administration.

Radionuclide angiography has also been used to assess the potential beneficial effect of coronary artery reperfusion utilizing intracoronary streptokinase. Reduto et al. successfully established reperfusion in 20 of 30 patients with totally occluded coronary arteries supplying their infarct regions [27]. No changes were noted in the radionuclide-determined left ventricular ejection fraction from the time of admission to discharge in the control population (46%−48%), nor in the streptokinase infusion failures (47%−49%). Although there was no change in the left ventricular ejection fraction in the 20 patients who underwent successful streptokinase infusion from the time of their admission to the period immediately following completion of streptokinase infusion, by the time of their hospital discharge these patients had appreciated a significant rise in their mean left ventricular ejection fraction, 46%−55% ($p=0.002$). The authors concluded that this late improvement was most likely secondary to delayed improvement in regional contractile function in the ischemic border zone. The authors also noted that this improvement was most impressive in the patients admitted with abnormal left ventricular function. Only one of the control patients and none of the streptokinase failures appreciated a significant increase in their individual ejection fraction from the time of admission to their discharge. However, all seven of the patients with depressed left ventricular function on admission who underwent successful reperfusion with streptokinase demonstrated a significant rise in their left ventricular ejection fraction, mean 32%−47% ($p=0.005$).

These two reports illustrate some of the potential difficulties that might be encountered when using radionuclide angiography to assess the efficacy of therapy. It is likely that the authors of the streptokinase study are correct in their hypothesis that the recovery of normal contractile function may be delayed in the ischemic border zones after reperfusion. Early repeat radionuclide angiography might therefore leave the practitioner to the erroneous assumption that he had not helped his patient. ST-segment mapping, thallium myocardial perfusion imaging, or other indices might have been more reliable in defining the immediate beneficial effects of the reperfusion. In the nitroglycerin study, both regional and global methods of analysis were used to demonstrate an enhanced systolic function following nitroglycerin. Regional ischemia may have been reduced by the drug's effects on increasing regional blood flow secondary to its direct action on the coronary circulation or indirectly by reducing venous return, left ventricular volume, and myocardial oxygen requirements. On the other hand, the observed increase in regional and global ejection fractions may have been, in part, secondary to the drug's effect on reducing the left ventricular afterload without significantly improving left ventricular ischemia or contractility. It is also possible that the observed increase in systolic function may have been accomplished at the expense of the ischemic border region.

Conclusion

Radionuclide angiography performed during the infarct period has increased our understanding of the infarct process and helped us to assess the effectiveness of treatment interventions that attempt to alter its natural history. These studies have illustrated the heterogeneity of left ventricular function in patients after acute infarction—even among those patients in similar clinical subsets. Until the exact role of radionuclide angiography has been determined, however, it should not be considered a routine study to be performed in the early phase of every patient's hospitalization. Most decision making will depend on traditional clinical parameters and on routine laboratory procedures such as electrocardiograms and chest x-rays. When the patient's status is uncertain or his course complicated or unstable, hemodynamic monitoring, radionuclide imaging, and, in an increasing number of patients, coronary arteriography may all be appropriate. In the future, it is likely that the continuing advancements in the field of nuclear imaging will enhance its importance in the care of the postinfarction patient.

References

1. Ross J Jr: Afterload mismatch and preload reserve: a conceptual framework for the analysis of ventricular function. Prog Cardiovasc Dis 18: 255–264, 1976.
2. Rackley CE: Quantitative evaluation of left ventricular function by radiographic techniques. Circulation 54:862–879, 1976.
3. MacGregor DV, Covell JW, Mahler F, Dilley RB, Ross J Jr: Relations between afterload, stroke volume, and descending limb of Starling's curve. Am J Physiol 227:884–890, 1974.
4. Stroebeck JE, Sonnenblick EH: Myocardial and ventricular function. Cardiovasc Rev Rep 4: 568–581, 1983.
5. Bodenheimer MM, Banka VS, Hermann GA, Trout RG, Pasdar H, Helfant RH: Reversible asynergy: histopathologic and electrographic correlations in patients with coronary artery disease. Circulation 53:792–796, 1976.
6. Ideker RE, Behar VS, Wagner GS, Starr JW, Starmer CF, Lee KL, Hackel DB: Evaluation of asynergy as an indicator of myocardial fibrosis. Circulation 57:715–725, 1978.
7. Falsetti HL, Marcus ML, Kerber RE, Skorton DJ: Quantification of myocardial ischemia and infarction by left ventricular imaging. Circulation 63:747–751, 1981.
8. Braunwald E, Kloner RA: The stunned myocardium: prolonged, postischemic ventricular dysfunction. Circulation 66:1146–1149, 1982.
9. Stack RS, Phillips HR III, Grierson DS, Behar VS, Kong Y, Peter RH, Swain JL, Greenfield JC Jr: Functional improvement of jeopardized myocardium following intracoronary streptokinase infusion in acute myocardial infarction. J Clin Invest 72:84–95, 1983.
10. Feild BL, Russell RO, Dowling JT, Rackley CE: Regional left ventricular performance in the year following myocardial infarction. Circulation 66: 679–689, 1972.
11. Palmeri ST, Harrison DG, Cobb FR, et al: A QRS scoring system for assessing left ventricular function after myocardial infarction. N Engl J Med 9:4–9, 1982.
12. Ohsuzu F, Boucher CA, Newell JB, et al: Relation of segmental wall motion to global left ventricular function in acute myocardial infarction. Am J Cardiol 51:1275–1281, 1983.
13. Wackers FJ, Berger HJ, Weinberg MA, Zaret BL: Spontaneous changes in left ventricular function over the first 24 hours of acute myocardial infarction: implications for evaluating early therapeutic interventions. Circulation 66:748–754, 1982.
14. Nemerovski M, Shah PK, Pichler M, et al: Radionuclide assessment of sequential changes in left and right ventricular function following first acute transmural myocardial infarction. Am Heart J 104:709–717, 1982.
15. Schelbert HR, Henning H, Ashburn WL, et al: Serial measurements of left ventricular ejection fraction by radionuclide angiography early and late after myocardial infarction. Am J Cardiol 38:407–415, 1976.
16. Steele P, Kirch D, Ellis J, et al: Prompt return to normal of depressed right ventricular ejection fraction in acute inferior infarction. Br Heart J 39:1319–1323, 1977.
17. Kostuk WJ, Ehsani AL, Kalriner JS, et al: Left ventricular performance after myocardial infarction assessed by radioisotope angiocardiography. Circulation 57:242–249, 1973.
18. Wynne J, Sayres M, Maddox DE, et al: Regional left ventricular function in acute myocardial infarction: evaluation with quantitative radionuclide ventriculography. Am J Cardiol 45:203–209, 1980.

19. Sanford CF, Corbett J, Nicod P, et al: Value of radionuclide ventriculography in the immediate characterization of patients with acute myocardial infarction. Am J Cardiol 49:637−644, 1982.

20. Rigo P, Murray M, Strauss HW, et al: Left ventricular function in acute myocardial infarction evaluated by gated scintiphotography. Circulation 50:678−684, 1974.

21. Page DL, Caulfield JB, Kastor JA: Myocardial changes associated with cardiogenic shock. N Engl J Med 285:133−137, 1971.

22. Weber KT, Ratshin RA, Janicki JS: Left ventricular dysfunction following acute myocardial infarction: a clinicopathologic and hemodynamic profile of shock and failure. Am J Med 54:697−705, 1973.

23. Geltman EM, Ehsani AA, Campbell MK, et al: The influence of location and extent of myocardial infarction on long-term ventricular dysrhythmia and mortality. Circulation 60:805−814, 1979.

24. Hirsowitz GS, Lakier JB, Marks DS, et al: Comparison of radionuclide and enzymatic estimate of infarct size in patients with acute myocardial infarction. J Am Coll Cardiol 1:1405−1412, 1983.

25. Epstein SE, Palmeri ST, Patterson RE: Evaluation of patients following acute myocardial function: indications for cardiac catheterization and surgical intervention. N Engl J Med 307:1487−1492, 1982.

26. Dunn RF, Botvinick EH, Benge W, et al: The significance of nitroglycerin-induced changes in ventricular function after acute myocardial infarction. Am J Cardiol 49:1719−1727, 1982.

27. Reduto LA, Freund GC, Gaeta JM, Smalling RW, Lewis B, Gould KL: Coronary artery reperfusion in acute myocardial infarction: beneficial effects of intracoronary streptokinase on left ventricular salvage and performance. Am Heart J 102:1168−1177, 1981.

26. TACHYARRHYTHMIAS DURING ACUTE MYOCARDIAL INFARCTION AND OPTIONS FOR THEIR ELECTRICAL MANAGEMENT

Archer Broughton

Tachyarrhythmias are common during the first few days following acute myocardial infarction, reflecting the unstable electrical properties of ischemic cardiac cells. In the conventional coronary care unit the control of these tachyarrhythmias by electrical means has usually involved emergency countershock for life-threatening episodes or the occasional use of overdrive pacing. The last decade has seen the emergence and refinement of electrophysiologic techniques allowing intracardiac recording and stimulation including the delivery of intravascular countershock. These more invasive techniques have not been widely applied in the setting of acute infarction, but the question arises as to their potential role. This chapter reviews the types of tachyarrhythmias observed in patients during acute myocardial infarction (AMI), and the electrical techniques available for diagnosis and management. The potential usefulness of newer approaches is discussed in the context of evidence from Duke University Medical Center regarding the spectrum of tachyarrhythmias detected in the coronary care unit of the 1980s.

Incidence of Tachyarrhythmias during Acute Myocardial Infarction: Previous Reports

The available data on the incidence of various supraventricular and ventricular tachyarrhythmias during the acute phase of myocardial infarction have been discussed in several recent reviews [1–3]. Although virtually every tachyarrhythmia has been reported [4–12], those most commonly observed have been sinus tachycardia, atrial flutter/fibrillation, ventricular tachycardia, and ventricular fibrillation.

Sinus tachycardia (>100/min) is common during the first few days of acute myocardial infarction (AMI). The reported incidence has ranged from 8% to 50%. [6–8, 13–19]. Inhospital mortality is increased. Management is almost always indirect and aimed at the underlying process, which has increased sympathetic tone. Factors such as unrelieved pain or anxiety, fever, left ventricular failure, hypovolemia, hypoxemia, anemia, pericarditis, and pulmonary emboli should be considered.

Atrial flutter and fibrillation have been reported in as many as 16% of patients with AMI [6–8, 14–17, 20]. Postmortem examination has detected necrosis of the sinus node and right atrium in some patients [21]. Atrial flutter is considered less common than atrial fibrillation, but the exact incidences remain in doubt since the rhythms interconvert in many patients, and their distinction is best based on atrial recordings. The ventricular response is typically rapid (>120/min) and may produce hemodynamic deterioration, with worsening of left ventricular failure or shock [9]. In-hospital mortality is increased in patients

R.M. Califf and G.S. Wagner (eds.), ACUTE CORONARY CARE: Principles and Practice. Copyright © 1985. Martinus Nijhoff Publishing, Boston/Dordrecht/Lancaster.

developing atrial flutter/fibrillation during AMI [14−16, 18, 22]. The worsening of prognosis reflects the underlying deleterious processes that provoke these arrhythmias and the adverse impact of tachycardia per se on the circulation and on myocardial oxygen delivery and consumption during AMI [23].

Other supraventricular tachycardias are less commonly encountered in AMI. These include junctional reentry or automatic tachycardias, and automatic atrial tachycardia. Digitalis toxicity should be considered when atrial tachycardia is accompanied by atrioventricular (AV) block [1]. Accelerated AV junctional tachycardia is associated with acute inferior infarction, because the right coronary artery supplies the AV nodal area in most patients [13, 21, 24−26]. This arrhythmia is usually transient and well tolerated since the rate ranges from 70 to 120/min [1].

Ventricular arrhythmias accompany almost every human AMI if isolated premature ventricular contractions are included in the analysis. Ventricular tachycardia (VT) was considered rare during human AMI before the advent of routine ECG monitoring [6, 7, 27]. However, analysis of continuously recorded ECG tapes has detected VT ($\geq$3 beats at a rate $\geq$120/min) in up to 73% of patients during the first 24 h [28]. Most episodes are unstable, usually terminating promptly but occasionally deteriorating into ventricular fibrillation. Sustained monomorphic episodes are rare [29] except where prior infarction has produced left ventricular (LV) aneurysm [30]. Coronary care data have generally indicated that all types of ventricular tachyarrhythmias decrease markedly over the first 24 h after hospitalization [12, 17, 31−33]. This includes premature beats and accelerated idioventricular rhythm, as well as the potentially lethal ventricular tachycardia and ventricular fibrillation. The risk of lethal arrhythmia is greatest at the outset, usually several hours before admission to a coronary care unit (see chapter 28). Up to 60% of the deaths during acute myocardial infarction occur within the first hour [19, 34, 35]. Death results from ventricular fibrillation in more than 90% of those who die suddenly [19, 36]. This initial high mortality greatly limits the extent that community AMI mortality can be lowered by inhospital coronary care.

EXPERIMENTAL OBSERVATIONS

Coronary artery occlusion in the dog is followed by two distinct phases of early ventricular arrhythmias as first shown by Harris [37]. Sudden total occlusion is followed by a brief, intense susceptibility to ventricular fibrillation lasting only 10 min. Loss of animals at the outset is avoided by more gradual "two stage" ligation so that ventricular arrhythmias then do not develop until after 4−8 h. Ventricular tachycardia is then the most prominent rhythm disturbance, attaining its highest incidence 10−20 h after occlusion and recurring for 2−4 days. The very early ventricular arrhythmias may reflect reentrant excitation within acutely ischemic and infarcting myocardium [38]. Recent findings [39] in the isolated heart, however, have supported Harris' original view [37] that the current of injury flowing at the border between ischemic and normal myocardium may be primarily responsible. The delayed arrhythmias appear to reflect abnormal automaticity and reentrant excitation within the subendocardial Purkinje network underlying infarcted myocardium [40, 41]. Similar mechanisms have also been alleged to operate within the overlying subepicardial myocardium [38].

Ventricular fibrillation (VF) during human AMI is frequently classified into primary and secondary categories, depending on whether it arises during uncomplicated AMI or in the setting of severe heart failure or shock. Primary VF is rarely fatal when direct current countershock is given promptly although the occasional patient requires multiple shocks [42]. Primary VF develops in 4%−9% of AMI patients who reach hospital [43−45]. The likelihood cannot usually be predicted from an analysis of the incidence of other ventricular arrhythmias [43−45] except in an occasional patient where a change in frequency of early cycle (R-on-T) ventricular ectopics is observed [46]. A primary VF rate as high as 30% may be applicable during the first hour after the onset of symptoms, but it is generally accepted that the incidence decreases "exponentially" with time, reaching a low level after 12 h [28]. Late initial episodes (>24 h after infarction), however, do occur and have been reported in up to 25% of patients with primary VF even where reinfarction was thought to be excluded [42].

Furthermore, according to Lie and colleagues [47], survivors of anterior infarction complicated by bundle branch block have a 35% incidence of late VF and should be monitored inhospital for six weeks.

Primary VF recurs in 20−30% patients, although the exact timing remains controversial [42−44]. VF always recurred with 12 h of infarction in one study unless reinfarction developed [44]. In a second study, however, later recurrences were reported in the absence of reinfarction [42]. The immediate and long-term outlook is much more optimistic with primary VF than with secondary VF. In a recent study [42], secondary VF recurred twice as often as primary VF and inhospital mortality was almost four times as great (85% vs 22%). The outlook remains poor for patients surviving secondary VF while survival rates following resuscitation from primary VF are generally comparable to those in patients without VF [28]. Campbell and colleagues [46] have documented a distinct bimodal distribution of ventricular arrhythmias during human AMI comparable to that observed during experimental infarction. During the first 4 h, all types of ventricular arrhythmias were frequent. Subsequently, the incidence of primary VF and R-on-T ectopic activity decreased rapidly and the incidence of VT and less premature (later cycle) ventricular ectopics increased.

Acute Myocardial Infarction Tachyarrhythmias: Duke University Medical Center Data

CHANGING TACHYARRHYTHMIA PATTERN: 1970−1982

Facilities for centralized ECG monitoring of all AMI patients have been available at Duke University Medical Center since the late 1960s (see chapter 37). Information on the tachyarrhythmias detected by arrhythmia surveillance personnel (monitor watchers) since 1969 has been stored in a computer-based data bank. Tachycardia was defined as >2 consecutive complexes at a rate >100/min. All patients were monitored for at least five days after the onset of transmural or subendocardial infarction. Those transferred from other hospitals after infarction were excluded

from this analysis. As can be seen from figure 26-1, the incidence of narrow complex tachycardia ("SVT") and broad complex tachycardia (presumed "VT") has fluctuated from year to year, with each of these arrhythmias being detected in about 20%−30% of patients. There seems little overall trend except perhaps toward more frequent broad complex runs in recent years. By contrast, the incidence of ventricular fibrillation has declined recently, both in patients experiencing their first infarct and in those with prior infarction. During 1971 and 1972, about 15% of patients in both groups developed ventricular fibrillation, both primary and secondary. A decade later, the incidence has fallen to 6% in patients hospitalized during first infarction, and fallen to 7.5% in patients undergoing second or subsequent infarction. The cause for the decline is not certain. A trend toward less severe coronary artery disease is one possibility. However, the proportion of patients with prior infarction has remained about one-third over the decade. The decline might reflect the use of routine lidocaine infusion from 1975 and 1976. In other recent studies, however, VF rates have been equally low in patients not receiving antiarrhythmic therapy [28, 48]. Previous investigators have not agreed on the value of prophylactic lidocaine during acute infarction [see chapter 32]. Apart from differences in dose, differences in baseline incidence of ventricular fibrillation may have clouded the issue. Thus, lidocaine has appeared of no value where the incidence of ventricular fibrillation in untreated patients was <5% [49, 50]. By contrast, an apparent strong protective effect was found in studies where the baseline incidence approached 10% [45, 51].

THE CURRENT SITUATION: AMI TACHYARRHYTHMIAS DURING 1981 AND 1982

Tachyarrhythmias were detected in about 40% of the Duke University AMI patients during 1981 and 1982. Multiple arrhythmias occurred in 12% of patients overall and in most of the patients developing VF (figure 26-2). VF developed in 16 (6.6%) of 241 patients undergoing first or subsequent AMI. The episode began as organized ventricular tachycardia in the majority (10 of 16), but not in all patients (figure 26-4D).

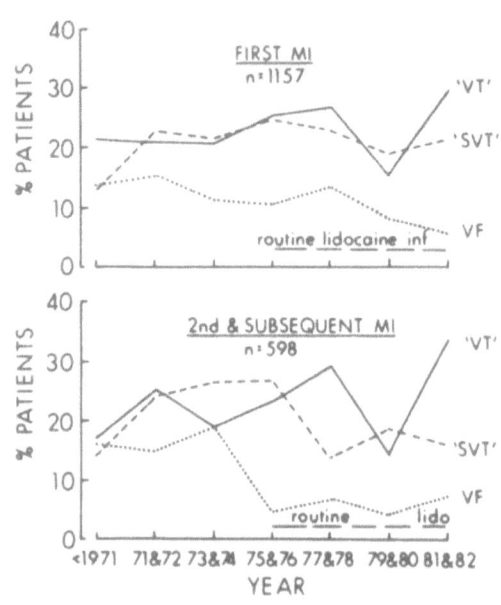

FIGURE 26-1. The incidence of various tachyarrhythmias during acute myocardial infarction (MI) at
Duke University Medical Center from 1969 to 1982.
Patients were monitored for the first five days at least
and have been grouped according to whether or not
there was a history of previous infarction. Lidocaine
was routinely infused in all patients with acute infarction from 1975/1976 onward. Tachyarrhythmia was
≥ 3 complexes, >100/min. "VT," broad complex
tachycardia; "SVT," narrow complex tachycardia; VF,
primary and secondary ventricular fibrillation.

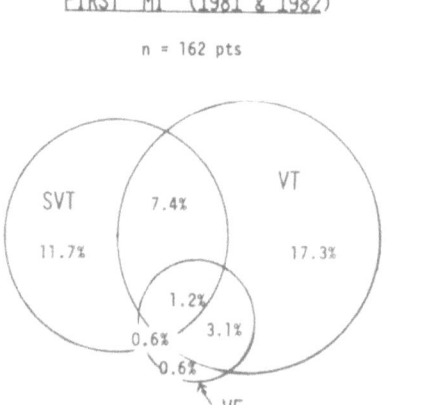

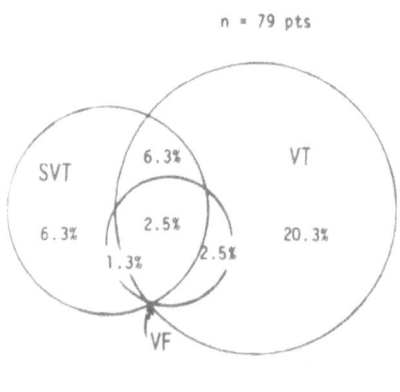

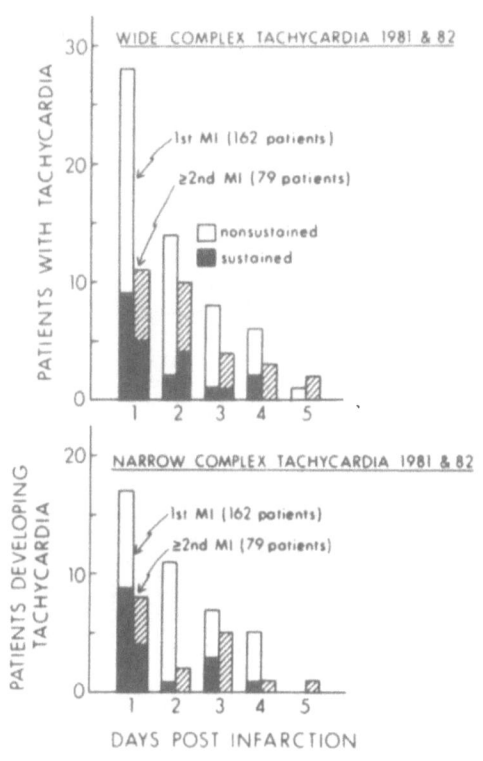

FIGURE 26-3. Time-dependent decrease in tachyarrhythmias after acute MI in Duke University Medical Center patients in 1981/1982. The height of the vertical bars shows the number of patients in which wide complex tachycardia (top panel) or narrow complex tachycardia (bottom panel) developed on each day. Bars are shaded light/dark to reflect the proportion of patients with nonsustained/sustained tachycardia.

VF occurred initially on day 1 in most patients (12 of 16), on day 2 in two, and was delayed beyond the first 48 h in the remaining two. Only five of 16 patients developed VF while on lidocaine in the absence of shock (VF occurred pre-lidocaine in five, during cardiogenic shock in four, and after lidocaine withdrawal in two).

The incidence of broad complex tachycardia

FIGURE 26-2. The distribution of the various tachyarrhythmias within patients with acute MI at Duke University Medical Center in 1981/1982. Abbreviations as in figure 26-1.

was highest on the day of infarction and declined with time (figure 26-3, top panel). Most episodes were nonsustained, terminating spontaneously within 1–60 s (figure 26-4C). Sustained episodes (requiring countershock) developed in about 30% of patients with broad complex tachycardia (first AMI: 13 of 47 patients with tachycardia; prior AMI: eight of 25 patients with tachycardia), but nearly half these sustained episodes occurred during cardiogenic shock. Most of the remaining "sustained" episodes degenerated promptly into VF. Stable broad complex tachycardia in the absence of cardiogenic shock was an infrequent finding (first AMI: three of 162 patients; prior AMI: one of 79 patients).

Narrow complex tachycardia (excluding sinus tachycardia; see figure 26-4B) developed in 20% of the AMI patients overall. The incidence was highest on the day of infarction and declined with time parallel to the incidence of broad complex episodes (figure 26-3, bottom panel). Most episodes were nonsustained, did not present a management problem, and could not be definitively classified from their rhythm strip appearance (figure 26-4A). Sustained episodes (requiring countershock, overdrive pacing, or drug treatment) developed in 17 (35%) of 48 patients with narrow complex tachycardia. Sustained episodes were atrial flutter or fibrillation in most patients (13 of 17), the remainder being unclassified supraventricular tachycardia. Stable narrow complex tachycardia in the absence of cardiogenic shock occurred more often than did stable broad complex episodes but remained uncommon (first AMI: seven of 162 patients; prior AMI: three of 79 patients). Esophageal recording and stimulation was used to diagnose and terminate atrial flutter in two patients (figure 26-5).

Electrical Management of Arrhythmias During Acute Infarction

TRANSTHORACIC COUNTERSHOCK

It has been known for many years that ventricular fibrillation is readily induced by passage of a small alternating current through the heart (see Hooker [52] and Lown [53] for detailed historical perspective). Application of even a 1-mA point-source current for 5 s readily induces the

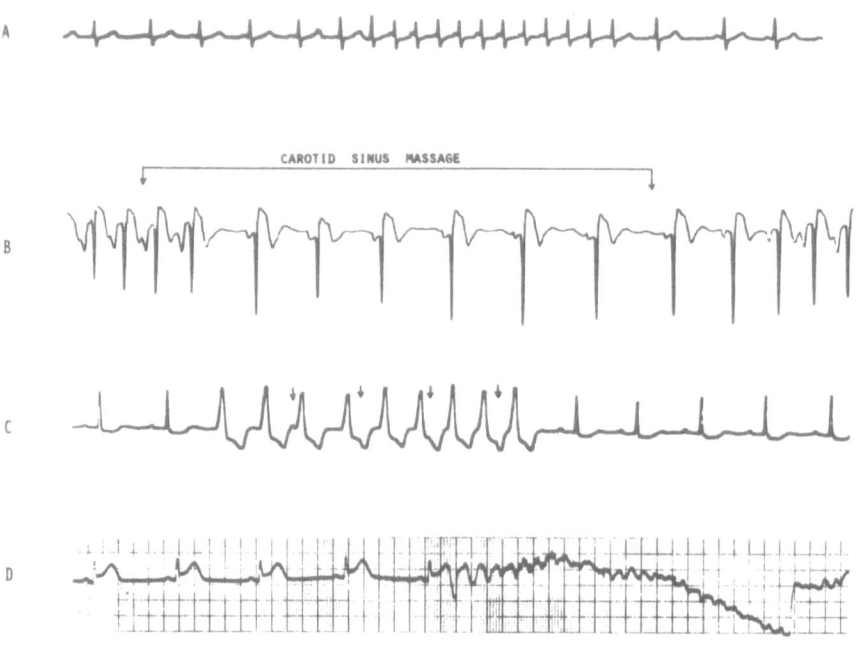

FIGURE 26-4. Examples of tachyarrhythmias during acute MI. (A) Nonsustained narrow complex tachy-cardia. (B) Automatic tachycardia of atrial origin (probably sinus tachycardia), which slowed during carotid sinus massage. (C) Nonsustained broad complex tachycardia with ventriculoatrial dissociation strongly suggesting ventricular origin. (D) Ventricular fibrillation.

arrhythmia [54]. Prevost and Battelli [55] were the first to report that ventricular fibrillation could also be terminated by the application of alternating current although much higher current was required than for induction. Subsequent investigation confirmed the antifibrillatory effect of high current, whether applied for 5 s or for as little as 0.1 s [54]. In 1947, Beck et al. [56] reported the first successful clinical application of alternating current countershock to the fibrillating human heart. Ordinary 110-V alternating current was momentarily applied to the exposed heart via two large electrodes to revert ventricular fibrillation of 35-min duration, on the second attempt. Subsequently, methods for closed-chest defibrillation were developed for hospital use. An important stimulus was the demonstration by Kouwenhoven et al. [57] that adequate circulation could be maintained during cardiac arrest by external cardiac massage until arrival of defibrillating equipment. Alternating-current (AC) defibrillators typically delivered about 5 A of 60-Hz current for a period of 0.25 s, which was applied in the direction of the long axis of the heart through electrodes on the chest [58−60].

Although Prevost and Battelli [55] observed

in 1899 that direct current (DC) could terminate ventricular fibrillation, this approach was initially neglected. While Guvich and Yuniev [61] found capacitor discharge highly effective, other investigators reported inconsistent and generally inferior results compared with those obtained with alternating current [62, 63]. However, the 1960s saw a renewed interest in DC countershock. This has been attributed, firstly, to the impression that VF during acute myocardial infarction was relatively resistant to AC countershock [64]. Secondly, the desire existed to extend countershock to the reversion of arrhythmias other than ventricular fibrillation. Alexander et al. [65] reported the first successful use of AC countershock to revert ventricular tachycardia in 1961. Subsequent studies showed the clear superiority of (DC) countershocks. Lown et al. [66] found that

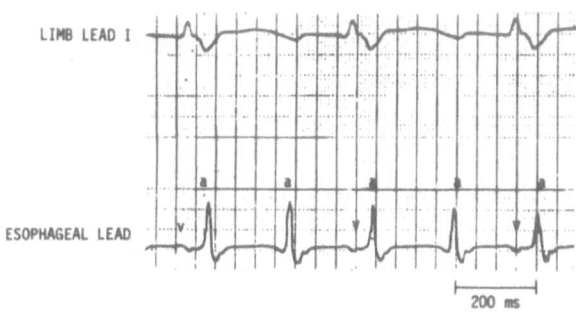

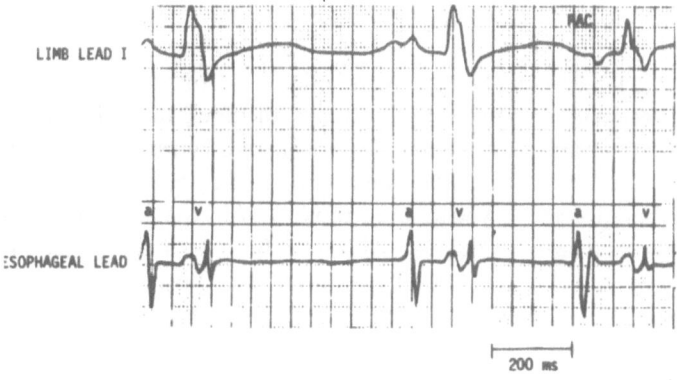

FIGURE 26-5. Sustained atrial flutter during acute MI. (Top panel) Esophageal recording shows organized atrial activity, cycle length 205 ms, with 2:1 ventricular response. (Bottom panel) Sinus rhythm with premature atrial contraction after termination of atrial flutter by esophageal stimulation (pacing cycle length 150 ms for 10 s, pulse width 9.9 ms, current 15 mA).

a DC unit was consistently more effective than the conventional AC unit in reverting ventricular tachycardia in the closed-chest dog. Deaths were confined to animals given AC shock. Ventricular fibrillation followed DC countershock in only 2% of dogs. As expected, the incidence of ventricular fibrillation varied inversely with AC voltage, but even discharges at the maximum 750 V caused VF in 13% of dogs. Lown and co-workers [67] showed it was possible to avoid VF entirely by the use of a properly synchronized capacitor discharge triggered to occur during the nonvulnerable phase of the cardiac cycle. A fur-

ther advantage of the DC unit was that only 1 A from the power line was required to store the countershock energy. AC defibrillators required as much as 70 A and were associated with power-line overload.

Considerable effort has been directed toward minimizing myocardial damage during DC countershock. Transient ECG changes are common after shock, but may reflect autonomic reflex changes and are not specific for myocardial damage [68, 69]. It has been established that shocks of high current and energy can directly damage the heart [70–72]. Experimentally, the incidence of death as well as the severity of myocardial damage increases with increasing shock strength and frequency [69, 70]. Tacker et al. [69] have demonstrated the presence of a wide safety margin between the threshold level for DC defibrillation (1 A/kg) in the dog, and the current level producing damage. No microscopic damage was detected until a threefold current overdose was delivered, and no gross lesions until a sixfold overdose. Deaths were limited to animals receiving a 12-fold overdose.

Capacitor discharge produces a voltage spike that decays exponentially from the initial peak value. Schuder et al. [73] demonstrated the detrimental effects of countershocks with long low-amplitude tails that refibrillate the heart. The shape and duration of the decay have been varied greatly in the search for optimal countershock waveforms. Myocardial damage has been related to excessive peak current [53]. Defibrillator designers have usually placed series inductance in the discharge circuit to round off the countershock waveform, reducing peak voltage and current, with negligible reduction in total energy delivered [11, 61, 66, 74–76]. Lown [53] identified several adverse characteristics of an unmodified condenser discharge that were eliminated in the "damped sinusoidal waveform" produced with series inductance. The adverse features that produced tissue damage and arrhythmia provocation during DC countershock were: (a) wavefront rise time <500 μs, (b) voltage >3000, (c) energy >400 J, and (d) absence of oscillatory ringing in the tail end of the wave. Schuder and colleagues [73] developed an alternative, "trapezoidal" countershock waveform by truncating the exponential capacitor discharge. The decrease in current during the pulse is described in terms of "tilt." This waveform is preferred in compact battery-powered systems since a bulky inductor is not required [77].

The fall in mortality among AMI patients following establishment of the coronary care unit can be credited almost entirely to the technique of transthoracic defibrillation. Inhospital mortality averaged 33% during the pre-coronary-care era, with rates ranging from 15% to 52% [78]. Interestingly, mortality did not decline with the introduction of centralized monitoring facilities per se, but only after the authority to initiate immediate defibrillation was invested in the nurse on duty [31]. This practice has reduced overall mortality into the range of 15%–25%, with the immediate risk in individual patients related to adverse factors such as advanced age, cardiomegaly, left heart failure, and shock, all indirect indicators of the extent of the underlying ventricular damage [79].

TRANSVENOUS COUNTERSHOCK

Mirowski and colleagues [80] showed over ten years ago in man that the energy required to terminate VF was reduced ten- to 20-fold when the countershock was delivered through an intravascular catheter within the ventricle. Defibrillation was accomplished with only 5–15 J in most patients. More recently, Zipes et al. [81] reported the successful use of even lower energy intravascular countershock (< 3 J) to terminate ventricular tachycardia in patients with a remote history of myocardial infarction. It is not clear whether the ease of termination was related to slow tachycardia rates in their patients who were on antiarrhythmic therapy. In earlier canine studies, 83% of tachycardias with cycle lengths >200 ms were terminated by ≤1-J countershocks synchronized to fall within the first 80% of the QRS [82]. However, faster tachycardias required higher energy shocks and VF resulted in some animals despite synchronized delivery. Yee et al. [83] have shown that transvenous countershock can be safely delivered by intensive-care nursing personnel for cardioversion and defibrillation in AMI patients and others with ventricular arrhythmias. Although it was not practicable to determine minimum energy levels, 94% of ventricular tachycardia episodes in six patients were successfully terminated by synchronized low-energy countershock (2.5–10 J). Only two-thirds of VF episodes could be terminated even with 40-J countershocks, but the study population was too small to permit adequate evaluation. Intracavitary delivery of countershock offers potential advantages over the conventional approach [83]: The countershock catheter can be used to record atrial and ventricular activity during tachycardia and to attempt conversion by burst pacing or ventricular extrastimuli. The catheter remains available for defibrillation if the tachycardia is accelerated and for pacing in the event of asystole. Delays while patient or defibrillator paddles are repositioned for countershock are avoided. Finally, the "lower" energy level of transvenous countershock may reduce myocardial damage. However, since only a fraction of the current during transthoracic shock actually passes through the heart, the transventricular current flow may not be reduced during intra-cavitary delivery of a comparably effective "low"-energy countershock.

PROGRAMMED VENTRICULAR STIMULATION AND PACING TECHNIQUES

Limited electrophysiologic evaluation is some-times justified to aid diagnosis and management of sustained or recurrent tachyarrhythmias in the setting of acute infarction. At the simplest level, atrial recordings may be used to clarify the AV relationship in the occasional broad complex tachycardia where the suspicion arises of supra-ventricular origin. AV dissociation strongly sup-ports ventricular origin whereas a one-to-one AV relationship is not helpful. A recording from the His bundle region is required to completely ex-clude supraventricular origin even in the pres-ence of AV dissociation [84]. Atrial catheter-ization has been of most frequent value in AMI patients when used to first document and then terminate atrial flutter by rapid pacing [85, 86]. Kerr and colleagues [87] have shown that these management goals can now be achieved less in-vasively, using the esophageal catheter for both atrial recording and stimulation (figure 26-5).

It has long been known that ventricular ar-rhythmias during complete heart block are sup-pressed by pacing the ventricles above their spon-taneous rate [88]. In 1964, Sowton et al. [89] showed that overdrive ventricular pacing (120/min) suppressed recurrent ventricular tachycar-dia and VF in some patients without heart block. Overdrive suppression of intractable ventricular tachyarrhythmias in AMI patients was subse-quently reported using both ventricular and atrial pacing [90, 91]. In some cases, high-paced heart rates were maintained for 1–2 weeks after infarc-tion. Atrial overdrive preserved atrial transport, but a stable pacing position was more difficult to maintain than during ventricular pacing. Ven-tricular overdrive was more effective in some patients, suggesting that the sequence of ven-tricular activation may play a role in overdrive suppression [86]. Suppression of ventricular ar-rhythmias by prolonged overdrive pacing is now rarely attempted because the success rate is low and because the substantial increase in myocar-dial oxygen consumption may increase infarct size [92]. The latter problems do not arise if overdrive pacing is reserved for ventricular tachy-cardia termination and not its suppression. Pac-ing rates as high as 250–300/min may be re-quired, but need only be maintained for 1–3 s. Alternatively, programmed ventricular extra-stimuli may be introduced. Previous studies suggest that ventricular stimulation including burst pacing may effectively terminate ventricu-lar tachycardia arising beyond the first week or so after AMI especially in patients with prior infarc-tion [29, 84–86]. This approach may accelerate the tachycardia, however [93], and requires that an intraventricular catheter (which could also cause ventricular arrhythmias) be left in situ. Tachycardia arising soon after AMI, especially during the first 24 h, appears refractory to ven-tricular stimulation [29], suggesting either an automatic mechanism or reentrant excitation pro-tected by factors such as distance from the stimu-lation site or entrance block [84, 85].

Conclusions

Tachyarrhythmias continue to be commonly en-countered in AMI patients, more than two dec-ades after the advent of intensive coronary care facilities. The future of transthoracic counter-shock as the mainstay of electrical management seems secure in the coronary care unit of the 1980s except in the case of sustained atrial flut-ter. This arrhythmia is best terminated by esoph-ageal pacing, avoiding the need for general anesthesia. Dividends for AMI patients in any widespread application of the newer invasive electrical techniques are likely to be very small. Most tachyarrhythmia episodes in hospitalized patients are self-terminating and require no im-mediate specific therapy even when of ventricular origin [28]. Many sustained tachyarrhythmias occur in the setting of cardiogenic shock, but are incidental to the primary problem of profound pump failure. Ventricular stimulation should be reserved for the very small proportion of AMI patients with recurrent sustained ventricular tachycardia after the first 24–48 h, many of whom will have a ventricular aneurysm as a result of previous infarction [30]. Since tachycardia may accelerate or degenerate into VF with ventricular stimulation, the ability to administer transvenous countershock via the same catheter would be advantageous. Further reduction in the mortality from primary VF during AMI will depend not on the provision of more sophisticated electrical techniques within coronary care units, but on the provision of adequate intensive prehospital care.

References

1. Chung EK: Tachyarrhythmias associated with acute myocardial infarction: diagnosis, frequency and significance. In: Brest AN, Wiener L, Chung EK, Kasparian H (eds) Innovations in the diagnosis and management of acute myocardial infarction. Philadelphia: FA Davis, 1975, p. 157.

2. Hindman MC, Wagner GS: Arrhythmias during myocardial infarction: mechanisms, significance and therapy. In: Castellanos A (ed) Cardiac arrhythmias: mechanisms and management. Philadelphia: FA Davis, 1980, p. 81.

3. Sloman JG, Hunt D, Sutton LD: Management of myocardial infarction. Rec Adv Cardiol 8:29, 1981.

4. Bashour FA, Jones E, Edmonson R: Cardiac arrhythmias in acute myocardial infarction. II. Incidence of the common arrhythmias with special reference to ventricular tachycardia. Dis Chest 51:520, 1967.

5. Hurwitz M, Elliot RS: Arrhythmias in acute myocardial infarction. Dis Chest 45:616, 1964.

6. Imperial ES, Carballo R, Zimmerman HA: Disturbances of rate, rhythm and conduction in acute myocardial infarction: a statistical study of 153 cases. Am J Cardiol 5:24, 1960.

7. Master AM, Dack S, Jaffe L: Disturbances of rate and rhythm in acute coronary artery thrombosis. Ann Intern Med 11:735, 1937.

8. Meltzer LE, Kitchell JB: The incidence of arrhythmias associated with acute myocardial infarction. Prog Cardiovasc Dis 9:50, 1966.

9. Mounsey P: Intensive coronary care: arrhythmias after acute myocardial infarction. Am J Cardiol 20:475, 1967.

10. Norris RM, Mercer CJ: Significance of idioventricular rhythm in acute myocardial infarction. Prog Cardiovas Dis 16:455, 1974.

11. Peleska B: Cardiac arrhythmias following condenser discharges and their dependence upon strength of current and phase of cardiac cycle. Circ Res 13:21, 1963.

12. Spann JF Jr, Moellering RC Jr, Haber E, Wheeler EO: Arrhythmias in acute myocardial infarction: a study utilizing an electrocardiographic monitor for automatic detection and recording of arrhythmias. N Engl J Med 271:427, 1964.

13. Chung EK: Principles of cardiac arrhythmias. Baltimore: Williams and Wilkins, 1971.

14. De Sanctis RW, Block P, Hutter AM: Tachyarrhythmias in myocardial infarction. Circulation 45:681, 1972.

15. James TN: Myocardial infarction and atrial arrhythmias. Circulation 24:761, 1961.

16. Jewitt DE, Balcon R, Raftery EB, Oram S: Incidence and management of supraventricular arrhythmias after acute myocardial infarction. Lancet 2:734, 1967.

17. Julian DG, Valentine PA, Miller GG: Disturbance of rate, rhythm and conduction in acute myocardial infarction: a prospective study of 100 consecutive unselected patients with the aid of electrocardiographic monitoring. Am J Med 37:915, 1964.

18. Lown B, Klein MD, Hershberg PI: Coronary and pre-coronary care. Am J Med 46:705, 1969.

19. Pantridge JF, Webb SW, Adgey AAJ, Geddes JS: The first hour after the onset of acute myocardial infarction. Prog Cardiol 3:173, 1974.

20. Cristal N, Perterburg I, Szwarcberg J: Atrial fibrillation developing in the acute phase of myocardial infarction: prognostic implications. Chest 70:1, 1976.

21. James TN: Pathogenesis of arrhythmias in acute myocardial infarction. Am J Cardiol 24:791, 1969.

22. Cristal N, Szwarcberg J, Grierson M: Supraventricular arrhythmias in acute myocardial infarction: prognostic implication of clinical setting; mechanism of production. Ann Intern Med 82:35, 1975.

23. Braunwald E: Control of myocardial oxygen consumption: physiologic and clinical considerations. Am J Cardiol 31:474, 1973.

24. James TN: The coronary circulation and conduction system in acute myocardial infarction. Prog Cardiovasc Dis 10:410, 1968.

25. Pick A, Dominquez P: Nonparoxysmal A-V nodal tachycardia. Circulation 16:1022, 1957.

26. Pick A, Langendorf R, Katz LN: A-V nodal tachycardia with block. Circulation 24:12, 1961.

27. Pick A: Cardiac arrhythmias associated with recent myocardial infarction. In: Likoff W, Moyer JH (eds) Coronary heart disease. New York: Grune and Stratton, 1963.

28. Campbell RWF: Treatment and prophylaxis of ventricular arrhythmias in acute myocardial infarction. Am J Cardiol 52:55C, 1983.

29. Wellens HJJ, Lie KI, Durrer D: Further observations of ventricular tachycardia as studied by electrical stimulation of the heart: chronic recurrent ventricular tachycardia and ventricular tachycardia during myocardial infarction. Circulation 49:647, 1974.

30. Wald RW, Waxman MB, Coney PN, Gunstensen J, Goldman BS: Management of intractable ventricular tachycardia after myocardial infarction. Am J Cardiol 44:329, 1979.

31. Killip T, Kimball JT: Treatment of myocardial infarction in a coronary care unit: a two year experience with 250 patients. Am J Cardiol 20:457, 1967.

32. Lawrie DM, Higgins MR, Godman MJ, Oliver MF, Julian DG, Donald KW: Ventricular fibrillation complicating acute myocardial infarction. Lancet 2:523, 1968.

33. Lown B, Fakhro AM, Hood WB, Thorn GW: The coronary care unit: new perspectives and directions. JAMA 199:188, 1967.

34. Bainton CR, Peterson DR: Deaths from coronary heart disease in persons fifty years of age and younger. N Engl J Med 268:569, 1963.

35. Gordon T, Kannel WB: Premature mortality from coronary heart disease: the Framingham study. JAMA 215:1617, 1971.

36. Cobb LA, Baum RS, Alvarez H, Schaffer WA: Resuscitation from out-of-hospital ventricular fibrillation: 4 years follow-up. Circulation 52:III-223, 1975.

37. Harris AS: Delayed development of ventricular ectopic rhythms following experimental coronary occlusion. Circulation 1:1318, 1950.

38. Lazzara R, El-Sherif N, Hope RR, et al: Ventricular arrhythmias and electrophysiological consequences of myocardial ischemia and infarction. Circ Res 42:740, 1978.

39. Janse MJ, Kleber AG: Electrophysiological changes and ventricular arrhythmias in the early phase of regional myocardial ischemia. Circ Res 49:1069, 1981.

40. Friedman PL, Steward JR, Wit AL: Spontaneous and induced cardiac arrhythmias in subendocardial Purkinje fibers surviving extensive myocardial infarction in dogs. Circ Res 33:612, 1973.

41. Horowitz LN, Spear JF, Moore EN: Subendocardial origin of ventricular arrhythmias in 24-hour-old experimental myocardial infarction. Circulation 53:56, 1976.

42. Logan KR, McIlwaine WJ, Adgey AAJ, Pantridge JF: Recurrence of ventricular fibrillation in acute ischemic heart disease. Circulation 64:1163, 1981.

43. El-Sherif N, Myerburg RJ, Scherlag BJ, Befeler B, Aranda JM, Castellanos A, Lazzara R: Electrocardiographic antecedents of primary ventricular fibrillation: value of the R-on-T phenomenon in myocardial infarction. Br Heart J 38:415, 1976.

44. Lie KI, Wellens HJJ, Durrer D: Characteristics and predictability of primary ventricular fibrillation. Eur J Cardiol 1:379, 1974.

45. Lie KI, Wellens HJJ, Van Capelle FJ, Durrer D: Lidocaine in the prevention of primary ventricular fibrillation: a double blind, randomized study of 212 consecutive patients. N Engl J Med 291:1324, 1974.

46. Campbell RWF, Murray A, Julian DG: Ventricular arrhythmias in first 12 hours of acute myocardial infarction: natural history study. Br Heart J 46:351, 1981.

47. Lie KI, Liem KL, Durrer D: Early identification of patients developing late in-hospital ventricular fibrillation after discharge from the coronary care unit. Am J Cardiol 41:674, 1978.

48. Campbell RWF, Achuff SC, Pottage A, Murray A, Prescott LF, Julian DG: Mexilitine in the prophylaxis of ventricular arrhythmias during acute myocardial infarction. J Cardiovasc Pharmacol 1:43, 1979.

49. Chopra MP, Thadani U, Portal RW, Aber CP: Lignocaine therapy for ventricular ectopic activity after acute myocardial infarction: a double blind trial. Br Med J 3:668, 1971.

50. Darby S, Bennett MA: Trial of combined intramuscular and intravenous lignocaine in prophylaxis of ventricular tachyarrhythmias. Lancet 1:817, 1972.

51. Wyman MG, Hammersmith L: Comprehensive treatment plan for the prevention of primary ventricular fibrillation in acute myocardial infarction. Am J Cardiol 33:661, 1974.

52. Hooker DR: On the recovery of the heart in electric shock. Am J Physiol 91:305, 1929.

53. Lown B: Electrical reversion of cardiac arrhythmias. Br Heart J 29:469, 1969.

54. Hooker DR, Kouwenhoven WB, Langworthy OR: The effect of alternating electrical currents on the heart. Am J Physiol 103:444, 1933.

55. Prevost JL, Battelli F: La mort par les courants

electriques—courants alternatifs a haute tension. J Physiol Pathol Gen 1:427, 1899.

56. Beck CS, Pritchard WH, Feil HS: Ventricular fibrillation of long duration abolished by electric shock. JAMA 135:985, 1947.

57. Kouwenhoven WB, Jude JR, Knickerbocker GG: Closed-chest cardiac massage. JAMA 173:1064, 1960.

58. Kouwenhoven WB, Jude JR, Knickerbocker GG, Chestnut WR: Closed chest defibrillation of the heart. Surgery 42:550, 1957.

59. Zoll PM, Linenthal AJ: Termination of refractory tachycardia by external countershock. Circulation 25:596, 1962.

60. Zoll PM, Linenthal AJ, Gibson W, Paul MH, Norman LR: Termination of ventricular fibrillation in man by externally applied countershock. N Engl J Med 254:727, 1956.

61. Guvich NL, Yuniev GS: Restoration of the heart rhythm during fibrillation by condenser discharge. Am Rev Soviet Med 4:252, 1947.

62. Guyton AC, Satterfield J: Factors concerned in electrical defibrillation of the heart, particularly through the unopened chest. Am J Physiol 167:81, 1951.

63. Kouwenhoven WB, Milnor WR: Treatment of ventricular fibrillation using a capacitor discharge. J Appl Physiol 7:253, 1954.

64. Nachlas MM, Bix HH, Mower MM, Siedband MP: Observations on defibrillators, defibrillation, and synchronized countershock. Prog Cardiovasc Dis 9:64, 1966.

65. Alexander S, Kleiger R, Lown B: Use of electric countershock in the treatment of ventricular tachycardia. JAMA 177:916, 1961.

66. Lown B, Neuman J, Amarasingham R, Berkovits BV: Comparison of alternating current with direct current electroshock across the closed chest. Am J Cardiol 10:223, 1962.

67. Lown B, Amarasingham R, Neuman J: New method for terminating cardiac arrhythmias: use of synchronized capacitor discharge. JAMA 182:548, 1962.

68. Pansegrau DG, Abboud FM: Hemodynamic effects of ventricular fibrillation. J Clin Invest 49:282, 1970.

69. Tacker WA Jr, Van Vleet JF, Geddes LA: Electrocardiographic and serum enzymic alterations associated with cardiac alterations induced in dogs by single transthoracic damped sinusoidal defibrillator shocks by varying strengths. Am Heart J 98:185, 1979.

70. Dahl CF, Ewy GA, Warner EP: Myocardial necrosis from direct current countershock: effect of paddle electrode size and time interval between discharges. Circulation 50:956, 1974.

71. Davis JS, Lie JT, Bentick DC, Titus JL, Tacker WA Jr, Geddes LA: Cardiac damage due to electric current and energy: light microscopic and ultrastructural observations of acute and delayed myocardial cellular injuries. In: Proceedings, Purdue cardiac defibrillation conference. Purdue University Engineering Experiment Station document no. 00147, 1975, p 27.

72. Warner ED, Dahl C, Ewy GA: Myocardial injury from transthoracic defibrillator countershock. Arch Pathol Lab Med 99:55, 1975.

73. Schuder JC, Rahmoeller GA, Stoeckle H: Transthoracic ventricular defibrillation with triangular and trapezoidal waveforms. Circ Res 19:689, 1966.

74. Balagot RC, Druz WS, Ramadan M, Lopez-Belio M, Jobgen E, Tomita M, Sadove M: A monophasic DC current defibrillator for ventricular defibrillation. J Thorac Cardiovasc Surg 47:487, 1964.

75. Detmer RA, Raush J, Fletcher E, Gordon AS: Ideal waveform and characteristics for direct current defibrillators. Surg Forum 15:249, 1964.

76. Mackay RS, Leeds SE: Effects of condenser discharges with application to tissue stimulation and ventricular defibrillation. J Appl Physiol 6:67, 1953.

77. Wessale JL, Bourland JD, Tacker WA, Geddes LA: Bipolar catheter defibrillation in dogs using trapezoidal waveforms of various tilts. J Electrocardiol 13:359, 1980.

78. Cohen LS: Early and late prognosis of myocardial infarction. In: Brest AN, Wiener L, Chung EK, Kasparian H (eds) Innovations in the diagnosis and management of acute myocardial infarction. Philadelphia: FA Davis, 1975, p 57.

79. Norris RM, Brandt PWT, Caughey DE, Lee AJ, Scott PJ: New coronary prognostic index. Lancet 1:274, 1969.

80. Mirowski M, Mower MM, Gott VL, Brawley RK: Feasibility and effectiveness of low energy catheter defibrillation in man. Circulation 47:79, 1973.

81. Zipes DP, Jackman WM, Heger JJ, Chilson DA, Browne KF, Naccarelli GV, Rahilly GT, Prystowski EN: Clinical transvenous cardioversion of recurrent life-threatening ventricular tachyarrhythmias: low energy synchronized cardioversion of ventricular tachycardia and termination of ventricular fibrillation using a catheter electrode. Am Heart J 103:789, 1982.

82. Jackman WM, Zipes DP: Low-energy synchro-

nous cardioversion of ventricular tachycardia using a catheter electrode in a canine model of subacute myocardial infarction. Circulation 66:187, 1982.

83. Yee R, Zipes DP, Gulamhusein S, Kallok MJ, Klein GJ: Countershock using an intravascular catheter in an acute care setting. Am J Cardiol (in press).

84. Josephson ME, Kastor JA, Horowitz LN: Electrophysiologic management of recurrent ventricular tachycardia in acute and chronic ischemic disease. In: Castellanos A (ed) Cardiac arrhythmias: mechanisms and management. Philadelphia: FA Davis, 1980, p. 35.

85. Josephson ME, Seides SF: Clinical cardiac electrophysiology. Philadelphia: Lea and Febiger, 1979, p 281.

86. Wellens HJJ, Bar FW, Gorgals AP, Muncharaz JF: Electrical management of arrhythmias with emphasis on the tachycardias. Am J Cardiol 41: 1025, 1978.

87. Kerr C, Gallagher JJ, Smith WM, Sterba R, German LD, Cook L, Kasell JH: The induction of atrial flutter and fibrillation and the termina-

tion of atrial flutter by esophageal pacing. Pace 6:60, 1983.

88. Haft JI: Treatment of arrhythmias by intracardiac electrical stimulation. Prog Cardiovasc Dis 16:539, 1974.

89. Sowton E, Leatham A, Carson P: The suppression of arrhythmias by artificial pacemaking. Lancet 2:1098, 1964.

90. Heiman DF, Helwig J: Suppression of ventricular arrhythmias by transvenous intracardiac pacing. JAMA 195:1150, 1966.

91. Moss AJ, Rivers RJ, Griffith LSC, et al: Transvenous left atrial pacing for the control of recurrent ventricular fibrillation. N Engl J Med 278: 928, 1968.

92. Sowton E: Overdrive pacing in tachycardias of AMI. In: Sandoe E, Flensted-Jensen E, Olesen KH, Astra AB (eds) Cardiac arrhythmias. Sodertalje, 1970, p 727.

93. Fisher JD, Matos JA, Kim SG: The sparkling joules of internal cardiac stimulation: cardioversion, defibrillation and ablation. Am Heart J 104:177, 1982.

V. CORONARY CARE: THE PREHOSPITAL PHASE

27. THE TIERED RESPONSE MOBILE INTENSIVE CARE SYSTEM IN THE MANAGMENT OF OUT-OF-HOSPITAL CARDIAC ARREST

Mickey S. Eisenberg

Lawrence Bergner

Alfred P. Hallstrom

The tiered response mobile intensive care system has been very successful in the management of out-of-hospital cardiac arrest. Communities utilizing such a system have reported high resuscitation rates, with as many as 60% of patients with cardiac arrest due to ventricular fibrillation being admitted to hospital [1]. This group of patients had a hospital discharge rate of 30%. This chapter discusses the development of tiered response systems and the factors accounting for successful resuscitation.

History

The ability to definitively treat out-of-hospital cardiac arrest was first described by Pantridge and Geddes in 1967 [2] (see chapter 25). This study described a mobile intensive care unit in

Research reported in this chapter was supported in part by grants (HS 02456 and HS 04000) from the National Center for Health Services Research. We are indebted to Linda Becker and Paul Litwin for help in data analysis, to Sheri Schaeffer for help in data collection, to Judy Prentice for assistance in preparation of the manuscript, and to Judith Pierce for making administrative arrangements for the study. We appreciate the cooperation of the King County paramedics and emergency medical technicians.

Belfast, Northern Ireland, that was designed to prevent death due to cardiac arrest. The basic premise of the program was for the mobile unit to reach an individual who had symptoms of myocardial infarction and have expert medical help in attendance so that, if a fatal arrhythmia should occur, appropriate treatment would be available. The system was initiated in response to recognized long delays from onset of symptoms to admission to a hospital. In their first report, the authors documented ten successful resuscitations; all ten patients were in ventricular fibrillation. Half of these patients were considered to be long-term "saves" [2]. In the United States the first mobile intensive care unit was activated in New York City [3]. The mobile unit was staffed by physicians and nurses and went beyond the Belfast unit by providing antiarrhythmic drugs so that major arrhythmias could be prophylactically treated.

The units in New York and Belfast were designed solely in response to acute coronary problems and were staffed with physicians or nurses. The concept of a mobile intensive care unit was expanded in 1970 in Miami with the creation of a more general, all-purpose mobile intensive care unit (MICU) [4]. In Miami, the MICU program was administered by the fire department and the unit staffed with highly trained paramedics. The vehicle utilized a telemetry system that could transmit a patient's electrocardiogram to a base hospital for interpretation by physicians [5]. Approximately the same time as the Miami program began, similar paramedic programs began in Columbus [6], Seattle [7], and Los Angeles [8]. Despite different training for the paramedics (from 400 to 1500 h) and different administrative arrangements, common denominator to all the programs was the ability of highly trained paramedic personnel (or in some instances, doctors or nurses [9]) to treat out-of-hospital emergencies. While training encompassed all types of emergencies, medical as well as trauma, the major emphasis was placed on the treatment of myocardial infarction and, specifically, cardiac arrest. To date, over 300 paramedic programs in the United States have been established [10].

Preceding the establishment of paramedic programs was the development of Emergency Medical Technicians (EMTs). The training of emergency medical technicians was stimulated by a concerted effort to prepare personnel and equip ambulances with appropriate equipment for dealing with trauma. The National Highway Safety Act (1966) authorized the Department of Transportation to set guidelines for emergency medical services and provided funds for the purchase of ambulances and equipment in support of emergency medical technician training programs [11]. The Department of Transportation established an 81 h course in conjunction with the National Academy of Sciences and the American Academy of Orthopedics to train ambulance and emergency personnel in basic life-support techniques. The course was designed to teach emergency care fundamentals such as maintenance of airway, control of external hemorrhage, administration of cardiopulmonary resuscitation (CPR), and immobilization of the patient with multiple injuries prior to transport to a hospital. A graduate of this training is designated an Emergency Medical Technician. It is estimated that 150,000 individuals have received emergency medical technician training.

The motive to combine EMT and paramedic services in a tiered response system (also known as a layered response system) came from the aware-ness that paramedics often arrived at the scene too late to resuscitate cardiac arrest patients. Paramedic units are significantly more expensive than EMT units and could not feasibly be substituted for all EMT units (see chapter 29). In addition to the cost of training and supporting paramedics, it is believed that there are too few calls that require the additional capabilities of paramedics and that their skills would depreciate in the absence of sufficient use.

Seattle and King County Tiered Response System

The opportunity to utilize the EMT and paramedics together created an efficient utilization of personnel. The tiered response emergency system in Seattle, WA, will serve as an example [7]. The emergency care system, operated by the Seattle Fire Department, and known locally as Medic I, provides coordinated EMT and paramedic response to a medical emergency. Simultaneous dispatching of an EMT aid unit and paramedic vehicle in apparent cardiac arrest cases assures the most rapid provision of basic and advanced medical care. Furthermore, an engine company with qualified EMTs on board may also be dispatched if it is closer to the scene of a possible cardiac arrest. Hence, it is not uncommon for a local engine company as well as an EMT aid unit, plus a paramedic vehicle, all to be dispatched to the scene, in effect, creating a triple-layered response system. To achieve the earliest possible initiation of CPR, the city of Seattle also embarked upon a massive training of citizens in CPR, known within the city as the Medic II program, and has, to date, trained over 25% of the population in cardiopulmonary resuscitation [12]. If the citizen who may have already started CPR is included, there exists a quadruple response system for the management of out-of-hospital cardiac arrest.

The tiered response system is a cost-efficient attempt to provide medical help rapidly. It is prohibitively expensive to train and staff sufficient numbers of paramedics so that they arrive at the scene within 4 min. Far more cost effective is to have already available fire department personnel providing the initial response followed by strategically located paramedic units that can arrive several minutes later. Thus, the first tier of EMTs extends the time in which the second tier of paramedics must arrive and still be effective. An important ingredient in utilization of a tiered response is a simultaneous dispatch of EMT and paramedic vehicles. In the city of Seattle, there are approximately nine aid units and 15 engine companies that provide basic EMT response and there are five paramedic vehicles. The average response time for the first arriving vehicle is 3 min and for the paramedic unit is 7 min.

The suburban areas around Seattle utilize a tiered response system patterned after the Medic I program. There are 45 EMT aid units scattered throughout 38 fire departments. Average response time for the EMT units is 4 min. In addition, there are eight paramedic vehicles with an average response time of 10 min. Hence, in a majority of situations, even when assuming that a citizen does not start CPR, a fire department vehicle staffed with EMT personnel arrives at the scene within 4 min and a mobile intensive care unit staffed with paramedic personnel arrives at the scene within 10 min.

We have had the opportunity to study the factors determining successful resuscitation from out-of-hospital cardiac arrest in the suburban area (population 600,000, 460 sq. miles) adjacent to Seattle in King County, WA. In a four-year evaluation study of paramedic services, sudden cardiac arrest was defined as "an unexpected non-traumatic death receiving out-of-hospital emergency care." The etiology was determined for each case of cardiac arrest. Approximately 80% of cases had underlying heart disease as the cause of cardiac arrest. The following discussion is based on the 1035 cardiac arrest cases owing to underlying heart disease [13].

Factors Accounting for Successful Resuscitation

Many factors determine whether an individual will live or die following out-of-hospital cardiac arrest. These factors can be conveniently grouped into fate factors and program factors. Fate factors are unpredictable circumstances surrounding the event or associated with the patient. Fate factors include the patient's age, sex, prior medical condition, rhythm at time of arrest, and whether the arrest was witnessed. The sex of the patient was

not predictive of survival, but age was related to outcome. Average age of patient discharged from the hospital was 61 years and those not discharged was 66 years ($p < 0.01$). Whether the collapse was directly witnessed or unwitnessed was also strongly predictive of survival. If the collapse was witnessed, 22% were discharged alive and with unwitnessed cardiac arrest, 4% were discharged ($p < 0.01$). For every cardiac arrest, the rhythm was determined immediately upon arrival of the paramedic vehicle. The average time from collapse to determination of rhythm was generally 10 min or less. As seen in figure 27-1, patients with ventricular fibrillation or ventricular tachycardia have a much higher likelihood of being resuscitated and discharged alive than those in other rhythms. Ventricular tachycardia represents a very small percentage of the cases (less than 2%).

Program factors, as opposed to fate factors, are determined to some degree by the system itself. The program factors associated with survival include factors that can be influenced by the design and operating characteristics of the emergency medical system. By examining some of the important system factors, it becomes apparent why tiered response emergency medical service system can be more effective than other configured emergency systems. Based upon our experience in King County, WA, the following program factors influence survival from cardiac arrest.

1. Type of emergency care available (EMT or EMT and paramedic)
2. Bystander initiation of CPR
3. Length from collapse to initiation of CPR
4. Length from time of patient collapse to provision of definitive care

The first factor, the type of service, was specifically studied in our service area. When the study began, portions of the study area had a single-tiered emergency system consisting of basic EMT services. Other portions of the study area had a tiered response system consisting of EMT and paramedic services. Comparing the outcomes of these two areas showed a dramatically greater survival for patients treated with EMT and paramedic services. Of all patients treated by EMTs, 6% were discharged alive from the hospital compared with 20% treated by EMTs and paramedics in a tiered response system (figure 27-2). These findings were confirmed in a before-and-after comparison as the tiered response was introduced elsewhere in the community.

Outcomes were also analyzed by whether bystander initiation of CPR occurred. Of patients receiving CPR initiated by bystanders, 25% were discharged compared with 10% of patients who did not receive bystander CPR (figure 27-3). The time from collapse to initiation of CPR is also strongly predictive of survival. If CPR was initiated within 4 min of collapse, 38% were discharged. If CPR was initiated more than 4 min after collapse, 13% were discharged (figure 27-4).

There was a striking association in outcome between the time from collapse to definitive care. As seen in figure 27-5, there is a linear relationship between the outcome and the time from collapse to definitive care. If the time was less than 6 min, 36% of patients were discharged. If time to definitive care was greater than 14 min, however, only 9% of patients were discharged.

The latter two factors, time from collapse to CPR and time from collapse to definitive care, are interactively predictive of survival. As seen in table 27-1, if both times are short, a very high discharge percentage occurs. If time to CPR exceeds 4 min and time to definitive care exceeds 8 min, only 10% of cardiac arrest patients survive.

Success of Tiered Response Systems

The two factors most predictive of survival—time from collapse to CPR and time from collapse to definitive care—suggest the reason that tiered response emergency medical systems are effective. The fact that an EMT vehicle can arrive at the scene rapidly and start CPR within 4 min of collapse allows the first component necessary for successful resuscitation to occur. The fact that the second tier of paramedics arrives in approximately 8–10 min allows the second important aspect of resuscitation, rapid provision of definitive care, to occur. The combination of these two factors, rapid onset of CPR and rapid provision of definitive care, is the essence of a successful emergency care system.

It should be apparent that a tiered response system is not the only option for achieving suc-

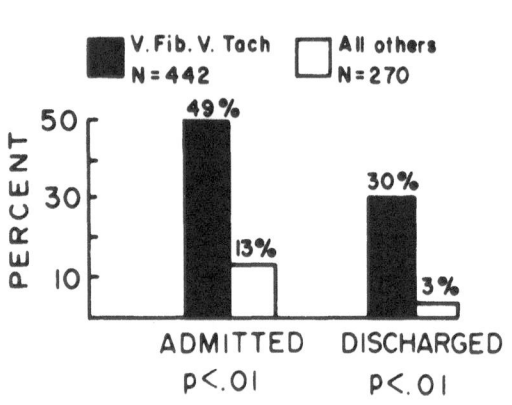

FIGURE 27-1. Rhythm causing cardiac arrest and outcome for patients with cardiac arrest due to heart disease.

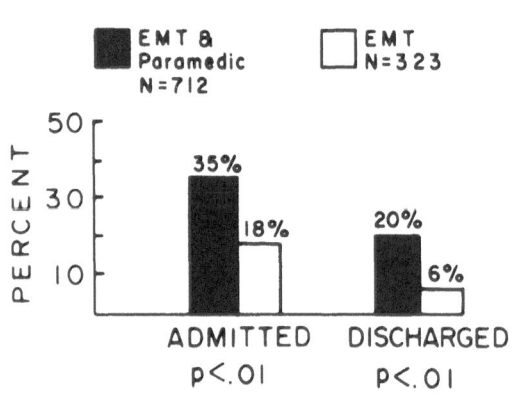

FIGURE 27-2. Type of service and outcome of cardiac arrests due to heart disease.

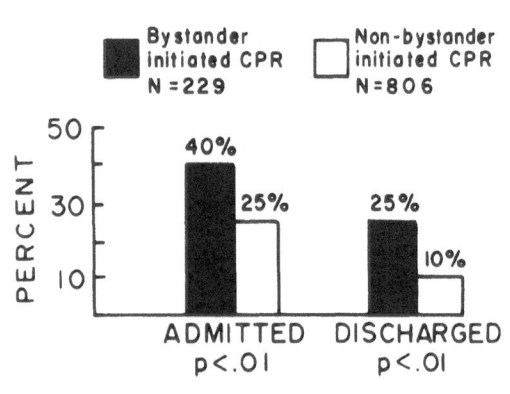

FIGURE 27-3. Bystander-initiated CPR and outcome for patients with cardiac arrest due to heart disease.

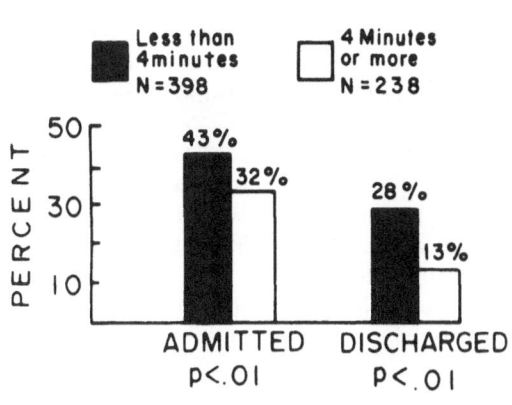

FIGURE 27-4. Time to initiation of CPR and outcome for cardiac arrests due to heart disease.

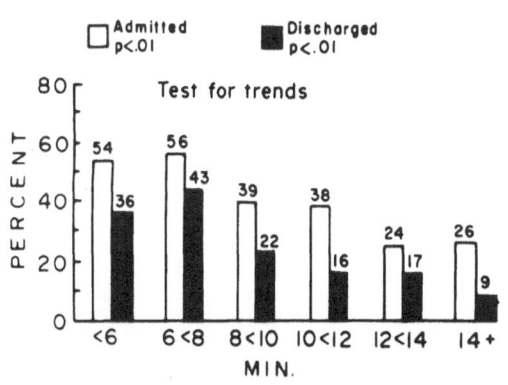

FIGURE 27-5. Time from collapse to definitive care and outcome of cardiac arrest due to heart disease.

TABLE 27-1. Percentage of patients discharged following cardiac arrest in relation to time to definitive care and time to initiation of CPR ($n = 645$)

		<8	≥8
Time to initiation of CPR (min)	< 4	$\dfrac{80}{198} = 40\%$	$\dfrac{35}{208} = 17\%$
	≥ 4	$\dfrac{12}{44} = 27\%$	$\dfrac{19}{195} = 10\%$

Time to definitive care (min)

cessful management of patients with out-of-hospital cardiac arrest. If there were sufficient paramedic resources such that they could arrive at the scene in 4 min and provide both CPR and definitive care within that time, then, of course, such a single-layer paramedic system would do as well if not better than a tiered response system. A variation on a single-tier paramedic system is a single-tier system utilizing EMTs trained to defibrillate. Such a system has been shown to be very effective [15]. Furthermore, it is reasonable to speculate that, if a community were completely trained in CPR and could start effective CPR at the time of collapse, there could perhaps not be a need for an EMT level response. If effective CPR were started immediately after collapse, followed by arrival of paramedics within 8–10 min, one could speculate that this could be as effective as a tiered response system.

In summary, the success of the tiered response system lies in its ability to deliver both CPR and definitive care rapidly through the appropriate utilization of personnel and equipment. Variations on this theme are likely to be effective as long as these two aspects can be achieved. A tiered response system is not magical, but it is effective and efficient.

References

1. Eisenberg M, Bergner L, Hearne T: Out-of-hospital cardiac arrest: a review of major studies and a proposed uniform report system. Am J Public Health 70:236–240, 1980.
2. Pantridge JF, Geddes JS: A mobile intensive care unit in the management of myocardial infarction. Lancet 2:271–273, 1967.
3. Grace WJ, Chadbourn JA: The mobile coronary care unit. Dis Chest 55:454–455, 1969.
4. Liberthson RR, Nagel EL, Hirschman JC, et al: Prehospital ventricular fibrillation: prognosis and followup course. N Engl J Med 291:317–320, 1974.
5. Nagel EL, Hirschman JC, Nussenfeld SR, et al: Telemetry–medical command in coronary and other mobile emergency care systems. JAMA 214:332–334, 1970.
6. Lewis RP, Stang JM, Fulkerson PK, et al: Effectiveness of advanced paramedics in a mobile coronary care system. JAMA 241:1902–1904, 1979.

7. Cobb LA, Baum RS, Copass MK: A rapid response system for out-of-hospital cardiac emergencies. Med Clin North Am 60:283−289, 1976.

8. Graf WS, Plin SS, Paegel BL: A community program for emergency cardiac care. JAMA 226:156−160, 1973.

9. Crampton RS, Aldrich RF, Gascho JA, et al: Reduction of pre-hospital, ambulance and community coronary death rates by the community wide emergency cardiac care system. Am J Med 58:151−155, 1975.

10. Romano TL, Eisenberg S, Frenandez-Caballero C, et al: Paramedic services: nationwide distribution and management structure. JACEP 7:99−102, 1978.

11. National Academy of Sciences, National Research Council, Division of Medical Sciences, Report: Accidental death and disability: the neglected disease of modern society. Washington DC, 1966.

12. Alvarez H, Cobb LA: Experiences with CPR training of the general public: proceedings of the national conference on standards for CPR and emergency cardiac care. American Heart Association, 1975.

13. Bergner L, Eisenberg M, Hallstrom A, et al: Evaluation of paramedic services for cardiac arrest. Hyattsville MD: National Center for Health Services Research (DHHS publication [PHS] 82-3310), 1981.

14. Eisenberg MS, Bergner L, Hallstrom A: Out-of-hospital cardiac arrest: improved survival with paramedic services. Lancet 1:812−815, 1981.

15. Eisenberg M, Copass M, Hallstrom A: Treatment of out-of-hospital cardiac arrest with rapid defibrillation by emergency medical technicians. N Engl J Med 302:1379−1383, 1980.

28. THE FIRST HOUR OF ACUTE MYOCARDIAL INFARCTION OBSERVED DURING MOBILE INTENSIVE CARE

A.A.J. Adgey

S.W. Webb

Between September 1970 and February 1973, we studied 294 patients with acute myocardial infarction (MI) who were seen and managed within 1 h of the onset of symptoms. The 294 patients were alive when first seen or were successfully resuscitated. In 111 (38%) of the 294 patients the interval between the onset of symptoms and initial observation was not greater than 30 min.

Of the patients, 257 (87%) were men and 37 (13%) were women. The ages of the men ranged from 24 to 80 (mean 56) and that of the women from 41 to 76 (mean 61).

The sites MI were anterior (138), diaphragmatic or posterior (147), combined anterior and diaphragmatic (2), and unknown because of left bundle branch block (7). Of the patients, 117 (40%) had had at least one previous documented myocardial infarction.

Of the 294 patients, 207 (70.5%) were observed outside of hospital by members of the mobile coronary care unit operating from the Royal Victoria Hospital, Belfast (table 28-1). The remaining 87 (29.5%) were first seen in the Royal Victoria Hospital, either because they developed the MI while in hospital (62) or because they reached the accident and emergency department within 1 h (25). All 25 patients who reached the accident and emergency department within 1 h did so without consulting their family doctor. The mobile coronary care unit was requested by a doctor for 111 patients (37.5%).

The doctor requested the mobile unit before seeing the patient in 35 (32%) of the 111 cases because the information he had received indicated the probability of myocardial infarction. A total of 82 patients (28%) were seen within 1 h by the mobile team after a call from a member of the public. The staff of an industrial medical center alerted the mobile unit for 14 patients (5%).

None of the 111 patients seen within 30 min had been given an analgesic prior to the initial observations; 33 (18%) of the 183 patients seen within the second half of the first hour had had an analgesic prior to the arrival of the mobile unit. Three patients were on beta-adrenoceptor-blocking drugs prior to the onset of the coronary attack and two were taking digitalis. Seven patients had a history of hypertension. Among the 271 patients who were not in ventricular fibrillation on arrival of the team, 17 (6%) had severe left ventricular failure or cardiogenic shock when first seen.

Five patients (2%) died outside hospital and the remaining 289 were admitted to the coronary care unit of the Royal Victoria Hospital, Belfast.

Incidence of Dysrhythmias

BRADYARRHYTHMIAS
Among the 248 patients in whom assessment was possible, 84 (34%) had a slow heart rate when

R.M. Califf and G.S. Wagner (eds.), ACUTE CORONARY CARE: Principles and Practice. Copyright © 1985. Martinus Nijhoff Publishing, Boston/Dordrecht/Lancaster.

TABLE 28-1. Site of initiation of coronary care in 294 patients seen within 1 h

Site	Source of referral	No. of patients	Total
Outside hospital	Doctor (usually family doctor)	111 (37.5%)	
	Lay person	82 (28%)	
	Industrial medical personnel	14 (5%)	207 (70.5%)
In hospital	Hospital personnel	62 (21%)	
	Self-referral to Accident & Emergency Room	25 (8.5%)	87 (29.5%)
		Total	294 (100%)

first seen. The incidence of bradyarrhythmia could not be assessed in 46 patients, either because of the absence of sinus rhythm (34) or because of therapy prior to the coronary attack (12). Bradyarrhythmia was most frequent among patients with diaphragmatic infarction. Fifteen (6%) had second- or third-degree atrioventricular (AV) block and all but one of these had a diaphragmatic infarction. In all patients with AV block complicating a diaphragmatic infarction within 4 h of the onset of symptoms, it was apparent within the first hour. A similar high incidence of bradyarrhythmia among patients seen within the first hour of acute MI has been recorded in Brighton [1].

TACHYARRHYTHMIAS

Of the 294, 171 (58%) had ventricular ectopics (greater than 5/min, R-on-T, salvos, multifocal) within the first hour of the onset of symptoms. Primary ventricular fibrillation (in the absence of significant left ventricular failure or cardiogenic shock) occurred in 28 (9.5%) of 294 within the first hour. Of the 28, 23 had ventricular fibrillation before the mobile team arrived. The sites of MI in the 23 patients were anterior (11), diaphragmatic (11), and unknown because of left bundle branch block (1). Those who developed ventricular fibrillation after the arrival of the team did so either in the absence of warning arrhythmias (figure 28-1) or with a very short

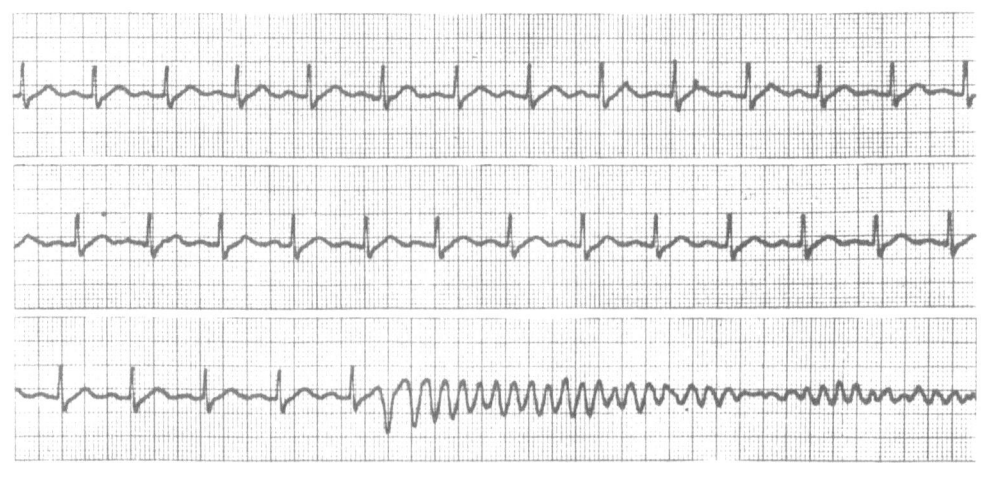

FIGURE 28-1. Development of primary ventricular fibrillation without warning dysrhythmias in a 37-year-old man during the first hour of an acute diaphragmatic infarction (continuous record).

time between the warning arrhythmias and ventricular fibrillation.

Sustained ventricular tachycardia occurred in only six (2%) of the 294 patients within the first hour. Two patients had continuous ventricular tachycardia when first seen (mean ventricular rate 205/min, mean systolic pressure 55 mmHg).

Patients who presented with ventricular fibrillation or ventricular tachycardia and those who were known to have chronic atrial fibrillation before infarction were excluded from the assessment of the incidence of supraventricular dysrhythmias. Among the 266 patients in whom assessment of the incidence was possible, four (1.5%) had a supraventricular dysrhythmia during the first hour. Atrial fibrillation was the most frequent of these occurring during this time period.

Autonomic Disturbance at the Initial Examination (see chapter 12)

Documentation of the autonomic disturbance when the patient was first seen was attempted. This was not possible in patients who presented with ventricular fibrillation, ventricular tachycardia, or supraventricular dysrhythmias and in those who had been on digitalis or beta-blocking agents prior to the onset of MI. Patients with a known history of hypertension and those showing left bundle branch block or combined anterior and posterior infarction were also excluded. Analysis of the incidence of autonomic disturbance was, therefore, confined to 240 of the 294 patients; 89 of the 240 patients were seen within 30 min. There was no significant difference in the age, sex, site of infarction, and number of patients with previous MI between the 89 patients seen within the first 30 min and the 151 patients seen within the second half of the first hour.

There is considerable evidence that acute MI is accompanied by an early rise in blood catecholamines [2]. This response probably results from nervous reflexes arising from the site and boundary of the infarct [3, 4]. Increased adrenaline secretion comes from the adrenal medulla while noradrenaline is probably released from the postganglionic sympathetic nerve endings in the heart [5]. Transient hypertension in the absence

of sinus tachycardia may be regarded as evidence of sympathetic overactivity, since a reflex sympathetic pressor response without alteration in heart rate has been described [6]. Patients with sinus tachycardia (heart rate ≥ 100) with or without transient hypertension (blood pressure $\geq 160/100$ mmHg) were also considered to show sympathetic overactivity.

Patients with sinus bradycardia (heart rate ≤ 60) or AV block (second or third degree) were considered to show parasympathetic overactivity. Transient hypotension (systolic blood pressure ≤ 100 mmHg) in the absence of bradycardia was also regarded as evidence of parasympathetic overactivity.

Of the 89 patients, 44 had anterior MI and 45 diaphragmatic or posterior MI. Sympathetic overactivity was observed in 19 (43%) and parasympathetic overactivity in 13 (30%) of the patients with anterior infarction. Therefore, only 12 (27%) of these patients had both normal heart rate and blood pressure when first seen.

Among the 45 patients with diaphragmatic or posterior MI, 12 (27%) showed sympathetic overactivity and 30 (67%) parasympathetic overactivity at the initial examination. Only three (7%) had both normal heart rate and blood pressure. When the 24 patients with previous infarction were excluded, evidence of parasympathetic overactivity was evident in 20 (95%) of the remaining 21.

The overall incidence of autonomic disturbance among patients with diaphragmatic or posterior MI (93%) was significantly greater than that (73%) among patients with anterior MI. This difference is due to the markedly higher incidence of parasympathetic overactivity in those with diaphragmatic location: 67% vs 30%.

The incidence of autonomic disturbance was significantly lower in the 151 patients seen within the second half of the first hour. Of the 89 patients seen within 30 min, 74 (83%) showed evidence of autonomic disturbance whereas only 85 (56%) of the 151 patients seen within the second half of the first hour showed this disturbance at the initial observation.

Of the 89 patients seen within 30 min, 36 (40%) had bradyarrhythmia at the initial examination whereas only 38 (25%) of those seen between 30 and 60 min had this dysrhythmia. Of the bradycardic patients seen during the first half hour, 47% also had profound hypotension (≤ 80 mmHg systolic), versus an incidence of 21% in the bradycardic patients seen during the second half hour.

The incidence of autonomic disturbance among patients seen within the second half hour showed that, in 27 (38%) of the 71 patients with anterior infarction and in 14 (17%) of the 80 with diaphragmatic infarcts, there was evidence of sympathetic overactivity. Also, 16% of the anterior infarct group and 42% of those with diaphragmatic infarcts had parasympathetic overactivity. Therefore, there were higher incidences of autonomic overactivity during observations of the first half hour (83%) than the second half hour (56%).

SIGNIFICANCE OF PARASYMPATHETIC OVERACTIVITY AND BRADYARRHYTHMIAS

The fundamental properties of the myocardium, namely, rhythmicity, conductivity, and contractility, may be suppressed by vagal overactivity. The important effects of vagal overactivity on the "booster pump" function of the atrium and on ventricular contractility should be noted. The liberation of acetylcholine in the atrial myocardium markedly inhibits atrial contractility even when the atrium is paced at a constant rate. The intrinsic contractility of the atrium is influenced by its contraction rate (the Bowditch effect), i.e., the slower the rate of the atrium, the less forcefully it contracts. The ventricle will contract more forcefully and expel a larger volume if the end-diastolic volume (fiber length) is increased. The stroke volume may fall by more than half when the ventricle is deprived of the atrial contribution as in AV dissociation either due to complete AV block or nodal rhythm. Thus, factors that depress atrial contractility can reduce stroke volume, cardiac output, and coronary perfusion pressure. During vagal hyperactivity, mean left atrial pressure has been shown to be higher for any given level of left ventricular end-diastolic pressure.

The level of the blood pressure accompanying bradycardia may depend on the ability of the damaged myocardium to compensate for the slow heart rate. This study shows that a fall in heart rate immediately after the onset of symptoms of acute myocardial infarction is frequently associated with a profound fall in blood pressure. Presumably the acutely damaged myocardium is unable to compensate for the reduction in heart rate by an increase in stroke volume causing a fall in cardiac output and systemic blood pressure. The vagal effect on the atrial contraction may also serve to diminish ventricular contractility. Also (see chapter 12), reflex parasympathetic activity may cause peripheral vasodilation, as in vasovagal syncope, and thus directly produce a hypotensive state.

The two other major aspects of bradycardia following acute MI are the effect on the ischemic zone surrounding the infarct and the relationship of the bradycardia to ventricular tachycardias.

The significance of bradycardia to the ischemic zone surrounding the infarct will depend on the frequency and magnitude of the accompanying fall in blood pressure. The mean systolic pressure of our patients was less than 70 mmHg. At this systolic pressure, blood flow through the ischemic zone is minimal and flow through the previously nonischemic myocardium is less than adequate. It has been shown that elevation of the arterial pressure increases coronary blood flow more than oxygen consumption. Conversely a fall in arterial blood pressure might be expected to reduce coronary blood flow more than oxygen consumption and thus lead to extension of the area of ischemic injury. Experimental evidence for the adverse effects of hypotension on the ischemic zone surrounding the infarct has been reported. Thus the fall in blood pressure that frequently accompanies early bradycardia may lead to an increase in the initial area of infarction and to an increased incidence of cardiogenic shock and pump failure.

It has been suggested that bradycardia may be a precursor of ventricular fibrillation and an important factor in the high early mortality from acute MI [7]. Malignant ventricular ectopics may appear in association with early bradycardia and hypotension and be abolished by increasing the heart rate and blood pressure. Early bradycardia and hypotension may lead to ventricular fibrillation (figure 28-2).

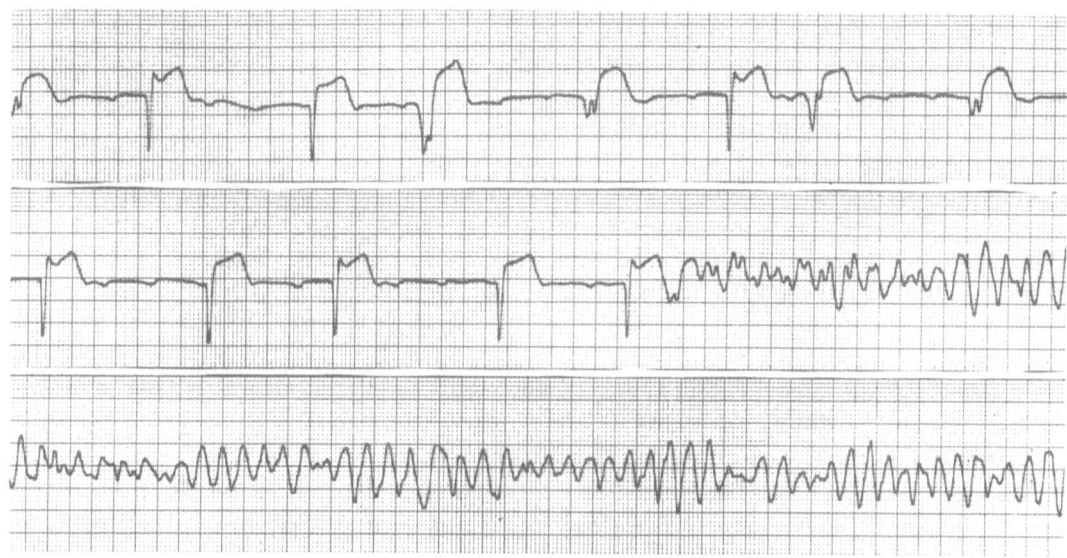

FIGURE 28-2. During the first hour of an acute dia-phragmatic infarction, complete AV block with the sudden development of ventricular fibrillation (continuous tracing).

EXPERIMENTAL EVIDENCE

The evidence regarding the relationship between bradycardia and ventricular dysrhythmias in the experimental situation is conflicting. When the myocardium is ischemic, ventricular ectopics are more frequent at slow heart rates [8]. Scherlag et al. [9] have shown in dogs that a key electrophysiologic feature associating bradycardia and ventricular arrhythmias in acute myocardial infarction is the continuous electrical activity in the ischemic zone. Thus, it may be presumed that the cardiac impulse survives in the ischemic zone beyond the refractory period of the previous beat to reenter the normal zone and induce single or repetitive excitations. Conversely, Epstein et al. [10] found that, when acute anterior myocardial ischemia was produced in the normotensive closed-chest dog, neither minimal spontaneous bradycardia nor moderate and sustained bradycardia from vagal stimulation resulted in an increase in serious ventricular dysrhythmias. Also, Kerzner et al. [11] found that, following experimental coronary occlusion, ventricular fibrillation was not induced by strong vagal stimulation. The application of these conflicting observations to the clinical setting requires considerable caution because there may be many differences between the experimental models and the patient with acute myocardial infarction. Corr et al. [12] have noted that the coronary arterial distribution in cats is more analogous to humans than that of dogs. The differences between the experimental animal and the clinical situations may be due to the simultaneous parasympathetic and sympathetic overactivity occurring in the patients.

SIGNIFICANCE OF SYMPATHETIC OVERACTIVITY AND TACHYARRHYTHMIAS

Tachycardia resulting from sympathetic overactivity may have an adverse effect on the ventricular fibrillation threshold. The magnitude of the infarct is likely to be affected adversely by tachycardia since the oxygen demand is increased in the absence of an increased oxygen supply.

Patient Management during the First Hour

VENTRICULAR FIBRILLATION

In all of the 23 patients with ventricular fibrillation before arrival of the mobile team, immediate DC shock was successful. Ten subsequently died, 9 h to eight days after resuscitation; 13 were long-term survivors, 12 of whom had normal cerebral function. A sharp precordial blow terminated primary ventricular fibrillation in two patients who developed this dysrhythmia after arrival of the mobile unit.

Because of the limitations of prolonged cardiopulmonary resuscitation, it is imperative that ventricular fibrillation is corrected immediately. We have found that 100 or 200 watt seconds stored energy was highly successful in correcting ventricular fibrillation. Since defibrillation with the least energy minimized the risk of myocardial damage, the lowest possible effective energy levels should be used. We suggest that the first (and, if required, the second) shock deliver 200 watt seconds stored energy. If both are unsuccessful, then 400 watt seconds stored energy should be used.

One paddle is placed immediately to the right of the sternum and under the right clavicle and the other on the anterior axillary line in the fifth left intercostal space. The paddles are covered by a saline electrode-jelly to obtain maximum reduction in transthoracic impedance. Both paddles are firmly held on the chest wall. Correction of metabolic acidosis with sodium bicarbonate is necessary. The maintenance of a stable rhythm may require lidocaine infusion. The wide spread availability of small inexpensive defibrillators is to be encouraged (figure 28-3).

CHEST PAIN

Pain may accentuate or, indeed, initiate autonomic disturbance. The majority of the pain fibers from the myocardium are located in the sympathetic system. Few, if any, are found in the vagi (see chapter 12).

Excess autonomic activity may subside when pain is relieved (figure 28-4). The ideal analgesic should have a rapid effect without causing nausea, vomiting, or significant adverse hemodynamic disturbance. Morphine is the drug most commonly employed. Administered intravenously, 10 mg will usually rapidly relieve pain and ease mental distress. Morphine causes venous dilatation, which pools the blood and diminishes return. Thus, it has a salutary effect on pulmo-

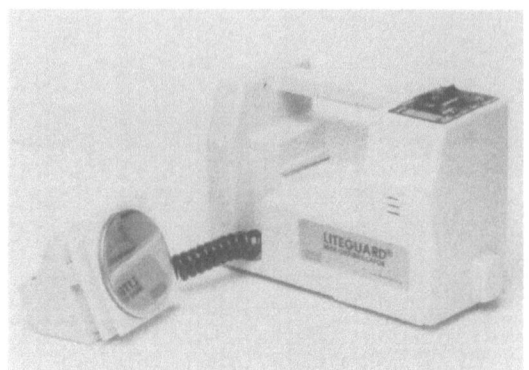

FIGURE 28-3. Small portable DC defibrillator.

nary congestion. While profound hypotension and bradycardia have been noted when the drug has been administered intravenously to the supine patient, this is most likely to occur when the patient is tilted or moved.

Nausea and vomiting are relatively common in patients with acute myocardial infarction. Since vomiting causes adverse circulatory effects, it is important that it be controlled quickly. Cyclizine (Marezine) has been used but this drug has been found to increase the heart rate, which is undesirable in patients with a normal or already increased heart rate. Metoclopramide monohydrochloride (Reglan) is a suitable alternative to cyclizine.

PARASYMPATHETIC OVERACTIVITY

Bradyarrhythmia does not require therapy unless the patient is hypotensive (figures 28-5 to 28-7) or there are associated ventricular dysrhythmias. Of the 240 patients, 35 (15%) were given atropine for bradyarrhythmia with hypotension. In 29 (83%) of the 35, the infarct was diaphragmatic or posterior. In 12 (34%), the bradyarrhythmia was AV block.

The effect of atropine in aliquots of $0.3-0.6$ mg in the 23 patients with sinus bradycardia and hypotension is shown in figure 28-8; 20 (87%) showed a prompt rise in heart rate and blood pressure. The mean heart rate in these patients rose from 53 to 86 beats/min and the mean systolic blood pressure from 82 to 125 mmHg. Patients in whom the blood pressure was unrecordable were assumed to have a systolic blood pressure not greater than 50 mmHg. The dose of

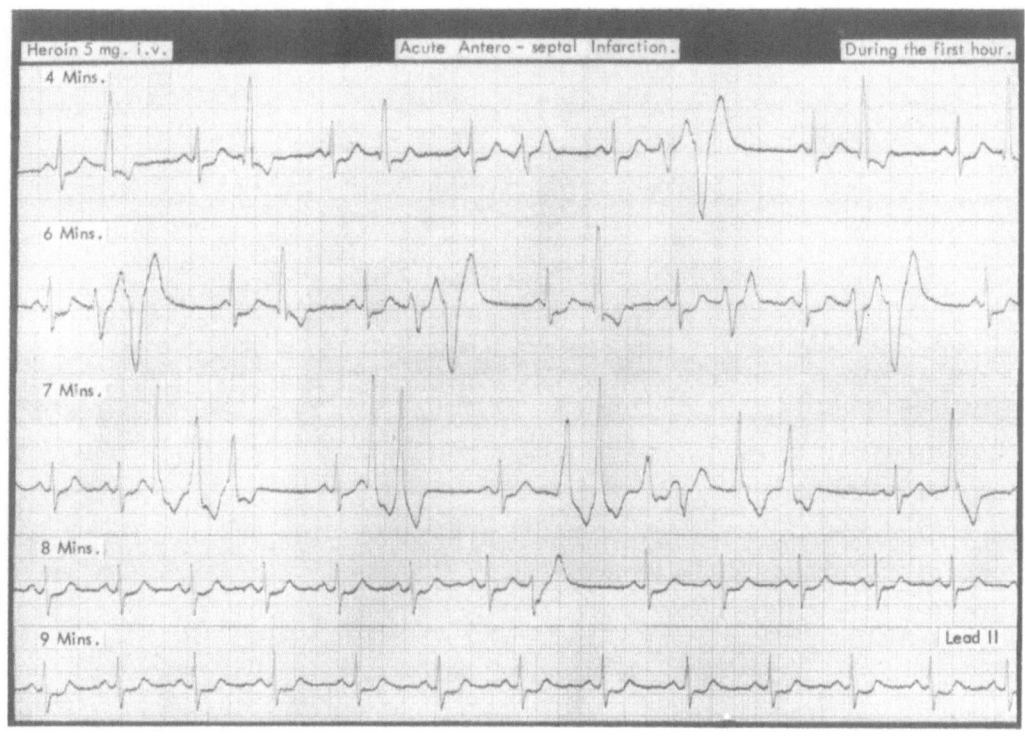

FIGURE 28-4. Record at an estimated 50 min after the onset of acute anterior infarction during severe chest pain. Heart rate 90/min with frequent salvos of ventricular ectopics; blood pressure 170/100 mmHg. At 9 min after the administration of diamorphine 5 mg intravenously, heart rate 80/min with disappearance of ventricular dysrhythmias; blood pressure 160/90 mmHg. No antiarrhythmic therapy was given.

atropine ranged from 0.3 to 1.2 mg (mean 0.7 mg). In four (20%) of the 20 patients, despite careful titration of the dosage, the heart rate after atropine exceeded 100 beats/min. The mean heart rate in these four patients rose from 51 to 111 beats/min and the mean systolic blood pressure from 85 to 143 mmHg. The mean atropine dosage ranged from 0.6 to 1.2 mg (mean 0.8 mg). Of the 20 patients, 19 survived, the one death being due to reinfarction.

If an overshoot in the heart rate (>100/min) occurs with atropine a beta-blocking agent should be administered intravenously, since tachycardia will be associated with a greater myocardial oxygen demand. If the tachycardia is not rapidly corrected by the beta-blocking agent, the increase in heart rate may trigger ventricular ectopics, tachycardia, or even fibrillation. Among the 23 patients with sinus bradycardia and hypotension, three (13%) failed to show a rise in blood pressure in association with the rise in heart rate from 51 to 72 beats/min (figure 28-8). Two of these patients died from cardiogenic shock and one from a ruptured ventricle.

Early complete AV block frequently responds to atropine, but the dosage required is usually greater than that required to correct sinus bradycardia. The effect of atropine in the 12 patients with complete AV block is shown in figure 28-9. Improvement in both AV conduction and blood pressure occurred promptly in eight (67%). The mean ventricular rate in these patients rose from 48 to 89 beats/min and the systolic blood pressure from 73 to 128 mmHg. The dose of atropine ranged from 0.6 to 2.8 mg (mean 1.4 mg). All had a diaphragmatic or posterior MI. Normal AV conduction was established in all eight patients, but complete AV block recurred in one, 16 h

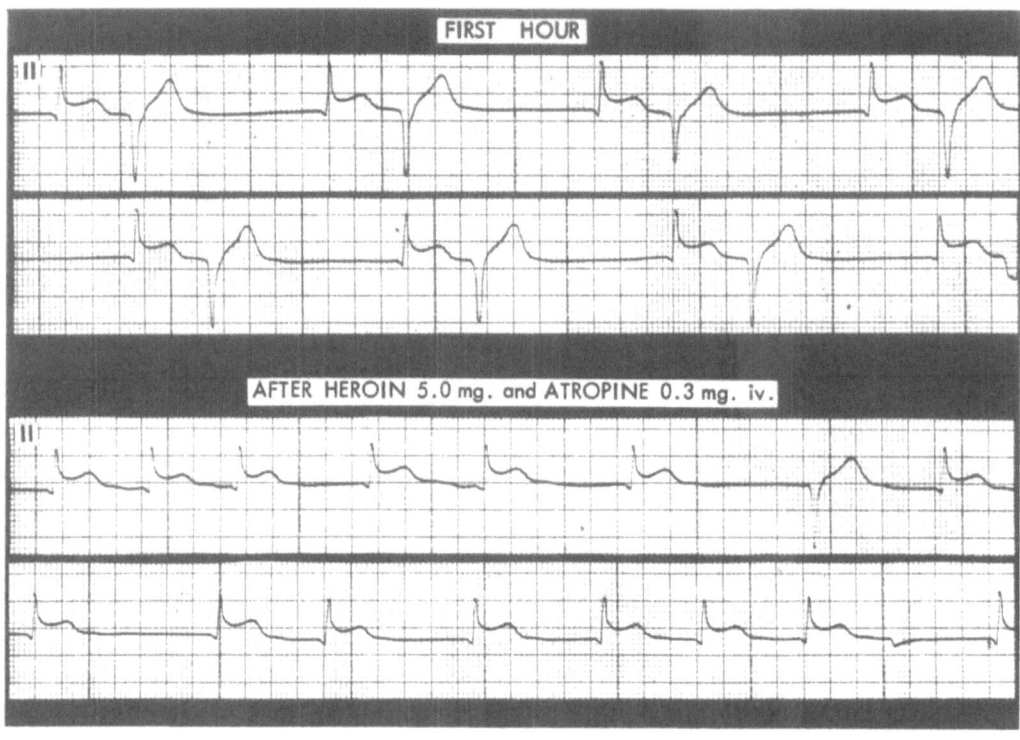

FIGURE 28-5. During first hour of acute diaphragmatic infarction, nodal bradycardia with ventricular bigeminy (BP 70/? mmHg) (lead-II ECG). After diamorphine 5 mg and atropine 0.3 mg intravenously, ventricular rate 60—70/min, probably atrial fibrillation, blood pressure 110/70 mmHg.

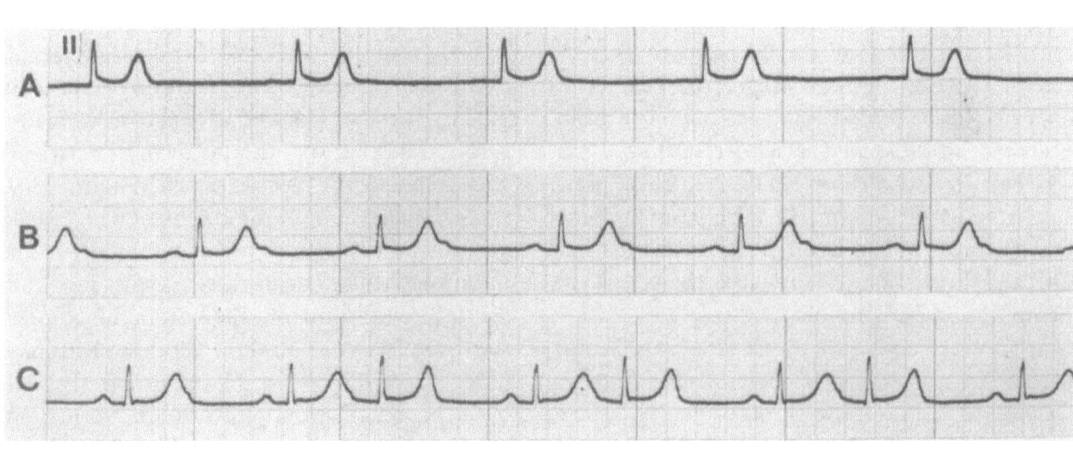

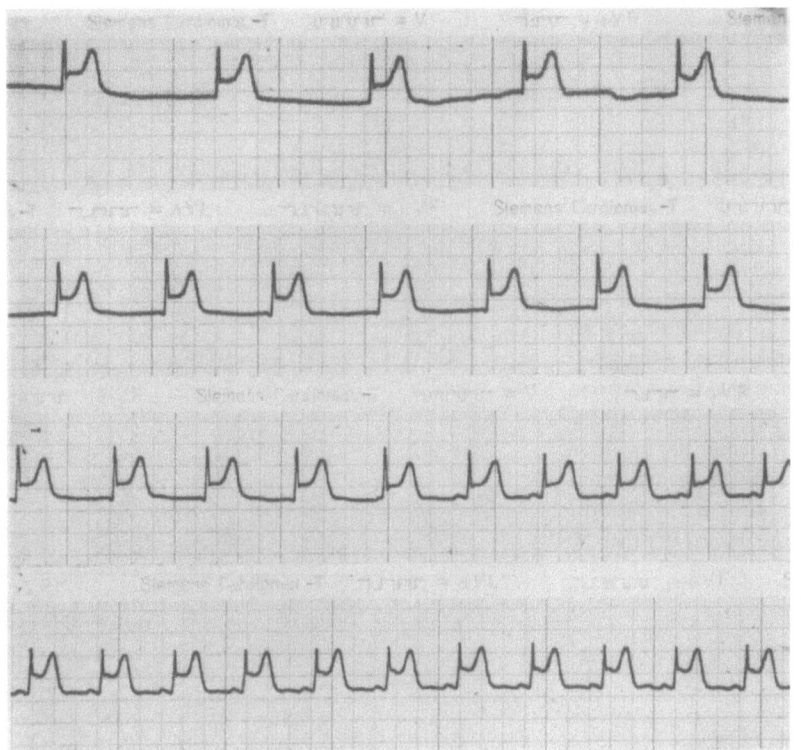

FIGURE 28-7. Effect of atropine on nodal bradycardia. (First tracing) Nodal bradycardia complicating acute diaphragmatic infarction; ventricular rate 42/min, blood pressure 60/? mmHg. (Second tracing) 1 min after atropine 0.6 mg, nodal rhythm, ventricular rate 60/min. (Third tracing) 1½ min after atropine 0.9 mg nodal rhythm, ventricular rate 75/min to sinus rhythm 88/min. (Fourth tracing) 2 min after atropine 1.2 mg, sinus rhythm 88/min, blood pressure 130/80 mmHg.

FIGURE 28-6. Record at an estimated 25 min after the onset of acute diaphragmatic infarction. (A) ?Sinus bradycardia, heart rate 43/min; systolic blood pressure 80 mmHg. (B) 1 min after atropine 0.6 mg intravenously; 2:1 AV block, atrial rate 100/min, ventricular rate 50/min. (C) 1 min after a total of atropine 1.2 mg; second-degree AV block (Wenckebach); blood pressure 140/80 mmHg.

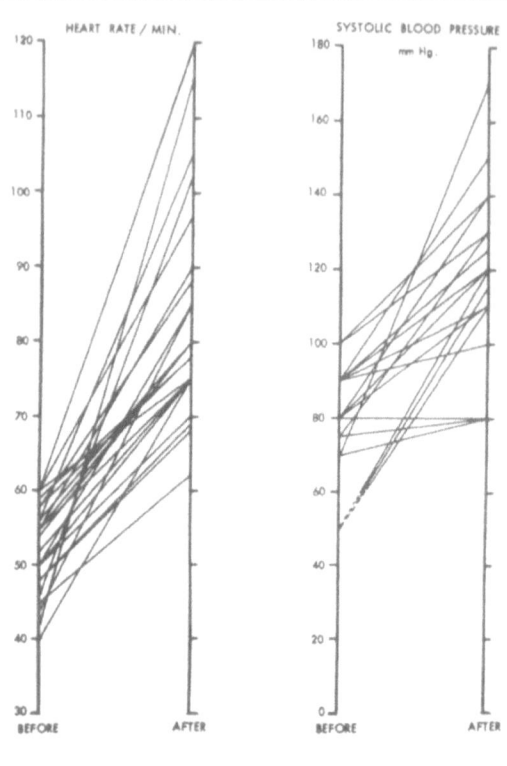

FIGURE 28-8. The effect of the intravenous administration of atropine in 23 patients with sinus bradycardia and hypotension. The systolic blood pressure rose from 80 to 120 mmHg in two patients, 90 to 100 in two patients, 90 to 120 in two patients, 100 to 140 in two patients, and 100 to 130 in two patients. Interrupted lines indicate patients whose blood pressure was unrecordable—assumed to be not greater than 50 mmHg.

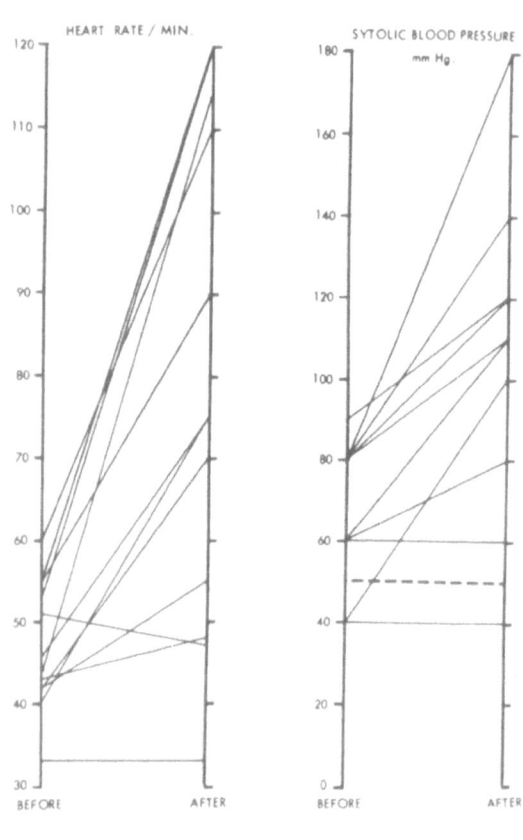

FIGURE 28-9. The effect of atropine in 12 patients with complete AV block accompanied by hypotension. In two patients the systolic blood pressure rose from 80 to 140 mmHg. Interrupted line indicates a patient whose blood pressure was unrecordable—assumed to be not greater than 50 mmHg.

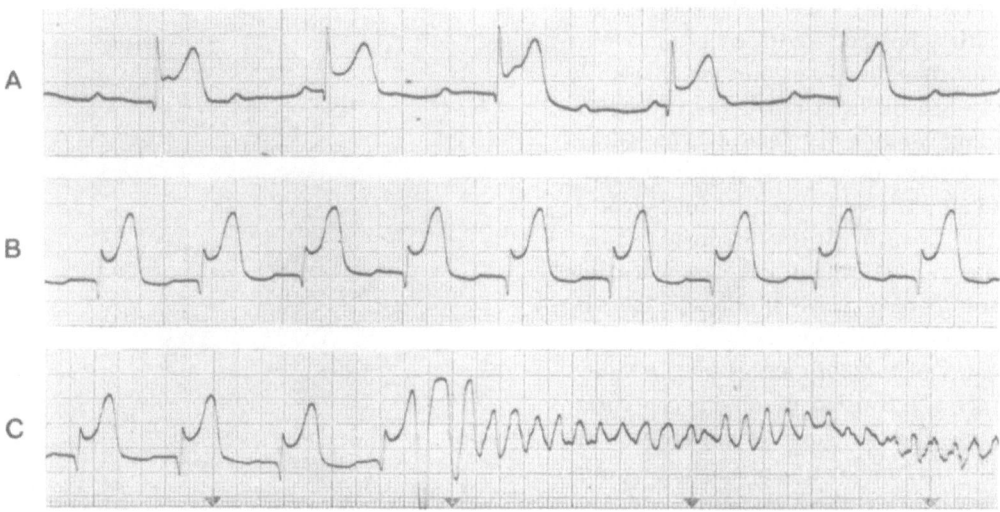

FIGURE 28-10. Record at an estimated 60 min after the onset of acute diaphragmatic infarction (lead 111). (A) Atrial rate 100/min, ventricular rate 42/min; systolic blood pressure 40 mmHg. (B) 2 min after atropine 1.5 mg intravenously; second-degree AV block, atrial rate 140/min, ventricular rate 70/min; systolic blood pressure 100 mmHg. (C) 4 min after atropine 1.5 mg intravenously; development of ventricular fibrillation.

later. The majority of patients with an acute diaphragmatic MI complicated by complete AV block within 1 h of the onset of symptoms and who respond to atropine do not require the insertion of prophylactic transvenous pacemakers. Sinus tachycardia (mean rate 115/min) occurred in three patients when normal AV conduction was established. One patient developed ventricular fibrillation in association with the increase in heart rate and blood pressure following atropine (figure 28-10), possibly due to reperfusion of the infarct. The blood pressure failed to rise in one patient despite the resumption of normal AV conduction, and atropine did not improve the AV conduction in the remaining three patients.

Thus, a rise in both heart rate and blood pressure was observed in 28 (80%) of the 35 patients with bradyarrhythmia and hypotension. Despite careful titration of the atropine dosage, however, a heart rate exceeding 100 beats/min occurred in seven (25%) of the 28.

SYMPATHETIC OVERACTIVITY

In the absence of heart failure, tachycardia due to sympathetic overactivity may be controlled by an appropriate beta-blocking drug, e.g., sotalol or practolol in boluses of 1 mg to a total of 10 mg or until a satisfactory reduction in heart rate has occurred.

The effect of practolol was studied in ten patients who presented with sinus tachycardia and in three in whom sinus tachycardia was unmasked by atropine. Eight of the ten patients who presented with sinus tachycardia were given 10 mg practolol intravenously. In the other two patients and in those in whom sympathetic overactivity was unmasked by atropine, only 5 mg of practolol was used.

Figure 28-11 shows the effect of practolol (10 mg) in eight patients who presented with sinus tachycardia. The mean heart rate was reduced significantly from 114 to 97 beats/min. A significant reduction in the heart rate was apparent within 2 min of giving the drug. There was a significant decrease in the mean systolic blood pressure from 145.5 to 132 mmHg with no alteration in the diastolic pressure.

VENTRICULAR ECTOPICS

Ventricular ectopics in a patient with a heart rate lower than 60 beats/min may be abolished (if clinically indicated) by raising the heart rate. An inappropriate rise in the heart rate may be avoided if atropine is given in aliquots of 0.3 – 0.6 mg intravenously. Ventricular ectopics in a patient with sympathetic overactivity and a heart rate greater than 100 beats/min are frequently abolished when the heart rate is reduced by the careful administration of a beta-blocking agent.

In the presence of a normal heart rate, however, lidocaine is used as the first-line agent in the control of ventricular ectopics in acute myocardial infarction. All the available evidence suggests that high blood levels of lidocaine must be present within the early minutes of MI if suppression of ventricular arrhythmias is to be achieved (see chapter 32). Satisfactory plasma concentrations during the first hour of therapy can be achieved by the combination of a bolus administered intravenously with a high infusion rate for a limited time. In view of the difficulty of maintaining the accuracy of a high infusion rate of lidocaine outside hospital, the usual regimen employed is a bolus of 100 mg intravenously followed by an infusion of 2 mg/min with careful monitoring of the heart rhythm. Frequently, refractory ventricular ectopics require additional boluses and/or an increase in the rate of infusion. Plasma levels greater than 3μg/ml have been recorded during the first hour of therapy following the combined administration of a bolus of lidocaine 100 mg intravenously and lidocaine 300 mg intramuscularly [13] (see chapter 56). The high plasma concentrations of lidocaine obtained were not associated with significant toxic effects.

Mexiletine is used for lidocaine-resistant ventricular ectopics (see chapter 32). This is given as a bolus of 200 mg administered over 3 min followed by infusions of 3 mg/min for 1 h, 1.5 mg/min for 3 h, and 1 mg/min thereafter.

At present we do not recommend prophylactic antiarrhythmic therapy for patients in the acute phase of MI.

VENTRICULAR TACHYCARDIA

Although sustained ventricular tachycardia is relatively uncommon immediately after the onset of acute MI, it is frequently accompanied by profound hypotension. The administration of antiarrhythmic agents in the presence of hypotension and metabolic acidosis may be hazardous.

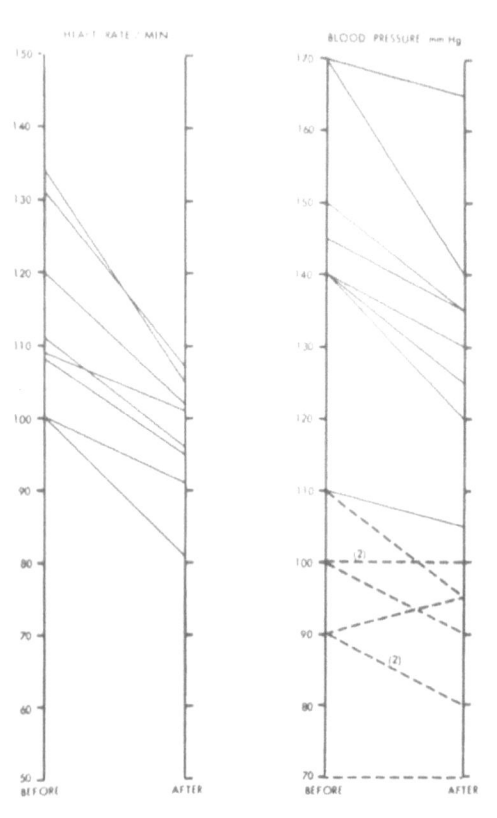

FIGURE 28-11. The effects on heart rate and blood pressure of practolol 10 mg intravenously in eight patients with sympathetic overactivity seen within the first hour. Figures in brackets indicate number of patients. Interrupted lines indicate diastolic blood pressure.

Ventricular tachycardia may be terminated by a sharp precordial blow (figure 28-12), but the majority require DC conversion and correction of the metabolic acidosis. Outside hospital, unsynchronized DC shock is frequently used. If ventricular fibrillation follows an unsynchronized shock, a further DC shock is given.

When ventricular tachycardia is not associated with significant hemodynamic embarrassment, lidocaine or mexiletine in boluses of 100 and 200 mg, respectively, may be successful in its correction.

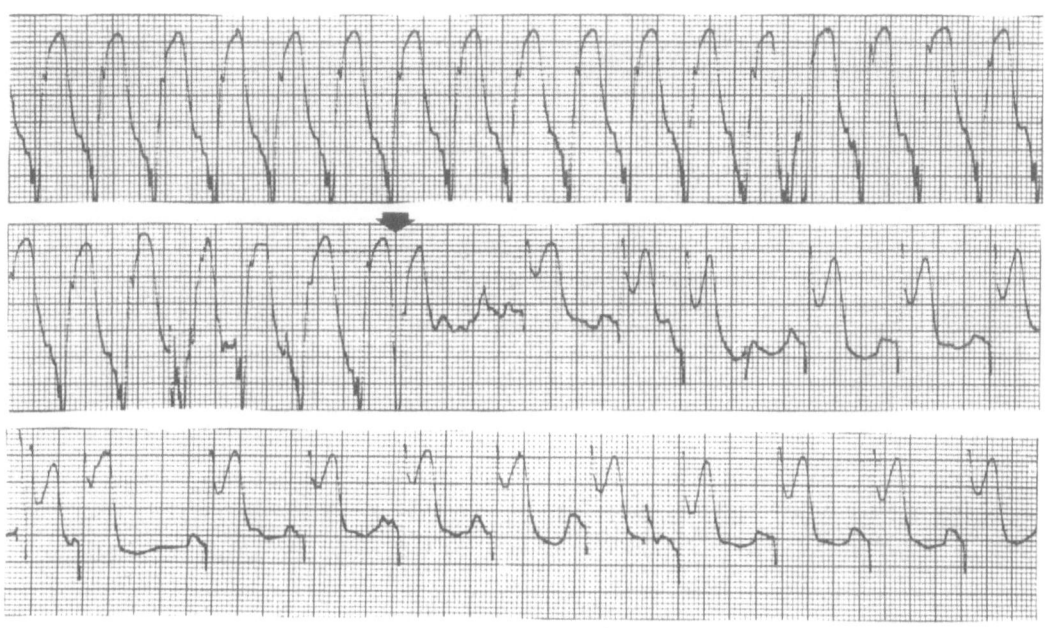

FIGURE 28-12. Ventricular tachycardia corrected by thump-version (arrow indicates chest thump).

SUPRAVENTRICULAR TACHYARRHYTHMIAS

The treatment depends on the hemodynamic situation. If the major problem is control of heart rate in the absence of left heart failure or profound hypotension, then after pain relief a beta-blocking agent may be given as described in (figure 28-13). Careful check on the blood pressure is maintained throughout the administration of the drug. If the heart rate is not reduced to ≤100 beats per minute after a total of 10 mg sotalol or practolol, no further beta-blocking agent should be given. Verapamil, which blocks the transmembrane influx of calcium through the "slow channel" and slows conduction through the AV node, may also terminate supraventricular tachyarrhythmias. It is administered in 1-mg boluses until a total of 5 − 10 mg have been given with careful supervision of the blood pressure. Care must be exerted when verapamil is administered after a beta-blocking agent has not achieved satisfactory control of the heart rate as the combination may precipitate significant and sudden slowing of the heart rate with resultant hypoten-

sion. If supraventricular tachyarrhythmias occur in the presence of left ventricular failure, the heart failure is treated first and, when satisfactorily controlled, there should be consideration of reduction in the heart rate. If the systolic blood pressure is <80 mmHg, with or without evidence of left ventricular failure, then immediate DC conversion should be performed. This is followed by attempted correction of the metabolic acidosis using sodium bicarbonate and the intravenous administration of a beta-blocking agent or digoxin to attempt to maintain sinus rhythm.

Mortality

Of the 294 patients, 278 were aged less than 70. There were seven deaths due to cerebral damage following inadequate resuscitation before arrival of the mobile team. The incidence of cardiogenic shock among the remaining 271 patients was 3.3% and the mortality (including prehospital deaths) prior to hospital discharge was 9.9%.

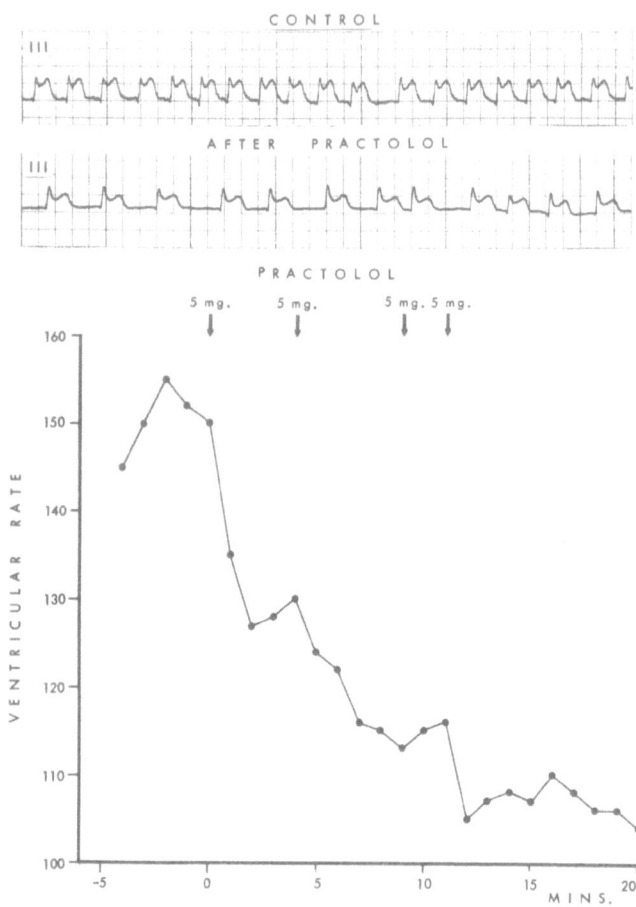

FIGURE 28-13. Effect of practolol 20 mg intravenously in a patient with atrial fibrillation during the first hour. (Control) Heart rate 145 – 155 beats/min; blood pressure 110/70 mmHg: ST-segment elevation 4.0 mm. (After practolol) Heart rate 105 beats/min; blood pressure 105/70 mmHg: ST-segment elevation 2.0 mm.

Conclusions

From this study of patients seen within the first hour of the onset of an acute MI, there is a high incidence of arrhythmias and autonomic disturbance with associated hemodynamic difficulties. The ultimate survival of ischemic tissue depends on the balance between oxygen demand and supply. Thus, complications of MI that increase oxygen demand or that reduce coronary blood flow will decrease oxygen tension in the ischemic area and cause further damage. Appropriate early pharmacologic intervention with relief of pain, stabilization of heart rhythm, and particularly correction of hypotension may limit the area of myocardial damage and thus the development of cardiogenic shock and pump failure. At present there is no simple approach to the correction of the autonomic disturbances and ventricular dysrhythmias seen early after acute MI. Careful titration of the dose of the necessary drugs is required.

References

1. O'Doherty M, Tayler DI, Quinn E, Vincent R, Chamberlain DA: Five hundred patients with myocardial infarction monitored within one hour of symptoms [submitted for publication, 1983].
2. Vetter NJ, Strange RC, Adams W, Oliver MF: Initial metabolic and hormonal response to acute myocardial infarction. Lancet 1:284, 1974.
3. Brown AM: Excitation of afferent cardiac sympathetic nerve fibres during myocardial ischaemia. J Physiol 190:35, 1967.
4. Malliani A, Schwartz PJ, Zanchetti A: A sympathetic reflex elicited by experimental coronary occlusion. Am J Physiol 217:703, 1969.
5. Staszewska-Barczak J: The reflex stimulation of catecholamine secretion during the acute stage of myocardial infarction in the dog. Clin Sci 41:419, 1971.
6. Peterson FD, Brown AM: Pressor reflexes produced by stimulation of afferent fibres in the cardiac sympathetic nerves of the cat. Circ Res 28:605, 1971.
7. Adgey AAJ, Geddes JS, Mulholland HC, Keegan DAJ, Pantridge JF: Incidence, significance and management of early bradyarrhythmia complicating acute myocardial infarction. Lancet 2:1097, 1968.
8. Han J, De Traglia J, Miller D, Moe GK: Incidence of ectopic beats as a function of basic rate in the ventricle. Am Heart J 72:632, 1966.
9. Scherlag BJ, Kabell G, Harrison L, Lazzara R: Mechanisms of bradycardia-induced ventricular arrhythmias in myocardial ischaemia and infarction. Circulation 65: 1429, 1982.
10. Epstein SE, Goldstein RE, Redwood DR, Kent KM, Smith ER: The early phase of acute myocardial infarction: pharmacologic aspects of therapy. Ann Intern Med 78:918, 1973.
11. Kerzner J, Wolf M, Kosowsky BD, Lown B: Ventricular ectopic rhythms following vagal stimulation in dogs with acute myocardial infarction. Circulation 47:44, 1973.
12. Corr PB, Pearle DL, Hinton JR, Roberts WC, Gillis RA: Site of myocardial infarction a determinant of the cardiovascular changes induced in the cat by coronary occlusion. Circ Res 39:840, 1976.
13. Sheridan DJ, Crawford L, Rawlins MD, Julian DG: Antiarrhythmic action of lignocaine in early myocardial infarction: plasma levels after combined intramuscular and intravenous administration. Lancet 1:824, 1977.

29. COST EFFECTIVENESS OF MOBILE INTENSIVE CARE UNIT FOR AN ENTIRE COMMUNITY

Sidney Goldstein

The mobile coronary care units (MCCU) have become an important part of many urban suburban and rural communities since their first use by Pantridge and Geddes in 1967 [1]. The ability to extend coronary care from the hospital coronary care unit to the community using mobile units captured the imagination of cardiologists the world over. In the years that followed, the logistics by which prehospital coronary care is provided to a community changed from a relatively slow physician-manned vehicle to a multitiered, rapid responding, paramedic-manned, intensive care unit. These units can now provide emergency cardiac care including cardiac defibrillation, external pacing, and endotracheal intubation within minutes of cardiac arrest. The spread of this system of prehospital cardiac care has been a result of the evangelical medical leadership of a handful of physicians and the development of electronic technology that permits portability of lifesaving equipment and telecommunications between paramedics in the field and medical consultants at the base hospital. The success of mobile MCCUs has passed from the anecdotal accounts of survivor to reports of hundreds of successfully resuscitated victims of out-of-hospital cardiac arrest.

This success has led to suggestions by some

authors that the overall decrease in community coronary heart disease mortality rates is at least partially a result of the MCCU [2, 3]. A decade after the report by Pantridge and Geddes, approximately 25% of the 297 emergency medical service projects that cover most of the United States have in place advanced life-support systems that include mobile MCCUs [4]. And yet, the precise cost effectiveness of these systems in terms of lives saved and dollars spent is not fully understood. It is difficult to establish a clear understanding of the cost and benefit of these units because they impact broadly upon emergency care in general. They affect not only cardiac care but also the care of trauma and other acutely ill individuals. The assessment of their benefit relative to other methods of coronary disease therapy has been compounded by a multiplicity of factors and therapeutic modalities coming into play at a time when coronary disease mortality itself has been decreasing for reasons that are not well understood. Although it is difficult to establish a clear statement of cost effectiveness in a community sense, for the individual survivor of out-of-hospital cardiac arrest it is dramatically obvious.

A number of factors impacting on the success of the MCCU must be understood before attempting to establish its true cost and benefit. Less than 10% of patients using the MCCU actually experience a cardiac arrest either before or during transit [4]. Life-threatening arrhythmias other

This work was supported in part by NHLBI R01-HL18800-08.

R.M. Califf and G.S. Wagner (eds.), ACUTE CORONARY CARE: Principles and Practice. Copyright © 1985. Martinus Nijhoff Publishing, Boston/Dordrecht/Lancaster.

than ventricular fibrillation or asytole occur in another 30% – 50% and require treatment in approximately one-half of these patients. It is clear, therefore, that the effect of the MCCU has wider effects other than just on the cardiac arrest victim. The resultant improvement of training and technology available in the MCCU has had a major impact on all emergency care.

The resuscitation and subsequent return to work of a previously healthy, fully employed person who experiences an out-of-hospital cardiac arrest is the simplest and most optimistic outcome. Unfortunately this describes a minority of the cardiac arrest victims. Many are symptomatic or chronically ill before their event. Others experience acute myocardial infarction either as a cause or result of cardiac arrest, leaving them with some residual cardiac dysfunction. In addition, emotional and socioeconomic factors may prevent a return to full employment. In one study [5], 40% of cardiac arrest victims were fully employed and 8% were working part time prior to arrest. Six months after their successful resuscitation, 21% were now working full time and 9% were working part time. It can, therefore, be appreciated that the achievement of these units is affected both by utilization in the community and the standards by which success is measured.

Community Factors

Foremost among the factors affecting success is the arrival time of the MCCU to the patient. The effect of arrival time on long-term survival is shown in figure 29-1 from data from our own study of out-of-hospital resuscitation [6]. Eisenberg et al. [7] also observed that long-term survival is related to arrival time of the MCCU (see chapter 27). Several studies indicate that over 50% of patients with cardiac arrests due to ventricular fibrillation can be resuscitated in the field if the MCCU arrives within 4 min of the event, and about 25% will be discharged from the hospital. Many less, and perhaps none at all, will be resuscitated if the event is characterized by ventricular asystole. The MCCU arrival time is related in part to the geography and the population density of the community and, therefore, rural and suburban communities are at a clear disadvantage.

Bystander administration of cardiopulmonary

resuscitation before definitive therapy can be initiated has improved survival. This has been particularly true when MCCU arrival times are long. The effect on resuscitation rate is less evident if the response time is less than 4 min [8, 9]. Thompson et al. [9] observed a twofold improvement in survival, from 21% to 43%, when bystander CPR was applied. The effect on survival to the hospital was negligible, but it did result in a decrease in cardiac and central nervous system sequelae of the arrest event. The community's use of the mobile MCCU also depends on the availability of an adequate alarm system. Nevertheless, even in communities where MCCUs are available, it is estimated that only 50% of patients actually use them. Those who use the MCCU are usually much more critically ill than nonusers [2] and have a higher incidence of serious inhospital complications. Socioeconomic community characteristics may also determine the use of the MCCU.

System Factors

The operations of the MCCU in various communities differ. Some are primary response systems and others are secondary responders. The primary response systems treat a broad variety of medical and surgical conditions in addition to cardiac arrest. It is, therefore, difficult to measure their effect, specifically upon successful resuscitation of cardiac arrest alone. They also make many more emergency runs. Cardiac runs represent approximately 10% of all emergency runs provided by primary response systems. The secondary responders, on the other hand, are called after the primary response team ascertains that a cardiac arrest or a significant cardiac event has occurred. They apply their expertise more specifically to the cardiac patient and their effect can be measured more directly in terms of successful resuscitation of cardiac arrest. Cardiac runs for secondary responders may represent as many as 50% of the MCCU calls. In Columbus, Ohio [2], the secondary response units saw approximately 57% of the acute myocardial infarction patients who did not experience sudden death and 59% of the coronary arrest patients. In addition to the different logistic application of the system, the training and control of paramedics vary widely. Some are trained for major resuscitation, includ-

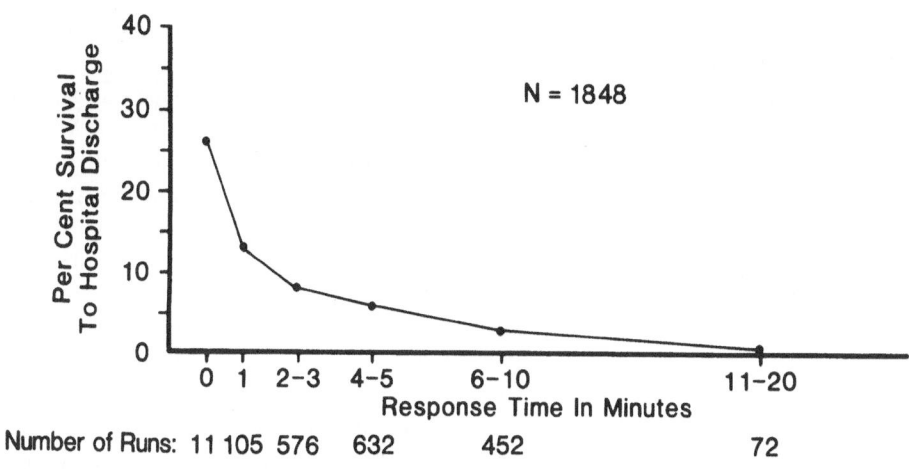

FIGURE 29-1. The relationship between arrival time of MCCU to ultimate hospital discharge.

ing endotracheal intubations, and others are limited both in terms of their expertise and the initiatives they can carry out. This further training not only results in improved success rate, but also adds to the expense of the program.

Pozen et al. [10] studied the accuracy of the paramedic and his medical control at the receiving hospital in correctly diagnosing and treating cardiac arrhythmias. When their diagnosis and treatment were evaluated subsequently by a cardiologist, only 39% of the life-threatening arrhythmias were correct, whereas 64% of those without life-threatening were correctly diagnosed. These incorrect responses may have adversely affected outcome, since the final mortality rate was 43% in the incorrectly treated group and only 20% in the correctly diagnosed and treated group.

As currently developed throughout the world, the MCCUs have adapted to the local health and emergency care systems because of economic, political, and medical pressures. Therefore, they are uniform neither in their design nor in their operation.

Evaluation of MCCUs

SUCCESS OF THE MCCU

The measurement of cost effectiveness of MCCUs can be estimated by considering both the ex-

pense associated with the system and the success achieved in terms of patient survival. Units that are primary responders are an integral part of an overall emergency care system. Those that are secondary responders stand somewhat apart from the ongoing emergency system and can be measured more directly by their effect on cardiac morbidity and mortality, and specifically on their ability to successfully resuscitate cardiac arrest victims.

The incidence of cardiac arrest in all MCCU runs is between 5% and 10%. Defibrillation is carried out in 7.1% − 10.6% of runs by cardiac-dedicated vehicles and in 0.2% − 1.8% of runs of regular ambulances [4]. Hospital discharge rates of those successfully defibrillated range between 6.7% and 30.8%, whereas the rates for those with asystole as the arrest rhythm approach zero [4]. The extent of neurologic damage of those discharged patients has been assessed by Nagel et al. [11], who reported that 12% of the patients discharged alive had significant central nervous system defects. Abramson et al. [12] observed that, in patients who lacked purposeful response to pain 10−15 min after resuscitation, 29% survived three months; of these 43% were awake, 36% had good cerebral function, and 25% regained previous cerebral status. Of the 40 patients who were resuscitated after 5 min of arrest, 15% recovered good cerebral function.

The long-term survival of resuscitated patients

is related not only to age, the use of CPR, and early resuscitation, but also the etiology of cardiac arrest [6]. Those with acute myocardial ischemia or infarction as their entry event have a one-year mortality rate of 15%. Patients with coronary heart disease, but without any evidence of associated acute ischemia or infarction (particularly the subgroup with high frequency of ventricular premature beats), are at very high risk of recurrent death, approaching 25% within one year [13].

If the effectiveness of units is evaluated in the broadest sense, they should be considered in relationship to all acute cardiac events occurring in the community. The incidence of acute cardiovascular events in the United States is approximately 1.5 deaths per 1000 persons [4]. As noted before, the mobile coronary care units are used in about 50% of the persons who experience such an event. In the ambulance, acute cardiovascular events represent 20% − 59.5% of all runs with a 10% − 33% mortality rate from initiation of emergency runs to hospital discharge [4]. Life-threatening arrhythmias occur in 30% − 52%, with about half of these patients receiving advanced medical and electrical intervention. The high degree of variability of these outcomes, however, makes it almost impossible to assess the true effect of the mobile coronary care units without considering their effect upon all of the acute cardiovascular events in the community.

COST OF THE MCCU

The expense of the MCCU has been studied in an attempt to establish the cost of saving a single life. Acton [14] estimated that the cost of saving a life, using a physician-attended MCCU, was approximately $14,000 per life saved in 1978 dollars. The cost of a life saved using an ambulance attended by nonphysician personnel trained to administer antiarrhythmic drugs was approximately $14,750. Cretin [15] developed a model to evaluate the cost of lives saved in a paramedic-staffed MCCU. She estimated that the cost was $3140−$6100 per life in 1975. In a study in Columbus, Ohio, by Lewis et al. [2], the estimated cost was approximately $1,038 in 1978. They estimated that 14.2 lives/100,000 population were saved annually by that MCCU's system. This cost assessment assumed that all the

suspect paramedic runs were true cardiac runs, but experience would suggest that this is not actually true.

A more careful study of the issue was carried out by Urban et al. [16] in King County, Washington. They had the opportunity to evaluate the lifesaving effect of adding a paramedic system to the usual community ambulance care. They evaluated the improvement in the number of lives saved and marginal or additional costs associated with the program. The community change in emergency care gave them the opportunity to compare simultaneously, over a three-year period, three different systems: (a) a paramedic system fully staffed with trained personnel, (b) an emergency system without paramedics, and (c) an experimental system in which paramedics were added in the latter part of the observation period. Table 29-1 shows the improvement of the rate of admission of cardiac arrest victims to the hospital observed between the early and late phases of the experimental system. It also can be seen that the admission rate was greater in the paramedic system when compared with the nonparamedic system. This was also reflected in the rate of discharge from the hospital of cardiac arrest victims resuscitated by the paramedic system of 55%, compared with that of the nonparamedic system of 33% ($P<0.01$). The estimated cost in 1978 associated with this improvement was $43,358 per cardiac arrest victim saved. Although this amount is higher than that of previous authors, it probably represents a more realistic cost estimate. Ornato et al. [17, 18] calculated that the statewide improvement in coronary mortality experienced in Nebraska was related to the MCCU system developed in that state. They concluded that, when one balances the expense of a MCCU system against income production and attending state revenue, units are cost effective.

These considerations raise the question of how much a life saved is worth. Beyond the emotional questions, there are certainly the economic questions of the likelihood of these individuals returning to active and productive work. We have already noted that approximately 20% of those individuals who were employed prior to their arrest returned to full employment. The calculation of this impact and the subsequent mortality rate in this population, of course, is difficult to

TABLE 29-1. Changes in admission rate of cardiac arrest victims in the different EMS systems

	Admissions per cardiac arrest		
	Early	Late	% Improved
Paramedic system	37.6	36.3	−1.3 ± 5.1
No paramedic system	11.3	24.1	12.8 ± 7.9
Experimental system	18.8	33.4	14.6 ± 3.8[a]

[a]$P < 0.001$.
Adapted from Urban et al. [16], with permission.

assess [19]. When a community embarks upon the assessment of the value of the establishment of an MCCU, it must be placed in relationship to other programs affecting coronary heart disease mortality. Acton [4] has approached this question in an idealized community of 100,000. The most cost-effective intervention would be a risk-factor screening and pretreatment program in which the net community benefit would be $300,000, assuming that 21 lives per year would be saved. Using the same measurements, the MCCU would have a net benefit of $197,000, assuming that 15.1 lives per year would be saved. The willingness to spend this amount of money is influenced by numerous political and emotional issues, but the electorate has voiced its decision by voting to provide funds for these programs in hundreds of communities across the land. In an attempt to deal with this issue by interviewing individuals in the community, Acton [4] reached a dollar amount of $28,000 per life saved that people would be willing to spend for such an intervention, an amount well within the assumed costs of the MCCU.

A survey of the changes in emergency medical care that have taken place in the last decade must support the fact that the impact on MCCUs has been dramatic and pervasive. Just as the impact of the coronary care unit cannot fully be estimated (see chapter 38) without appreciating the changes in the hospital cardiac care in general, so too must one appreciate the improvement of emergency medical care as a result of the MCCU. To fully evaluate these systems in the community, one must study the community as a whole. In this setting, the moments between life and death are fleeting and the imperatives of providing medical care to the dead and dying often makes it difficult to assess the mechanisms of the provision of medical care. Nevertheless, it is clear that as the MCCUs developed, emergency care also vastly improved. As a result, the care of the acutely ill cardiac patient has been vastly improved. The cost and benefit of these changes may never be fully measured or appreciated. Their impact, however, on medical care has been in the past, and will be in the future, immense.

References

1. Pantridge J, Geddes J: A mobile intensive care unit in the management of myocardial infarction. Lancet 2:271, 1967.
2. Lewis R, Lanese R, Stang J, Chirikos T, Keller M, Warren J: Reduction of mortality from prehospital myocardial infarction by prudent patient activation of mobile coronary care system. Am Heart J 103:123, 1982.
3. Crampton R, Aldrich R, Gascho J, Miles J, Stillerman R: Reduction of prehospital, ambulance and community coronary death rates by the community-wide emergency cardiac care system. Am J Med 58:151, 1975.
4. The effect of emergency medical systems on prehospital cardiovascular care. Department of Transportation, DOT HS 805204, April 1981.
5. Bergner L, Eisenberg M, Hallstrom A, Cobb L: Health status of survivors of out-of-hospital cardiac arrest. Circulation 66:II-350, 1982.
6. Goldstein S, Landis J, Leighton R, Ritter G, Vasu C, Lantis A, Serokman R: Characteristics of resuscitated out-of-hospital cardiac arrest victims with coronary heart disease. Circulation 64:977, 1981.
7. Eisenberg M, Hallstrom A, Bergner L: Long-term survival after out-of-hospital cardiac arrest. N Engl J Med 306:1340, 1982.
8. Lund I, Skulberg A: Cardiopulmonary resuscitation by lay people. Lancet 1:702, 1976.
9. Thompson R, Hallstrom A, Cobb L: Bystander-initiated cardiopulmonary resuscitation in the management of ventricular fibrillation. Ann Intern Med 90:737, 1979.
10. Pozen M, D'Agostino R, Sytkowski P, Schneider R, Berezin M, Bremer L, Riggen R: Effectiveness of a prehospital medical control system: an analysis of the interaction between emergency room physician and paramedic. Circulation 63:442, 1981.
11. Nagle R, Gangola R, Picton-Robinson I: Factors

influencing return to work after myocardial infarction. Lancet 2:454, 1971.

12. Abramson N, Safar P, Detre K, Monroe J, Kelsey S, Reinmuth O, Synder J, Mullie A, Hedstrand U, Tammisto T, Lund I, Breivik H, Lind B, Jastremski J: Neurological function in CPR survivors. Circulation 66:II-350, 1982.

13. Temesy-Armos P, Goldstein S, Landis J, Leighton R, Ritter G, Vasu C, Lantis A, Serokman R, Wolfe R: Complex ventricular premature depolarizations as a predictor of mortality in survivors of out-of-hospital cardiac arrest. Am J Cardiol 49:928, 1982.

14. Acton J: Evaluating public programs to save lives: the case of heart disease. Rand Corporation report R930 RC. Santa Monica CA: Rand Corporation, 1973.

15. Cretin S: Cost—benefit analysis of treatment and prevention of myocardial infarction. Health Serv Res 12:174, 1977.

16. Urban N, Bergner L, Eisenberg M: The costs of suburban paramedic program in reducing deaths due to cardiac arrest. Med Care 19:379, 1981.

17. Ornato J, Craren E, Nelson N, Smith H: The economic impact of CPR and emergency cardiac care (ECC) programs. Circulation 66:II-349, 1982.

18. Ornato J, Craren E, Nelson N, Smith H: The impact of emergency cardiac care (ECC) on the reduction in mortality from myocardial infarction (MI). Circulation 66:II-349, 1982.

19. Vetter N, Pocock S, Julian D: Measuring the effect of a mobile coronary care unit upon the community. Br Heart J 41:418, 1979.

VI. CORONARY CARE: THE POSTADMISSION PHASE

30. OPTIMAL IDENTIFICATION OF THE PATIENT WITH ACUTE MYOCARDIAL ISCHEMIA IN THE EMERGENCY ROOM

Harry P. Selker

Michael W. Pozen[†]

Ralph B. D'Agostino

Although angina pectoris was meticulously described more than 200 years ago by Heberden [1] and the presentation of myocardial infarction was first reported 50 years ago by Herrick [2], accurate identification of acute ischemic heart disease (AIHD) in the emergency room (ER) remains a task that challenges the skill of the most seasoned clinician. In the United States, for each coronary care unit (CCU) patient in whom AIHD is confirmed, two patients are admitted with this as an ER diagnosis. There are great costs to patients and to the medical reimbursement system resulting from the large number of false-positive AIHD diagnoses and the resulting CCU overuse. Since each year in this country more than 1.5 million patients with suspected AIHD are admitted to CCUs, even a modest improvement in admitting practices would yield substantial savings. Additionally, many patients would be spared the needless physical and psychological side effects resulting from unnecessary admission to intensive care units. This chapter reviews studies that have attempted to optimize AIHD diagnostic accuracy in the ER setting.

Over the past two decades there have been two opposing pressures that have, along with clinical judgment, influenced physicians' diagnostic and triage decisions for ER patients suspected of having AIHD. With the recognition that CCU care might prevent early arrhythmia-related mortality associated with acute infarction [3], physicians have tended to overdiagnose AIHD and overadmit patients to CCUs. More recently, this tendency has been reinforced by the availability in the CCU of special instrumentation and procedures aimed at protecting endangered myocardium. The conscious strategy of maintaining high diagnostic sensitivity so that any errors are in the direction of overdiagnosis has had the intended effect: of all patients with acute infarction who seek attention in ERs, generally the diagnosis is missed in less than 5%. In contrast, mistakes in the other direction, CCU admission for presumed AIHD for patients who actually do not have the disease, occur ten times more frequently; typically 50% of patients admitted to CCUs turn out not to have had infarction [4–10]. In recent years, with the wide proliferation of coronary units, the costs of large numbers of apparently needless CCU admissions have caused interest in improving diagnostic specificity. To date, however, overadmission has not been effectively reduced.

In this discussion, AIHD is considered to in-

[†]Deceased

R.M. Califf and G.S. Wagner (eds.), ACUTE CORONARY CARE: Principles and Practice. Copyright © 1985. Martinus Nijhoff Publishing, Boston/Dordrecht/Lancaster.

clude new onset or unstable angina pectoris as well as acute infarction. For the purposes of ER triage, the diagnosis of AIHD better identifies patients for CCU admission than does the diagnosis of acute myocardial infarction alone. This is in part because of the difficulty in differentiating prospectively new onset or unstable angina pectoris from infarction, and in part by intent, since it is hoped that CCU admission helps reverse ischemia. In fact, for patients with AIHD with prolonged chest pain but without infarction, the medium and long-term mortality may be as poor or worse than for those who actually have a myocardial infarction [11,12].

In general terms, there are two kinds of studies that have sought to improve the identification of AIHD in ERs. Most work has been aimed at identifying the most diagnostically significant features of the clinical presentation. The smaller and more recent group of studies involve newer tests and computer-based or mathematical-modeling approaches. Both groups of work are selectively reviewed below, and the Boston City Hospital prospective trial using an AIHD predictive instrument [9] will be described in some detail.

Essentially, each of these studies suffers from some problem in study design, and their interpretation is hampered by lack of representativeness and comparability of data. One primary cause of this is "inclusion bias", i.e., nonrepresentativeness of study subjects caused by the use of different study inclusion criteria that miss some particular group of patients with AIHD. For example, if the chief complaint of substernal pressurelike chest pain is used as sole requisite for study inclusion, many patients whose myocardial infarctions present atypically will be excluded. Alternatively, if the entry criteria for chief complaint include any location and any character of chest pain, epigastric pain, arm pain, shortness of breath, dizziness, or palpitations, a study will include a large number of patients without AIHD. One well-validated set of entry criteria is the Imminent Myocardial Infarction Rotterdam (IMIR) criteria that capture more than 90% of all patients with AIHD who seek medical care [13]. These criteria include male patients 30 years of age and older and female patients 40 years of age

and older presenting with a chief complaint of chest pain, jaw or left arm pain, shortness of breath, or changed angina pectoris pattern, in association with specified corroborating aspects of the past medical history.

Another important source of bias in these clinical studies is nonrepresentativeness of the patient populations and medical practices at the study centers. Thus, even if standardized criteria such as the IMIR set are used, the actual incidence of AIHD among patients presenting to different ERs will vary considerably between hospitals, depending on their catchment area and referral roles in their communities. Unless a study includes a number of hospitals that span a wide range of settings and teaching levels, it will have bias derived from the particular patient distribution seen at the study sites. At the Boston City Hospital ER, for example, the diagnoses for 856 consecutive patients fulfilling the IMIR criteria were distributed as follows: 17% AIHD, 24% other cardiac disease, 8% chest pain of unknown cause, and 51% noncardiac disease [9].

Even more likely to have unrepresentative patient profiles are studies done in non-ER settings, such as intensive care units. An example of how an unrepresentative study sample might cause misleading conclusions is found in a recent study of two-dimensional echocardiography for diagnosing acute infarction in the ER. The test's diagnostic sensitivity and specificity for infarction were 94% and 84% respectively; the test misdiagnosed only seven of 80 patients [14]. Since the study subjects were patients admitted to an intensive care unit, as would be expected, about half had acute infarction. When this study's data are adjusted to a 15% incidence of infarction typical of the ER setting, the predictive value of a positive (abnormal) test is 52%; i.e., in an ER, of all patients with chest pain who have abnormal echocardiograms, only about half would actually have acute infarction. Thus, what at first appeared to be an excellent test turns out to be no better than current performance when projected to the ER population. (The definitions of sensitivity, specificity, and their use in analyzing diagnostic performance are illustrated later in this chapter in the review of the Boston City Hospital AIHD predictive instrument trial.)

Diagnostic Value of Presenting Clinical Features

There has been considerable investigation of the diagnostic features of clinical presentations in the ER. Although specific predictive values can be assigned to each symptom, sign, and ECG finding, these values are of limited usefulness because of problems in representativeness discussed above. Nonetheless, certain of these results do reinforce and perhaps improve our clinical senses.

Data from an English study are fairly representative of the chief complaints of patients suffering from acute myocardial infarction: 82% presented with chest pain; 12% with syncope, sudden shortness of breath, or collapse; and the remaining 6% with a variety of complaints [15]. In a study of hospitalized patients with myocardial infarction and patients who died suddenly before hospitalization, however, about two-thirds of patients with acute infarctions experienced prematory symptoms in the preceding few weeks including, in order of frequency, chest pain, fatigue or weakness, dyspnea, general malaise, anorexia/nausea, and arm and other pain [16]. In a cross-sectional study of a British community, 40% of patients dying suddenly or unexpectedly from coronary disease had complained of unusual tiredness in the weeks prior to their demise, and there was a surprisingly high frequency of rather "atypical" chest-pain complaints in the preceding weeks [15]. One would expect that the chief complaints of patients presenting to ERs would be biased in favor of more dramatic and recognizable symptoms because the less specific and less noticeable ones may be less likely to prompt a patient to seek ER care. These data regarding those dying outside the ER are consistent with this hypothesis.

In Sweden, Säwe studied 191 patients admitted to the CCU, and found that the clinical features most correlated with infarction were a pressure or constricting character of chest pain, radiation to both arms or to the neck and jaw, pain of greater than 1-h duration and, most predictive, the interpretation of acute infarction on ECG [17]. Another Scandinavian study of patients admitted to the CCU also found longer duration of chest pain and the presence of arm or neck radiation correlated with later documentation of AIHD [18]. In a retrospective study of CCU admissions done in Montreal, duration of chest pain of longer than 30 min, diaphoresis, and ischemic changes on ECG were the best predictors of AIHD [19]. In England, Short studied 456 patients with acute chest pain that their general practitioner thought was not severe enough to warrant hospitalization but had nonetheless asked for cardiologic consulation [20]. He attempted to identify the signs and symptoms with the highest predictive value for AIHD, and particularly for myocardial infarction. In patients with a prior history of ischemic heart disease, those unlikely to have acute ischemia included those whose pain was affected by breathing, twisting, or bending, those whose chest pain had a different epicenter from previous AIHD, and those whose ECG was normal or unchanged from previously. The clinical signs that predicted infarction best were dyspnea, shock, bradycardia, tachycardia, the ECG findings of ST elevation (however slight), and deterioration from a previous ECG. For patients with no previous history of ischemic heart disease the discriminating symptoms, signs, and ECG abnormalities were the same, with the additions that the presence of the pain in more than one place also made AIHD unlikely, and ECG ST-segment depression and T-wave inversion were also predictive of infarction.

As is well known to ER clinicians, esophageal reflux and motility disorders and musculoskeletal pain are common masqueraders of AIHD. In a study of all patients discharged from a CCU with undetermined causes of chest pain, over half had esophageal dysfunction [21]. When these patients' presenting complaints were compared with those of patients without AIHD, those with esophageal disorders were likely to complain of a lump in their throat, acid taste, overfullness after eating, a hacking cough, and chest pain awakening at night, and were less likely to report effort-related chest pain, or a history of nitroglycerin use or reliable chest-pain relief with its use. Eliminating the next most common masquerader, musculoskeletal pain, may occasionally be difficult. Indeed, in an interesting, although limited, case-control study of the time-honored practice of attempting to duplicate chest pain by chest wall pressure, musculoskeletal chest pain was more often elicitable in patients with than in those without AIHD [22].

Chest pain in the presence of valvular disease can pose a diagnostic dilemma, particularly in patients with aortic stenosis. Although the absence of chest pain makes coronary artery disease unlikely, its presence does not necessarily confirm it (see chapter 31). In a study of patients referred for valve replacement, of those with "typical anginal" chest pain, 64% had coronary artery disease, while among those with "atypical" chest pain, 29% had significant coronary artery disease [23].

A past history of medication use for coronary disease increases the likelihood that the current chest pain is AIHD. Not surprisingly, in the Boston City Hospital predictive instrument study, a history of nitroglycerin was found to be one of the most powerful predictors of AIHD [9]. Nonetheless, nitrates can cause dramatic relief of chest pain from esophageal spasm [24] and thus the details of the history must be noted.

In addition to the presenting clinical features, knowledge of a patient's coronary artery disease risk factors are diagnostically helpful. From the Framingham study we know that a person's risks of developing ischemic heart disease are increased by being male, having advancing age, a smoking habit, hypertension, hypercholesteremia, glucose intolerance, ECG abnormalities, a type-A personality, a sedentary life style, and a family history of early coronary heart disease [25]. Although the exact risk values published in the American Heart Association's Coronary Risk Handbook [26] are not specifically applicable because they are derived from incidence estimates in asymptomatic populations, ER patients who are in the Handbook's higher-risk groups certainly do have higher likelihoods of having coronary artery disease. A patient's pretest likelihood of having coronary disease greatly affects the probability that a patient with an abnormal test result or a complaint of chest pain truly has AIHD [27]. For example, a 30-year-old man with no coronary risk factors who complains of central chest pain is much less likely to actually have AIHD than a 60-year-old man with hypertension and diabetes who describes exactly the

same type of chest pain. Similarly, ST-segment abnormalities in the ECG of the 30-year-old will be much less likely to represent AIHD than identical ST abnormalities in the 60 year old's ECG. This kind of reasoning, long-used intuitively by clinicians, and formally stated in Bayesian analysis, is employed in some predictive instruments of coronary disease [28], though not yet in the ER setting.

Technically Based Diagnostic Aids

Although the studies reviewed above do provide insight into the clinical indicators of AIHD, there are problems in actually using their data as interventions that can be tested for effect on AIHD diagnostic and triage practices. To be useful and generally applicable, a diagnostic aid must be testable in a clinical setting, and its effectiveness must be demonstrated by a prospective clinical trial that includes a wide range of settings. Unfortunately, to date, most available investigation in this area falls short in at least one of these respects. Recently several technically based methods for improving AIHD diagnosis have been devised that are more easily tested in the clinical setting. As will be reviewed below, these divide generally into two approaches: those based on specific diagnostic tests of myocardial function or damage, and those using computer-based mathematical modeling analysis of the clinical presentation to supplement physicians' diagnostic judgment.

MYOCARDIAL ASSAYS AS DIAGNOSTIC AIDS
Eisenberg and colleagues studied the likely usefulness of having "stat" creatinine kinase (CK) tests available in the ER [6]. Among 80 patients with chest pain seen in the Hospital of the University of Pennsylvania ER, if abnormal CK results had been used as admission criteria, one patient who had been sent home with a myocardial infarction would have been admitted; however, 11 patients appropriately sent home without infarction would have been admitted, and five patients appropriately admitted for infarction would have been sent home. The lack of utility of immediate CK assay results in the ER was confirmed by results of a similar study at Montreal General Hospital [18], and by a study

done in a private community hospital in Phoenix [30]. Additionally, using a somewhat different type of retrospective analysis, Goldman et al. found that in multivariate modeling of ER diagnostic decision making, the availability of cardiac enzymes did not improve diagnostic accuracy [31].

As already discussed, two-dimensional echocardiography is a sensitive and relatively specific test for infarction [31] but, as outlined earlier, since it has not been tested in the ER setting, its usefulness there remains undetermined. Similarly, although thallium-201 scintigraphy may aid recognition of AIHD in the CCU, particularly in patients without prior infarction, its usefulness in the ER must be proved [32].

MATHEMATICAL MODELS AS
DIAGNOSTIC AIDS

Analysis of medical decision making suggests that an ideal AIHD diagnostic aid would supplement ER physicians' diagnostic specificity without disrupting their already desirably high diagnostic sensitivity. Rather than depend on a single assay result to improve CCU admission practices, some workers have attempted to harness computer-based mathematical modeling to improve ER decision making. Using computer analysis, Säwe devised a discriminant function to predict infarction based on nine clinical variables derived from his earlier work [17]. In a prospective trial of 191 CCU patients [29], his function missed no diagnosis of infarction, but correctly identified only 16% of patients who did not have infarction, thus being of limited practical value in reducing CCU admissions. The variables in his model, along with their respective weights for descriminant analysis, are: +11 for an ECG suggestive of acute infarction; +7 for extension of pain to the jaw; +6 for unstable angina; +5 for radiation of chest pain to the arms; +4 for a history of smoking; +2 for pulse pressure less than 60 Torr; −3 for duration of chest pain less than 1 h; −6 for arrhythmic sensations; and −8 for a respiratory rate less than 16/min.

Goldman et al. developed a computer-based decision protocol based on recursive partitioning using nine variables that categorize ER patients as being likely or unlikely to be having acute infarction [33]. The variables used in his

model were: at the first split node, the presence or absence of ST elevation or new Q waves on the ECG; at the next nodes, the nature of and timing of the patient's chest pain; and at subsequent nodes, the patient's age and prior history of similar pain or coronary disease. When tested in the care of 468 patients at the Brigham and Women's Hospital, this protocol performed as well as ER physicians correctly classifying patients as having myocardial infarctions. In a hypothetical experiment, when both the physicians' and the protocol's diagnoses were combined, the diagnostic specificity for acute infarction was 7% better than either alone, though no better in diagnostic sensitivity. Whether this improvement would occur in practice, however, remains unknown pending a prospective trial of the protocol's actual use in the clinical setting.

Using a somewhat different approach, reasoning that a single numerical probability value might be easily incorporated into physicians' clinical decision-making processes, researchers at the Boston City Hospital developed a mathematical instrument to provide the ER physician with a patient's likelihood of having AIHD [9]. The methodology and analysis used in the development and prospective trial of the instrument are illustrative of recent directions in this type of research, and thus are described in some detail below.

The study included all patients seen at the Boston City Hospital ER during the study's duration who fulfilled the IMIR criteria. In the study's first phase, the AIHD predictive instrument was developed from data on 925 patients seen in the ER between October 1976 and 1977. From 105 variables available to ER physicians, including clinical presentations, past history, physical findings, ECGs, sociodemographic characteristics, and coronary disease risk factors, a stepwise logistic regression equation was developed that used only nine of the 105 original variables. This mathematical instrument provides a prediction of a patient's likelihood of having AIHD expressed as a number between 0.0 and 1.0. When programmed into a handheld calculator, the instrument requires less than 20 s of computation time. The nine clinical features required for input are, in order of their relative weights in the predictive function, the presence or absence of the following: any ECG ST-segment abnormality; ECG T-wave peaking or inversion; patient's report of chest pain localized to the middle or lower substernal area; history of myocardial infarction; ECG ST-segment elevation or depression of 1 mm or more; patient's report of dyspnea; patient's report of chest pain or pressure as the most important presenting symptom; history of angina pectoris or nitroglycerin use; and any ECG T-wave abnormality.

The study's second phase was a prospective trial of the predictive instrument's effect on CCU admitting practices in which the ER physicians received the instrument's probability only during every other month of the ten month trial. During the experimental months (401 patients), the research assistant simply handed the physician a piece of paper with the probability written on it before the physician's admission or discharge decision. The physician was free to incorporate the probability into decision making, or to ignore it altogether. During the control months (455 patients), the probability was calculated in the same manner; however, the physician was not given the value.

For data analysis, each patient was assigned a final diagnosis by a physician who reviewed, in a blinded fashion, the serial ECGs, cardiac enzymes, and ER and hospital records. Emergency room physicians' initial AIHD diagnoses were compared with final diagnoses and classified as follows: "true positive" if both the ER and final diagnoses were AIHD, "false positive" if the ER diagnosis was AIHD but the final diagnosis was not, "false negative" if the ER diagnosis was not AIHD but the final diagnosis was, and "true negative" if neither the ER nor the final diagnosis was AIHD.

A number of measures were used to assess the ER physicians' diagnostic performance. The "false-positive diagnosis rate" was calculated as

$$\frac{\text{false positives}}{\text{false positive} + \text{true positives}}$$

The "false-negative diagnosis rate" was used to assess physicians' inappropriate discharges from the ER and was defined as

$$\frac{\text{false negatives}}{\text{false negative} + \text{true negatives}}$$

Note that we have used what we term the false-positive *diagnosis* rate and the false-negative *diagnosis* rate, which are different from the commonly used "false-positive rate" and "false-negative rate." The false-positive diagnosis rate tells us, out of all patients receiving *positive* diagnoses, what proportion actually *did not* have acute ischemia. The false-negative diagnosis rate tells us, out of all patients receiving *negative* diagnoses, what proportion actually *did* have ischemia. Since patients are admitted to the CCU based on a positive or negative diagnosis of AIHD, these false diagnosis rates are of primary importance, since they assess unnecessary admissions to the coronary unit and mistaken ER discharges to home. Other conventional measures used to assess diagnostic performance included "diagnostic accuracy," defined as

$$\frac{\text{true positive} + \text{true negatives}}{\text{true pos.} + \text{false pos.} + \text{true neg.} + \text{false neg.}}$$

"sensitivity," defined as

$$\frac{\text{true positives}}{\text{true positives} + \text{false negatives}}$$

and "specificity," defined as

$$\frac{\text{true negatives}}{\text{false positives} + \text{true negatives}}$$

The above-defined diagnostic classifications and rate calculations were used to compare diagnostic performances in the experimental and control periods. As shown in table 30-1, during the experimental periods the diagnostic accuracy rate increased from 83% to 91% ($p < 0.005$), and the specificity improved from 80% to 92% ($p < 0.005$), while there was no significant change for sensitivity. The false-positive diagnosis rate decreased from 51% to 33% ($p < 0.01$) while, importantly, the false-negative diagnosis rate remained unchanged at 3%.

TABLE 30-1.Emergency room acute ischemic heart disease diagnostic performance with and without the use of the predictive instrument (rates expressed as percent)

	Experimental months	Control months	Significance level
Diagnostic accuracy	91	83	$p < 0.005$
False-positive diagnosis rates	33	51	$p < 0.01$
False-negative diagnosis rates	3	3	NS
Sensitivity	86	90	NS
Specificity	92	80	$p < 0.005$

NS, not significant

TABLE 30-2.Comparison of patient disposition: experimental and control months (data given as percent)

Patient disposition	Experimental months (n = 401)	Control months (n = 455)
Coronary care unit	14	26
Ward	30	33
Discharged	56	41

TABLE 30-3.False-positive diagnostic rate classified by probability of acute ischemic heart disease

	Probability less than 50%		Probability greater than 50%	
	Experimental months	Control months	Experimental months	Control months
True positives (no. of patients)	18	25	39	46
False positives (no. of patients)	12	57	16	18
Total (no. of patients)	30	82	55	64
False-positive diagnosis rate (%)	40	70	29	28
	$p < 0.01$		Not significant	

In terms of actual CCU admitting practices, as shown in table 30-2, during the control periods 26% of all patients with (IMIR) symptoms suggestive of AIHD were admitted to the CCU, whereas during the experimental periods this dropped to 14%, a 46% reduction of CCU admissions ($p < 0.001$). Among patients admitted to the CCU, the ratio of true-positive to false-positives increased from 1.7 to 1.0 during the control periods to 3.9 to 1.0 during the experimental periods. Thus the use of the predictive instrument reduced the number of CCU admissions by reducing the number of false-positive admissions.

Further analysis was done to try to determine which patients benefited most from the use of the instrument. Considering at false-positive diagnosis rates, patients were stratified by whether they had a high or low probability of having AIHD. The data in table 30-3 show that, for patients with less than 50% likelihood of having AIHD, the false positive diagnosis rate was 70% during the control months and fell to 40% during the experimental periods, a 43% reduction ($p < 0.01$). For patients with greater than 50% likelihood of having AIHD, there was no significant change. Thus the predictive instrument was most helpful for correctly diagnosing patients with less definite signs and symptoms of AIHD, while physician judgment alone was sufficient to diagnose correctly AIHD in patients whose probabilities exceeded 50%. In clinical terms, for patients presenting to the ER with clear-cut signs of AIHD, the addition of any diagnostic aid is probably superfluous. However, most ER patients with chest pain have symptoms suggestive, but not diagnostic, of AIHD. These patients represent the vast majority of those admitted to CCUs for presumed AIHD, only later to have the diagnosis "ruled out." It is for these patients, who form the great preponderance of ER patients with chest pain, that the use of the instrument causes the greatest improvement in physicians' diagnostic and admission decisions.

Conclusions

As reviewed in this chapter, strategies to improve the accuracy of ER diagnosis and triage of AIHD have included identification of the clinical factors most highly predictive of AIHD, rapid access to cardiac enzymes, two-dimensional echocardiography, thallium-201 scintigraphy, and computer-based methods. Except for the AIHD predictive instrument trial at Boston City Hospital, however, none has been shown prospectively to reduce CCU overadmission of non-AIHD patients.

The Boston City Hospital predictive instrument gives the ER physician a simple numerical probability of a patient's likelihood of having AIHD. This probability, derived from nine clinical features of the patient's presentation, can be obtained from a programmable calculator within 20 seconds and provides more information than any single available diagnostic test. The instrument is designed to complement a physician's judgment rather than stand alone. Indeed, since ER physicians miss few diagnoses of AIHD, but do tend to overdiagnose AIHD, the instrument's predictive characteristics are specifically constructed to help identify patients with truly low likelihood of having AIHD.

The AIHD predictive instrument has recently been tested in a multicenter trial that included ER settings ranging from major urban teaching centers to rural nonteaching hospitals and these

results should be available soon [34]. If the instrument is effective in this clinical trial, it should be ready for general use. If widely used in hospital emergency rooms, it would seem likely to reduce unnecessary CCU admissions and thus to have substantial medical and financial benefit.

Added in Proof: Multicenter and Predictive Instrument Trial Results

While this manuscript was in press, the results of the *Multicenter AIHD Predictive Instrument Trial* were published [34]. The structure of the trial was analogous to the above-described Boston City Hospital study, but included six New England hospitals, two urban major teaching centers, two medical-school-affiliated teaching hospitals in smaller cities, and two nonteaching hospitals in rural locations. In the study's first phase, from data on 2,801 patients seen in the emergency rooms in the six hospitals, a new AIHD predictive instrument was developed that was applicable to all the study hospitals (and very similar to the original Boston City Hospital instrument). In the second phase, a prospective clinical trial, the predictive instrument was tested in the care of 2,320 patients seen over an eleven-month period in the emergency rooms in the six hospitals.

The impact of multicenter predictive instrument was very similar to that seen in the Boston City Hospital study. When given the probability of AIHD generated by instrument, physicians' diagnostic specificity for AIHD improved, without deterioration of sensitivity, and their false-positive diagnosis rates decreased without any increase in false-negative diagnosis rates. Among patients without AIHD, the number of CCU admissions decreased by 30%, without any increase in missed diagnoses of acute ischemia. Reflecting this, the proportion of CCU admissions dropped from 44% to 33% for patients without AIHD.

The multicenter results suggested that if the AIHD predictive instrument is applied widely in this country, it could reduce CCU admissions by 250,000 per year, and thus should have very substantial medical and financial benefits.

References

1. Heberden W: Some account of a disorder of the breast. Med Trans R Coll Phys Lond, 1772.
2. Herrick JB: Clinical features of sudden obstruction of the coronary arteries. JAMA 59:2015–2020, 1912.
3. Lown B, Fakhro AM, Hood WB Jr, Thorn GW: The coronary care unit: new perspectives and directions. JAMA 199 156–166, 1967.
4. Bloom B, Peterson O: End results, costs, and productivity of coronary care units. N Engl J Med 288:77–78, 1973.
5. Schor S, Behar S, Modan B, et al: Disposition of presumed coronary patients from an ER: a follow-up study. JAMA 236:941– 943, 1976.
6. Eisenberg JM, Horowitz LN, Busch R, et al: Diagnosis of acute myocardial infarction in the ER: a prospective assessment of clinical decision making and the usefulness of immediate cardiac enzyme determination. J Community Health 4: 190–198, 1979.
7. McGuinness JB, Begg TB, Semple T: First electrocardiogram in recent myocardial infarction. Br Med J 2:451–453, 1976.
8. Schroeder JS, Lamb IH, Hu M: The pre-hospital course of patients with chest pain: analysis of the prodromal, symptomatic, decision-making, transportation, and ER periods. Am J Med 64: 742–748, 1978.
9. Pozen MW, D'Agostino RB, Mitchell JB, et al: The usefulness of predictive instrument to reduce inappropriate admissions to the coronary care unit. Ann Intern Med 92:238–242, 1980.
10. Fuchs R, Scheidt S: Improved criteria for admission to cardiac care units. JAMA 246:2037–2041, 1981.
11. Lopes MG, Spivak AP, Harrison DC, Schroeder JS: Prognosis in coronary care unit noninfarction cases. JAMA 228:1558–1562, 1974.
12. Schroeder JS, Lamb IH, Harrison DC: Patients admitted to the coronary care unit for chest pain: high risk subgroup for subsequent cardiovascular death. Am J Cardiol 39:829–832, 1977.
13. Van der Does E, Lubsen J, Pool J, et al: Acute coronary events in a general practice: objectives and design of the Imminent Myocardial Infarction Rotterdam Study. Heart Bull 7:91–98, 1976.
14. Horowitz RS, Morganroth J Parrotto C, et al: Immediate diagnosis of acute myocardial infarction by two-dimensional echocardiology. Circulation 65:323–329, 1982.
15. Kinlen LJ: Incidence and presentation of myocardial infarction in an English community. Br Heart J 35:616–622, 1973.
16. Alonzo AA, Simon AB, Feinleib M: Prodromata of myocardial infarction and sudden death. Circulation 52: 1056–1062, 1975.
17. Säwe U: Pain in acute myocardial infarction: a study of 137 patients in a coronary care unit. Acta Med Scand 190:79–81, 1971.
18. Ahnve S: Noninfarctional cases without previously known ischemic heart disease admitted to a coronary care unit. Eur J Cardiol 9:307–318, 1979.
19. Nattel S, Warnica JW, Ogilvie RE: Indications for admission to a coronary care unit in patients with unstable angina. CMA J 122:180–184, 1980.
20. Short D: Diagnosis of slight and subacute coronary attacks in a community. Br Heart J 45: 299–310, 1981.
21. Areskog M, Tibbling L, Wranne B: Oesophageal dysfunction in non-infarction coronary care unit patients. Acta Med Scand 205:279–282, 1979.
22. McElroy JB: Angina pectoris with coexisting skeletal chest pain. Am Heart J 66:296–300, 1963.
23. Paquay PA, Anderson G, Diefenthal H, et al: Chest pain as a predictor of coronary artery disease in patients with obstructive aortic valve disease. Am J Cardiol 38:863– 869, 1976.
24. Orlando RC, Bozymski EM: Clinical and monometric effects of nitroglycerin in diffuse esophageal spasm. N Engl J Med 289:23–25, 1973.
25. Gordon T, Sorlie P, Kannel WB: Coronary heart disease, atherothrombotic brain infarction, intermittent claudication—a multivariate analysis of some factors related to their incidence: Framingham study, 16-year follow-up. Sect 27, US Govt Print Office, 1971.
26. American Heart Association: Coronary risk handbook. Dallas: American Heart Association, 1973.
27. Rifkin RD, Hood WB Jr: Bayesian analysis of electrocardiographic exercise testing. N Engl J Med 297:681–686, 1979.
28. Diamond GA, Staniloff HM, Forrester JS, et al: Computer-assisted diagnosis in the noninvasive evaluation of patients with suspected coronary artery disease J Am Coll Cardiol 1:444–455, 1983.
29. Säwe U: Early diagnosis of acute myocardial infarction with special reference to the diagnosis of the intermediate coronary syndrome: a clinical study. Acta Med Scanda (Suppl) 520:1–76, 1972.

30. Seager SB: Cardiac enzymes in the evaluation of chest pain. Ann Emerg Med 9:346–349, 1980.
31. Goldman L, Cook EF, Weisberg M: Incremental value of the EKG and enzymes in the evaluation of ER patients with acute chest pain. Clin Res 31:233A, 1983.
32. Wackers FJT, Lie KI, Liem KL, et al: Potential value of thallium-201 scintigraphy as a means of selecting patients for the coronary care unit. Br Heart J 41:111–117, 1979.
33. Goldman L, Weinberg M, Weisbert M, et al: A computer-derived protocol to aid in the diagnosis of ER patients with acute chest pain. N Engl J Med 307:588–596, 1982.
34. Pozen MW, D'Agostino RB, Selker HP, et al: A predictive instrument to improve coronary-care-unit admission practices in acute ischemic heart disease: a prospective multicenter clinical trial. N Engl J Med 310:1273–1278, 1984.

31. ACHIEVING PAIN RELIEF WITH PHYSIOLOGIC MANAGEMENT AND ANALGESIC AGENTS DURING ACUTE MYOCARDIAL INFARCTION

Robert Lester

The initial management of chest pain in patients with acute myocardial ischemia or infarction has been aimed at relief of the pain rather than modification of the physiologic determinants of the pain. General supportive measures including analgesia, sedation, and oxygenation have been routinely employed whether the patient has only a suspected myocardial infarction or has an obvious large evolving infarction. Recently interventions have been developed that may favorably affect the balance between myocardial oxygen supply and demand. Beta-blockers, nitroglycerin, calcium channel blockers, intraaortic balloon counterpulsation, and thrombolytic therapy commonly have a beneficial effect on the chest pain. The purpose of this chapter is to develop a physiologic approach to the management of chest pain complicating acute infarction by focusing on the effects of interventions on the myocardial oxygen demand/supply ratio.

The mechanisms of pain production and the clinical features of chest pain will first be considered along with an analysis of the principal determinants of myocardial oxygen consumption. Thereafter, guidelines for controlling pain will be presented. Discussions of calcium channel blockers and beta-blockers, mechanical circulatory assistance, and thrombolysis have intentionally been omitted since these are presented elsewhere in this book.

Myocardial Oxygen Balance

Myocardial oxygen supply is governed by coronary blood flow, the oxygen-carrying capacity of arterial blood, and the amount of oxygen extracted from the blood by the heart. Since both the oxygen content of arterial blood and the myocardial oxygen extraction ratio are essentially fixed, the only mechanism whereby myocardial oxygenation can satisfy demands is through an augmentation in coronary blood flow. The normal coronary circulation has the capacity to dilate to reduce arteriolar resistance, thereby enabling flow to be maintained commensurate with metabolic need. In contrast, coronary occlusive disease compromises this response and prevents epicardial vessel dilatation at the site of stenosis. Moreover, coronary stenosis renders the myocardium more vulnerable to systemic hypotension and may alter regional perfusion by stimulation of collateral flow [1]. The net result of these effects is that ischemia may be perpetuated in a cascade fashion unless prompt intervention is initiated. Unless coronary occlusion is directly eliminated, the physiologic relief of chest pain in patients with acute ischemia must be effected by therapy that decreases myocardial oxygen consumption.

Myocardial oxygen utilization is primarily determined by heart rate, contractility, and systolic wall stress. The latter varies directly with changes in ventriclar thickness, ventricular diameter, and systolic blood pressure. Thus, when tachycardia, increased blood pressure, ventricular dilatation, or enhanced contractility occurs, myocardial oxygen consumption increases. Each of these responses may, in patients with fixed coronary stenoses, precipitate chest pain due to acute ischemia. Hence, the ability to favorably modulate these parameters so that myocardial oxygen supply is balanced with demand determines the capabilities of the various clinical interventions in relieving this ischemic chest pain.

Pathogenesis of Cardiac Pain

The clinical recognition and management of chest pain is aided by a knowledge of the mechanism of pain impulse generation and transmission [2, 3]. The precise neuroanatomic basis for cardiac pain in general, and that related to acute myocardial ischemia in particular, is incompletely understood. However, it is known that both the atria and ventricles are richly innervated with sympathetic sensory fibers (see chapter 12). There are two networks of fibers: one is perivascular and encircles the coronary arteries in their adventitia; the other is paravascular and courses adjacent to the blood vessels in subepicardial tissue. This latter network terminates in unmyelinated freebranching nerve endings between the muscle fiber layers. Afferent nerve fibers from the heart connect to the spinal cord through the cardiac nerves, the upper five thoracic sympathetic ganglia, the white rami communicantes, and finally the first through fifth thoracic dorsal roots. Impulse transmission then occurs to the thalamus and cerebral cortex. The convergence of impulses from somatic thoracic structures in the ascending spinal neurons is likely responsible for the phenomenon of referred cardiac pain.

The sympathetic afferent fibers are both myelinated and unmyelinated and respond to mechanical and chemical stimulation. The current concept of pain maintains that, with myocardial ischemia and infarction, pain-producing substances are elaborated. These by-products of ischemic metabolism include potassium, hydrogen ions, lactate, and plasma kinins, the latter of which is thought to be activated by kallikrein. The receptors at the free ends of unmyelinated sympathetic afferent fibers are excited by these substances and transmit pain impulses to the spinal cord and cerebral cortex as outlined earlier. Stasis of blood flow secondary to coronary occlusion augments the concentration of these substances and potentiates nociception.

The clinical expression of chest pain involves a complex interplay of factors. In addition to cellular hypoxia, pain generation depends upon the frequency, density, and distribution of neuronal receptor stimulation. Increases in cardiac sympathetic nerve activity may not necessarily participate in pain production but, rather, may trigger excitatory reflexes manifesting as hypertension and tachycardia. From these observations, it has been proposed that receptors must attain a threshold level of stimulation in order to activate the sequence of nociceptive pathways. Moreover, the cortical recognition and processing of these stimuli is variable and likely contingent upon conditioned responses. Hence, these considerations may help to explain why patients experiencing acute myocardial ischemia and infarction demonstrate considerable disparity in their clinical expression of chest pain.

Coronary Prodrome

It is estimated that one-half of the mortality associated with acute myocardial infarction occurs prior to hospital admission [4–7]. Since most of these fatalities occur within the first hour of symptoms [7], a reduction in mortality is contingent upon out-of-hospital recognition of these individuals either before or within minutes of the acute event. In this regard, the history remains of paramount importance in alerting both patient and physician that coronary care should be initiated.

The reported incidence of prodromal symptoms prior to infarction or sudden death ranges from 10% to 60% [8], thus underscoring the importance of early recognition of warning symptoms when they are present. Solomon et al. [9] observed prodromal symptoms in 65% of patients admitted to the coronary care unit with acute myocardial infarction. Chest pain was present in

91% of cases and most individuals were noted to have preexisting angina. Alonzo et al. [10] studied antecedent symptoms in a population of 169 hospitalized patients with acute myocardial infarction and compared them with symptoms in 138 individuals who died prior to admission. Although two-thirds of subjects in both groups reported some warning symptoms, only 27% of the hospitalized cohort and 36% of the out-of-hospital group had consulted a physician. The mean duration of symptoms was 29 days in those who were admitted but only 10½ days in those who died before hospitalization. Older and chronically ill patients were more likely to seek medical attention than younger individuals. Stowers and Short [8] analyzed the prevalence of antecedent symptoms in the two-month period prior to acute myocardial infarction in 180 patients: 68% had prodromal symptoms (most commonly, chest pain), but only 21% with warning symptoms sought a physician's consultation. Furthermore, of one-third of those who visited a physician, they received only reassurance, thus emphasizing that delay in recognition of symptoms may occur at the patient or physician level.

In those with prodromal symptoms, chest pain is the commonest presenting feature [8–10]. A prior history of angina pectoris or precipitation by exercise are variable features. The pain of acute infarction typically persists for half an hour or longer. It is variable in intensity, although usually severe, and is not relieved by rest or sublingual nitroglycerin. It is commonly substernal in location and may radiate to both sides of the thorax, back, shoulders, arms, neck, and jaw. The quality of pain may be described as squeezing, oppressive, crushing, viselike, or choking. Patients occasionally mention a feeling of someone sitting or standing on the chest. Occasionally the discomfort may originate in the epigastrum and mimic a gastrointestinal disorder. In those with preexisting angina the pain is similar in quality and location but lasts longer, is more intense, and unresponsive to routine antianginal medications. Associated symptoms include diaphoresis, palpitations, breathlessness, a sensation of impending doom, and nausea and vomiting, the latter features being more characteristic of inferoposterior infarction.

It is important to appreciate that chest pain is not invariably present in patients with acute myocardial infarction. Painless infarcts have been reported in as many as 50% of patients with fatal and 30% of patients with nonfatal coronary events [11]. Painless infarcts have been reported to occur more often in diabetics, blacks, and in those with either atrial fibrillation or hypertension [11–14]. They are also more prevalent in patients with chronic hypoperfusion and low cardiac output who may be obtunded and therefore not acknowledge pain. Atypical presentations of acute infarction may include new-onset pulmonary edema, syncope, peripheral arterial embolism, sudden mania or psychosis, cardiac dysrhythmias, and a cerebrovascular accident [15].

The longer the interval between the occurrence of symptoms and time of questioning, the less likely is chest pain to be mentioned. The Western Collaborative Group Study [11] found a 30% prevalence of silent myocardial infarction in nonfatal cases, whereas Margolis et al. [12] documented a 17% prevalence of silent myocardial infarction in the Framingham series. This latter study revealed that silent infarction was rare in persons with prior angina, but not uncommon in those with hypertension or diabetes. Similar findings were confirmed by Medalie and Goldbourt [13], who also noted age and cigarette smoking to be correlated with unrecognized infarction. Finally, Uretsky and colleagues [14] found that 25.5% of patients admitted to the hospital with acute coronary events mentioned no pain. Their inhospital mortality was 50% compared with a similar group with antecedent pain whose mortality was 18%.

From the above discussion it is apparent that retrosternal chest pain is both an insensitive and nonspecific indicator of acute myocardial infarction. Patients with typical pain may prove to have acute coronary insufficiency or one of several noncardiac conditions that simulate acute infarction. Similarly, prodromal symptoms including chest pain may be absent in those with infarction documented by laboratory techniques. It is frequently difficult for both the patient and physician to determine whether acute myocardial infarction is occurring. Both should therefore maintain a high index of suspicion and move rapidly to initiate coronary care whenever prodromal symptoms are observed.

Management of Cardiac Pain

GENERAL MEASURES

In a patient with suspected myocardial infarction, one of the first therapeutic goals is to relieve chest pain. This is important not only for the comfort of the patient, but also to lessen the frequency of deleterious cardiovascular effects associated with enhanced autonomic nervous system activity. Increased sympathetic tone directly increases systemic blood pressure, heart rate, and the contractile state of the myocardium, all contributing to increased myocardial work and metabolic demands. In addition, elevated levels of circulating catecholamines may potentiate cardiac arrhythmias, particularly ventricular tachycardia or ventricular fibrillation [16, 17]. Maintenance of a quiet environment coupled with sedative hypnotics is a useful therapeutic measure.

As an adjunct in pain relief, coincident with admission to the coronary care unit the patient should be placed at bedrest for the first 24–48 h. Those individuals with an uncomplicated course may be permitted to use the bedside commode from time of admission. Enforced rest, particularly in bed, for uncomplicated patients beyond 48 h may predispose to complications. These include pulmonary emboli, decubitus ulcers, atelectasis, constipation, stress ulcers, impaired intake of fluids, and deconditioning. Avoidance of such complications is essential and limited activity should be initiated as soon as possible.

OXYGEN THERAPY

Patients with acute myocardial infarction often demonstrate arterial hypoxemia. This has been attributed to increased physiologic pulmonary dead space and to ventilation–perfusion abnormalities caused by left ventricular failure [18, 19]. Although decreased partial pressures of oxygen are most commonly observed in patients with infarction complicated by congestive heart failure, hypoxemia also occurs in individuals without clinically apparent left ventricular dysfunction [20]. For these reasons, the routine use of oxygen in all patients with acute myocardial infarction has been advocated.

Support for this approach comes from the experimental work of Maroko et al. [21], who have shown a reduction in infarct size with acute coronary occlusion in dogs treated with 40% oxygen inhalation. Clinically, Madias et al. [22] have demonstrated a reduction in both the magnitude and extent of ST-segment elevation in patients with anterior wall infarction exposed to 100% oxygen within 12 h after hospital admission. Discontinuation of oxygen was attended by a reduction in the electrocardiographic markers of ischemic damage.

The precise mechanism for oxygen's beneficial effect on cardiac muscle damaged by ischemia is uncertain although the major action appears to be a reduction in myocardial work. Oxygen is proposed to reduce the indices of myocardial contractility by enhanced oxygen delivery to border zones of ischemic tissue surrounding areas of irreversible cell injury [23, 24]. Salutary effects on ischemic muscle may also be mediated by hyperoxygenated blood coursing through collaterals and improved oxygen transport peripherally [25].

Several studies have noted possible detrimental hemodynamic effects of oxygen therapy in patients with myocardial infarction. In patients with arterial desaturation (S_AO_2 <90%), administration of oxygen increased oxygen transport to the tissues by augmenting cardiac output as well as oxygen content [24]. In individuals with no or only mild hypoxemia (S_AO_2 >90%), oxygen inhalation leads to an increase in systemic vascular resistance with a rise in systolic pressure and a lowering of cardiac output [26, 27].

In view of the possible adverse effects of oxygen therapy in patients without significant hypoxemia, it may be more prudent to restrict supplemental oxygen use to those patients with documented arterial desaturation (S_AO_2 <90%) by blood gas measurements at the time of admission to the coronary care unit. If blood gas determinations are not feasible, supplemental oxygen should be prescribed for all patients with acute ischemia or infarction. Withholding oxygen from patients with unsuspected hypoxemia is probably more hazardous than using it in patients without arterial hypoxemia.

Oxygen delivery should be effected either by nasal prongs at flow rates of $2-4$ l/min, or by mask designed to achieve $30\%-40\%$ inspired concentration. Due to the unproven efficacy of higher inspired oxygen concentrations and their potential for pulmonary toxicity, therapeutic interventions with concentrations greater than 40% are not routinely advised. Repeat blood gas analysis should be made to confirm the adequacy of therapy. Oxygen may be discontinued after correction of ventilation—perfusion abnormalities or after $24-48$ h when activity has been liberalized. Patients with severe hypoxemia and pulmonary edema or cardiogenic shock may require endotracheal intubation and high concentrations of inspired oxygen to achieve satisfactory oxygen saturations. Finally, caution should be exercised in treating patients with chronic obstructive pulmonary disease since mechanical ventilation may be needed if their hypoxic drive is eliminated (see chapter x). Precise oxygen delivery devices such as the ventimask should be considered in this population to reduce the risk of respiratory depression and impaired ventilation.

NITROUS OXIDE

Nitrous oxide is the oldest and most widely prescribed agent for inhalation-induced analgesia. It was first prepared in 1776 by Joseph Priestley and later combined with oxygen in 1868 as an anesthetic mixture for generalized pain relief. In 1881, Kilkovich introduced nitrous oxide for the treatment of anginal pain. Sporadic reports of its use followed until 1966, when it was employed in England for management of coronary pain and has been widely used in this capacity ever since.

In high concentrations, nitrous oxide produces surgical anesthesia and, in lower concentrations $(30\%-50\%)$, analgesia, amnesia, and alterations in consciousness. Its effectiveness as an analgesic has been favorably compared with morphine. Its actions are rapid and reversible and it is conducive to self-administration and is well tolerated [28]. It is especially beneficial in those with mild chest pain [29] and may be useful during recurrent prolonged bouts of discomfort. For these reasons, it has gained enthusiastic acceptance in Europe for relieving chest pain associated with myocardial ischemia and infarction [29, 30].

Nitrous oxide has been shown to exert a bene-

ficial effect on the balance between myocardial oxygen supply and oxygen demand [31, 32]. Lichtenthal et al. [31], who employed $30\%-50\%$ concentrations of nitrous oxide in normal volunteers and in patients with acute myocardial infarcts, found that mean blood pressure and heart rate declined while left ventricular performance indices were unchanged. Wynne and co-workers [32] investigated the effects of 50% nitrous oxide inhalation during cardiac catheterization in 30 patients, of whom 25 had coronary artery disease. Preangiographic measurements of hemodynamics and left ventricular performance using micromanometer-tipped catheters were secured. A small reduction in left ventricular stroke volume and dP/dT were noted and heart rate and the pressure—rate product declined significantly. There was no appreciable change in ejection fraction. The favorable cardiac effects of nitrous oxide are, therefore, related to its diminishing myocardial oxygen requirements. This response is thought to be mediated by a reduction in cardiac sympathetic stimulation due to the drug's sedative properties.

Despite the salutary actions of nitrous oxide, universal acceptance has not occurred and its routine use is not encouraged for several reasons. Its role in patients receiving morphine is limited because of a prominent fall in cardiac index when the two drugs are used concurrently [34]. Its clinical applicability is compromised because of untoward and often unpredictable effects including excessive sedation, respiratory depression, nausea and vomiting, and occasionally agitation and excitation. Therefore, more extensive investigation into the hemodynamic and clinical effects of nitrous oxide in patients with acute ischemia and infarction is required.

NARCOTIC ANALGESIA

Narcotic analgesic agents are essential in controlling chest discomfort during acute infarction. A variety of drugs have been utilized and include meperidine, pentazocine, butorphanol, nalbuphine, and morphine. This latter agent remains the preferred drug of choice except in patients with documented morphine hypersensitivity. It is the most potent analgesic agent currently available and has a long record of proven efficacy in acute coronary syndromes [35—37]. It should be administered intravenously in doses of 2−5 mg repeated every 5−10 min until sedation and relief of pain are witnessed or untoward effects ensue. Significant individual variability in dosing is well recognized with some patients requiring a cumulative dose as high as 2−3 mg/kg.

Morphine's beneficial effects are related to its reduction in autonomic nervous system activity [38−40]. Anxiety and restlessness are blunted by the combined withdrawal of sympathetic tone and augmentation of vagal tone. This in turn leads to increased venous capacitance, with a reduction in preload, and decreased arteriolar resistance, with a decline in afterload. Consequently, there is a reduction of oxygen consumption, myocardial work, and cardiac energy needs [38]. In contrast to the dog model, morphine does not increase coronary vascular resistance in humans and thus coronary blood flow is maintained. Moreover, a protective effect against malignant ventricular tachyarrhythmias has been documented [42].

Most individuals tolerate morphine well, although occasional patients may experience nausea or vomiting requiring treatment with antiemetics. Systemic hypotension has also been recorded that may be corrected by maintaining the individual in the supine position and elevating the legs [43]. If this proves insufficient, cautious infusion of fluids will usually restore filling pressures and raise the blood pressure. Hypotension may also occur in conjunction with bradycardia. This problem is more prevalent in patients with inferoposterior infarction, particularly with right ventricular involvement, and in those with intravascular volume depletion who are relying upon an elevated systemic vascular resistance to maintain blood pressure. In these circumstances, heightened vagal tone is potentiated by morphine and, atropine, in doses of 0.5 mg up to 2 mg intravenously, may be needed to abolish the drug's vagotonic influence.

Morphine reduces the work of breathing and respiratory rate via its sedative properties. A decrease in ventilation and a mild degree of hypoxemia are commonly encountered and should be routinely expected after its use [44]. Accentuation of underlying arterial hypoxemia might ensue and produce ventricular dysrhythmias. This underscores the importance of continuous ECG

monitoring and suggests that periodic measurement of arterial blood gases may be helpful. Marked respiratory depression, which is a feature of all narcotic agents, is a rare complication of morphine, especially in those with severe pain or pulmonary edema. In the even that significantly impaired ventilation is encountered, Narcan in doses of 0.4 mg intravenously at 5-min intervals to a maximum of 1.2 mg should be employed and is an effective opiate antagonist.

Meperidine, because of its atropinelike properties, has been preferred by some physicians particularly in patients with inferoposterior infarction and those with bradycardia or atrioventricular block. It reportedly produces less respiratory depression and nausea than does morphine. In our experience the incidence of side effects is equivalent to morphine and, since it is less effective as an analgesic, it offers no major advantage. Pentazocine and butorphanol may both increase systemic vascular resistance and myocardial metabolic demands and are therefore not recommended. Nalbuphine has been proposed as an alternative to morphine because of its equivalent analgesic potency and reduced propensity for respiratory depression. Although seemingly attractive, its acceptance should await further clinical evaluation of its cardiovascular effects during acute myocardial infarction.

NITROGLYCERIN

Since its introduction in 1879 for relief of angina, nitroglycerin has remained the cornerstone of therapy for chest pain secondary to coronary artery disease. It is a rapidly acting agent that is metabolized in the liver by the enzyme glutathione organic nitrate reductase. The metabolites of hepatic degradation have no significant vasoactive properties [45].

Nitroglycerin is a generalized vascular smooth muscle relaxant that acts at specific receptor sites in the vessel wall. Its proposed mechanism of vascular relaxation has recently been reviewed [46]. Vessel relaxation may occur by either a reduction of intracellular calcium or dephosphorylation of myosin light chains. Nitroglycerin inhibits thromboxane A_2 synthesis and enhances prostacyclin production, thereby leading to cyclic-AMP formation. This latter substance promotes vascular smooth muscle relaxation by lowering intracellular calcium. A second pathway by which nitrates produce vasodilation is through generation of cyclic GMP, a regulator of vascular smooth muscle calcium concentration.

The dominant effect of nitroglycerin is an increase in venous capacitance due to dilatation of veins and venules [47]. As a consequence, venous return to the right heart is decreased and left ventricular end-diastolic volume and stroke volume are reduced. In the systemic circulation, nitroglycerin mediates a fall in vascular resistance unless reflex vasoconstriction is pronounced. The same reduction in resistance is also seen in the pulmonary vasculature. There is no significant change in total coronary blood flow nor any direct effects on myocardial contractility or heart rate [48].

In response to the hemodynamic effects of nitroglycerin, reflex mechanisms may be activated that theoretically might increase myocardial oxygen consumption. A decline in stroke volume and blood pressure triggers arterial baroreceptors, which lead to increased sympathetic discharge manifesting as an increase in heart rate and cardiac contractility. Alternatively, the reduction in systolic wall stress engendered by lowering of preload and afterload may diminish myocardial demands. The net influence of nitrates on myocardial metabolic oxygen consumption therefore depends upon which of these effects predominate. The beneficial action of nitroglycerin in relieving chest pain associated with myocardial ischemia presumably occurs because of a net decrease in cardiac energy needs.

Several additional mechanisms have been suggested to explain the favorable effects of nitrates on the chest pain of myocardial ischemia. This agent may dilate intracoronary collateral channels and redistribute coronary blood flow with improved subendocardial perfusion in the ischemic zone [49]. Total transmural coronary blood flow is unchanged due to autoregulation of arteriolar flow in the setting of ischemia. Moreover, nitrates may produce vasodilation at the site of epicardial coronary stenosis, thereby improving antegrade flow and oxygen supply [50]. Finally, reversal of coronary artery spasm may also play a role in enhancing oxygen delivery [51].

During experimental acute myocardial infarction, favorable observations have been recorded following nitroglycerin administration. These include a reduction in ischemic injury, an improvement in segmental and global ventricular function, and a protective effect against ischemia-induced ventricular fibrillation [52]. As a result of these reports, a series of clinical investigations have been undertaken to evaluate the drug's safety and efficacy during acute myocardial infarction.

Clinical Studies. Kim and Williams [53] have studied the therapeutic benefit of large-dose sublingual nitroglycerin in patients with acute infarction. Using a mean total dose of 24 mg, they documented a reduction or resolution of chest discomfort in 13 of 15 subjects after 30 min. Furthermore, there was a significant decline in appearance and magnitude of Q waves on the electrocardiogram compared with a control group given morphine sulfate, thereby suggesting a reduction in infarct size. A related investigation employing intravenous nitroglycerin was recently reported by Roberts [48]: 85 patients with acute myocardial infarction were randomized prospectively to either nitrates or placebo administered within 12 h of admission. Patients receiving nitroglycerin were titrated to a hemodynamic end point (10% decrease in systolic pressure or systolic pressure of 95 mmHg) or a total dose of 200 μg/min and received the drug for 24 h. He noted a 36% reduction in estimated infarct size in patients with inferior infarction, but no appreciable effect in the cohort with anterior infarction. Infarct size was estimated by creatine kinase enzyme and isozyme analysis. The drug was well tolerated, with 7% of patients developing hypotension that was readily reversed. Flaherty and co-workers [49] assessed the effects of intravenous nitroglycerin on mortality and preservation of ischemic myocardium in 104 patients with acute infarction. A prospective randomized study design was used. They cited a beneficial myocardial protective effect only in those with small-to moderate-sized infarctions and only if treatment was initiated within 10 h from the onset of symptoms. Mortality, infarct extension, and the incidence of left ventricular failure were also lowered in the subgroup given nitroglycerin. Hypotension, rapidly corrected by cessation of therapy, occurred in 9% of patients.

In spite of these encouraging reports, the routine use of nitroglycerin in all patients with acute infarction is not recommended. A number of important and controversial issues require further clarification by clinical studies: the role of nitrates in modifying ischemic injury, their effects on ventricular function, better definition of the optimal dose and times of initiation and duration of therapy, and assessment of effectiveness in those with and without left ventricular failure. Currently, nitroglycerin should primarily be limited to patients (a) whose chest pain is not readily responsive to bedrest, oxygen, and narcotic analgesics, (b) who have left ventricular failure, and (c) who show evidence of coronary vasospasm.

Intravenous nitroglycerin is preferred over other routes of administration because of the drug's short half-life and ease of titration to desired clinical or hemodynamic end points [54]. In addition, it may be effective when sublingual dosing regimens have failed and offers the advantage of allowing patients to rest and sleep uninterrupted during use [55]. An initial dose of 10 μg/min is advocated with 10-μg/min increments every 5 min as needed for pain relief. Doses beyond 400 μg/min are seldom required. If pain is not controlled at this level of support, cardiac catheterization and supplemental interventions should be entertained. In our experience, the combination of a normal ECG during pain and refarctoriness to a 400-μg/min infusion of nitroglycerin is strongly predictive of insignificant coronary occlusive disease.

Well-recognized side effects of nitroglycerin include pulsatile headache, lightheadedness, nausea and vomiting, flushing, and palpitations. However, the most serious complication resulting from nitrate therapy is hypotension. Blood pressure typically drops a small degree in the supine position, but may fall profoundly if the patient is upright. Restoration of an adequate pressure can usually be effected by maintaining the patient in the supine position and elevating the legs. Hypotension is frequently accompanied by bradycardia due to sinus slowing or to high-degree AV block, and by syncope. Individuals with either anterior or inferoposterior infarctions may develop these complications. Come and Pitt [56] found seven episodes of severe systemic arterial hypotension and absolute or relative bradycardia in five out of 54 subjects with acute infarction given nitroglycerin. The mechanism for this response is uncertain. These investigators theorized that bradycardia was vagally mediated since it improved with atropine, that hypotension caused normal baroreceptor responses to fail to increase heart rate, or that sympathoinhibitory reflexes were activated. The disturbances in blood pressure and cardiac rhythm that may follow nitroglycerin use emphasize the importance of careful and continuous monitoring of these variables during drug administration.

Postinfarction Pain

The chest pain associated with acute myocardial infarction typically resolves within 24 h from the time of admission to the coronary care unit. Persistance or recurrence of pain after this period requires careful evaluation since both ischemic and nonischemic disorders may be responsible. This latter category includes pericarditis, which is often seen with Q-wave infarction; pleuritis, either secondary to Dressler's syndrome or less commonly, pulmonary embolism; costochondritis; aortic dissection, usually in conjunction with hypertension; and gastrointestinal disease, especially esophageal motility syndromes.

Postinfarction angina and threatened infarct extension, however, remain the foremost considerations in patients with recurrent chest pain. It may be difficult to diagnose true infarct extension although it tends to involve more severe pain, new ECG changes, signs of left ventricular failure, and reelevation of serum enzymes [57]. Postinfarction angina may have a higher incidence in those with non-Q-wave myocardial infarction [58].

The occurrence of postinfarction angina is an ominous prognostic event [59] and frequently heralds an unstable course characterized by infarct extension, left ventricular decompensation, and malignant ventricular tachyarrhythmias. In one study, Chaturvedi et al. [60] documented a 12% incidence of recurrent chest pain within 48 h after acute myocardial infarction. In this cohort, the three-month mortality was 25%. Schuster et al. [61] observed a 17% incidence of angina in association with ST-T-wave abnormalities within ten days of acute infarction and a 57% six-month mortality in this subgroup. On the basis of these reports and our own experience, we favor prompt cardiac catheterization in these high-risk patients with an orientation toward either intraaortic balloon support, percutaneous transluminal coronary angioplasty, or myocardial revascularization. Aggressive medical therapy with intravenous nitroglycerin, beta-blockers, and calcium channel blockers is recommended to help stabilize the patient, but these should not obviate the need to perform coronary angiography even if chest pain is eliminated.

References

1. Hood WB Jr: Pathophysiology of ischemic heart disease. Prog Cardiovasc Dis 14:297, 1971.

2. Malliani A, Lombardi F: Consideration of the fundamental mechanisms eliciting cardiac pain. Am Heart J 103:575, 1982.

3. Gorlin R: Pathophysiology of cardiac pain. Circulation 32:138, 1963.

4. Gordon T, Kannel WB: Premature mortality from coronary heart disease: the Framingham study. JAMA 215:1617, 1971.

5. Kuller L, Libenfeld A, Fisher R: Epidemiological study of sudden and unexpected deaths due to arteriosclerotic heart disease. Circulation 34:1056, 1966.

6. McNeilly RH, Pemberton J: Duration of last attack in 998 fatal cases of coronary artery disease and its relation to possible cardiac resuscitation. Br Med J 3:139, 1968.

7. Pantridge JF, Adgey AAJ, Geddes JS, Webb SW: Acute coronary attack. New York: Grune and Stratton, 1975.

8. Stowers M, Short D: Warning symptoms before major myocardial infarction. Br Heart J 32:833, 1970.

9. Solomon HA, Edwards AL, Killip T: Prodromata in acute myocardial infarction. Circulation 45:463, 1969.

10. Alonzo A, Simon AB, Feinlieb M: Prodromata of myocardial infarction and sudden death. Circulation 52:1056, 1975.

11. Rosenman RH, Friedman M, Jenkins CD, et al: Clinically unrecognized myocardial infarction in the Western Collaborative Group Study. Am J Cardiol 19:776, 1967.

12. Margolis JR, Kannel WB, Feinlieb M, Dauber TR, McNamara PM: Clinical features of unrecognized myocardial infarction—silent and symptomatic: eighteen years follow-up. The Framingham study. Am J Cardiol 32:1, 1973.

13. Medalie JH, Goldbourt V: Unrecognized myocardial infarction: five year incidence, mortality and risk factors. Ann Intern Med 84:526, 1976.

14. Uretsky BF, Farquhar DS, Besezin AF, Hood WB: Symptomatic myocardial infarction without chest pain: prevalence and clinical course. Am J Cardiol 40:498, 1977.

15. Bean WB: Masquerade of myocardial infarction. Lancet 1:1044, 1977.

16. Harris AS, Otero H, Bocage AJ: The induction of arrhythmias by sympathetic activity before and after occlusion of a coronary artery in the canine heart. J Electrocardiol 4:34, 1971.

17. Maling HM, Moran NC: Ventricular arrhythmias induced by sympathetic amines in unanesthetized dogs following coronary artery occlusion. Circ Res 5:409, 1957.

18. Fillmore SJ, Shapiro M, Killip T: Arterial oxygen tension in acute myocardial infarction: serial analysis of clinical state and blood gas changes. Am Heart J 79:620, 1970.

19. Hardy WE, Ayres SM, Keyloun V, et al: Causes of hypoxemia and alkalosis in acute myocardial infarction. Clin Res 16:370, 1968.

20. Valencia A, Burges HJ: Arterial hypoxemia following acute myocardial infarction. Circulation 40:641, 1969.

21. Maroko PR, Radvany P, Braunwald E, Hale SL: Reduction in infarct size by oxygen inhalation following acute coronary occlusion. Circulation 52:360, 1975.

22. Madias JE, Madias NE, Hood WB Jr: Precordial ST segment mapping-effects of oxygen inhalation on ischemic injury in patients with acute myocardial infarction. Circulation 53:411, 1976.

23. Ishikawa K, Sarma R, Getzen JH, McNair JD, Cosby FS: Fall in myocardial contractility following 100% oxygen breathing in patients with and without coronary artery disease [abstr]. Circulation (Suppl 4) 48:IV-180, 1973.

24. Sukumalchantra Y, Levy S, Danzig R, Rubins, Alpern H, Swan HJC: Correcting arterial hypoxemia by oxygen therapy in patients with acute myocardial infarction. Am J Cardiol 24:838, 1969.

25. Saijen JJ, Sheldon WF, Howitz O, Kuo PT, Peirce G, Zinsser HF, Mead J Jr: Studies of coronary disease in the experimental animal. II. Polaro-graphic determinations of local oxygen availability in the dog's left ventricle during coronary occlusion and pure oxygen breathing. J Clin Invest 30:932, 1951.

26. Thomas M, Malmerona R, Shillingford J: He-

modynamic effects of oxygen in patients with acute myocardial infarction. Br Heart J 27:401, 1965.

27. Wolk MJ, Scheidt S, Killip T: Heart failure complicating acute myocardial infarction. Circulation 45:1225, 1972.

28. Thal ER, Montgomery SJ, Atkins JM, Roberts BG: Self-administered analgesia with nitrous oxide. JAMA 242:2418, 1979.

29. Stern MS, Katz RL, McElroy CR, Shine KI: Nitrous oxide and oxygen in acute myocardial infarction. Circulation (Suppl 2) 58:171, 1978.

30. Kerr F, Brown MG, Irving JB, Hoskins MR, Ewing DJ, Kirby BJ: A double-blind trial of patient-controlled nitrous oxide/oxygen analgesia in myocardial infarction. Lancet 1397, 1975.

31. Lichtenthal P, Philip J, Gloss LJ, Gabel R, Lesch M: Administration of nitrous oxide in normal subjects. Chest 72:316, 1977.

32. Wynne J, Mann T, Alpert JS, Green LH, Grossman W: Haemodynamic effects of nitrous oxide administered during cardiac catheterization. JAMA 243:1440, 1980.

33. Parbrook G: Therapeutic uses of nitrous oxide. Br J Anaesth 40:365, 1968.

34. Eisele JH: Nitrous oxide administration and hemodynamics. Chest 72:271, 1977.

35. Lee G, De Maria AN, Amsterdam EA: et al: Comparative effects of morphine, meperidine and pentazocine on cardio-circulatory dynamics in patients with acute myocardial infarction. Am J Med 60:949, 1976.

36. Alderman EL: Analgesics in the acute phase of myocardial infarction. JAMA 229:1646, 1974.

37. Lal S, Savidge RS, Ghabra GP: Cardiovascular and respiratory effects of morphine and pentazocine in patients with myocardial infarction. Lancet 1:379, 1969.

38. Rouby JJ, Eurin B, Glaser P, et al: Hemodynamic and metabolic effects of morphine in the critically ill. Circulation 64:53, 1981.

39. Zelis R, Mansour EJ, Capone RJ, et al: The cardiovascular effects of morphine: the peripheral capacitance and resistance vessels in human subjects. J Clin Invest 54:1246, 1974.

40. Ward JM, McGrath RL, Weil JV: Effects of morphine on the peripheral vascular response to sympathetic stimulation. Am J Cardiol 29:659, 1972.

41. Leaman DM, Nellis SH, Zelis R, Field JM: Effects of morphine sulfate on human coronary blood flow. Am J Cardiol 41:324, 1978.

42. DeSilva RA, Verrier RL, Lown B: The effects of

psychological stress and vagal stimulation with morphine on vulnerability to ventricular fibrillation in the conscious dog. Am Heart J 95:197, 1978.

43. McIntyre KM, Lewis AJ: Textbook of advanced cardiac life support, ch 8. American Heart Association, 1981.

44. Weil MH, Anderson GJ: Thirteenth Bethesda conference: emergency cardiac care. Am J Cardiol 50:365, 1982.

45. Abrams J: Nitroglycerin and long-acting nitrates. N Engl J Med 302:1234, 1980.

46. Zelis R: Mechanisms of vasodilation in first North American conference on nitroglycerin therapy. Am J Med 74:3 − 12, 1983.

47. McGregor M: Pathogenesis of angina pectoris and role of nitrates in relief of myocardial ischemia in first North American conference on nitroglycerin therapy. Am J Med 74:21 − 27, 1983.

48. Roberts R: Intravenous nitroglycerin in acute myocardial infarction in first North American conference on nitroglycerin therapy. Am J Med 74:45 − 52, 1983.

49. Flaherty JT, Becker LC, Bulkley BH, Weiss JL, et al: A randomized prospective trial of intravenous nitroglycerin in patients with acute myocardial infarction. Circulation 68:576, 1983.

50. Brown BG, Bolson E, Petersen RB, Pierce CD, Dodge HT: The mechanisms of nitroglycerin action: stensosis vasodilation as a major component of the drug response. Circulation 64:1089, 1981.

51. Rentrop P, Blanke H, Hassck KR, et al: Selective intracoronary thrombolysis in acute myocardial infarction and unstable angina pectoris. Circulation 63:307, 1981.

52. Epstein SE, Kent KM, Goldstein RE, Boser JS, Redwood DR: Reduction of ischemic injury of nitroglycerin during acute myocardial infarction. N Engl J Med 292:29, 1975.

53. Kim YI, Williams JF: Large dose sublingual nitroglycerin in acute myocardial infarction: relief of chest pain and reduction of Q wave evaluation. Am J Cardiol 49:842, 1982.

54. Carfman GD, Heinsimer JA, Lozner EC, Fung HL: Intravenous nitroglycerin in the treatment of spontaneous angina pectoris: a prospective randomized trial. Circulation 67:276, 1973.

55. Mikolich JR, Nicoloff NB, Robinson PH, Logue RB: Relief of refractory angina with continuous intravenous infusion of nitroglycerin. Chest 77:375, 1980.

56. Come PC, Pitt B: Nitroglycerin induced severe

hypotension and bradycardia in patients with acute myocardial infarction. Circulation 54:624, 1976.

57. Alpert JS, Braunwald E: Pathological and clinical manifestations of acute myocardial infarction. In: Braunwald E (ed) Heart disease, ch 36. 1980.

58. Madigan NP, Rutherford BD, Frye RL: The clinical course, early prognosis and coronary anatomy of subendocardial infarction. Am J Med 60:634, 1976.

59. Epstein SE, Palmieri ST, Patterson RE: Evalua-

tion of patients after acute myocardial infarction: indications for cardiac catheterization and surgical intervention. N Engl J Med 307:1487, 1982.

60. Chaturvedi NC, Walsh MJ, Evans A, Munro P, Boyle DM, Barber JM: Selection of patients for early discharge after acute myocardial infarction. Br Heart J 36:533, 1974.

61. Schuster EH, Bulkey BH: Early post-infarction angina: ischemia at a distance and ischemia in the infarct zone. N Engl J Med 305:1101, 1981.

32. THE USE OF INTRAVENOUS ANTIVENTRICULAR ARRHYTHMIC AGENTS DURING ACUTE MYOCARDIAL INFARCTION

W. Wayne Stargel

Philip A. Routledge

Galen S. Wagner

The use of intravenous antiarrhythmic drugs in the setting of acute myocardial infarction is aimed at either preventive therapy (i.e., prophylaxis of ventricular fibrillation) or the treatment of documented atrial and ventricular arrhythmias. This chapter focuses on the rationale for both prophylactic and therapeutic use of intravenous antiarrhythmic agents in the management of ventricular tachyarrhythmias occurring in this acute clinical problem.

Rationale for Prophylactic Therapy

Ventricular fibrillation is the leading cause of sudden death following acute myocardial infarction. The incidence of ventricular fibrillation is approximately 3% — 10% in patients admitted to the coronary care unit with myocardial infarction but without clinical cardiac failure [1, 2], and this arrhythmia accounts for the majority of deaths prior to hospitalization [3]. The incidence of primary ventricular fibrillation (ventricular fibrillation without cardiac failure) decreases with time, with 60% — 90% of cases occurring within the first 6 h [1, 2] (see chapter 28). Therefore, early intervention is required if prophylactic therapy is to be beneficial. The abilities to pre-

vent ventricular fibrillation with medication and promptly treat with DC shock have had the greatest impact on reducing inhospital morbidity and mortality associated with acute myocardial infarction.

Coronary care units were first developed to decrease the incidence of sudden death in patients with myocardial infarction. The initial focus of therapy was prompt cardiopulmonary resuscitation and defibrillation when ventricular fibrillation occurred. Subsequently, the goal changed from treatment to prevention with prophylactic antiarrhythmics, the prototype being lidocaine.

One of the first studies of lidocaine prophylaxis by Lown et al. [4] documented that ventricular fibrillation did not occur in any of the 130 patients with acute myocardial infarction treated with lidocaine after "warning arrhythmias" had been documented. These warning arrhythmias consisted of (a) R-on-T phenomenon, (b) greater than 5 PVCs/min, (c) multiform configuration, and (d) 2 or more consecutive PVCs. These warning arrhythmias were initially considered to be important predictors of risk for ventricular fibrillation. However, subsequent studies showed that ventricular fibrillation frequently occurred without prior warning arrhythmias [5, 6].

R.M. Califf and G.S. Wagner (eds.), ACUTE CORONARY CARE: Principles and Practice. Copyright © 1985. Martinus Nijhoff Publishing, Boston/Dordrecht/Lancaster.

An important concern is the capability of the detection system used in coronary care units to monitor for warning arrhythmias. Several studies have shown that the coronary care unit staff does not adequately detect warning arrhythmias [7−9]. Even when the warning arrhythmias are detected, there may be insufficient time to administer prophylactic therapy.

These inabilities of (a) warning arrhythmias to accurately predict ventricular fibrillation, and (b) monitoring techniques to adequately detect warning arrhythmias, have prompted several investigators to advocate prophylactic use of intravenous lidocaine for all patients suspected of having an acute myocardial infarction [10−12].

Value of Prophylactic Lidocaine in the Hospital Phase

Numerous studies have attempted to show benefit of lidocaine prophylaxis, but most have had poor study design [13, 14]. Lie et al. [15], however, in a well-designed trial, demonstrated a distinct advantage of lidocaine prophylaxis in the prevention of ventricular fibrillation. This was a double-blind, randomized, placebo-controlled study that included 212 patients admitted within 6 h from the time of acute onset of chest pain. The group treated with lidocaine consisted of 107 patients who were administered a 100-mg bolus, followed by a maintenance infusion of 3 mg/min for 48 h. The placebo group received a continuous infusion of 5% dextrose in water. Both control and treatment groups were comparable in sex, age, site, and extent of infarction. There were no patients with either primary ventricular fibrillation or death in the lidocaine-treated group; in contrast, in the control group there were nine patients with primary ventricular fibrillation and one death. Four of the nine patients who experienced primary ventricular fibrillation demonstrated no warning arrhythmias, whereas 57 of the 96 control patients who did not develop ventricular fibrillation experienced warning arrhythmias.

Previous studies [16, 17] have reported that patients resuscitated from cardiac arrest had excellent short-term and long-term prognosis. This prompted the assumption that patients could be routinely resuscitated from episodes of ventricular fibrillation without adverse sequelae, thus eliminating the need for prophylactic antiarrhythmic agents. Conley et al. [18], however, studied myocardial infarct patients with cardiac arrests due to primary ventricular tachycardia or fibrillation, and reported that only 59% survived hospitalization, compared with an 88% survival rate in patients who did not experience cardiac arrest. This observation has recently been confirmed by Wyman et al. [19]. These studies further documented an increased long-term mortality rate in patients with a cardiac arrest. Cardiopulmonary resuscitation is also complicated by significant morbidity (i.e., fractured ribs, lacerated liver, increased infarct size, pneumothorax, hypoxic brain damage, and psychological trauma).

Therefore, numerous factors indicate that lidocaine prophylaxis in hospitalized patients with suspected myocardial infarction may be beneficial: (a) the inability to predict who will have ventricular fibrillation, (b) the increased short- and long-term mortality in patients experiencing cardiac arrest, (c) the morbidity of cardiopulmonary resuscitation, and (d) the ability of lidocaine to prevent primary ventricular fibrillation.

Value of Prophylactic Lidocaine in the Prehospital Phase

The greatest incidence of ventricular fibrillation occurs within the first few hours of onset of myocardial infarction and, therefore, the majority of deaths from ventricular fibrillation occur outside the hospital [3]. This has prompted the development of preventive programs designed to ensure the earliest possible administration of prophylactic lidocaine (see chapter 56). These preventive programs have examined the benefit of lidocaine administered intramuscularly in the first 6 h in hospital [20] or in the prehospital phase either by paramedical personnel [21, 22] or patient self-administration [23]. One prehospital program [21] reported a beneficial effect of 300 mg of lidocaine administered intramuscularly. This was a double-blind placebo-controlled study that involved 269 patients with suspected myocardial infarcts. During the first 2 h after the intramuscularly administered lidocaine there were three deaths among 156 patients, compared with eight deaths in 113 patients treated with placebo. Unfortunately, however, the discrepancy between the numbers in the treatment and placebo groups casts some doubt on the adequacy of randomization of this study.

In contrast, another double-blind, randomized study [20] showed no benefit of intramuscular lidocaine in 300 patients with acute myocardial infarcts. This study reported that six of 147 patients experienced ventricular fibrillation treated with lidocaine, compared with four of 153 control subjects given intramuscular saline. Although 300 mg of lidocaine had been administered, the plasma concentration was only 1.4 ± 0.7 mcg/ml (mean ± standard deviation) in those patients experiencing ventricular fibrillation. This suggested the need for higher intramuscular doses of lidocaine to obtain therapeutic concentrations.

A more recent study [22] examined paramedic administration (automatic injector) of higher doses (400 mg) of lidocaine intramuscularly in the prehospital phase of myocardial infarction. This double-blind, randomized placebo-controlled study examined 7504 patients with suspected myocardial infarction. The lidocaine-treated group consisted of 3191 patients of whom six patients experienced ventricular fibrillation. In contrast, the placebo group of 3224 patients demonstrated 16 patients with ventricular fibrillation. This study also reported termination of ventricular tachycardia in six of nine patients treated with lidocaine, and none of five patients treated with placebo. These results are encouraging and suggest that prophylactic lidocaine may offer benefits to the patient at high risk for prehospital ventricular fibrillation.

Lidocaine Pharmacokinetics

It is important to understand lidocaine pharmacokinetics to ensure safe and effective use [24]. The therapeutic range of lidocaine has been considered to be 1.5−5.0 mcg/ml, but there may be considerable overlap between the therapeutic and toxic plasma concentrations. Some patients may experience central nervous system toxicity with plasma concentrations as low as 3 mcg/ml, while other patients may require plasma concentrations of 8−10 mcg/ml to control their arrhythmias. Since the plasma concentration needed for effec-

tive prophylaxis is not known, the design of a dosage regimen should be aimed at achieving a concentration within the "therapeutic range" of 1.5−5.0 mcg/ml.

Lidocaine plasma concentrations decline in a biphasic pattern after intravenous administration. There is an initial rapid decline ("distributive phase") wherein plasma concentration decreases with a half-life of 4−12 min. This occurs because of rapid equilibration between plasma and highly perfused tissues (i.e., liver, lungs). Subsequently, the slower decline is referred to as the "elimination phase" and has a half-life of approximately 120 min. This slower elimination phase represents the removal of lidocaine from the body, primarily regulated by hepatic metabolism.

Plasma concentrations after a loading dose of lidocaine are inversely related to the volume of distribution (plasma concentration = $\frac{\text{loading dose}}{\text{volume of distribution}}$). Factors known to decrease the volume of distribution will require adjustments in the loading dose to avoid high plasma concentrations and possible toxicity. This is best illustrated by patients with cardiac failure who have a lower volume of distribution and therefore require smaller loading doses of lidocaine. The reduction in the volume of distribution in cardiac failure may partially be explained by decrease in tissue perfusion, which results in an overall decrease in tissue drug uptake.

Following a loading dose of lidocaine, patients are given a continuous infusion to maintain adequate plasma concentrations. During maintenance infusion of lidocaine the pharmacokinetic process of "clearance" is primarily responsible for elimination and accumulation. Clearance of lidocaine is predominately dependent upon hepatic metabolism, with less than 10% being excreted as unchanged drug by the kidney. The hepatic metabolism of lidocaine is primarily dependent upon hepatic blood flow, and factors known to decrease this flow will decrease the clearance of lidocaine (i.e., cardiac failure, beta-blocking agents, and cimetidine).

Lidocaine Dosing Regimens

Lidocaine regimens should consist of a loading dose to achieve a rapid therapeutic effect, fol-

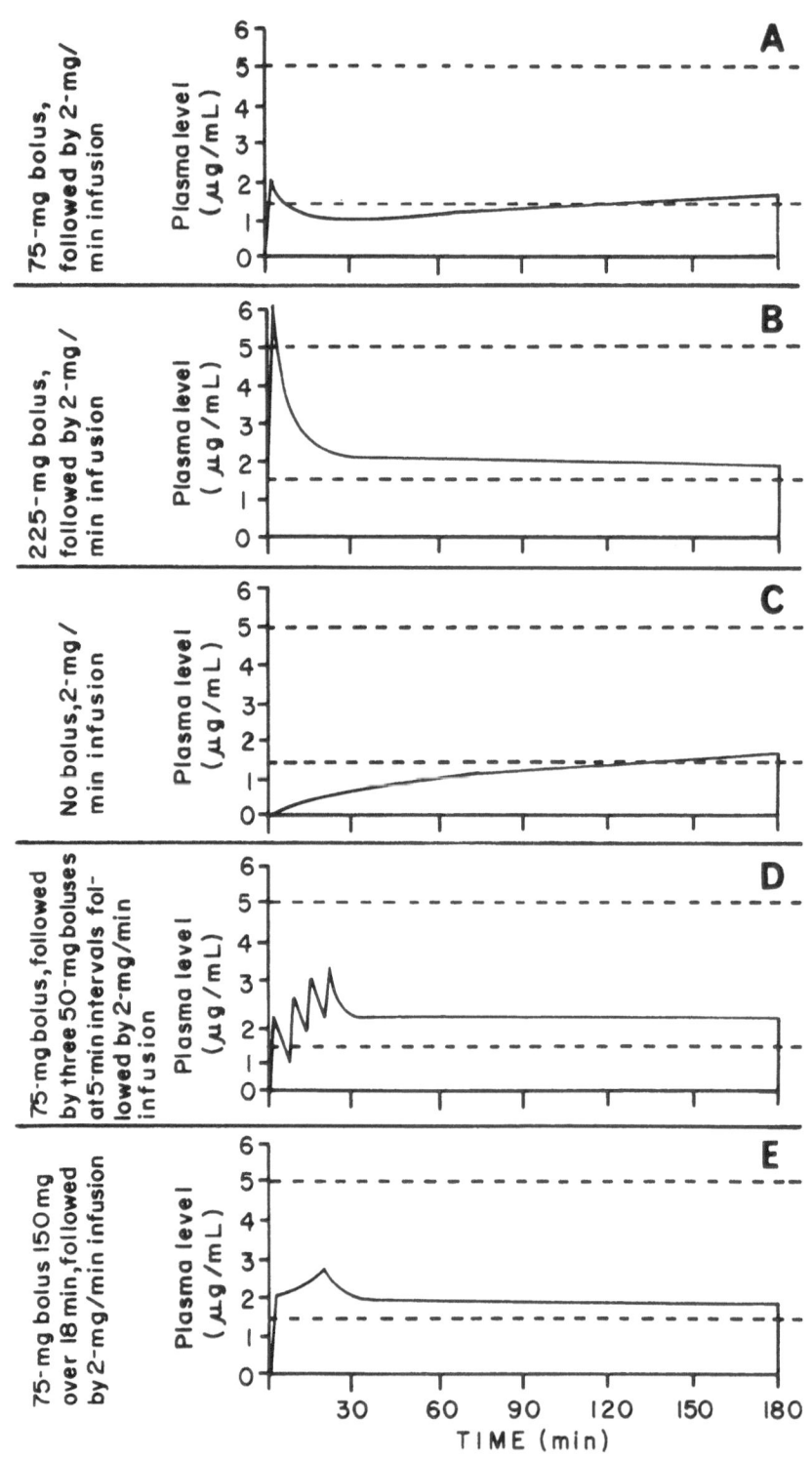

FIGURE 32-1 (A–E). Lidocaine plasma levels after various dosage regimens: ------ upper and lower limits of the therapeutic range of lidocaine; _____ plasma levels simulated from the dosage regimens accompanying each panel

lowed by a continuous infusion to maintain adequate plasma concentrations. Although numerous dosage regimens have been proposed for intravenous administration of lidocaine, certain pitfalls in regimen design may result in either toxicity or ineffective therapy. One of the most common recommended dosage regimens consists of a single intravenous bolus of 75—100 mg followed by a maintenance infusion of 2 mg/min (figure 32-1A). This regimen will usually rapidly achieve a therapeutic plasma concentration (1.5—5.0 mg/ml) after the initial bolus. Because of the fast distributive phase (half-life 4—12 min), however, the concentration will then fall below the minimum effective concentration. This drop in plasma concentration within the first hour may have accounted for the labeling of patients as "resistant to lidocaine." A regimen designed to administer an initial larger bolus to saturate the body tissues is not possible because of the high incidence of central nervous system toxicity (figure 32-1B). Initiating a continuous infusion of 2—4 mg/min without a loading dose is equally unacceptable, due to the delay of obtaining therapeutic plasma concentrations (figure 32-1C). A continuous infusion of lidocaine will take approximately 4—5 half-lives (8—10 h) to achieve a steady state and will, therefore, result in subtherapeutic concentrations during those initial hours when the incidence of ventricular fibrillation is the highest.

These considerations prompted the development of several methods designed to rapidly achieve and maintain therapeutic plasma concentrations. One such regimen consists of administering a loading dose of 225 mg over 20 min, followed by a continuous infusion of 2 mg/min. The loading dose may be administered by two methods: (a) 75-mg bolus given over 2 min followed by 50-mg boluses (over 1 min) administered at 5-min intervals, for a total of 225 mg over 20 min (figure 32-1D), or (b) 75-mg bolus (over 2 min) followed by 150-mg infusion administered over 18 min (8.33 mg/min) (figure 32-1E). Although both regimens are effective in obtaining adequate plasma concentrations, method (b) has been reported to cause less central nervous system toxicity [25]. However, regimen (b) may be too complex for routine administration. Therefore, the multiple-bolus regimen (a) may be the clinical method of choice.

The initial maintenance infusion of lidocaine (usually 2 mg/min) has been recommended to be continued for 36—48 h following onset of acute myocardial infarction [11]. Even this duration of prophylactic therapy may be excessive, however, since the majority of instances of primary ventricular fibrillation occur within the initial 24 h [1]. When the decision has been made to institute postinfarction antiventricular arrhythmia therapy, lidocaine maintenance infusion should be continued until adequate plasma concentrations of an oral agent have been obtained. When lidocaine is discontinued, no "tapering" of the drop is required, and it is important to observe a "lidocaine-free" period via continuous ECG monitoring before this monitoring, and "acute coronary care" in general, is discontinued.

Other Antiarrhythmic Agents for Prophylaxis of Primary Ventricular Fibrillation

Several agents other than lidocaine have been examined in the prophylaxis of primary ventricular fibrillation during acute myocardial infarction. These include phenytoin, disopyramide, tocainide, mexiletine, oxprenolol, and atenolol. None of these drugs has been shown to be effective in prophylaxis, although some have reduced the incidence of other ventricular tachyarrhythmias. Lidocaine therefore remains the only antiarrhythmic agent presently available that has been proven to be effective for prophylaxis of ventricular fibrillation.

Antiarrhythmic Agents in the Treatment of Established Arrhythmias

PROCAINAMIDE

Procainamide is a widely used antiarrhythmic agent in the treatment of both supraventricular and ventricular arrhythmias. It is generally reserved in the setting of acute infarction for the patient with ventricular arrhythmias refractory to lidocaine, or with lidocaine intolerance. The "therapeutic range" of procainamide has been reported to be 4—10 mcg/ml [26], but recent studies suggest some patients may require higher plasma concentrations for refractory arrhythmias [27]. The significance of this "therapeutic range" has been further complicated by an active metabolite of procainamide produced by the liver called N-acetylprocainamide (NAPA). Although some investigators have suggested adjustments in the dose of procainamide based on the concentration of NAPA, its contribution to the antiarrhythmic effects of procainamide remains unclear [28].

Procainamide plasma concentrations decline after intravenous administration in a biphasic pattern similar to those of lidocaine. The rapid distributive phase of procainamide has a half-life of approximately 5 min, and is the result of equilibration between plasma and highly perfused tissues (i.e., brain, heart, kidney). The slower elimination phase represents the removal of procainamide from the body. Elimination of procainamide is controlled about equally by both renal and hepatic mechanisms. The acetylation of procainamide (to NAPA) in the liver is under genetic control, with patients being classified as "fast acetylators" or "slow acetylators." Generally the North American population is bimodally distributed with half the population being fast and half being slow acetylators of procainamide. Slow acetylators will have higher procainamide concentrations in relation to NAPA, while fast acetylators will have higher NAPA concentrations than procainamide. Since the therapeutic effects of NAPA are uncertain [28], fast acetylators may or may not require additional procainamide dosages to attain the desired therapeutic effects.

Acetylation capability is clinically important primarily in the presence of renal insufficiency when prolonged procainamide infusion is maintained. NAPA is 80%−85% eliminated unchanged by the kidneys, with a half-life of 6 h with normal renal function. Therefore, rapidly acetylating patients with renal failure may have marked accumulation of NAPA with half-life prolonging to as long as 40 h, and may experience toxic effects. All patients with renal failure should receive decreased procainamide dosage. Because of the potential for extremely high NAPA levels, the procainamide dosage should be markedly decreased in rapid acetylators with renal failure.

Intravenous administration of procainamide was initially reported to produce serious side effects (i.e., profound hypotension, heart block,

arrhythmias) because of too rapid administration. Two regimens have been proposed for the safe administration of procainamide: a series of short infusions, or a loading infusion followed by a maintenance infusion.

One method commonly used is to administer 100-mg boluses of procainamide over 2-min periods every 5 min until (a) adequate control of the arrhythmia, (b) side effects, or (c) a cumulative dose of 1000 mg is reached [26]. This is generally followed by a maintenance infusion of 2 mg/min. Another approach is to administer 17 mg/kg over 1 h, followed by a continuous infusion of 2.8 mg/kg/h [29]. Both the loading and maintenance doses should be reduced by one- to two-thirds, depending on the degree of heart failure. However, only the maintenance infusion should be reduced in patients with renal insufficiency because they have a normal volume of distribution. Due to the large variability in procainamide pharmacokinetics, general dosage recommendations are difficult and most often inaccurate. Therefore, close monitoring of the patient's plasma procainamide levels, hemodynamics, and electrocardiogram is required.

BRETYLIUM

Bretylium is a quarternary ammonium compound which has been documented to be useful in both preventing and treating ventricuar tachycardia and ventricular fibrillation. Although generally reserved for the treatment of ventricular arrhythmias refractory to both lidocaine and procainamide, bretylium should be considered early in the treatment of patients with recurrent ventricular fibrillation. The therapeutic range for bretylium has not been studied as adequately as that of other antiarrhythmics. Therefore most dosage regimens are empiric with some patients requiring relatively large doses.

Bretylium plasma concentrations decline in a biphasic pattern after intravenous administration. The initial rapid decline (distributive phase) has a half-life of approximately 30 min, the slower decline (elimination phase) has a half-life that is dependent upon the patient's renal function. Patients with normal renal function have an elimination half-life of approximately 7−10 h, whereas patients with end-stage renal failure may have a half-life of greater than 80 h [30]. Bretylium is primarily excreted unchanged, and a recent study showed a strong correlation between bretylium and creatine clearances. Although adjustment of the dose of bretylium is recommended for patients in renal insufficiency, there is little information available on how to accomplish this goal.

In patients with ventricular fibrillation it is recommended to administer an undiluted rapid intravenous bolus of 5 mg/kg followed by electrical defibrillation. If ventricular fibrillation persists, the bretylium dose may be increased to 10 mg/kg and repeated as necessary. In patients treated for refractory ventricular tachycardia, a bretylium dose of 5 − 10 mg/kg should be diluted in 50 ml and administered over approximately 10 min. Faster intravenous administration may result in nausea and vomiting. If the ventricular tachycardia does not respond to the initial dose, another dose of 5 − 10 mg/kg can be repeated in 30 − 60 min and, if necessary, subsequent boluses may be tried. If the ventricular arrhythmia is controlled by bretylium, several methods are available for maintenance therapy. The first is to give the effective dose every 6 − 8 h. Another method is to administer bretylium by a continuous infusion of 1 − 2 mg/min. Until further information is available on adjustments of bretylium in various conditions (i.e., renal failure), the dosage regimen is only guided by clinical response and toxicity. The toxicities of bretylium primarily involve the cardiovascular system. Bretylium is a postganglionic adrenergic blocking drug that produces a biphasic pattern of events on the cardiovascular system after intravenous administration. The first phase after intravenous administration is an increase in heart rate and blood pressure. This is a result of the initial release of catecholamines from the adrenergic neuron, and is generally short-lived (approximately 20 min). This is followed by the second phase, during which postural hypotension is the most common adverse effect. This occurs as a result of peripheral vascular adrenergic blockade. The other common side effect is nausea and vomiting that can occur from too rapid intravenous administration.

PHENYTOIN

Phenytoin is an anticonvulsant with electrophysiologic effects on the heart similar to those of lidocaine. It has limited value in the treatment of ventricular tachyarrhythmias after myocardial infarction [31]. Because of phenytoin's low therapeutic to toxic ratio, the loading dose of 15 mg/kg should be given very slowly at a rate not exceeding 50 mg/min. Because of the alkaline pH of the solution, great care should be taken to avoid perivascular extravasation or accidental intraarterial administration. Thereafter, the drug is normally given orally, 95% of the dose being metabolized by the liver. The clearance of phenytoin is dose dependent and variable between individuals so that the maintenance dose must be individually adjusted with a therapeutic plasma concentration range (10 − 20 mcg/ml) being helpful in avoiding long-term toxicity. Adverse effects of acute intravenous administration are respiratory arrest, hypotension, asystole, heart block, and ventricular fibrillation, which are more likely when the drug is administered too rapidly.

MEXILETINE

Mexiletine has not yet been approved in the United States, but has been shown to abolish ventricular arrhythmias when given to patients with acute myocardial infarction [32]. In this study, mexiletine was effective in over half the patients who had not responded to lidocaine. Because of its very large distribution volume (about 400 l in the adult) and its long elimination half-life (10 − 20 h), it is necessary to give a loading dose before the maintenance infusion. One recommended regimen is to give 100 − 250 mg over 5 − 10 min, then 250 mg (as a 0.1% solution) over 1 h, 125 mg/h for 2 h, and finally the maintenance infusion. Since the average plasma drug clearance is approximately 450 ml/min, the average maintenance infusion required to keep the patient within the therapeutic range (0.75 − 2.0 mcg/ml) is 500 mcg/min (0.5 mg/min). Mexiletine is primarily (80% − 90%) cleared via hepatic metabolism. Clearance may be increased in patients receiving phenytoin and rifampin because of the effects of these agents in enhancing the hepatic metabolism of mexiletine. Clearance is likely to be decreased in patients with liver disease and in cardiac failure.

Mexiletine has a narrow therapeutic ratio and adverse effects have been reported involving the gastrointestinal system (e.g., nausea and vomiting), the central nervous system (e.g., tremor, ataxia, and convulsions) and cardiovascular system (e.g., hypotension, bradycardia, complete heart block, and worsening of left ventricular function). The drug should therefore be used with caution in patients with sinus node dysfunction, conduction defect, bradycardia, or hypotension. Judicious use of plasma-level monitoring may help to avoid adverse effects that are in part concentration related.

TOCAINIDE

Tocainide, another experimental agent in the United States, has also been shown to be effective in suppressing ventricular arrhythmias in patients with acute myocardial infarction [33]. It is an analogue of lidocaine with similar activity but, because of its high bioavailability (about 100%), it can also be administered orally during chronic therapy. A recommended tocainide loading regimen would be 500−750 mg over 15−20 min intravenously followed immediately by 600−800 mg orally. If continuous intravenous maintenance therapy is required, the range of plasma clearances (115−170 ml/min) indicates that an infusion rate of 1 mg/min maintains most patients within the therapeutic range of 4−10 mcg/ml [33]. However, loading is not necessary, and initiation of the daily oral maintenance will rapidly achieve therapeutic plasma concentrations; 60% of the administered dose is cleared by hepatic metabolism to metabolites that appear to have little antiarrhythmic activity. There is little information concerning factors affecting the hepatic clearance of the drug so it should be used with caution in patients with severe liver disease or cardiac failure; 40% of the drug is cleared by renal elimination of unchanged drug, which occurs by active tubular secretion as well as by glomerular filtration. Urinary alkalinization, by reducing the passive reabsorption of tocainide from the renal tubular fluid, can reduce the renal clearance of the drug. In moderate severe renal failure (creatinine clearance below 30 ml/min), a 25% reduction in dose is recommended. The drug is approximately 50% protein bound in plasma and it is unlikely therefore that marked variability in the percentage of drug in the free form will occur.

Adverse effects of tocainide are similar to those occurring with lidocaine, but tend to be less severe. They include tremor, dizziness, paresthesia, convulsions, nausea and vomiting, bradycardia, and hypotension. Very rarely lupus erythematosuslike syndrome, rash and fever, hepatitis, transient neutropenia agranulocytosis, or fibrosing alveolitis may occur. The gastrointestinal and neurologic adverse effects are often related to high plasma concentrations and may be minimized by monitoring the plasma levels.

References

1. Lawrie DM, Higgins MR, Godman MJ, Oliver MF, Julian DG, Donald KW: Ventricular fibrillation complicating acute myocardial infarction. Lancet 2:523−528, 1968.
2. Morgensen L: Ventricular tachyarrhythmias and lignocaine prophylaxis in acute myocardial infarction. Acta Med Scand (Suppl) 513:1−29, 1970.
3. Pantridge JF, Adgey AAJ: Pre-hospital coronary care: the mobile coronary care unit. Am J Cardiol 24:666−673, 1969.
4. Lown B, Fakhro AM, Hood WB, Thorn GW: The coronary care unit: new perspectives and direction. JAMA 199:188−198, 1967.
5. Lie KI, Wellens HJJ, Downar E, Durrer D: Observations on patients with ventricular fibrillation complicating acute myocardial infarction. Circulation 52:755−759, 1975.
6. El-Sherif N, Myerburg RJ, Scherlag BJ, Befeler B, Aranda JM, Castellanos A, Lazzara R: Electrocardiographic antecedents of primary ventricular fibrillation: value of the R-on-T phenomenon in myocardial infarction. Br Heart J 38:415−422, 1976.
7. Romhilt DW, Bloomfield SS, Chou TC, Fowler NO: Unreliability of conventional electrocardiographic monitoring for arrhythmia detection in coronary care units. Am J Cardiol 31:457−461, 1973.
8. Ryden L, Waldenstrom A, Holmberg S: The reliability of intermittent ECG sampling in arrhythmia detection. Circulation 52:540−545, 1975.
9. Lindsay J Jr, Bruckner NV: Conventional coronary care unit monitoring: non-detection of transient rhythm disturbances. JAMA 232:51−53, 1975.
10. Ribner HS, Isaacs ES, Frishman W: Lidocaine prophylaxis against ventricular fibrillation in

acute myocardial infarction. Prog Cardiovasc Dis 21:287–313, 1979.

11. Noneman JW, Rogers JF: Lidocaine prophylaxis in acute myocardial infarction. Medicine 57: 501–515, 1978.

12. Harrison DC: Should lidocaine be administered routinely to all patients after acute myocardial infarction? Circulation 58:581–584, 1978.

13. Bennett MA, Wilner JM, Pentecost BL: Controlled trial of lignocaine in prophylaxis of ventricular arrhythmias complicating myocardial infarction. Lancet 2:909–911, 1970.

14. Bleifeld W, Merx W, Heinrich KW, Effert S: Controlled trial of prophylactic treatment with lidocaine in acute myocardial infarction. Eur J Clin Pharmacol 6:119–126, 1973.

15. Lie KI, Wellens HJ, Van Capelle FJ, Durrer D: Lidocaine in the prevention of primary ventricular fibrillation. N Engl J Med 291:1324–1326, 1974.

16. Dupont B, Flensted-Jensen E, Sandoe E: The long-term prognosis for patients resuscitated after cardiac arrest. Am Heart J 78:444–449, 1969.

17. Geddes JS, Adgey AAJ, Pantridge JF: Prognosis after recovery from ventricular fibrillation complicating ischemic heart disease. Lancet 2:273–275, 1967.

18. Conley MJ, McNeer JF, Lee KL: Cardiac arrest complicating acute myocardial infarction: predictability and prognosis. Am J Cardiol 39: 7–12, 1977.

19. Wyman MG, Cardinale M, Goldreyer BN, Cannom DS: Primary ventricular may be hazardous to your health [abstr]. Circulation (Suppl 3) 68: 107, 1983.

20. Lie KI, Liem KL, Louridtz WJ, Janse MJ, Willebrands AF, Durrer D: Efficacy of lidocaine in preventing primary ventricular fibrillation within 1 hour after 300 mg intramuscular injection. Am J of Cardiol 42:486–488, 1978.

21. Valentine PA, Frew JL, Mashford ML, Sloman JG: Lidocaine in the prevention of sudden death in the prevention pre-hospital phase of acute infarction. N Engl J Med 291:1327–1331, 1974.

22. Koster RW, Dunning AJ: Pre-hospital prevention of ventricular fibrillation in acute myocardial infarction [abstr]. Circulation (Suppl 3) 68: 275, 1983.

23. Capone RJ, Visco J, Curwen E, Van Every S: Patient activated pre-hospital system for prevention of coronary death [abstr]. Circulation (Suppl 4) 64:188, 1981.

24. Benowitz NL, and Meister W: Clinical pharmacokinetics of lignocaine. Clin Pharmacokinet 3: 177–201, 1978.

25. Stargel WW, Shand DG, Routledge PA, Barchowsky A, Wagner GS: Clinical comparison of rapid infusion and multiple injection methods for lidocaine loading. Am Heart J 102:872–876, 1981.

26. Giardina EGV, Heissenbuttel RH, Bigger JT Jr: Intermittent intravenous procainamide to treat ventricular arrhythmias: correlation of plasma concentration with effect on arrhythmia, electrocardiogram, and blood pressure. Ann Intern Med 78:183–193, 1973.

27. Greenspan AM, Horowitz LN, Spielman SR, Josephson ME: Large dose procainamide therapy for ventricular tachyarrhythmia. Am J Cardiol 46:453–462, 19801.

28. Roden DM, Reele SB, Higgins SB, Wilkinson GR, Smith RF, Oates JA, Woosley RL: Antiarrhythmia efficacy, pharmacokinetics and safety of N-acetylprocainamide in human subjects: comparison with procainamide. Am J Cardiol 46: 463–468, 1980.

29. Lima JJ, Conti DR, Goldfarb AL, Golden LH, Jusko WJ: Pharmacokinetic approach to intravenous procainamide therapy. Eur J Clin Pharmacol 13:303–308, 1978.

30. Josselson J, Narang PK, Adir J, Yacobi A, Sadler JH: Bretylium kinetics in renal insufficiency. Clin Pharmacol Ther 33:144–150, 1983.

31. Wit AL, Rosen MR, Hoffman BF: Electrophysiology and pharmacology of cardiac arrhythmias. VIII. Cardiac effects of diphenyl hydantoin. Am Heart J 90:397, 1975.

32. Campbell NPS, Chaturvedi NC, Kelly JG, Strong JE, Shanks RG, Pantridge JF: Mexiletine in the management of ventricular dysrhythmias. Lancet 2:404–407, 1973.

33. Nyquist O, Forssell G, Nordlander R, Schenck-Gustufson K: Hemodynamic and antiarrhythmic effets of tocainide in patients with acute myocardial infarction. Am Heart J 100:1000–1005, 1980.

33. THE CLINICAL USE OF
THROMBOLYTIC AGENTS

David S. Grierson

Robert M. Califf

Galen S. Wagner

Thrombolytic therapy for patients with acute myocardial ischemia and infarction is undergoing such a rapid evolution that the evaluation of currently available clinical results may not apply to clinical practice in the near future. The procedure itself, as well as ancillary drugs and criteria for patient selection, are changing for both intravenous and intracoronary streptokinase administration. New thrombolytic agents are being developed that may dramatically alter clinical practice. The management of the patient after successful thrombolysis is also evolving rapidly. Despite these factors that limit the relevance of past studies, the clinician must make decisions about current patients with available data. Furthermore, a review of previous studies will enable the reader to interpret future studies more easily. In this chapter, the generic problems with clinical trials of thrombolytic therapy are outlined, and the current results of trials involving intracoronary and intravenous streptokinase are reviewed. Finally, the clinical application of thrombolytic therapy at Duke University Medical Center is outlined.

Methodologic Considerations

A major problem with the evaluation of clinical trials involving streptokinase, especially by the intracoronary route, is the variability in the technique used [1]. Table 33-1 lists the major aspects of technique in which differences exist. Recent trends have included more frequent use of mechanical recanalization, higher total doses and concentrations of drug, continued infusion after clot lysis, and infusions using selective catheters. In addition, different approaches to the use of supporting drugs such as heparin, intravenous and intracoronary nitroglycerin, and calcium channel blockers have been advocated by particular investigators. With intravenous therapy, a clear trend toward more rapid infusion of higher doses of thrombolytic agents is evident. Unfortunately, the impact of these variations in technique upon outcome cannot be estimated, since no controlled studies comparing one method to another are available.

Perhaps even more important than the technique of the thrombolytic procedure is the approach to the patient after successful reperfusion (table 33-2). Varying approaches to the duration and intensity of anticoagulation may affect recurrent infarction and/or complication rates. Most investigators are using antiplatelet agents, although the particular drugs and dosages are variable (see chapter 16). Some investigators are performing angioplasty during the same procedure as streptokinase administration [2], others consider angioplasty later, while others do not perform repeat angiography in the absence of objective evidence of ischemia on functional testing or recurrent symptoms. Similar differences

R.M. Califf and G.S. Wagner (eds.), ACUTE CORONARY CARE: Principles and Practice. Copyright © 1985. Martinus Nijhoff Publishing, Boston/Dordrecht/Lancaster.

with respect to the application of coronary artery bypass grafting are found [3]. Finally, the relative benefit of beta-blocking drugs in patients after thrombolytic therapy is not known. All studies of these drugs in post myocardial infarction (MI) patients reported to date have involved non-reperfused patients.

In addition to differences in the procedure and post-procedure care, the particular protocol used to identify and enter patients could have a dramatic effect on outcome. Animal studies have clearly established the importance of time to reperfusion and collateral flow as the primary determinants of the amount of myocardium salvaged [4]. When patients present for coronary care late after the onset of symptoms or when the delay from identification of the patient to initiation of thrombolytic therapy is prolonged, the therapeutic effect should be diminished. When the status of the arterial occlusion is not established by pretreatment cardiac catheterization, one must assume that 15%−30% of patients have patent vessels prior to thrombolytic therapy [5].

Table 33-3 lists the commonly used end points in clinical trials of streptokinase therapy. The rationale for the use of ventricular function as an end point is clear: if perfusion has a favorable effect on patient outcome, the mechanism for this benefit should be the salvage of myocardium. Attempts to measure the amount of "myocardium salvaged" make a measure of presumed myocardium in jeopardy in the acute state, usually with thallium-201 perfusion imaging [6]. After therapy the amount of myocardium remaining viable and perfused compared with the amount that was in jeopardy can be assessed. Measurement of estimated final infarct size in a treated group compared with a control group with radionuclide angiography or cardiac catheterization remains the most common method of assessing therapeutic efficacy. However, little improvement in global left ventricular function has been identified in the available studies [7]. Stack et al. [8] and Sheehan et al. [9] have demonstrated significant improvement in function in the region supplied by the recanalized artery despite no improvement in global function. These investigators suggest that the lack of improvement in global function is not due to

TABLE 33-1. Intracoronary streptokinase: sources of variability in methods

Intracoronary nitroglycerin (NTG)
Mechanical recanalization
Dosage
Infusion rate
Duration of infusion
Selective vs subselective infusion
Supporting drugs (heparin, NTG, nifedipine)

TABLE 33-2. Successful intracoronary streptokinase variables in postintervention care

Anticoagulation
Antiplatelet agents
Angioplasty
Coronary artery bypass grafting
Beta-blockers

TABLE 33-3. End points of thrombolytic trials

"Amount salvaged"
Thallium, *positron emission tomography (PET) *Nuclear magnetic resonance (NMR)
"Infarct size"
Enzyme, QRS change
Global left ventricular function (catheterization, radionuclide angiography)
Regional left ventricular function (catheterization, radionuclide angiography)
Imaging of infarcted or nonperfused tissue (thallium, *NMR, *PET, *antimyosin antibody)
Death
Recurrent infarction
Functional status
Angina, exercise capacity, disability, "quality of life"

*Not yet clinically available.

failure to attain the therapeutic goal of myocardial salvage, but rather that improved function in the jeopardized region is masked by a reduction in the compensatory hypercontractility in the uninvolved regions (see chapter 34). These favorable findings on ventricular function may not necessarily result in better functional status or lower mortality, especially when residual stenoses are present with the subsequent risk of reinfarction. Difficulty in interpretation may arise when treated patients appear to be improved with respect to one end point (ventricular function) and worsened with respect to another end point (mortality or recurrent infarction).

The remainder of the chapter considers the results of controlled trials of thrombolytic drug administration. Trials in which the control group is composed of patients who either refused the treatment or were excluded for medical reasons are discussed. Although such studies may yield valid results in other situations [10, 11], the clinical variablility of acute MI diminishes their usefulness in this context. Baseline inequalities in patient characteristics that can not be properly characterized or adjusted for may lead to an apparent treatment effect when none exists.

Intravenous Streptokinase in Acute Myocardial Infarction: Clinical Trials

The initial use of intravenous streptokinase in acute myocardial infarction was reported by Fletcher, Alkjaersig, and Sherry in 1959 [12]. Even in this initial study, the changes of earlier peaking in enzymes and rapid evolution of the QRS changes on the ECG in some patients were noted. The mechanisms of these occurrences, however, were not completely understood. During the 1960s and 1970s, numerous European trials compared intravenous streptokinase to anticoagulation with heparin and/or warfarin. During this time, interest in thrombolytic therapy of acute myocardial infarction had diminished in the United States. The reasons for this trend were enumerated in an editorial by Sherry [13]. There were conflicting results in the early intravenous streptokinase trials, some of which were probably due to inadequacies in trial design. Most importantly, these early trials enrolled patients up to 72 h after the onset of symptoms. According to current understanding of the pathophysiology of infarction and reperfusion, this time frame would bias the studies against streptokinase therapy. More detailed reviews are provided by Simon et al. [14] and Duckert [15].

In 1982, Stampfer et al. reviewed eight of these randomized trials of intravenous streptokinase [16]. A weighted relative risk ratio was calculated and defined as the proportion of patients who died in the treatment groups divided by the proportion of patients who died in the control groups. Three of the eight trials had sufficient numbers of patients to demonstrate independently a statistically significant advantage for survival in the streptokinase groups. No trial showed a significant advantage for the control groups. In pooling the results of all eight trials, the relative risk ratio for death was 0.80 (with 95% confidence limits of 0.68−0.95) for the streptokinase groups, an approximately 20% reduction in early mortality by streptokinase therapy. When a subset of the six trials that enrolled patients within 24 h and gave similar dosing regimens of streptokinase was analyzed, the relative risk ratio was 0.74 (with 95% confidence limits of 0.62−0.89). Although there are problems with pooling of data [17], including the fact that trials without positive results are often unreported, it appeared that intravenous streptokinase resulted in reduced mortality in patients with acute MI.

The most recent of these trials, performed before early catheterization in myocardial infarction had gained wide acceptance, was the European Cooperative Study [18]. In this study, 315 patients, stratified into medium- and high-risk prognostic groups and treated in coronary care units, were randomized within 12 h of symptom onset to intravenous streptokinase or placebo. The high-risk group required three of the following five criteria: systolic blood pressure below 90 mmHg, heart rate above 120 beats/min, respiration rate above 25/min, central venous pressure above 15 cm of water, and more than 5 ventricular premature beats per minute. The medium-risk group had one or two of the above criteria or one of the following: older age group, second or subsequent infarction, heart rate below 60 or greater than 100 beats/min, more than 5 premature ventricular or supraventricular beats per minute, a QRS duration of 0.12 s or longer, second- or third-degree atrioventricular block, and atrial flutter or fibrillation. The low-risk groups were those patients not fulfilling the above criteria. The mortality at 21 days was 12% in the streptokinase group and 18% in the control group. By six months, the mortality was 16% in the streptokinase group and 31% in the control group ($p < 0.01$). The mortality in the nonrandomized low-risk group was 6%.

During the 1970s, observations reported by De Wood et al. [19] and Rentrop et al. [20] documented the etiologic role of coronary thrombosis in acute myocardial infarction and showed that acute coronary angiography could be performed with low morbidity and mortality. De Wood et al. [19] further documented that fewer patients had occlusive thrombi as time from symptom onset to catheterization increased. Rentrop et al. [20] demonstrated that acute recanalization could be accomplished by pharmacologic or mechanical techniques. These observations stimulated renewed interest in intravenous thrombolytic therapy with streptokinase. Schroder used "intermediate" doses (500,000 U over 30 min) [21] in patients with angiographically documented complete arterial occlusions. Reperfusion occurred within 1 h in 11 (52%) of the 21 patients. However, other investigators have not achieved similar results. Rogers et al. achieved reperfusion in only one of ten patients [22], and Saltups et al. in three of ten patients, using this 500,000 U dose [23].

Intravenous streptokinase has more recently been given in higher doses of 850,000–1,700,000 U over 30–60 min. Spann et al. [24] initially reported that they achieved angiographically documented thrombolysis in six (46%) of 13 patients with the 850,000 U dose. Despite increasing the dose to 1,500,000 U over 1 h, they achieved a similar reperfusion rate (48%) in 31 patients. Neuhaus et al. treated 39 patients with 1,700,000 U of streptokinase over 60 min. Angiographic reperfusion occurred in 24 (62%) by an average of 48 min after the initiation of the infusion [25]. Rogers et al. [26] administered 1,500,000 U over 45 min to 15 patients, but did not perform acute angiography. The CK peak occurred at less than 16 h in 64%, suggesting successful reperfusion. Maddahi et al. [27] attained evidence via thallium scanning of reperfusion in 42 (95%) of 44 patients who received two consecutive intravenous infusions of 750,000 U of streptokinase over 15–30 min separated by a 30-min interval. These patients also did not undergo acute angiography. At this time, the reperfusion rate using intravenous streptokinase appears to be between 46% and 95%. The highest incidence documented angiographically is 62%. The correlation between the various methods of determining reperfusion has not yet been established.

Intracoronary Streptokinase in Acute Myocardial Infarction

Great enthusiasm was generated for the use of intracoronary streptokinase after the initial report by Rentrop et al. [20] and subsequent studies by Mathey et al. [28] and Reduto et al. [29], which showed improvement in global left ventricular function in some patients who were successfully reperfused with intracoronary streptokinase in the early hours of myocardial infarction. However, these initial studies were uncontrolled and a need for randomized controlled trials of intracoronary thrombolytic therapy was evident [30].

The importance of controlled trials is highlighted by two recent studies that observed the "natural history" of either left ventricular ejection fraction or CK-MB levels during acute MI. Wackers et al. [31] showed that 19 (56%) of 34 patients with MI, who were studied with serial gated cardiac blood pool imaging over 24 h, had substantial spontaneous changes in ventricular function. These changes ranged from a 32% increase to a 14% decrease in ejection fraction. Of the patients, 11 showed improvement and eight deteriorated. Ong et al. [32] studied 52 patients by serial CM-MB determinations and by admission and discharge radionuclide ejection fractions. Patients were divided into two groups based on the rate of early rise of CK-MB values. The group of 24 patients with rapid CK-MB increases had a significant increase (10%) in ejection fraction during their hospitalization whereas those without such rapid increases showed no net ejection fraction change. The authors interpreted these results to support the view that spontaneous reperfusion occurs in a group of patients with acute MI, and that this event is associated with an improvement in ejection fraction. These two studies demonstrate that the course of acute MI may be associated with spontaneous reperfusion and with diverse changes in ventricular function.

Currently, five randomized controlled trials of

TABLE 33-4. The five randomized controlled trials of intracoronary streptokinase that have been published

		University of Michigan [33]	University of Utah [34]	The Netherlands[a] [35]	George Washington University [36]	Western Washington Trial [7]
Entry criteria for chest-pain duration		<6 h	<4 h	<4 h	<4 h	<12 h
Number of patients randomized		40	50	173	43	250
Randomization pre- or postcatheterization		Post	Post	Pre	Pre	Post
Subtotal occlusion randomized		No	Yes	Yes	No	Yes
Controls cathed		Yes	No	No	Yes	Yes
Reperfusion rates	SK	60%	79%	79%	68%	68%
	Cont	10%	DK	DK	17%	12%
Hours to treatment (mean)		5.4	4	DK	4	4.6
Heparin		No	Yes	DK	Yes (if reperfused)	Yes
Antiplatelet agents		Yes	Yes	DK	No	No
Treatment effect on ventricular function[b]		No change	Improved	DK	No change	No change
Mean follow-up (months)		10	1	10	11	6
Mortality	SK	5% } NS	4% } NS	12% } NS	18% } NS	3.7% } P = 0.0025
	Cont	20%	15%	13%	11%	17.7%

[a] Reported in abstract form.
[b] Global ejection fraction by RNA.
DK, don't know; NS, not statistically significant; SK, streptokinase; Cont, control.

intracoronary streptokinase have been published and are reviewed here (table 33-4).

THE MICHIGAN STUDY

Khaja et al. [33] randomized 40 patients with acute myocardial infarction who entered the hospital within 6 h of the onset of chest pain. Only patients who showed persistent total coronary occlusion after intracoronary nitroglycerin were randomized and all patients underwent acute angiography. Of 305 patients with acute MI during the study period, only 25% were admitted within 6 h of symptom onset. The only significant baseline inequality was that more patients in the control group had either three-vessel or left main disease than in the treatment group (7 vs 1). Initial angiographic ejection fractions were similar (treatment $48 \pm 14\%$, control $47 \pm 15\%$). The streptokinase group received a 15,000 U intracoronary bolus followed by an infusion of 500 U/min to a total dose of 250,000 U.

Thrombolysis occurred in 12 (60%) of 20 streptokinase patients and two (10%) of 20 control patients ($p < 0.05$). The immediate post-intervention angiographic ejection fractions were unchanged from pretreatment (treatment $51 \pm 14\%$, control $49 \pm 12\%$). No differences were found when regional wall motion was analyzed.

In both groups, serial ECGs and CK enzymes were performed and three radionuclide ventriculograms were done. The times to peak CK activity differed when the data were analyzed according to the presence or absence of reperfusion. Although the absolute peak enzyme levels were similar, peak enzyme activity occurred at 17 ± 8h vs 24 ± 8h in reperfused vs non-reperfused patients. Radionuclide ventriculograms were done at $1-3$ days in 32 patients, at $8-16$ days in 29 patients, and at $3-7$ months in 22 patients. The early ejection fraction determination was $45 \pm 15\%$ in the treatment group and $36 \pm 12\%$ in the control group, and no significant changes occurred in the sequential radionuclide studies. When the groups were analyzed on the basis of reperfusion vs non-reperfusion, no differences in ejection fraction were found. On the day after catheterization, both groups received aspirin and dipyridamole. One patient in the streptokinase group underwent bypass surgery versus five in the control group. There were five deaths (treatment, 1; control, 4) among the 40 patients at a mean follow-up of ten months. All of the deaths occurred in non-reperfused patients. Three deaths occurred in the hospital. The death in the streptokinase group occurred 1 h after the procedure. The two inhospital deaths in the control group were the patients with left main disease: one of a recurrent infarction and one after bypass surgery. Two late deaths occurred in the control group. Two deaths occurred in the catheterization laboratory: one streptokinase patient who was not reperfused and one patient in shock who died during ventriculography before randomization. The authors concluded that intracoronary thrombolytic therapy was applicable to only a small percentage of patients with acute MI and appeared to show no major clinical benefit.

THE UTAH STUDY

Anderson et al. [34] studied 50 patients with acute MI who entered the hospital within 4 h of chest-pain onset. Patients were randomized before catheterization. The treatment group underwent catheterization and received intracoronary streptokinase whether total or subtotal occlusions were found. The control group had routine CCU (coronary care unit) care without catheterization. Two-thirds of the treatment group had anterior infarctions and, in the control group, half were anterior and half were inferior. Treatment consisted of an intravenous heparin bolus (5000 U) and intracoronary nitroglycerin followed (in those with total occlusion) by intracoronary streptokinase at a mean rate of 5000 U/min (3000−7000 U) until reperfusion occurred. The infusion was then continued at a mean rate of 3000 U/min (2000−4000 U) for an additional 30−60 min in the total occlusion subset. Subtotal occlusion was treated with the heparin and nitroglycerin followed by 100,000 U of streptokinase. Treatment patients received three days of intravenous heparin followed by antiplatelet therapy with aspirin and dipyridamole for three months. Control patients received subcutaneous heparin until ambulation, then similar antiplatelet therapy. Ventricular function was assessed by two-dimensional echocardiograms on admission, day 1, and day 10, and by gated radionuclide ventriculograms on days 1 and 10.

Total coronary occlusion was present in 20 of the 24 streptokinase patients and was unchanged after intracoronary nitroglycerin. The streptokinase was begun an average of 4 h after symptom onset and perfusion was "re-established or maintained in 19 patients." The mean time to recanalization of totally occluded vessels was 30 min (range $2-100$ min) with an average dose of streptokinase of 215,000 U (range 100,000−390,000 U).

The radionuclide ejection fractions on day 1 were similar in the two groups (treatment $43 \pm 11\%$, control $42 \pm 13.3\%$). By day 10, the ejection fractions in the 23 surviving streptokinase patients were $47 \pm 9\%$ vs $39 \pm 12\%$ in the 22 surviving control patients ($p < 0.05$). The ejection fraction increased a mean of $4 \pm 5\%$ in the treated group compared with a decrease of $3 \pm 8\%$ in the control group. A similar improvement in echocardiographic regional wall motion in the streptokinase group was observed. Although the peak CK enzyme levels were similar in both groups, the time to peak CK was earlier in the streptokinase group (13 ± 6 h) than in the control group (22 ± 4 h). Maximum Killip class was higher in the control group (2.1 vs 1.4) and pain relief was more rapid in the streptokinase group as assessed by morphine requirement.

Analysis of the ECGs showed greater relative R-wave preservation and a lesser Q-wave development in the streptokinase group. Systemic lytic effects occurred in the streptokinase group as assessed by a prolonged thrombin clotting time in 94%, a shorter euglobulin lysis time in 80%, and a decline in fibrinogen in 76%. In 16 patients who were reperfused, repeat angiography at ten days showed persistent vessel patency in all and an angiographic ejection fraction of $60 \pm 14\%$ compared with the baseline angiographic ejection fraction of $55 \pm 14\%$ ($p < 0.02$). Coronary bypass surgery was performed in seven streptokinase patients and two control patients at an average of seven days ($1-12$ days). This practice may confound the interpretation of the mean late radionuclide and echocardiographic analyses of ventricular function. Five in-hospital deaths occurred: one in the streptokinase group and four in the control group—all were due to pump failure. The authors concluded that streptokinase therapy leads to significant clinical improvement.

THE NETHERLANDS STUDY

Simoons et al. [35] randomized 173 patients admitted within 4 h of symptom onset to intracoronary streptokinase or conventional treatment. This work has only been presented in abstract form at the time of this writing. Ten of the 86 patients randomized to streptokinase refused the procedure, but were included in the total streptokinase group. Of 76 catheterized patients, 75% had total coronary occlusion and recanalization was achieved in 79% of these. Immediate angioplasty was attempted in 23 patients and was successful in 19. Three control and eight streptokinase patients had no elevation of CK levels. The overall mortality at a median follow-up of ten months was 11 of 87 control vs 10 of 86 streptokinase patients. The incidences of recurrent infarction, subsequent angina, and need for coronary bypass surgery were similar. Three of the deaths in the streptokinase group occurred in the ten patients who did not undergo the procedure. None of the 19 patients with successful angioplasty died. The authors concluded that they could not demonstrate that thrombolytic therapy resulted in an improved clinical course.

THE GEORGE WASHINGTON STUDY

Lieboff et al. [36] studied 55 patients who presented within 4 h of the onset of chest pain. Randomization to intracoronary streptokinase occurred before catheterization and all patients underwent the acute catheterization. However, 12 patients had only subtotal occlusions, received only intracoronary nitroglycerin, and were analyzed separately. Patients randomized to streptokinase received intracoronary nitroglycerin followed by a continuous infusion of streptokinase at $2000-4000$ U/min for 75 min (mean total dose 240,000 U). The control group received intracoronary nitroglycerin every 15 min and was observed angiographically for a total of 90 min. No patient had angioplasty. Of the 40 patients with initial total occlusions, 22 received streptokinase and 18 were controls. Reperfusion occurred in 15 (69%) of 22 streptokinase patients and in three (17%) of 18 control patients. The average time to reperfusion was $4\frac{3}{4}$ h in these 18 reperfused patients. CK peaked at 11 h in the reperfused patients and at 23 h in those without reperfusion. The patients who initially had incomplete occlusion had CK curves indistinguishable from those who had initial occlusion and successful reperfusion.

Global ejection fractions by radionuclide ventriculography were performed within 3 h of catheterization and at $10-14$ days. Six patients underwent bypass grafting after day 10, but all of the late radionuclide scans were performed before the surgery. The mean initial ejection fractions were not significantly different (treatment 46%, control 42%). At two weeks, there was a mean decrease of 2.8% in the streptokinase group and a decrease of 0.4% in controls. When reperfused versus nonreperfused patients were compared, there were also no ejection fraction differences. However, the most interesting finding was that the group of nine patients who initially had subtotal occlusions and were not randomized had an improved ejection fraction at two weeks (53% vs 46% on admission).

Of the 15 reperfused streptokinase patients, 11 underwent repeat catheterization at $12-14$ days and five of these had reoccluded despite continuous intravenous heparin therapy. In all five patients, >90% residual stenosis was present after acute reperfusion. One of the patients with

reocclusion had experienced hematuria and a discontinuation of heparin, and three had periods
of subtherapeutic anticoagulation.

At a mean follow-up of 11 months, six of 55
patients had died. There was one inhospital death
in the control group due to reinfarction on day 4,
and two inhospital deaths in the streptokinase
group, both after bypass surgery for recurrent
angina. One control and two streptokinase patients died after discharge. The authors concluded (a) that clinically important benefits from
streptokinase therapy should not be expected
when treatment begins at or after 4 h from the
onset of symptoms, and (b) that patients who
have subtotal occlusions initially may have had
early spontaneous thrombolysis and associated
improvement in ventricular function.

THE WESTERN WASHINGTON STUDY
Kennedy et al. [7], in the largest randomized
trial, studied 250 patients with acute myocardial infarcts: 134 patients received intracoronary
streptokinase and 116 patients were controls. All
patients were catheterized and randomized within 12 h of the onset of symptoms. The study
was performed in 11 community hospitals and
three university hospitals. Treatment patients received intracoronary nitroglycerin followed by
4000 U/min of streptokinase to a total dose of
250,000−350,000 U. Control patients were
returned to the CCU. Both treatment and control groups received intravenous heparin during
hospitalization and reperfused patients received
Coumadin for three months. In each hospital, the
randomization was stratified within four subgroups: anterior or inferior infarct location and
symptoms of less than 3 or 3−12 h. A gated
blood pool scan was performed as soon as possible
after catheterization (0−48 h) and at two weeks
in all patients; 55 patients (22%) were randomly
assigned within the first 3 hours and 195 patients
(78%) between 3 and 12 h. The mean time from
symptoms to hospitalization was 134 min, but
an average of 276 min elapsed between symptom
onset and the completion of angiography and
randomization. The average dose of streptokinase
was 286,000 ± 77,800 U over 72 ± 24 min.
Of the 134 streptokinase patients, 108 had total
occlusion and 68% of these were reperfused. Of
the 116 control patients, 12% had spontaneous

reperfusion during angiography. During the first
30 days, mortality was 3.7% for the streptokinase group and 11.2% for controls ($p = 0.02$).
At six months, no further deaths had occurred in
the streptokinase group, but the mortality in the
control group had increased to 14.7% ($p = 0.0025$).

The angiographic ejection fractions on admission were 50 ± 13% in the streptokinase group
and 49 ± 13% in controls. The initial radionuclide ejection fractions were 47 ± 17% in the
streptokinase group and 46 ± 15% in controls.
No significant difference in the ejection fractions
were found at discharge (average 15 days). Mortality was related to the location of infarction. In
the anterior infarction group, 18.9% of controls
and 7.9% of streptokinase-treated patients died.
Among those with inferior infarction, the control
mortality was 4.8% and none died in the streptokinase group. Complications of angiography
occurred in 14 % of the treatment group and
7.8% of the control group. Bleeding occurred in
5% of the treatment group and 1% of control ($p = 0.05$). The authors concluded that the major
benefit of therapy occurred in the patients with
anterior infarcts. The mechanism by which mortality was reduced was unclear, however, as global ventricular function was not significantly
changed by treatment.

INTRACORONARY STUDIES: CONCLUSION
In summary, only one of the trials has shown a
significant affect of intracoronary streptokinase
on mortality. Significant benefits of reperfusion
on global left ventricular function have been
shown in one other trial. Three of the five trials
have concluded that intracoronary streptokinase
does not appear to cause significant clinical benefit. In all of these trials, the average time to
treatment has been 4 h or more. Because of the
complex logistics and the cost of moving patients
rapidly through the emergency system to the
catheterization laboratory, the numbers of patients who can be reperfused more quickly by the
intracoronary route will be low. Whether specific
subgroups of patients are more likely to benefit
from the procedure, particularly when coupled
with mechanical recanalization, is a matter for
future research. From our current understanding
of the pathophysiology of ischemic myocardial

necrosis, it appears that although treatment begun after 4−6 h of ischemia may improve regional myocardial function, it may not consistently produce clinically beneficial effects. Whether more rapid thrombolysis with intravenous therapy can lead to improved myocardial salvage and more convincing clinical improvement remains to be determined.

As discussed by Furberg [37], the small numbers of patients in each study greatly reduce the probability that a difference in clinical outcome could be detected, even if it existed (type-II error). The positive result from the Western Washington trial raises a number of questions about the interpretation of clinical trials. Should the results of one well-designed and well-executed randomized trial be accepted as definitive, when other trials have different results? When multiple small trials are performed with the same design, what is the probability that one trial will find positive results by chance? Until these issues are resolved, the results of the randomized trials must be regarded as inconclusive. While we wait for a larger randomized trial with adequate study design, the available trials must be placed in the context of other knowledge from observational studies and the basic laboratory.

Current Practice at Duke Medical Center

SELECTION OF PATIENTS

While almost all observers agree that more careful studies must be done, the likelihood that a definitive trial will be available in the near future is small because of the rapidly evolving technique and variability in treatment strategies. Therefore, the only firm conclusion about selection of patients for thrombolytic therapy is that the recommendations will change, and that no definite criteria can be established at this time. In general, however, the factors that should be considered are listed in table 33-5. According to current understanding, the most critical factors for selecting patients most likely to benefit from therapy are the amount of myocardium jeopardized by the occluded vessel and the duration of the occlusion [38]. For this reason, only patients with ST elevation on ECG are considered, since

TABLE 33-5. Factors supporting choice of thrombolytic therapy for MI

Time from symptom onset
<3 h: strongly supports therapy
>6 h: strongly discourages therapy
Unless symptoms have waxed and waned
Large amount of myocardium at risk
ST elevation present
Anterior MI
Large number of leads with ST elevation
Inferior MI with anterior ST depression or apical
(V_5, V_6) ST elevation
Hemodynamic compromise

many patients with ischemic chest pain but without ST elevation do not have an MI. Patients with anterior MI and ST elevation in multiple leads are given priority due to the usual larger size of anterior MI and the probable relationship between the amount of jeopardized myocardium and the number of leads with ST elevation [39]. Patients with inferior MI are considered for thrombolytic therapy at our institution only if ST-segment changes are also present in the precordial leads or if hemodynamic compromise is present. The mortality and morbidity from inferior MI without these complicating factors is low enough that no treatment could be expected to alter outcome significantly. Although patients with hemodynamic instability are at high risk of complications during the procedure, they may gain the most by salvage of myocardium.

The time course of infarction is quite variable, probably depending on the presence or absence of total occlusion of the infarct-related vessel and the extent of collateral flow. If thrombolytic therapy salvages myocardium, the earlier the clot is lysed, the more myocardium should be saved. Our policy is to consider thrombolytic therapy strongly in patients seen within 3 h of the onset of symptoms, and to withhold thrombolytic therapy if the duration of symptoms has exceeded 6 h. Patients with symptoms that wax and wane over a long period of time are also considered for acute catheterization. These patients often have thrombus almost totally occluding the vessel with intermittent total occlusion.

TABLE 33-6. Characteristics of streptokinase, urokinase, and plasminogen activator

	Streptokinase (SK)	Urokinase (UK)	Tissue plasminogen activator (TPA)
Source	Lancefield group-C streptococci	Kidney cell cultures	Gene from melanoma cell line
Mechanism	Not direct Combines with plasminogen SK-PG complex active	Direct activation of PG	Activates only PG bound to fibrin
Half-life	11−17 min (antibody) 80−90 min (activator)	10−15 min	5−8 min
Side effects	Bleeding, hypotension, fever, anaphylaxis, serum sickness	Bleeding	Bleeding ?? Few expected
Hemostatic changes	↓ Fibrinogen ↓ Plasminogen ↓ Plasmin inhibitors ↓ Factor V, VIII coagulation activity ↓ PT, PTT, TCT	Same as SK	?? Few expected
Monitoring	PTT or TCT to assure a "Lytic state"	PTT or TCT to assure a "Lytic state"	Theoretically not required
Advantages	Available Cheapest	Available	? Faster clot lysis No effect on clotting Short duration of action Enables safer invasive procedures after infusion stopped
Disadvantages	Affects clotting factors Antibody resistance Prolonged risk of bleeding	Affects clotting factors Prolonged risk of bleeding Expensive	? Availability

PG, Plasminogen; PT, prothrombin time; PTT, partial thromboplastin time; TCT thrombin clotting time.

SELECTION OF AGENT

Table 33-6 contrasts the characteristics of streptokinase, urokinase, and tissue plasminogen activator (TPA) (see chapter 7). Although urokinase has the advantage of being a direct activator, its cost makes streptokinase the preferable agent. If TPA performs as well in large-scale human trials as in preliminary animal and human studies, it should become the agent of choice due to its fibrin specificity. This characteristic should lead to a lower risk of bleeding after the therapy has been given since clotting factors and hemostatic integrity are not affected, as they are by streptokinase and urokinase. Until this promising agent can be fully evaluated in the clinical situation, streptokinase remains the agent of choice.

METHOD OF ADMINISTRATION: COMMUNITY HOSPITAL

Streptokinase has not yet been approved for intravenous (IV) use in the United States. Until approval is obtained, physicians wishing to use IV streptokinase should develop a protocol for approval by the local institutional review board. This practice will lead to more uniform, and thus more safe, use of the drug and should provide a mechanism for evaluating the complications and results of therapy.

If streptokinase is to be used in the community

hospital, a mechanism should be developed as part of the protocol to evaluate rapidly and thoroughly the patient with suspected acute infarction. The history should be oriented toward detection of contraindications to streptokinase therapy as well as to the usual cardiac history. Except for active internal bleeding and high-risk intracerabral processes, other contraindications are relative (table 33-7). The risk of drug administration must be weighed against the potential benefits of reperfusion. If serious bleeding occurs during thrombolytic therapy with streptokinase, the treatment should include: (a) discontinuation of streptokinase; (b) replacement of blood loss with packed red blood cells or whole blood; (c) replacement of fibrinogen and coagulation factors with fresh frozen plasma, and; (d) reversal of the fibrinolytic state with AMICAR (epsilon aminocaproic acid) as an intravenous loading dose of 5 g over 1 h followed by a 1 g/h infusion for 2–4 h.

Once the candidate for reperfusion is identified using the history and 12-lead ECG, sublingual nitroglycerin (NTG) should be administered to exclude Prinzmetal's angina. Routine baseline laboratory values (see chapter 37) including a PTT and perhaps a thrombin clotting time should be drawn. If pain relief and ST-segment resolution do not occur with NTG, our current recommendation is that 1.5 million U of streptokinase be given over 30–60 min.

TABLE 33-7. Contraindications to streptokinase therapy

Absolute
  Active internal bleeding
  High risk of intracerebral bleeding (severe uncontrolled hypertension, recent stroke, intracranial metastases)
Relative (high risk)
  Major surgery or deep biopsy within ten days
  Recent serious trauma
  Thoracentesis, paracentesis
Relative (unknown risk)
  Postpartum period
  Menses
  Diabetic retinopathy
  Postcardiopulmonary resuscitation
  Intracardiac thrombus (as in chronic atrial fibrillation with mitral valve disease)

Other routine care for myocardial infarction should be given as usual. The patient should be monitored for arrhythmia especially carefully initially because of the possibility of reperfusion arrhythmia.

The PTT can be checked shortly after drug administration to assure a lytic state and should be followed serially every 4 h until it drops to twice control. At this point we recommend the initiation of heparin therapy (1000 U/h without a bolus) for a period of 2–3 days with dose adjustment to maintain this PTT. We then recommend the initiation of treatment with aspirin and dipyridamole. The practitioner must be aware that little scientific rationale currently exists for the choice of one anticoagulation regimen over another at this time and that the preferred therapy will change as evidence accumulates. Many experts in this area recommend heparinization for up to one week followed by Coumadin therapy for 3–6 months [40].

In the absence of angiographic documentation of reperfusion, the practitioner may wish to follow the 12-lead ECG and CK-MB enzymes every 8 h for several days. The patient with reperfusion can be characterized by rapid resolution of ST segments and rapid Q-wave development on the ECG. The CK enzyme curve of reperfused patients shows a more rapid peak compared with non-reperfused patients.

Since many patients will have a tight residual stenosis after reperfusion, careful attention must be given to the evaluation of the patient for residual jeopardized myocardium (see chapter 13). We currently recommend that, at a minimum, these patients should undergo an exercise test prior to hospital discharge. Others prefer routine angiography, although the Western Washington study [6] has reported few cardiac events in the follow-up of their patients who did not have routine catheterization at the time of discharge after intracoronary thrombolysis. Furthermore, Harrison et al. [41] have demonstrated that lesions which appear critical immediately after thrombolysis may regress, implying that there is early persistence of thrombus in many patients after successful thrombolysis. Until further evidence is available, we also treat our post-reperfusion patients with beta-blocking drugs (see chapter 17).

METHOD OF ADMINISTRATION:
MEDICAL CENTER

Practitioners with rapid access to a cardiac catheterization laboratory are now faced with a variety of options for initial treatment of patients with MI. Our current practice is to identify patients rapidly as outlined above and to proceed immediately to the cardiac catheterization laboratory. A team should consist of at least two cardiologists, a laboratory technician, and registered nurse in order to guarantee patient safety when intracoronary thrombolysis is attempted. Immediate backup support from respiratory therapy, pharmacy, intraaortic balloon pump, and laboratory personnel also should be available. In hemodynamically unstable patients, right heart catheterization can be performed by one cardiologist while another performs the left heart catheterization. Central venipunctures should be avoided if possible, so the basilic vein or external jugular vein approaches are preferred for right heart catheterization.

Most angiographers initially visualize the coronary arteries least likely to be obstructed [42]. The 12-lead ECG can be used to decide whether to use the right or left coronary catheter first. When the obstructed artery is found, a bolus of 200–400 μg of NTG is given directly into the artery to relieve any spasm that may be present (see chapter 5). If no change is observed after NTG, streptokinase is given as a bolus of 20,000 U followed by an infusion of 4000 U/min. For distal lesions, a subselective catheter may be introduced to ensure that the drug reaches the thrombus. Some of our angiographers prefer to move rapidly to mechanical recanalizaion in an effort to reduce the time to reperfusion. A 0.021–0.028-inch guidewire can often be advanced through the clot. If patency is achieved, the infusion is continued for 30–60 min in accordance with the generally recognized phenomenon that the vessel is prone to spasm and rethrombosis immediately after thrombolysis [1, 40, 42] or until a total dose of 400,000 U is used.

If a high-grade proximal lesion remains after antegrade flow has been restored, our current practice is to proceed with immediate PTCA. Reocclusion rates in this situation have not been adequately documented yet, but little additional time and expense is involved in angioplasty once intracoronary thrombolytic therapy has been given. The patient is then returned to the CCU with the same protocol as outlined for patients given intravenous streptokinase.

Because of the evidence outlined in this chapter, we are currently considering a protocol of starting IV streptokinase immediately in the emergency room. The femoral artery sheath for catheterization can be placed before the drug is administered, so that the chances of major bleeding complications are minimized. This initial step of early drug administration would save 60–90 min of time during which the rate of myocardial necrosis appears to be rapid.

Especially with the advent of TPA, the possibility exists that intracoronary thrombus can be lysed without creation of a systemic lytic state, as suggested by the recent reports by Van de Werf et al. [43, 44]. These investigators have reported the use of TPA in animals and man without significant alteration in levels of circulating fibrinogen or alpha-2 antiplasmin. If these findings are confirmed in larger populations, invasive procedures can be considered immediately after thrombolysis without significant risk of bleeding. Only careful observation of clinical practice and controlled trials will lead to a more rational plan for the timing of intervention to alter the structure of the underlying coronary anatomy.

References

1. Cowley MJ: Methodologic aspects of intracoronary thrombolysis. Circulation (Suppl 1) 68:90–95, 1983.

2. Meyer J, Merx W, Schmitz H, Erbel R, Kiesslich T, Dorr R, Lambertz H, Bethge C, Krebs W, Bardos P, Minale C, Messmer BJ, Effert S: Percutaneous transluminal coronary angioplasty immediately after intracoronary streptolysis of transmural myocardial infarction. Circulation 66: 905–913, 1982.

3. Mathey DG, Rodewald G, Rentrop P, Leitz K, Merx W, Messmer BJ, Rutsch W, Bucherl ES: Intracoronary streptokinase thrombolytic recanalization and subsequent surgical bypass of remaining atherosclerotic stenosis in acute myocardial infarction: complementary combined approach effecting reduced infarct size, preventing reinfarction, and improving left ventricular function. Am Heart J 102:1194–1201, 1981.

4. Jennings RB, Reimer KA: Factors involved in salvaging ischemic myocardium: effect of reperfusion of arterial blood. Circulation (Suppl 1) 68:25−36, 1983.

5. Smalling RW, Fuentes F, Matthews MW, Freund GC, Hicks CH, Reduto LA, Walker WE, Sterling RP, Gould KL: Sustained improvement in left ventricular function and mortality by intracoronary streptokinase administration during evolving myocardial infarction. Circulation 68: 131−138, 1983.

6. Beller GA: Myocardial imaging with thallium-201 for assessment of regional myocardial perfusion and viability after intracoronary thrombolytic therapy. Circulation (Suppl 1) 68:70−76, 1983.

7. Kennedy JW, Ritchie JL, Davis KB, Fritz JK: Western Washington randomized trial of intracoronary streptokinase in acute myocardial infarction. N Engl J Med 309:1477−1482, 1983.

8. Stack RS, Phillips HR, Grierson DS, Behar VS, Kong Y, Peter RH, Swain JL, Greenfield JC: Functional improvement of jeopardized myocardium following intracoronary streptokinase infusion in acute myocardial infarction. J Clin Invest 72:84−95, 1983.

9. Sheehan FH, Mathey DG, Schofer J, Hans-Joachim K, Dodge HT: Effect of interventions in salvaging left ventricular function in acute myocardial infarction: a study of intracoronary streptokinase. Am J Cardiol 52:431−438, 1983.

10. Rosati RA, Lee KL, Califf RM, Pryor DB, Harrell FE Jr: Problems and advantages of an observational data base approach to evaluating the effect of therapy on outcome. Circulation (Suppl 2) 65:27−32, 1982.

11. Hlatky MA, Lee KL, Harrell FE Jr, Pryor DB, Califf RM, Mark DB, Rosati RA: Tying clinical research to patient care by use of an observational database. Stat Med (in press).

12. Fletcher AP, Alkjaersig N, Sherry S: The maintenance of a sustained thrombolytic state in man. I. Induction and effects. J Clin Invest 38:1096−1110, 1959.

13. Sherry S: Personal reflections on the development of thrombolytic therapy and its application to acute coronary thrombosis. Am Heart J 102: 1134−1139, 1981.

14. Simon TL, Ware JH, Stengle JM: Clinical trials of thrombolytic agents in myocardial infarction. Ann Intern Med 79:712−719, 1973.

15. Duckert F: Thrombolytic therapy in myocardial infarction. Prog Cardiovasc Dis 21:342−350, 1979.

16. Stampfer MS, Goldhaber SZ, Yusuf S, Peto R, Hennekens C: Effect of intravenous streptokinase on acute myocardial infarction: pooled results from randomized trials. N Engl J Med 307: 1180−1182, 1982.

17. Goldman L, Feinstein AR: Anticoagulants and myocardial infarction: the problems of pooling, drowning and floating. Ann Intern Med 90:92−94, 1979.

18. European Cooperative Study Group for streptokinase treatment in acute myocardial infarction: Streptokinase in acute myocardial infarction. N Engl J Med 301:797−802, 1979.

19. De Wood M, Spores J, Notske R, Mouser LT, Burroughs R, Golden MS, Lang HT: Prevalence of total coronary occlusion during the early hours of transmural myocardial infarction. N Engl J Med 303:897−902, 1980.

20. Rentrop P, Blanke H, Karsch KR, Kaiser H, Kostering H, Leitz K: Selective intracoronary thrombolysis in acute myocardial infarction and unstable angina pectoris. Circulation 63:307−317, 1981.

21. Schroder R: Systemic versus intracoronary streptokinase infusion in the treatment of acute myocardial infarction. J Am Coll Cardiol 1:1254−1261, 1983.

22. Rogers WJ, Mantle JA, Hood WP, Baxley WA, Whitlow PL, Reeves RC, Soto B: Prospective randomized trial of intravenous and intracoronary streptokinase in acute myocardial infarction. Circulation 68:1051−1061, 1983.

23. Saltups A, Boxall J, Ho B: Intracoronary versus intravenous streptokinase in acute myocardial infarction. Circulation 68:III-119, 1983.

24. Spann JF, Sherry S, Carabello BA, Denenberg BS, Mann RH, McCann WD, Gault JH, Gentzler RD, Belber AD, Maurer AH, Cooper EM: Coronary thrombolysis by intravenous streptokinase in acute myocardial infarction: acute and follow-up studies. Am J Cardiol 53:655−661, 1984.

25. Neuhaus KL, Kostering H, Tebbe U, Sauer G, Kreuzer H: High dose intravenous streptokinase infusion in acute myocardial infarction. Z Kardiol 70:791, 1981.

26. Rogers WJ, Hood WP, Reeves RC, Whitlow PL: Randomized trial of intracoronary versus intravenous streptokinase in acute myocardial infarction. J Am Coll Cardiol 3:525, 1984.

27. Maddahi J, Weiss T, Geft I, Shah PK, Berman D, Swan HJC, Ganz W: Coronary thrombolysis with intravenous streptokinase salvages jeopardized myocardium in evolving myocardial infarction in assessment by quantitative thallium-201

imaging. Circulation 68:III-120, 1983.

28. Mathey DG, Kuck KH, Tilsner V, Krebbver HJ, Bleifield W: Nonsurgical coronary artery recanalization in acute transmural myocardial infarction. Circulation 63:489−497, 1981.

29. Reduto LA, Smalling RW, Freund GC, Gould KL: Intracoronary infusion of streptokinase in patients with acute myocardial infarction: effects of reperfusion on left ventricular performance. Am J Cardiol 48:403−409, 1981.

30. Muller JE, Stone PH, Markis JE, Braunwald E: Let's not let the genie escape from the bottle— again. N Engl J Med 304:1294−1296, 1981.

31. Wackers FJ, Berger HJ, Weinberg MA, Zaret BA: Spontaneous changes in left ventricular function over the first 24 hours of myocardial infarction: implications for evaluating early therapeutic interventions. Circulation 66:748−754, 1982.

32. Ong L, Reiser P, Coromilas J, Scherr L, Morrison J: Left ventricular function and rapid release of creatine kinase MB in acute myocardial infarction: evidence for spontaneous reperfusion. N Engl J Med 309:1−6, 1983.

33. Khaja F, Walton JA, Brymer JF, Lo E, Osterberger L, O'Neill WW, Colfertt T, Weiss R, Lee T, Kurian T, Goldberg AD, Pitt B, Goldstein S: Intracoronary fibrinolytic therapy in acute myocardial infarction: report of a prospective randomized trial. N Engl J Med 308:1305−1311, 1983.

34. Anderson JL, Marshall HW, Bray BE, Lutz JR, Frederick PR, Yanowitz FG, Datz FL, Klausner SC, Hagan AD: A randomized trial of intracoronary streptokinase in the treatment of acute myocardial infarction. N Engl J Med 308:1312−1318, 1983.

35. Simoons ML, Fiorette P, Brand M, Serruys PW, Krauss XH, Remme T, Wall EE, Verheugt F: Randomized trial of thrombolysis with streptokinase in acute myocardial infarction. Circulation 68:III-120, 1983.

36. Lieboff RH, Katz RJ, Wasserman AG, Bren GB, Schwartz H, Varghese PJ, Ross AM: A randomized, angiographically controlled trial of intracoronary streptokinase in acute myocardial infarction. Am J Cardiol 53:404−407, 1984.

37. Furberg C: Clinical value of intracoronary streptokinase. Am J Cardiol 53:626−627, 1984.

38. Rentrop P, Smith H, Painter BA, Holt J: Changes in left ventricular ejection fraction after intracoronary thrombolytic therapy: results of the registry of the European Society of Cardiology. Circulation (Suppl 1) 68:55−60, 1983.

39. Corsa AT, Hindman NB, Califf RM, McKinnis RA, Wagner GS: The ability of initial quantitative epicardial injury to predict infarct size estimated by QRS score. JACC (in press).

40. Little WC: Thrombolytic therapy of acute myocardial infarction. Curr Probl Cardiol 8:1−47, 1983.

41. Harrison DG, Ferguson DW, Kioschos JM, Marcus ML, White CW: Inapparent persistent thrombi following "successful" streptokinase reperfusion during acute myocardial infarction. Circulation (Suppl 2) 66: 335, 1982.

42. Ports TA: Thrombolytic therapy for acute myocardial infarction. In: Scheinman MM (ed) Cardiac emergencies. Philadelphia: WB Saunders, 1984, pp 59−73.

43. Van de Werf F, Bergmann SR, Fox KA, De Geest H, Hoyng CF, Sobel BE, Collen D: Coronary thrombolysis with intravenously administered human tissue-type plasminogen activator produced by recombinant DNA technology. Circulation 69:605−610, 1984.

44. Van de Werf F, Ludbrook PA, Bergmann SR, Tiefenbrunn AJ, Fox KA, DeGeest H, Verstraete M, Collen D, Sobel BE: Coronary thrombolysis with tissue-type plasminogen activator in patients with evolving myocardial infarction. N Engl J Med: 310:609−613, 1984.

34. METHODS FOR DETECTING SALVAGE OF JEOPARDIZED MYOCARDIUM FOLLOWING INTRACORONARY THROMBOLYSIS IN ACUTE MYOCARDIAL INFARCTION

Richard S. Stack

Robert K. Stack

Several studies have recently shown that coronary recanalization can be accomplished in a majority of patients with acute myocardial infarction by using intracoronary streptokinase [1−5] (see chapter 6). The ability to salvage significant amounts of jeopardized myocardium by using this technique, however, has only recently been established [6, 7]. Most studies have relied on analysis of the global left ventricular ejection fraction to assess myocardial function following reperfusion. However, the global ejection fraction represents an average of the contractile performances of all segments of the left ventricular myocardium. Although diminished contractile performance in the ischemic area may be reflected in a diminished global ejection fraction, hyperdynamic compensatory changes in the uninvolved regions will influence the ejection fraction in the opposite direction. If a significant improvement occurred in the contractile function of the jeopardized myocardium following reperfusion, it is likely that the hyperdynamic compensatory wall motion of the uninfarcted myocardium would return toward normal. This could result in an unchanged or even decreased global ejection fraction following coronary reperfusion despite sig-

nificant functional improvement in the region of the jeopardized myocardium. This chapter reviews a recent study that used quantitative angiographic techniques to analyze sequential changes over time in the regional wall motion of both the ischemic segment and the uninvolved compensatory segments following intracoronary streptokinase infusion in patients with acute myocardial infarction.

Design of the Study

Twenty-four consecutive patients with acute myocardial infarction who were admitted within 6 h of the onset of symptoms were studied [7]. There were 21 men and three women with a mean age of 55 years. The diagnosis of acute myocardial infarction was determined by the presence of persistent ST-segment elevation of greater than 2 mm in two or more leads on the electrocardiogram, associated with a typical precordial pain pattern. The usual exclusion criteria for the administration of streptokinase were observed, including age greater than 75 years. Patients with chronic congestive heart failure were excluded because of the difficulty in assessing the

R.M. Califf and G.S. Wagner (eds.), ACUTE CORONARY CARE: Principles and Practice. Copyright © 1985. Martinus Nijhoff Publishing, Boston/Dordrecht/Lancaster.

influence of acute coronary reperfusion on regional wall motion.

Biplane left ventriculograms in the 30° right anterior oblique and 60° left anterior oblique projections were obtained. All ventriculograms were recorded using a 35-mm camera at 60 frames per second following the power injection of 45 cc of renografin. On coronary arteriography, all patients demonstrated total occlusion of the proximal coronary artery that perfused the infarcted area, with the exception of one patient who showed minimal filling of the distal vessel. Each patient received an intracoronary bolus of 300 μg of nitroglycerin followed by repeat injection with contrast to exclude focal spasm as the sole etiology of the transmural injury. Streptokinase (Kabikinase) was administered into the occluded coronary artery as a 20,000-U bolus over 2 min. This was followed by a constant infusion of 4000 U/min until a total dose of 350,000 U was administered. Vessel patency was assessed every 15 min. The entire dose of 350,000 U of streptokinase was infused regardless of whether or not recanalization was established.

Intravenous heparin was begun at a rate of 1000 U/h when the partial thromboplastin time fell to less than twice normal. At 24 h after the initial study, cardiac catheterization including coronary arteriography and left ventriculography was repeated in 19 of the 24 patients. A repeat catheterization study was performed from the opposite femoral artery in 15 patients before discharge from the hospital.

Six patients developed local hematomas, one of which required surgical evacuation. One additional patient had an unexplained decrease in hematocrit requiring transfusion. All bleeding complications occurred while the patients were on full-dose heparin therapy. All but one occurred more than 24 h after the streptokinase infusion was completed (a length of time associated with a return of plasma fibrinogen levels to the normal range in most patients following administration of intracoronary streptokinase) [8].

REGIONAL WALL MOTION ANALYSIS

Regional wall motion was analyzed in the right anterior oblique projection by using a quantitative angiographic technique [9, 10]. Cineangiograms from all patients were coded and placed in random order. The left ventricular silhouette from each film was projected onto a rear projection screen and was traced onto clear plastic sheets at end-diastole and end-systole by a single blinded observer. These traces were then digitized by a second blinded observer using a sonic digitizing device interfaced to a PDP 11/45 computer (Digital Equipment Corporation). This digitized information was then used to calculate the ejection fraction, according to the method of Kennedy et al. [11], using biplane ventricular volume determinations as described by Dodge et al. [12]. Quantitative regional wall motion analysis was performed as follows: A longitudinal axis is constructed connecting the middle of the aortic valve plane and the apex of the heart for both the end-diastolic and end-systolic silhouettes. The midpoint of this axis is then determined by the computer and radii are constructed from the midpoint to the edge of the ventricular silhouette at 15° intervals (figure 34-1). The percent shortening of each radius is calculated according to the formula: % shortening = (diastolic length − systolic length)/(diastolic length) × 100. Radial axes 1 and 21–23 were not included in the analysis because they overlie aortic and mitral valve structures. Normal values for radial shortening had been derived from 58 previous patients with normal coronary arteriograms and left ventriculograms [10]. Abnormal radial shortening in the study group was defined quantitatively as percent shortening greater than 2 standard deviations (SD) below the normal mean. The ischemic zone (jeopardized region) in each patient was identified as the longest continuous asynergic segment found in any of three studies as defined by abnormal radial shortening in the distribution of the occluded vessel. The remaining normal or hyperdynamic (greater than 2 SD above the normal mean) radii comprised the compensatory region.

Results of the Study

Fifteen patients (62%) were reperfused during the initial study within 6 h of the onset of symptoms. Twelve patients had anterior and 12 had inferior wall infarctions indicated by ECG. Nine had single-vessel disease and 15 had multivessel involvement. Among the patients who were not

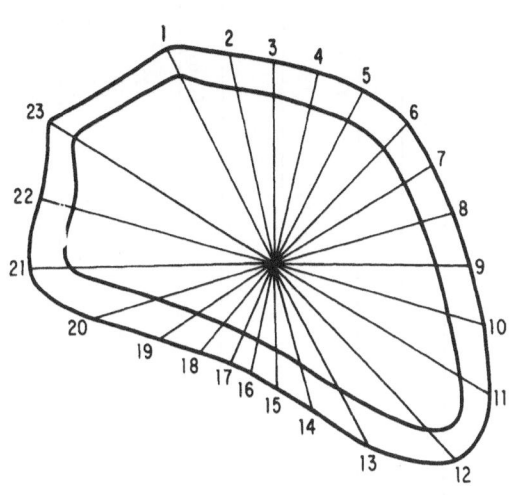

FIGURE 34-1. The 23 radii constructed for evaluation of regional wall motion in the right anterior oblique ventriculogram are identified. The center is located at the midpoint of the longitudinal axis of the ventricle and there are 22° between each of the radii (the 24th radius would bisect the aortic valve).

successfully recanalized, one died following streptokinase infusion before left ventriculography could be performed. Five patients who were shown to have coronary occlusion at the end of the acute study were found to be recanalized at the time of the 24-h study. Four of these five patients were restudied before discharge from the hospital and two were found to have reocclusion. One patient was reperfused during the acute study but reoccluded before the predischarge study. One patient demonstrated persistent occlusion during each of the three studies. The mean time from the onset of symptoms to the infusion of streptokinase for all patients was 4.4 ± 1.2 h. Among the patients who were recanalized acutely, the mean time from the onset of symptoms to reperfusion was 4.8 ± 0.9 h. The average time from the beginning of the infusion to successful recanalization was 34 ± 18 min with a range of 15−75 min.

A total of four patients died, all within the first week after the acute infarction. Two of the patients were successfully reperfused acutely and two were not. Angiography was performed in three of the patients, all of whom had ejection fractions of less than 21%. The mean radial

shortening was below the normal range in both the jeopardized region (7 ± 8%) and the compensatory region (13 ± 6%).

The mean data for all patients with both acute and subsequent studies are shown in the upper panel of table 34-1. In the patients who were acutely reperfused, there was a significant improvement in the region of the jeopardized myocardium, although there was no change in the global ejection fraction (EF). In the patients who were not initially reperfused, there was no improvement in the EF or in the segmental function of the ischemic zone, nor was there a decrease in the amount of compensatory wall motion. There was no significant change in heart rate, mean systemic arterial pressure, or left ventricular end-diastolic pressure in either the reperfused or nonreperfused groups between the acute and subsequent studies.

The lower panel of table 34-1 shows the mean data for patients from all three studies. In patients who were acutely reperfused, there was no significant change between the acute and 24-h studies in either the EF or fractional shortening of the ischemic or compensatory regions, but there was a marked increase of the mean radial shortening in the region of the jeopardized myocardium (into the normal range) between the 24-h and predischarge studies. Among the patients who were not reperfused acutely, there was no significant change in either the EF or the segmental function of the jeopardized or compensatory regions between the acute and 24-h studies. There was also no significant change between the 24-h and the predischarge studies in these patients.

All acutely reperfused patients who showed improvement in global EF (greater than or equal to 5%) between the acute and subsequent studies are shown in figure 34-2A. Radial shortening in the ischemic segment is plotted using solid lines. There was improvement in contractile function between the acute and subsequent studies in the region of the jeopardized myocardium in each patient. Mean radial shortening in the compensatory region is shown for each patient, using interrupted lines.

Patients who were reperfused, but showed no improvement or a decrease in the global EF between the acute and subsequent studies, are shown in figure 34-2b. The uniform improvement in

TABLE 34-1. Acute and subsequent studies

	EF			%RS Jeop			%RS Comp		
	Acute	24°	p	Acute	24°	p	Acute	24°	p
Opened (n = 9)	45 ± 8	48 ± 5	0.35	9 ± 4	17 ± 4	0.01**	37 ± 10	34 ± 10	0.06
Closed (n = 6)	37 ± 11	33 ± 9	0.18	10 ± 3	6 ± 2	0.06	32 ± 17	27 ± 10	0.58

All three studies

	EF			p values		%RS Jeop			p values		%RS Comp			p values	
	1st	2nd	3rd			1st	2nd	3rd			1st	2nd	3rd		
Opened (n = 8)	44 ± 7	40 ± 8	48 ± 6	0.07	0.03	8 ± 4	8 ± 3	18 ± 5	0.52	0.01¶	37 ± 10	32 ± 8	35 ± 9	0.07	0.72
Closed (n = 4)	41 ± 5	38 ± 6	35 ± 5	0.58	0.58	10 ± 3	5 ± 4	5 ± 2	0.10	1.00	37 ± 10	32 ± 8	35 ± 9	0.07	0.72

EF, ejection fraction; %RS Jeop, mean % radial shortening in jeopardized region; %RS Comp, mean % radial shortening in compensatory region; 1st, acute; 2nd 24°; 3rd, predischarge.
[a]$p < 0.05$; [b]$p < 0.025$.

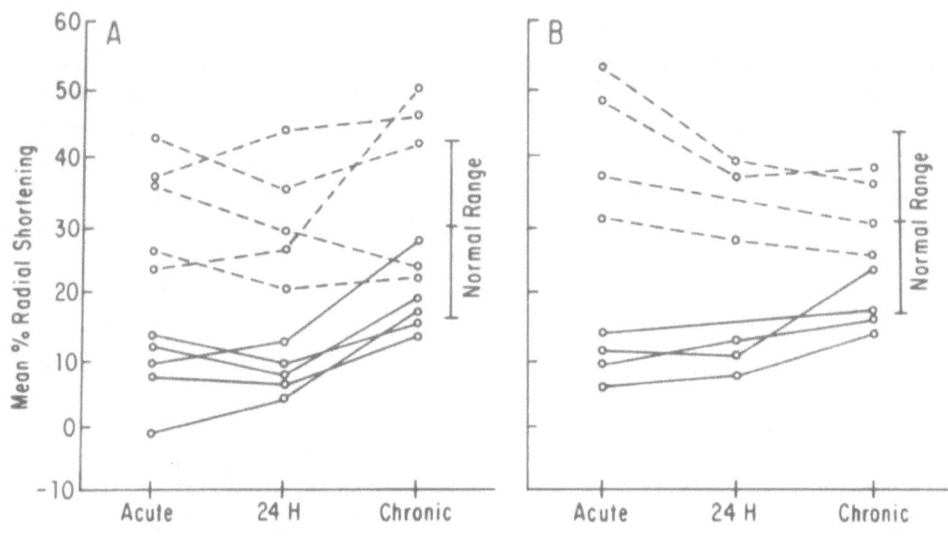

FIGURE 34-2. The changes in percent radial shortening in both the ischemic (solid lines) and compensatory (dashed lines) regions is indicated for all nine patients who received all three studies. The five who had improvement in global EF are indicated in A and those four with no improvement in B. There is similar improvement in the ischemic regions in both groups, but a decrease in the compensatory regions in group B.

the region of the jeopardized myocardium is again demonstrated despite the absence of improvement in the EF. There was a decrease in the degree of compensatory wall motion in the uninvolved region in each patient between the acute and subsequent studies.

The radial shortening data in the ischemic zone among the patients who were not successfully recanalized during the acute study are indicated by the solid lines in figure 34-3. The patency status during each study is indicated by an open circle to indicate late opening of the infarct-related coronary artery. There was no improvement in the contractile function of the jeopardized myocardium in any of these patients despite the frequent occurrence of late spontaneous recanalization. The mean radial shortening in the compensatory region is shown for each patient, using interrupted lines.

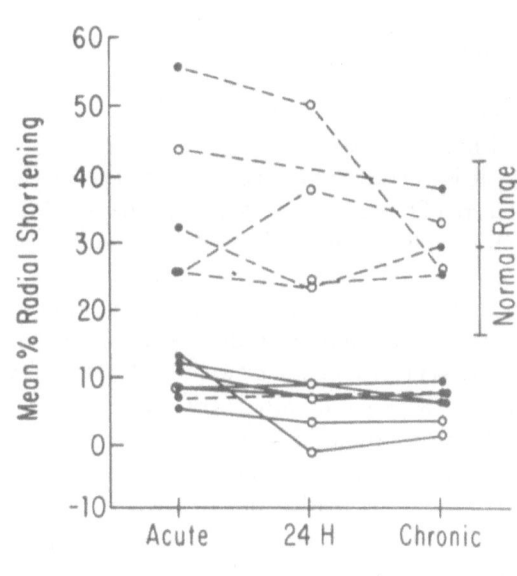

FIGURE 34-3. The changes in percent radial shortening in both the ischemic (solid lines) and compensatory (dashed lines) regions is indicated for the six patients who were not reperfused. Open circles indicate that the involved artery was patent at that study and the solid circles indicate occluded arteries. There was no improvement in shortening in the ischemic regions in any of the patients.

Discussion

The technique used in this study [7] for quantitative analysis of regional wall motion utilizes multiple radii that sample segmental wall motion at 15° intervals around the ventricular silhouette. This method determines the systolic and diastolic radial lengths independently and thus corrects for heart motion artifact. The normal range of fractional shortening for each radius was determined using a large number of normal patients who were shown to have no evidence of heart disease at cardiac catheterization [10].

All of the patients who were reperfused within 6 h of the onset of symptoms improved the mean radial shortening in the region of the jeopardized myocardium. In 56% of these patients, the segmental function in the jeopardized region was returned to the normal range by the time of the predischarge catheterization study. Despite their improvement in segmental function, however, 44% of the reperfused patients showed either no improvement or a decrease in global EF between the acute and predischarge studies. Failure of the global EF to improve despite a significant return of function in the jeopardized region was due to a decrease in the amount of compensatory wall motion in the uninvolved region in each patient within 24 h after reperfusion.

It is important to consider the time course of return of function in myocardium that has been profoundly ischemic. There was no improvement of segmental function in the ischemic region of acutely reperfused patients at 24 h in the group of patients with all three studies. A significant improvement in regional as well as global performance, however, occurred between the 24-h and subsequent studies. Previous experimental studies have documented a delayed functional recovery within the borders of the jeopardized myocardium. Theroux et al. [13] studied segmental function following a 2-h temporary occlusion using ultrasonic crystals in awake dogs. These investigators showed that there was a delayed functional improvement at 2–4 weeks at the center and (more markedly) at the margins of the ischemic zone. Puri [14] found a 60% recovery of segmental function at two weeks in dogs after a 3-h occlusion. The mechanism of delayed functional recovery after reperfusion is not known. One explanation could be that some of the myocytes in the region of the jeopardized myocardium become intensely ischemic, but are able to survive in the absence of blood flow until the time of reperfusion. Restoration of blood flow into the infarcted area could possibly promote hypertrophy of these cells, allowing partial recovery of the involved region. Other explanations could be either a delayed repletion of myocardial ATP stores in the ischemic region or prolonged abnormality in local calcium activity [15] (see chapter 3).

This study was designed to compare changes in global and segmental function among patients who were acutely reperfused and those who either could not be reperfused within 6 h of the onset of symptoms or who demonstrated late reocclusion of the infarct-related vessel. The patients who were not initially perfused demonstrated a wide spectrum of late recanalization as well as late reocclusion of the infarct-related coronary artery. However, functional changes in the region of the ischemic myocardium within this group were consistent and differed markedly from the changes in the patients who were acutely reperfused. There was no improvement in the mean radial shortening in the region of the jeopardized myocardium at 24 h or at the time of the predischarge catheterization in any of the patients who could not be recanalized within 6 h of the onset of symptoms. There was also no significant reduction in the degree of compensatory wall motion between the acute and 24-h or the 24-h and predischarge studies. None of the four patients with late recanalization showed improvement in segmental function in the ischemic region compared with the acute study, suggesting that late reperfusion does not result in significant salvage of function of the jeopardized myocardium. This is consistent with previous histologic studies in dogs that showed little or no salvage of ischemic myocardium following 6 h of temporary occlusion [16, 17]. Because of differences in species, mechanism of occlusion, and degree of collateral flow, the length of time available for successful reperfusion in man may differ from that of the dog model.

The study reported in this chapter illustrates the complexity of evaluating the effects of thrombolytic therapy in acute myocardial infarction. Days and even weeks may be required for transiently ischemic myocardium to regain normal function. Meanwhile, compensation by non-ischemic myocardium may invalidate global measurements for estimating either damage or recovery. Currently, methods other than direct injection of contrast agents into the left ventricle have not been proven to assess regional function accurately. Thus, an invasive study remote from the acute intervention may be the only valid method available for detecting salvage of jeopardized myocardium in patients with acute myocardial infarction.

References

1. Rentrop P, Blancke H, Karsch KR, Kaiser H, Kostering H, Leitz K: Selective intracoronary thrombolysis in acute myocardial infarction and unstable angina pectoris. Circulation 63:307–316, 1981.

2. Reduto LA, Smalling RW, Freund GC, Gould KL: Intracoronary infusion of streptokinase in patients with acute myocardial infarction. Am J Cardiol 48:403–409, 1981.

3. Mathey DG, Kuck KH, Tilsner V, Krebber HJ, Bleifield W: Nonsurgical coronary artery recanalization in acute transmural myocardial infarction. Circulation 63:489–497, 1981.

4. Lee G, Amsterdam EA, Low R, Joye JA, Kimchi A, DeMaria AN, Mason DT: Efficacy of percutaneous transluminal coronary recanalization utilizing streptokinase thrombolysis in patients with acute myocardial infarction. Am Heart J 102:1159–1167, 1981.

5. Rentrop P, Blanke H, Karsch KR: Effects of nonsurgical coronary reperfusion on the left ventricle in human subjects compared with conventional treatment. Am J Cardiol 49:1–8, 1982.

6. Markis JE, Malagold M, Parker JA, Silverman KJ, Barry WH, Als AV, Paulin S, Grossman W, Braunwald E: Myocardial salvage after intracoronary thrombolysis with streptokinase in acute myocardial infarction. N Engl J Med 305:777–782, 1981.

7. Stack RS, Phillips HR III, Grierson DS, Behar VS, Kong Y, Peter RH, Swain JL, Greenfield JC

Jr: Functional improvement of jeopardized myocardium following intracoronary streptokinase infusion in acute myocardial infarction. J Clin Invest 72:84–95, 1983.

8. Mandelkorn J, Wolf NM, Singh S, Bentivoglio L, Meister SG: Systemic thrombolytic effect of intracoronary streptokinase [abstr]. Circulation 64:IV-191a, 1981.

9. Ideker RE, Behar VS, Wagner GS, Starr JW, Starmer CF, Lee KL, Hackel DB: Evaluation of asynergy as an indicator of myocardial fibrosis. Circulation 57:715–720, 1978.

10. Behar VS: Contrast ventriculography. In: Wagner GS (ed) Quantification of ischemic and infarcted myocardium. The Hague: Martinus Nijhoff, 1982, pp 173–197.

11. Kennedy JW, Baxley WA, Figley MM, Dodge HT, Blackmon JR: Quantitative angiography. I. The normal left ventricle in man. Circulation 34:272–278, 1966.

12. Dodge HT, Hay RE, Sandler H: An angiographic method for directly determining left ventricular stroke volume in man. Circ Res 11:739–746, 1962.

13. Theroux P, Ross J, Franklin D, Kemper WS, Sasayama S: Coronary artery reperfusion. III. Early and late effects on regional myocardial function and dimensions in conscious dogs. Am J Cardiol 38:599–606, 1976.

14. Puri PS: Contractile and biochemical effects of coronary reperfusion after extended periods of coronary occlusion. Am J Cardiol 36:244–251, 1975.

15. Braunwald E, Kloner RA: The stunned myocardium: prolonged, postischemic ventricular dysfunction. Circulation 66:1146–1149, 1982.

16. Reimer KA, Lowe JE, Rasmussen MM, Jennings RB: The wavefront phenomenon of ischemic cell death. I. Myocardial infarct size vs duration of coronary occlusion in dogs. Circulation 56:786–794, 1977.

17. Reimer KA, Jennings RB: The wavefront phenomenon of myocardial ischemic cell death. II. Transmural progression of necrosis within the framework of ischemic bed size (myocardium at risk) and collateral flow. Lab Invest 40:633–644, 1979.

35. THE ROLE OF SURGERY IN UNSTABLE ANGINA PECTORIS AND ACUTE MYOCARDIAL INFARCTION

Marcus A. De Wood

Ronald P. Grunwald

William P. O'Grady

Michael L. Hinnen

Gerald R. Hensley

J. Paul Shields

Short-term studies indicate that coronary bypass surgery is an effective form of therapy for patients with unstable angina pectoris because symptoms of myocardial ischemia are usually relieved and exercise tolerance is improved [1−5]. Until recently there have been few long-term studies examining the mortality, morbidity, and functional status subsequent to surgical therapy for either unstable angina pectoris or acute myocardial infarction [5−9] and no general agreement has been reached regarding the current role of this surgical treatment. This chapter examines both short- and long-term results with combined medical and surgical therapy.

Definitions

A variety of terms have been used to describe unstable angina pectoris: accelerated angina pec-

This work was supported in part by the Deaconess and Sacred Heart Research Foundations, Max Baer Heart Fund (Washington Fraternal Order of Eagles), and the Inland Empire Heart Research Foundation.

toris, impending myocardial infarction, preinfarction angina, coronary insufficiency, crescendo angina, and the intermediate coronary syndrome. As implied by the different nomenclature, patients with varying clinical degrees of anginal severity have been included in these categories. In patients treated at Sacred Heart and Deaconess Medical Centers, the patient population with "unstable angina pectoris" includes only those patients with (a) progressive rest pain, (b) ST- and T-wave abnormalities on the electrocardiogram (ECG) obtained in the coronary care unit, and (c) normal preoperative total CK and MB-CK activity. These patients had progressive pain despite conventional medical therapy that consisted of nitrates and, if indicated, beta-blockade. The majority of patients were managed before the widespread clinical application of calcium channel blockers.

The definition of unstable angina used in the report by Rahimtoola et al. [5] included three categories of patients: (a) rest pain warranting admission to the coronary care unit, (b) persistent anginal pain within three months of an acute myocardial infarction, and (c) the onset of anginal pain within six months after coronary surgery that was of increasing severity, duration, or frequency in spite of medical therapy. In the National Unstable Angina Study [3], patients were considered to have "unstable angina" when they had either new-onset angina or a changing pattern of previously stable angina severe enough to warrant admission to the intensive care unit to rule out myocardial infarction. Patients with an infarction within the previous three months were excluded as were patients older than 70 years of age. All patients were required to have transient ECG changes during at least one episode of pain, and patients with ECG or enzymatic evidence of evolving myocardial infarction were excluded. In the study by Mulcahy et al. [10], the diagnosis of unstable angina was made when patients had typical cardiac pain requiring admission to the cardiac care unit and ST- and T-wave changes on the ECG without evidence for myocardial necrosis on serial ECGs and cardiac isozymes.

Two varieties of myocardial infarction are included in this review. *Nontransmural myocardial infarction* is defined as chest pain in conjunction with ST- and T-wave abnormalities *not* progressing to abnormal Q waves on the ECG, but *with* documented elevation of total CK activity (preoperatively in surgical patients). *Transmural myocardial infarction* is defined as chest pain in conjunction with persistent ST-segment elevation that usually progressed to abnormal Q waves on the ECG, and with abnormal preoperative total CK activity.

Unstable Angina Pectoris

Between 1973 and 1981, 1012 patients underwent coronary artery bypass surgery at the Sacred Heart and Deaconess Medical Centers for unstable angina pectoris. During the follow-up period (1973–1983), survivors were contacted by questionnaire and by personal telephone contact, if needed. The patients were classified according to both the extent of coronary occlusive disease (one-, two-, or three-vessel disease) and left ventricular function as measured by the global left ventricular ejection fraction dichotomized at 50%.

Table 35-1 demonstrates this experience. Forty

TABLE 35-1. The annual hospital mortality and patient flow for the period described.
Overall the short-term mortality for the unstable angina group was 2.17% (22 of 1012).

Unstable angina pectoris annual hospital mortality		
1973	0/50	(0%)
1974	1/84	(1.19%)
1975	2/135	(1.48%)
1976	1/127	(0.78%)
1977	3/151	(1.98%)
1978	4/108	(3.70%)
1979	5/150	(3.33%)
1980	5/146	(3.42%)
1981	1/61	(0.16%)
Total	22/1012	(2.17%)

patients were lost to follow-up and were not included in subsequent analyses. The mean duration of follow-up was 4.8 years. The annual hospital mortality is also indicated in table 35-1: 2.2% (22 of 1012) for the eight-year period. The group's one-year mortality was 4.3% and the total follow-up mortality was 13.2%. This mortality rate is somewhat less than that reported from the surgery group from the early period (1972) of the unstable angina trial sponsored by the National Institutes of Health [3], but it is comparable to the experience described during the last four years (1973–1976) of the trial. These results are also very similar to those reported by Rahimtoola et al. [5].

THE INFLUENCE OF THE EXTENT OF CORONARY DISEASE

The effect of the number of diseased vessels on survival in patients with unstable angina pectoris in the present series is depicted in figure 35-1. Of the 1012 patients, only 225 (22%) had single-vessel coronary disease. The mortality of these patients was 2.2% (5 of 225) inhospital and 3.8% at one year. The mortality rose to 9.8% during the ten-year follow-up period. This inhospital mortality is slightly higher than that of the surgical group from the National Institutes of Health study group [3] (0%), while it is slightly lower than the mortality of their medically treated patients (6%). The results are similar to the

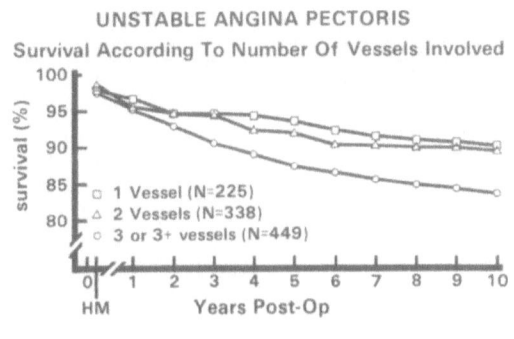

UNSTABLE ANGINA PECTORIS
Survival According To Number Of Vessels Involved

□ 1 Vessel (N=225)
△ 2 Vessels (N=338)
○ 3 or 3+ vessels (N=449)

FIGURE 35-1. The survival (ordinate) and the years relative to the years postoperatively in the patient cohorts defined by one-, two-, and three-vessel disease. As is shown, one- and two-vessel involvement behaves with a similar mortality over the years while triple-vessel disease was associated with the highest mortality.

recently published short- and long-term mortality data of Rahimtoola et al. [5].

Two-vessel disease was demonstrated in 338 (34%) of the study population. The hospital mortality was 1.2% (4 of 338), and the one-year mortality was 4.7%. The cumulative ten-year mortality of this group (11.5%) was also very similar to the results reported by Rahimtoola et al. [5]. These hospital mortality figures are similar to those of the surgical group from the NIH study (2%) and are somewhat lower than the 4% mortality in their medical group [3].

The remaining 449 patients (44%) had three-vessel coronary disease. They had a hospital mortality of 2.9% (13 of 449) (figure 35-1) and a one-year mortality of 4.8% was observed. The ten-year follow-up mortality was 16.3%. This inhospital mortality is lower than that of 10% in the NIH study for their surgically treated patients. The reasons for this mortality difference are unclear, but sample size may be an important factor. Similarly low inhospital and ten-year mortality rates were observed in the study by Rahimtoola et al. [5], which had a similar sample size. The long-term mortality in the present study appears to be somewhat more favorable than that reported using conventional medical therapy with [4] or without [9, 10] angiographic evaluation. Despite these apparent differences in mortality, rigorous evaluation of medical versus surgical therapy requires either concurrently treated controls or randomized treatment.

THE INFLUENCE OF LEFT VENTRICULAR EJECTION FRACTION ON SURVIVAL

Until recently [5], few studies have examined the influence of baseline left ventricular performance on short- or long-term mortality in patients treated surgically for unstable angina pectoris. Because many of the ventricular silhouettes could not be accurately defined in our population, left ventricular ejection fraction was determined in 724 of the 1012 patients (figure 35-2): 584 patients demonstrated global ejection fraction of 50% or greater while 140 patients demonstrated left ventricular dysfunction, defined as a global ejection fraction less than 50%.

The hospital mortality in patients with an ejection fraction of 50% or more was 1.2% (7 of 584). This figure rose to only 2.6% at one year. The group with normal left ventricular ejection fraction maintained a low cumulative mortality of 11% over the ten-year follow-up period. By contrast, the mortality of patients with depression of left ventricular performance was greater. The inhospital mortality was 3.6% (5 of 140) and this rose to 9.3% at one year. The total mortality during the ten-year follow-up was 20% (28 of 140). Thus, left ventricular performance was a major determinant of short- and long-term mortality in this series of patients with unstable angina pectoris. These data support the recently published findings of Rahimtoola et al. [5], who demonstrated similar survival rates for "normal" and "abnormal" left ventricular function, although the level that was considered normal was not specifically defined in their study. Similar results with regard to left ventricular function in the overall group of patients with coronary artery disease have been reported by the Coronary Artery Surgery Study [11].

RELIEF OF ANGINA PECTORIS

Our data suggest that the relief of angina pectoris is not a short-term phenomenon. Instead, coronary artery bypass surgery appears to be exceptionally effective in the relief of angina because of improved myocardial perfusion and relief of ischemia [12].

These data were not compared with results derived from aggressive therapy with calcium channel blockers. However, a recent randomized study [13] to evaluate short-term effects of nifedipine in unstable angina pectoris suggested that one-third of the treated population will eventually require coronary artery bypass surgery. Furthermore, the mortality in patients treated nonsurgically was 9% (8 of 91) at four months. Detailed baseline characteristics are not available for a direct comparison of these patients with ours, but these data suggest that surgical therapy may provide benefit even when calcium channel blockers are available. Importantly, randomized studies of unstable angina pectoris have shown that at least 40% of patients treated with medical therapy will develop disabling angina again during the follow-up period [1, 3, 12, 14]. In comparison, less than 10% of the surgically treated patients in our study reported major angina pectoris with limitation of function (figure 35-3).

CLINICAL IMPLICATIONS

The study by Gazes and co-workers in 1973 [9] indicated a much higher mortality with medical therapy than more recently managed medical groups [1, 3, 12, 13]. The reasons for this decline in medical mortality are not known, but the recent availability of angiographic definition of the nature and extent of coronary disease and left ventricular function has allowed for better characterization of the patient populations in recent years. Nevertheless, one of the factors associated with high mortality during the ten-year follow-up in the series reported by Gazes et al. [9] was persistent angina in the hospital. Mulcahy et al. [10] have reported that persistent angina in the hospital was the chief predictor of poor outcome in their series of patients. These findings emphasize the importance of angiographic definition of the extent of coronary disease during the early course of unstable angina pectoris.

It is important to note (figure 35-1) that the majority of patients in the present series demonstrated multivessel disease and that only 22% had single-vessel involvement. The study by Rahimtoola et al. [5] also indicated that approximately 80% of patients with unstable angina

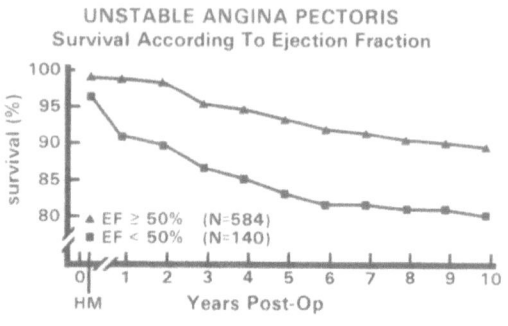

FIGURE 35-2. The results in patient groups dichotomized at a global ejection fraction of 50%. As is shown, an ejection fraction of less than 50% was associated with a relatively adverse outcome presumably because of preexisting myocardial damage.

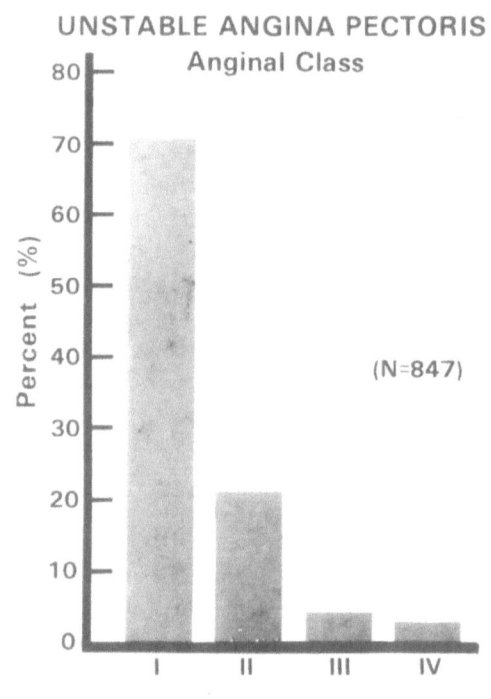

FIGURE 35-3. The anginal class in the patients with unstable angina pectoris who could classify their anginal status (see text for classification) by questionnaire. As is shown, most patients had satisfactory long-term anginal relief with fewer than 10% reporting symptoms of any major proportion.

who are referred to surgery have multivessel disease. The high prevalence of multivessel disease may be secondary to the selection of patients with extensive disease for surgery by the involved clinicians. Although recent advances in medical therapy, such as calcium channel blockers and percutaneous transluminal coronary angioplasty, may allow more patients initially to be treated medically, the majority of evidence indicates that a high percentage of patients will eventually need surgical therapy.

Thus, although unstable angina pectoris may not be a surgical emergency, we attempt to promptly arrange surgery for patients who demonstrate failure of aggressive medical therapy, especially if two- and three-vessel disease is present. Likewise, urgent surgical intervention is applied in selected situations, such as the presence of significant left main coronary stenosis. Because coronary anatomy and left ventricular function are determined early in the course of unstable angina, and because surgery can be applied urgently if indicated, a low mortality rate can be attained. Persistent chest discomfort, as described by Gazes et al. [9], is not permitted to continue, because this symptom complex suggests that ongoing ischemia will lead to more difficult clinical problems with the potential for an unfavorable outcome unless prompt, aggressive treatment is initiated.

OCCURRENCE OF MYOCARDIAL INFARCTION AND REOPERATION
The occurrence of documented myocardial infarction following coronary bypass surgery for unstable angina pectoris was low during the ten-year follow-up period (11.6%). Reoperation due to progression of disease in the native circulation or reccurrence of disease in bypass grafts was necessary in 63 patients (6.45%). This incidence of approximately 1% per year is consistent with the report by Rahimtoola et al. [5]. They reported a reoperation rate of 1.2% per year for the first five years after the first operation, and 2.2% per year for the second five years. Since these patients are attaining prolonged survival, however, the importance of reoperation will increase during longer follow-up.

Acute Myocardial Infarction

OVERVIEW
One of the major factors responsible for contractile impairment during early "transmural myocardial infarction" is the high incidence of complete coronary occlusion [15, 16]. Morbidity and mortality are related to the magnitude of myocardium lost. Autopsy and angiographic data suggest that "subendocardial myocardial infarction" (without ST-segment elevation or Q-wave formation) is frequently associated with high-grade stenosis, but not with total coronary occlusion.

Medical therapy directed at preservation of jeopardized ischemic myocardium by reducing myocardial oxygen demand has not appeared to result in substantial salvage [17, 18]. Recent clinical studies have been directed toward the fundamental issue of restoration of blood flow during the early phases of evolving myocardial infarction. Mechanisms of restoration of blood flow have included surgical reperfusion [6—8] and nonsurgical thrombolysis [16] with and without mechanical manipulation of the coronary arteries [19] (see chapters 6 and 8). The remainder of this chapter focuses on surgical myocardial revascularization for acute myocardial infarction.

RATIONALE FOR SURGICAL REPERFUSION
The primary goal of the restoration of blood flow distal to the point of coronary occlusion is to protect marginally perfused ischemic areas that might otherwise progress to frank infarction with permanent loss of function. Successful early surgical reperfusion has been demonstrated to be associated with improvement in global and regional left ventricular function [20]. If early surgical reperfusion is successful, it should also be accompanied by reduction in mortality compared with medical therapy. Furthermore, lower mortality should be observed in early treatment groups relative to patients undergoing later surgical therapy, since all basic experiments have shown that the amount of myocardium salvaged is proportional to the rapidity with which reperfusion is accomplished (see chapter 2).

PILOT STUDIES EXAMINING MORTALITY IN MATCHED MEDICAL AND SURGICAL COHORTS

As shown in table 35-2, we compared two groups of patients with acute myocardial infarcts between 1972 and 1976 [6]. The first group was comprised of 200 patients aged 65 years or less who were given conventional medical therapy. The inhospital mortality and long-term mortality of these patients were compared with 187 patients undergoing surgical reperfusion for an evolving transmural myocardial infarction. The two groups were comparable in average age, the incidence of previous myocardial infarcts, the frequency of initial abnormal elevation of total CK activity, the location of infarction by the ECG, and the number of vessels with significant (i.e., ≥70%) stenosis by autopsy or catheterization. A drawback with the study is that the definition of coronary anatomy was possible in only 70% of ptients given conventional therapy. The clinical classification of heart failure (Killip class [21]) was not significantly different except for a higher incidence of cardiogenic shock in the surgically treated group. Thus, in most respects, the baseline characteristics of the groups were similar.

SHORT- AND LONG-TERM MORTALITY

We subsequently evaluated the short- and long-term mortality of the two groups in the presence and absence of cardiogenic shock (table 35-3). When patients in Killip class IV were included, the hospital mortality of the conventional therapy group was 11.5% (23 of 200). There were an additional 18 deaths, bringing the total mortality to 20.5% (41 of 200) during the mean follow-up period of 36 months. Importantly, 55 of the survivors underwent elective coronary artery bypass surgery later without a death. In the surgical group the hospital mortality was 5.8% (11 of 187). There were 11 additional deaths, or a total mortality of 11.7% (22 of 187) during a mean follow-up of 37 months.

Cardiogenic shock is a high-risk clinical situation that is caused by dysfunction of an excessive area of myocardium, unless associated with a

TABLE 35-2. The clinical characteristics of groups I and II on entry into the study. As is shown, there were no major significant differences (apart from the higher incidence of cardiogenic shock in the surgical treatment group) between the two groups.

	Group I (n = 200)	Group II (n = 187)
Age (yr) (mean ± SD)	53.2 ± 8.1	52.7 ± 9.1
Incidence of previous MI	28 (14%)	30 (16%)
Patients with abnormal (>90 IU) elevation of total CK activity on initial sampling	119 (59.5%)	110 (58.8%)
Area of infarction (ECG)		
Anterior	73 (36.5%)	88 (47.0%)
Anterolateral	29 (14.5%)	14 (7.5%)
Inferior	74 (37.0%)	72 (38.5%)
Inferoposterior	11 (5.5%)	8 (4.3%)
Lateral	6 (3.0%)	2 (1.1%)
Uncertain	7 (3.5%)	3 (1.6%)
Vessels with CAD (no.)		
1	38 (27.4%)	59 (31.5%)
2	57 (41.0%)	67 (35.8%)
3	44 (31.6%)	61 (32.6%)
Clinical class (Killip)		
I	123 (61.5%)	112 (59.9%)
II	60 (30%)	48 (25.6%)
III	10 (5%)	9 (4.8%)
IV	7 (3.5%)	18 (9.6%)

TABLE 35-3. The inhospital, long-term, and total mortality in the conventional (group I) and surgical (group II) treatment groups with and without inclusion of patients who were in Killip class IV (cardiogenic shock) on entry into this study. As is shown, the mortality was exceptionally low with early reperfusion. The difference was less marked with class-IV patients excluded in the conventional therapy group because of the selection process and attempts to eliminate bias against the conventional therapy group on study entry. Nevertheless, mortality was lower both with and without class IV excluded with surgical reperfusion. The difference is widened with clinical class-IV patients excluded.

		Mortality		
	Patients (no.)	Inhospital	Long-term	Total (18−56 mo)
Class IV included				
Medical group (I)	200	23 (11.5%)	18 more deaths	41 (20.5%)
Surgical group (II)	187	11 (5.8%)[a]	11 more deaths	22 (11.7%)[b]
Class IV excluded				
Medical group (I)	193	18 (9.3%)	17 more deaths	35 (18.1%)
Surgical group (II)	169	2 (1.2)[c]	10 more deaths	12 (7.1%)[d]

[a]$p<0.08$. [b]$p<0.03$. [c]$p<0.003$. [d]$p<0.005$.

mechanical defect (see chapter 45) such as a septal defect, mitral regurgitation, or right ventricular infarction. Since it seems unlikely that any therapy can limit mortality in the presence of such excessively damaged myocardium, we compared the two cohorts not in shock. When Killip class-IV patients were excluded, the mortality of the conventional group was 9.3% (11 of 193) in hospital and 18.1% (35 of 193) during follow-up. By contrast, the mortality of the group undergoing surgical reperfusion was 1.2% (2 of 169) inhospital and 7.1% (12 of 169) during the follow-up period. These data strongly support the concept that surgical reperfusion can be performed with low mortality and suggest that the results are more favorable in the absence of cardiogenic shock. Importantly, the conventional therapy group contained fewer patients with cardiogenic shock (see table 35-2) on study entry because many patients in shock were excluded to avoid a bias against the conventional therapy group.

MORTALITY OF THE EARLY (WITHIN 6 h OF SYMPTOM ONSET) SURGICAL REPERFUSION GROUP RELATIVE TO THE CONVENTIONAL THERAPY GROUP
Myocardial infarction is a regional disease that ultimately affects the global performance of the heart. If early reperfusion can limit the extent of infarction, short- and long-term mortality should be altered. Accordingly, we analyzed short- and long-term mortality subsequent to early reperfusion and compared the results with mortality in patients receiving conventional therapy. Of the 100 patients placed on cardiopulmonary bypass within 6 h, the mortality was 2% in hospital and 6% at an average follow-up of 36 months (figure 35-4). By contrast, the patient cohort given conventional therapy demonstrated an 11.5% hospital mortality, and 20.5% long-term mortality. Both the short-term and long-term results, therefore, indicate that early reperfusion was associated with significant differences in mortality. These observations, therefore, supported the concept derived from animal experiments that the degree of success with reperfusion varies inversely with the time interval from the onset of occlusion to the restoration of coronary blood flow [22–24] (see chapter 2).

Because infarction of the anterior wall of the heart involves larger portions of jeopardized heart muscle than inferior wall infarction, we have focused on patients with anterior transmural infarcts. Selinger and co-workers [25] have demonstrated that even large anterior transmural infarcts can be successfully treated by early surgical reperfusion. Our group has also found that short-term mortality in patients given medical therapy is substantially higher than in those treated by surgical reperfusion during anterior transmural myocardial infarction [26]. These results suggest that surgical therapy is beneficial, but the absence of detailed coronary anatomic and left ventricular function measurements in the medically treated group does not allow us to make a rigorous therapeutic comparison in which baseline factors can be adequately controlled for. A well-controlled clinical trial now seems indicated.

MORTALITY PATTERNS WITH EARLY VERSUS LATE REPERFUSION
In a later series, patients with transmural anterior and inferior infarcts were divided into groups receiving early (within 6 h) or late (longer than 6 h) reperfusion [26]. A total of 291 patients were placed on cardiopulmonary bypass within 6 h, while 149 patients were placed on cardiopulmonary bypass longer than 6 h from symptom onset. In the group receiving early reperfusion, the short-term mortality was substantially lower than in the group receiving late reperfusion (11 of 291, 3.8%, versus 12 of 149, 8.0%; $p=0.05$). Further analysis indicated that the long-term outlook was far less favorable in the patient group receiving late reperfusion. The group of patients receiving early reperfusion maintained a lower long-term total mortality (24 of 291, 8.2%) than the group receiving later reperfusion (31 of 149, 21.0%) ($p < 0.01$) (figure 35-5).

The recent observations which indicate that both global and regional left ventricular function are improved if patients are treated early rather than late [20] provide further support for the concept that early reperfusion is superior to later reperfusion. Importantly, the only patients who experienced significant improvement in function with late reperfusion were those who demonstrated either adequate collateral blood flow or antegrade flow through the infarct-related vessel.

Clinical Implications

The data presented in this chapter demonstrate that reperfusion for both unstable angina pectoris and acute myocardial infarction can be performed with acceptably low mortality. Our results suggest that surgical therapy for unstable angina appears to offer a major advantage for patients with two- and three-vessel disease, especially in the presence of disabling chest pain. An addi-

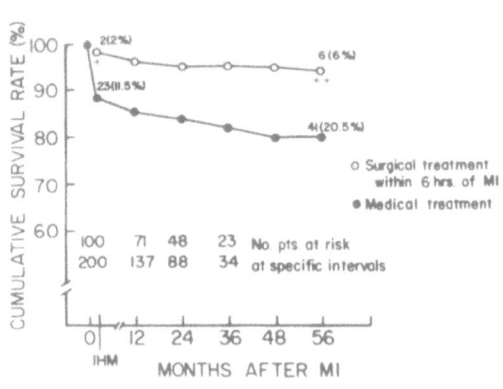

FIGURE 35-4. The mortality between the surgically treated group who underwent reperfusion within 6 h of transmural myocardial infarction (*open* circles) compared with conventional therapy. As is shown, there are major mortality differences both at study entry and in the long term. This Figure provided courtesy of the American Journal of Cardiology and the authors.

tional important factor was baseline left ventricular function. Compromised left ventricular function continues to be associated with unfavorable outcome even in the presence of a technically successful operation.

Regarding acute myocardial infarction, multiple problems arise when data regarding surgical reperfusion are based on patients who were not randomized. The data in this chapter may produce valuable information regarding long-term survival, ventricular function, and operative mortality. Moreover, our results are exceptionally attractive when compared with studies of conventional therapy in this community [6]. True perspectives on the value and limitations of surgical revascularization or other types of reperfusion should be evaluated in a controlled randomized trial.

In our community, medical and surgical management of coronary heart disease (acute and chronic) is viewed as complementary and not competitive. With this approach the mortality has remained low. Perhaps this is so because the nature and extent of the disease process is determined angiographically and the regions at risk and the potential for future clinical problems are defined and often treated prior to their occurrence.

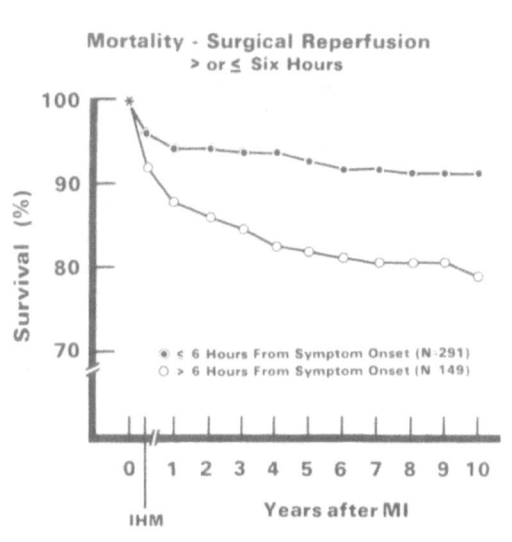

FIGURE 35-5. The mortality for the transmural myocardial infarction group divided into subgroups receiving early (within 6 h) or late (longer than 6 h)
reperfusion. Inhospital mortality for the early reperfusion group was significantly lower than that for the
late reperfusion group. This trend continued in the
ten-year follow-up period. The mortality of patients
operated upon within 6 h of symptom was 3.8% (11 of
291), but was 8% (12 of 149) in the late reperfusion
group. Likewise the long-term outlook was less favorable for the late reperfusion group, as is demonstrated.
Courtesy of the authors, *Circulation*, and the American
Heart Association.

References

1. Selden R, Neill WA, Ritzmann LW, Okies JE,
   Anderson RP: Medical versus surgical therapy for
   acute coronary insufficiency: a randomized study.
   N Engl J Med 293:1329−1333, 1975.
2. Boncheck LI, Rahimtoola SH, Anderson RP, et
   al: Late results following emergency saphenous
   vein bypass grafting for unstable angina. Circulation 50:972−977, 1974.
3. Russel RO Jr, Moraski RE, Kouchoukos N, et al:
   Unstable angina pectoris: National Cooperative
   Study Group to compare surgical and medical
   therapy. II. In-hospital experience and initial
   follow-up results in patients with one, two, and
   three vessel disease. Am J Cardiol 42:839−848,
   1978.
4. Bertolasi CA, Tronge JE, Capreno CA, et al:
   Unstable angina: prospective and randomized

5. Rahimtoola SH, Nunley D, Grunkemeier G,
   Tepley J, Lambert L, Starr A: Ten-year survival
   after coronary bypass surgery for unstable angina.
   N Engl J Med 308:676−681, 1983.
6. De Wood MA, Spores J, Notske RN, et al:
   Medical and surgical management of myocardial
   infarction. Am J Cardiol 44:1356−1364, 1979.
7. Phillips SJ, Zeff RH, Kongtahorn C, et al: Surgery for evolving myocardial infarction. JAMA
   248:1325−1328, 1982.
8. De Wood MA, Spores J, Berg R Jr, et al: Acute
   myocardial infarction: a decade of experience with
   surgical reperfusion in 701 patients. Circulation
   68:II-8−12, 1983.
9. Gazes PC, Mobley EM Jr, Paris HM Jr, Duncan
   RC, Humphries GB: Preinfarctional (unstable)
   angina: a prospective study—ten-year follow-up.
   Circulation 48:331−337, 1973.
10. Mulcahy R, Daly L, Graham I, et al: Unstable
    angina: natural history and determinants of prog-
    nosis. Am J Cardiol 48:525−528, 1981.
11. Kennedy JW, Kaiser GC, Fisher LD, Fritz JK,
    Myers W, Mudd JG, Ryan TJ: Clinical and
    angiographic predictors of operative mortality
    from the collaborative study in coronary artery
    surgery (CASS). Circulation 63:793−802, 1981.
12. Neill WA, Ritzmann LW, Okies JE, Anderson
    RP, Selden R: Medical vs. urgent surgical ther-
    apy for acute coronary insufficiency: a ran-
    domized study. In: Rahimtoola SH (ed) Coronary
    bypass surgery. Philadelphia: FA Davis, 1977,
    pp 179−87.
13. Gerstenblith G, Ouyang P, Achuff SC, et al:
    Nifedipine in unstable angina: a double-blind,
    randomized trial. N Engl J Med 306:885−889,
    1982.
14. Conti CR, Hodges M, Hutter A, et al: Unstable
    angina: a national cooperative study comparing
    medical and surgical therapy. In: Rahimtoola SH
    (ed) Coronary bypass surgery. Philadelphia: FA
    Davis, 1977, pp 167−178.
15. De Wood MA, Spores J, Notske R, et al: Preva-
    lance of total coronary occlusion during the early
    hours of transmural myocardial infarction.
    N Engl J Med 303:897, 1980.
16. Mathey DG, Kuch KH, Tilsner V, Krebber HJ,
    Bleifeld W: Nonsurgical coronary artery recana-
    lization in acute transmural myocardial infarc-
    tion. Circulation 63:489, 1981.
17. Rude RE, Muller JE, Braunwald E: Efforts to
    limit the size of myocardial infarcts. Ann Intern
    Med 95:736−761, 1981.
18. Goldman L, Cook F, Hashimoto B, Stone B,

Muller J, Loscalzo A: Evidence that hospital care for acute myocardial infarction has not contributed to the decline in coronary mortality between 1973–1974 and 1978–1979. Circulation 65: 936, 1982.

19. Meyer J, Merx W, Schmitz H, et al: Percutaneous transluminal coronary angioplasty immediately after intracoronary streptolysis of transmural myocardial infarction. Circulation 66: 1000, 1982.

20. De Wood MA, Heit J, Spores J, Selinger SL, Rudy LW, Hensley GR, Shields JP: Anterior transmural myocardial infarction in man: the effects of surgical reperfusion on global and regional left ventricular function. J Am Coll Cardiol 1:1223–1234, 1983.

21. Killip T III, Kimball JT: Treatment of myocardial infarction in a coronary care unit: a two year experience with 250 patients. Am J Cardiol 20:457, 1967.

22. Costantini C, Corday E, Lang T, et al: Revascularization after 3 hours of coronary arterial occlusion: effects on regional cardiac metabolic function and infarct size. Am J Cardiol 36:368–384, 1975.

23. Maroko PR, Libby P, Ginks WR, et al: Coronary artery reperfusion. I. Early effects on local myocardial function and the extent of myocardial necrosis. J Clin Invest 51:2710–2723, 1972.

24. Ginks WR, Sybers HD, Maroko PR, Covell JW, Sobel BE, Ross J Jr: Coronary artery reperfusion. II. Reduction of myocardial infarct size at one week after the coronary artery occlusion. J Clin Invest 51:2717–2723, 1972.

25. Selinger SL, Berg R Jr, Leonard JJ, Grunwald RP, O'Grady WP: Surgical treatment of acute evolving anterior myocardial infarction. Circulation (Suppl 2) 64:II-28, 1981.

26. De Wood MA, Spores J, Rudy LW, Grunwald R, Shields JP: Relationship of mortality and regional wall motion in anterior myocardial infarction treated by early surgical reperfusion. J Am Coll Cardiol 1:592, 1983.

VII. CORONARY CARE: THE CORONARY CARE UNIT

36. THE EVOLUTION OF CARE OF PATIENTS WITH UNSTABLE ANGINA AND MYOCARDIAL INFARCTION

Michael Thomas

Clinical practice provides a rather ruthless assessment of the real value of any medical innovation, and fortunately the medical practice that becomes accepted as routine has usually been well tried. Unfortunately, new thinking and new techniques are not easily seen in perspective at the time of introduction and we are obliged to explore many areas from which only a minority of ideas bear fruit. From an opposite viewpoint, accepted routine practice sometimes discourages critical new thought, because the originators and first work become obscure, and because the very nature of routine discourages unsettling criticism. The evolution of the care of patients with unstable angina pectoris and myocardial infarction illustrates the uncertain path of medical progress. Dramatic advances have occurred, but "penicillins are rare" and the revolution that has taken place represents the very many different ways in which improvements are brought about. New attitudes, techniques, drugs, and surgical expertise have all made their point—and the successive generations of medical, nursing, and paramedic support personnel have refined their practical skills and training.

Overriding all these considerations is the necessity to appreciate when we don't understand and to reassess continually the quality of evidence relating to methods of clinical care. A recognition of ignorance is not always an agreeable exercise, but it was in such a spirit that the research-orientated special care unit for patients with acute

ischemic heart disease came about in the early 1960s. At this time in Britain, thinking in cardiology was dominated by concern for patients with rheumatic valve disease and intricate congenital malformations. It was only in moments of irony that the future of the vast majority of cardiac patients, suffering from ischemic heart disease, was considered. These individuals were fated to become ill at any time of the day or night, usually far away from centers of cardiac expertise, without any chance of informed, effective intervention. Even in academic teaching circles, where such patients were regularly evaluated, ischemic heart disease competed most unfavorably for constructive thought, allocation of facilities, and exposure of the considerable problems.

The first commitment to investigate deeply the illness and treatment of the individual patient suffering from acute ischemic heart disease was at the Postgraduate Medical School, Hammersmith Hospital, London. A very small single-bed unit dedicated to those problems was set up as a pilot scheme [1]. To those involved at the time, the intrinsic interest of such patients was considerable, but the far-reaching implications took longer to appreciate.

The facilities were basic, but careful preliminary work in validating methods of measuring cardiac output and intraarterial and intracardiac pressures in acutely ill patients enabled reliable repetitive measurements to be made without disturbing the patients. Apart from ethical considerations, it is very important that the effects of the illness, rather than the investigation, were recorded. The serial measurements of naturally occurring changes in the circulation over several days of acute myocardial infarction, together with continuous magnetic tape records of the naturally occurring arrhythmias, were made in all patients as a routine. For about three years, hemodynamic and ECG data were collected in a series of patients. The first presentations and published papers aroused considerable interest and seeded several other sources of work [2].

The problems of manual analysis of hemodynamic data were oppressive and the real time assessment of taped ECG records was demanding. In the course of this period it became apparent that the "pilot" role of the unit was largely exhausted. Many offshoots of interest required their own facilities: the effects of drug treatment on arrhythmias and hemodynamics; the use of drugs in a preventive sense; and, of especial note, the contribution of changes in autonomic tone and circulating catecholamines influencing illness and treatment. There seemed to be no prospect of doing all this in the local circumstances.

The concept of units dedicated to a patient study in depth attracted the interest of the National Institutes of Health. In the mid-1960s, a team representing the NIH visited the Hammersmith Hospital, London. During the visit the discussions were very much directed toward the basic changes taking place in the heart and circulation of the patient suffering acute myocardial ischemia and infarction, but the broader clinical implications for the patients admitted to the hospital, or cared for at home, or struck down by chest pain or cardiac arrest at work, were also widely discussed. No declaration was made at the time, but shortly afterward the Myocardial Infarction Research Unit (MIRU) program, through the aegis of the National Institutes of Health, was set up in the United States.

Local interests at Hammersmith concentrated on the contribution of autonomic drive to the illnesses associated with acute and subacute myocardial ischemia. The various clinical syndromes were followed by circulation measurements and matched adrenaline and nor-adrenaline studies

[3]. The wide variety of neurosympathetic responses were documented in detail; and the possible therapeutic use of specific beta-adrenergic-blocking drugs being developed in Britain by ICI Pharmaceuticals was anticipated.

Without conscious appreciation, the evolution of the medical care for the patient with acute ischemic heart disease became dominated by the requirements to deal with the "inevitable" consequences of acute myocardial ischemia. Easily provable benefit was to be had from the treatment of life-threatening cardiac arrhythmias by drugs and DC shock treatment. The success in treating cardiac arrest through ventricular fibrillation rapidly increased with better instant action where monitoring alert was given and the technical benefits of development in DC apparatus [4], largely through the determined efforts of Dr. Bernard Lown. Improved cardiac pacing techniques and the use of antiarrhymic drugs also gave credibility to the "coronary care unit." But once again the limitations of even these successes had to be recognized. Prevention of the causal mechanisms, primarily the atherosclerotic coronary stenosis, through dietary or other interference did not seem likely to reduce materially the inexorable fate of thousands of patients predictably falling ill year by year. Treatment of angina pectoris was potentially much improved by the prescription of beta-blocking agents, but ultimately severe angina often escaped the limiting properties of such drugs, with restriction in life style, loss of work, heart attacks, and death. An historically inevitable, but non-the-less fantastic, leap forward came with the introduction of selective coronary arteriography [5] by Dr. Mason Sones and his colleagues together with the now classic surgical procedure of coronary bypass by Dr. Favaloro and the Cleveland team [6]. Even now the impetus given by these developments cannot be overemphasized. The radiologic benefits allow surgeons a precise knowledge of the anatomy of the vessels to be dealt with, and have also given the physician a key to a much improved understanding of the consequences of ischemic heart disease on a regional myocardial basis. Small areas of myocardium count less than large areas. Infarction of upper ventricular septal muscle, involved in early ventricular electrical activation, and larger areas of muscle, gives more lethal consequences than more peripheral smaller lesions. In broad prognostic terms the fewer arteries severely diseased, the better the outlook. Early intimation of such concepts, made possible by the selective technique now in everyday use for routine patient evaluation, was implicit in regional coronary studies by Dr. Richard Gorlin's group [7].

Coronary bypass surgery is now so well established in regular strategic decisions for the patient with angina pectoris that national assessments of costs on a public health scale are serious undertakings. The value to a particular patient, properly selected and successfully operated, must also be given prominence. For most patients with angina pectoris, whose symptoms are incompletely solved by beta-blockade and other treatment, the symptomatic benefits, given correct selection, are quite simply fantastic. Longer-term prognostic outlook after coronary surgery, including the ability and wish to return to work, now provides occupation for those enticed by such analysis.

All this is history; and taking stock, at the time the contributors to this book are writing, is a salutary exercise. The primary prevention of coronary atherosclerotic plaques, for all its appeal, does not seem likely to influence the bulk of ischemic heart disease within the next decade. Inevitably there will be some reduction in heart-attack rate as those most motivated, or most fearful, stop smoking, eat less, take more exercise, and take care of their personal lives. For the most part, educating our children at the teenager period stands a better chance of significantly deferring coronary arterial degeneration, but there is much circumstantial evidence that success in altering accepted habits in later life may not come easily. It seems certain that myocardial infarction will continue to occur. In Britain, one major question has been whether to treat such patients at home or in special care units. There are arguments in each direction. The clinical trials purporting to test the hypothesis that home care is as good for the patient as hospital care are now open to serious criticism as often the more obviously ill patients have been selectively removed from the randomization in order to guarantee SCU care in potentially lethal circumstances. It seems clear that many undeclared factors come into this dilemma. Equally clear is the point that cardiac arrest at home, without mobile SCU support, is almost certainly untreatable, whereas SCU facilities very likely allow recovery in presence of instant resuscitation and adequate myocardial function.

Separate from the benefits of arrhythmia control and cardiac resuscitation is the growing interest in the management of the infarct itself. Experimental work has provided great insight into the factors determining acute myocardial ischemia. In man, knowledge of the intimate anatomy and physiology of the acute infarct, using modern radionuclide techniques has been a fascinating new contribution. The function, regional and general, of the infarcted heart can also be described with useful accuracy by noninvasive ultrasound and Doppler methods. The major argument for use of these systems is the availability of fair quantification without seriously disturbing the patient. Some guidance in treatment can be had from the results, but the accuracy required for the small changes evident in the most seriously ill patients sometimes defeats the possibilities available.

The question of providing SCU care for the specific purpose of minimizing the amount of heart tissue lost by ischemia remains highly controversial. Patients do show some lessening of the signs of infarction with beta-blockade [8] and other interventions, but whether this really alters their subsequent natural history through avoidance of further attacks, less heart failure, or less chance of sudden death is not at all clear. Lowering the oxygen consumption of the myocardium, by whatever safe means, would seem to be sensible thinking in highly activated patients with tachycardia and reactive hypertension. Proof that we should organize our structure of clinical management for all patients around that consideration is awaited. Demonstration that beta-blockade over a period of two years after myocardial infarction does help the survival outlook by about 25% is at hand [9]. This means that one or two extra patients per year in each 100 patients treated will survive if beta-blockade is routinely undertaken except where risks are anticipated.

Whether we can pick out those patients most likely to benefit by noninvasive methods is an important question [10].

We are now at a stage where treatment of the patient with ischemic heart disability satisfies many in terms of our understanding and the presently available drugs and surgical treatment. The prospect of delivering such treatment to all patients at the appropriate time finally involves political and financial elements to a degree unlikely to be influenced by the innovators in medical science. Any reappraisal of the present medical situation must accept the increasing difficulty of generating new ideas on the one hand, and, on the other, the practical and financial barriers to carrying them through to the patient. One reality is the enormous cost of satisfying new "safety" testing of new drugs before use in man. In the case of biologic malfunction particular to man, for example, the many variations in heart failure and high blood pressure, the actual value of a new agent cannot be assessed until considerable development costs have been incurred. Failure at the clinical stage implies a loss of all development finance. Where drugs for minority patient groups, or special clinical syndromes, are concerned, the financial realities may become prohibitive under present legislation.

The defense against these new problems and difficulties has always been a willingness to think harder, to continually reassess old conclusions, and to offer new ideas. In such endeavor we hope that many specialist writers in this book will make their contribution.

References

1. Shillingford JP, Thomas M: Organisation of unit for intensive care and investigation of patients with acute myocardial infarction. Lancet 2:113, 1964.
2. Shillingford JP, Thomas M: Haemodynamic effects of acute myocardial infarction in man. Prog Cardiovasc Dis 9:571, 1967.
3. Valori C, Thomas M, Shillingford JP: Free noradrenaline and adrenaline urinary excretion in relation to clinical syndromes following myocardial infarction. Am J Cardiol 25:605, 1967.
4. Lown B, Amarasingham R, Neuman J: New method for terminating cardiac arrhythmias: use of synchronised capacitor discharge. JAMA 182: 548, 1962.
5. Sones F, Shirey EK: Cine coronary arteriography. Mod Concepts Cardiovasc Dis 31:735, 1962.
6. Favaloro RG: Saphenous vein graft in the surgical treatment of coronary artery disease: operative technique. J Thorac Cardiovasc Surg 58:178, 1969.
7. Elliott WC, Gorlin R: The coronary circulation, myocardial ischaemia and angina pectoris II. Mod Concepts Cardiovasc Dis 35:117, 1966.
8. Pelides LJ, Reid DS, Thomas M, Shillingford JP: Inhibiton by b-blockade of the ST segment elevation following acute myocardia infarction in man. Cardiovasc Res 6:295, 1972.
9. Prevention of myocardial reinfarction: what is the role of beta blockers? Prim Cardiol Suppl 1, 1982.
10. Linden RJ, Mary DASG: Limitations and reliability of exercise electrocardiography tests in coronary heart disease. Cardiovasc Res 16:675–710, 1982.

37. ORGANIZATION AND ADMINISTRATION OF THE CARDIAC CARE UNIT

Wanda Bride

Marguerite English

Robert M. Califf

A cardiac care unit is designed to accommodate critically ill patients with specific needs. Patients with a broad spectrum of problems such as unstable angina, acute myocardial infarction arrhythmia, cardiogenic shock, aortic dissection, pericarditis, tamponade, and cardiomyopathy must be cared for. Because of this varied population and because of the rapid evolution of complex technical treatment strategies, highly educated and trained nurse professionals are needed. This chapter is intended to aid in the design and administration of such a specialized and complex unit.

Unit Design

The design of the cardiac care unit (CCU) should balance the competing goals of (a) allowing optimal observation of, and rapid nursing access to, patients and (b) maintaining privacy for the patient. The Joint Commission of Accreditation of Hospitals (JCAH) requirements for CCUs include the capability of observing all patients from a central nursing station. Private rooms with doors with glass areas that permit observation without entering the rooms provide the most acceptable compromise. Curtains inside the patient rooms can allow privacy when needed by the nurse or desired by the patient. The nursing and

physician staffs should assume that patients prefer to have the curtains closed when they are examined or otherwise exposed.

The rooms should be bright and well lighted. Lighting should be adjustable so that it is soft for patient use, but bright for personnel use. A private sink and bedside commode for each room are desirable. A clock or calender should be present in each room to help the patient remain oriented to time and place, while a television and radio can also provide diversion and reduce stress for particular patients. Restful pictures and windows are also desirable features in a CCU room. The goal is to maintain a sense of continuity with the external environment, thereby reducing patient anxiety.

Several factors must be considered when the number of beds for the CCU is determined. First, the size of the community and the number of distant referrals should be evaluated into the institution. Then, medical guidelines for both patient admission to and transfer from the CCU should be developed. These criteria should be established by the medical director and the nursing leadership group. Any patient with an unstable chest-pain pattern should be evaluated for possible admission to the CCU, whether or not acute myocardial infarction is documented. Finally, the mix of patients should be considered.

R.M. Califf and G.S. Wagner (eds.), ACUTE CORONARY CARE: Principles and Practice. Copyright © 1985. Martinus Nijhoff Publishing, Boston/Dordrecht/Lancaster.

Centers dealing with complex patients will need more beds per admission than community hospitals because of the longer duration of stay.

Ideally, a CCU should be compact so that patient rooms can be reached quickly in emergencies and patients can be observed easily by the staff. A small, close-knit unit provides an atmosphere conducive to good working relationships, teamwork, and togetherness. With the increasing centralization of tertiary care referral centers and the expanding indications for intensive cardiac care, many units have become quite large. Some desirable features of "smallness" can be maintained in these circumstances by dividing the unit into subunits or wings with decentralized nursing substations. This design enables nurses to work together and spend more time with the patients.

The modern CCU either must be located close to areas in which technical procedures can be performed or the facilities for these procedures must be available in the CCU. Under ideal circumstances, the emergency room and the CCU should be in close proximity to minimize transport time. Fluoroscopy is essential for many common CCU procedures, including complicated right heart catheterization and pacemaker insertion. The availability of portable bedside fluoroscopy reduces the risk and discomfort involved in moving critically ill patients to centrally located, fixed fluoroscopy equipment. In centers with the capability for cardiac catheterization, cardiac surgery, and electrophysiologic testing, access to these facilities via specific avenues of transport must be carefully planned. Ample space should be available throughout the route to move patient-connected equipment and to perform resuscitation.

Equipment in Patient Room

The patient rooms must be large enough to contain life-support equipment such as a ventilator and diagnostic radiology or nuclear medicine equipment. In many centers, artificial circulatory support devices such as the intraaortic balloon pump must also have allocated space. In addition, access to the patient should be available on at least three sides. To accommodate this equipment, at least eight electrical outlets with three different circuits, two oxygen outlets, two compressed air outlets, and two vacuum outlets are necessary. These outlets should be in a central location away from the floor and near the head of the bed for both access and safety. An ECG monitor must be available for every CCU bed. The monitor should be mounted on the wall or ceiling so that it can be seen easily and does not provide a hazard for the patient.

Central Arrhythmia Surveillance System

Patient arrhythmia monitoring can be accomplished in several ways:

1. Bedside monitoring only.
2. Monitoring in a central area observed by unit personnel.
3. Monitoring in a central area using computerized arrhythmia detection.
4. Monitoring in a central area observed by unit personnel with computer assistance.

A system of simple bedside monitoring with alarms set is clearly not preferable. Alarms that are loud enough to alert nursing personnel will cause undue patient anxiety and arrhythmias cannot easily be observed and analyzed without causing patients concern. A central arrhythmia surveillance area is an essential aspect of any CCU. This area might also serve to monitor non-CCU patients via telemetry. Dedicated phone lines can connect the CCU central surveillance area with the nursing stations on the wards of the telemetered patients. In a small unit, it might not be necessary or possible to assign a specific person as a "monitor watcher." In larger units, such an individual is essential. The experience at Duke indicates that a single "monitor watcher" can observe up to 24 patients. Nurses need not be used; rather, specifically trained individuals can be employed after a two-week training period that consists of classroom teaching as well as "hands on" experience with a preceptor. A methodical system of evaluating performance and continuing education is recommended. These "monitor watchers" must also be trained in communicating with the CCU nurses and physicians.

Human observation alone has been shown to miss many arrhythmias that are documented by tape. Therefore, even the best nonautomated system will serve only to detect sustained arrhythmias and document the rhythm at specified intervals. Efficiency will be improved by providing at least $10-15$ s of "memory" for each ECG channel. Accurate quantification of arrhythmias will require use of a continuous ambulatory taping system. Maximal "online" surveillance will require some form of computerized arrhythmia detection system.

Many computer systems are now available with options ranging from simple heart rate detection to computerized interpretation and storage with quantitative recall. All require some form of human involvement to edit the significant amount of "false positive" detection. The relative merits of the various systems will not be discussed here. Currently the Duke CCU central surveillance system handles 48 patients concurrently with two trained Central Surveillance Technicians (CST) without computer assistance. Each CST is given a 30-min meal break and at least a 15-min break every 4 h by a CCU nurse.

A method for quality control is a critical element in any CCU monitoring. Ambulatory monitoring tapes can be used intermittently to evaluate the performance of each CST. A CCU nurse should supervise the central surveillance system to detect problems and maintain quality assurance. A physician should be responsible for reviewing critical strips. A logbook can be kept with a running record on each patient, documenting important arrhythmias for each monitored patient. Arrhythmia monitoring is a critical aspect of the CCU since arrhythmia detection and treatment probably accounts for the major effect of CCUs on patient outcome (see chapter 38).

Equipment and Medications

Because of the instability of the cardiac patient, emergency equipment should be readily available in the CCU. Such equipment should include a defibrillator (with synchronous mode for cardioversion), pacemaker wires and generators, and intubation equipment. A number of different defibrillators are now available. Factors that should be considered before purchase include weight, size, recorder capabilities, and efficiency and simplicity of operation. Pacemaker wires and generators should be matched to the preference and skills of the physicians who will be performing the procedures. In medical centers, consideration should be given to the availability of atrial pacing wires and atrioventricular sequential generators. A supply of essential medications for emergency use should be stored adjacent to the defibrillator on an emergency cart. The medication box should be sealed to ensure that all of the essential medications will be available when an arrest occurs. After the supplies are used during an arrest, the supplies can be restacked and the box resealed.

All emergency equipment should be checked each shift for mechanical failure. Emergency carts should be inspected to check the expiration dates of sterile equipment and medications. Table 37-1 shows a list of standard equipment kept on an emergency cart. Furthermore, electrical equipment should be evaluated monthly by personnel trained in medical electronics to ensure its safe use.

Administration: Nursing Leadership

The nursing leadership group should consist of the head nurse, one or more assistant head nurses, and a nurse clinician to develop and organize inservice education. The functions of this group can be divided into several critical areas: (a) writing, reviewing, and updating all pertinent policies, procedures, and standing orders; (b) orienting both new and experienced nursing personnel about these procedures; and (c) supervising the nursing personnel to ensure that patient-care procedures are properly performed.

Leadership should be capable and willing to perform counseling or disciplinary action when necessary. Of equal importance, positive evaluations should be given on a regular basis when the job is done well. A crucial aspect of nursing leadership in a busy CCU is the basic nursing ability of the leaders. These nurses should be respected by the staff for their abilities to accurately assess and efficiently care for the CCU patient. Thus, a combination of practical nursing talent and administrative ability is required for success in CCU nursing administration. The nursing leadership serves as the liaison between

TABLE 37-1. Standard equipment kept on an emergency cart

TOP OF CART
Isuprel setup
    1—D5W 500cc   1—10-cc syringe
    1—minidrip tubing   1—no. 20 needle
    2 amps isuprel
Abbojects
    4—Bicarb   3—Calcium
    3—Epinepherine   3—Atropine
    4—Xylocaine
Needle Box
5—Heparin Flushes
ECG paste
Pacer Pack
    Generator   Betadine swabs
    Gloves (large and medium)   4 × 4's
    Transthoraxic pacer kit   10-cc syringe
    Pink tape

TOP LEFT DRAWER
ECG paste
3-cc syringes
10-cc syringes
50-cc syringes
Needles: nos. 19, 20, 22, and, 25
5—Intracardiac needles
1—Pericardial needle
Alcohol swabs
Labels

TOP RIGHT DRAWER
2—Vials lidocaine (2 g)
5 amps adrenalin
5 amps atropine
5 amps calcium chloride
5 amps dilantin
4 amps dopamine
3 amps bretylium
5 amps isuprel
5 amps levophed
2—Vials: pronestyl and dobutamine (ea.)
1—Vial normal saline and water (ea.)
5 amps xylocaine (100 mg)
5—ABG setups
    Heparin and tips

SECOND LEFT DRAWER
Suture removal set
Generator
Gloves (large and medium)
Transthoraxic pacer kit
Pink tape
Betadine swabs
4 x 4's
10-cc syringe

SECOND RIGHT DRAWER
1—Shirley Trach no. 6
Needle electrodes
ET tubes nos. 6, 7, 8, and 9
Laryngoscope with 2 blades
10-cc syringe
Airways
Scissors
Kelley clamp
1—Y connector
1—1st connector
Pink tape

TABLE 37-1. *(Continued)*

FIRST LONG DRAWER
1—NS 1000 cc
2—D5W 500 cc
2—Buretols (Soluset)
2—Venotubes
1—Minidrip tubing
1—Macrodrip tubing
2—Tourniquets
1—Scalpel
2—no. 14 Angiocath 5½"
2—nos. 16 and 18—4" long dwell
2—nos. 16, 18, and 20—2½" long dwell
1" and 2" tape
2—Stopcocks
4—Stopcock covers

SECOND LONG DRAWER
2—no. 16 salem sumps
Suction catheters
    2—nos. 14 and 16 plastic
    2—nos. 14 and 16 red rubber
3—Deseret sets
4—Lube jelly
1—Balectrode pacing kit
Introducer and guide wire

LOWER LEFT DRAWER
6—Bicarb abbojects
Back paddles
Cardioversion cables
Extra ECG paste

LOWER RIGHT DRAWER
Flashlight
AMBU bag with mask
1—Flow meter
2—Oxygen connecting tubes
1—Suction connecting tube
2—Wingnut adaptors
1—Suction bottle

ER BOX
Puritan setup (on top)
Oxygen setup
Connecting tubing
Mask and prong
Suction setup

BAG
AMBU bag setup
Airways

the CCU and all other areas of the hospital—physicians, other nursing staff, radiology, dietetics, environmental services.

Together with the physician leadership, the nursing leadership should develop forms so that critical data can be recorded accurately and stored. These forms should include a nursing admission sheet (figure 37-1), a standard order sheet (figure 37-2), and flow sheets for hemodynamic monitoring (figure 37-3) and patient care (figure 37-4). The nursing admission sheet should contain space for critical information that the physician often does not record adequately: temperature, height, weight, allergies. In addition, a checklist can be included to ensure that

patients and families are properly oriented to the CCU (bottom of figure 37-1). Since most CCU patients will have a common set of orders, the standard order sheet can save time and prevent inadvertent omission of routine orders. Standard order sheets do increase the risk, however, that an adjustment will not be made when appropriate in dosage or administration of a therapy. Therefore, when a standard order sheet is used, the nursing staff should be vigilant about such issues as the adjustment of lidocaine dose for heart failure or hepatic failure. Compared with other intensive care units in which most patients require one-to-one nursing, the CCU often has less critically ill patients who predominantly need only rhythm

DUKE UNIVERSITY MEDICAL CENTER
CCU NURSE ADMISSION SHEET

Form 841

Name:_____ Age:_____ Date:_____ Time:_____

Mode Of Transportation:_____ Admitted To:_____ From:_____ Religion:____

Chief Complaint:_____
(Location, Duration and Intensity Of Pain)

Known Allergies And Types Of Reactions: _____

Physical Exam

Blood Pressure: Rt. Arm_____   Pulses: Apical_____Regular_____
                Lt. Arm_____   Radial_____Irregular_____

Respiration:_____ Breath Sounds:_____ Edema: Present_____ Where_____
                                                    Absent_____

Temperature:_____ Weight:_____ Height:_____ Rhythm Strip:_____

Conditions of Skin: Warm   Dry   Cool   Moist   Cold   Clammy
Color of Skin: Pink   Cyanotic   Mottled   Pale   Normal
Neck Veins: Distended _____   Peripheral Pulses: Present_____
              Flat_____   Absent_____

O₂ _____L/m Cannula   Mask   IV   Heparin Lock_____

Past History

Previous MI_____ Angina_____ Diabetes_____ Arrhythmia_____ TB_____
When_____ Hypertension_____ Glaucoma_____ Ulcers_____ Emphysema_____

Other_____
Medications Taken At Home: (Drug, Dose and Frequency)

Explanation Of: Clothing/Valuable Disposal:
Monitor____ O₂ Outlet____   ____Kept in room
TV_____ Telephone____   ____Given to family
Intercom____ Visitors____   ____Locked on unit
Activity____ Diet_____   ____Sent to Business Office
I/O_____

              Family Member To Notify:_____

              Phone Number:_ _____   Admitting Nurse:_____

Figure 37-1. Standard nursing admission sheet.

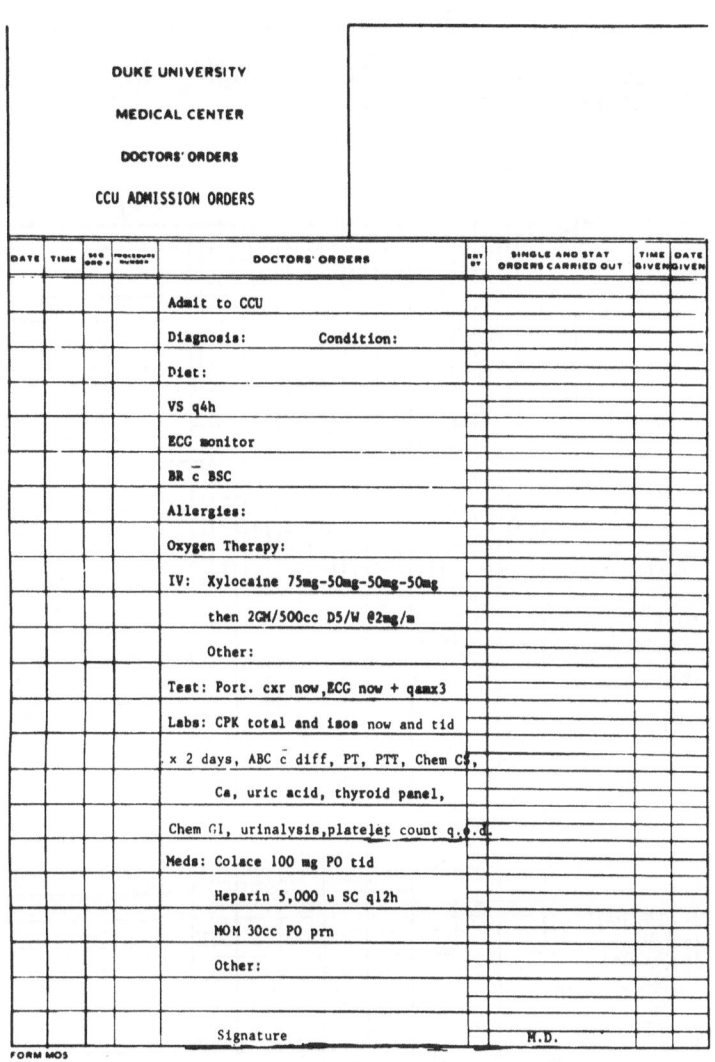

DUKE UNIVERSITY

MEDICAL CENTER

DOCTORS' ORDERS

CCU ADMISSION ORDERS

DATE	TIME	MD ORD #	PROCEDURE NUMBER	DOCTORS' ORDERS	ERT BY	SINGLE AND STAT ORDERS CARRIED OUT	TIME GIVEN	DATE GIVEN
				Admit to CCU				
				Diagnosis: Condition:				
				Diet:				
				VS q4h				
				ECG monitor				
				BR c̄ BSC				
				Allergies:				
				Oxygen Therapy:				
				IV: Xylocaine 75mg-50mg-50mg-50mg				
				then 2GM/500cc D5/W @2mg/m				
				Other:				
				Test: Port. cxr now, ECG now + qamx3				
				Labs: CPK total and isos now and tid				
				x 2 days, ABC c̄ diff, PT, PTT, Chem C$,				
				Ca, uric acid, thyroid panel,				
				Chem GI, urinalysis, platelet count q.o.d.				
				Meds: Colace 100 mg PO tid				
				Heparin 5,000 u SC q12h				
				MOM 30cc PO prn				
				Other:				
				Signature	M.D.			

FORM MOS

Figure 37-2. Standard admission order sheet for patient with unstable ischemic syndrome.

monitoring. For this reason we have found that the use of two different nursing flow sheets is helpful: a complex sheet for hemodynamic monitoring and a simpler sheet for patients requiring less intensive care. In the near future, commercially available programs will also be in use to record such data on computer. The advantage of these systems will be the rapid calculation of the hemodynamic profile, accurate drip rates, and potentially even suggested changes in ventilator settings or drip rates.

Physician Director

Because of the nature of the patient population and the rapidly evolving, highly technical therapy, a competent physician director of the CCU is necessary. In conjunction with the head nurse, the physician director should be involved in the daily operation of the unit. Policies, procedures, and standing orders should be written, reviewed, and approved by the physician director as well as and the nursing leadership. The director func-

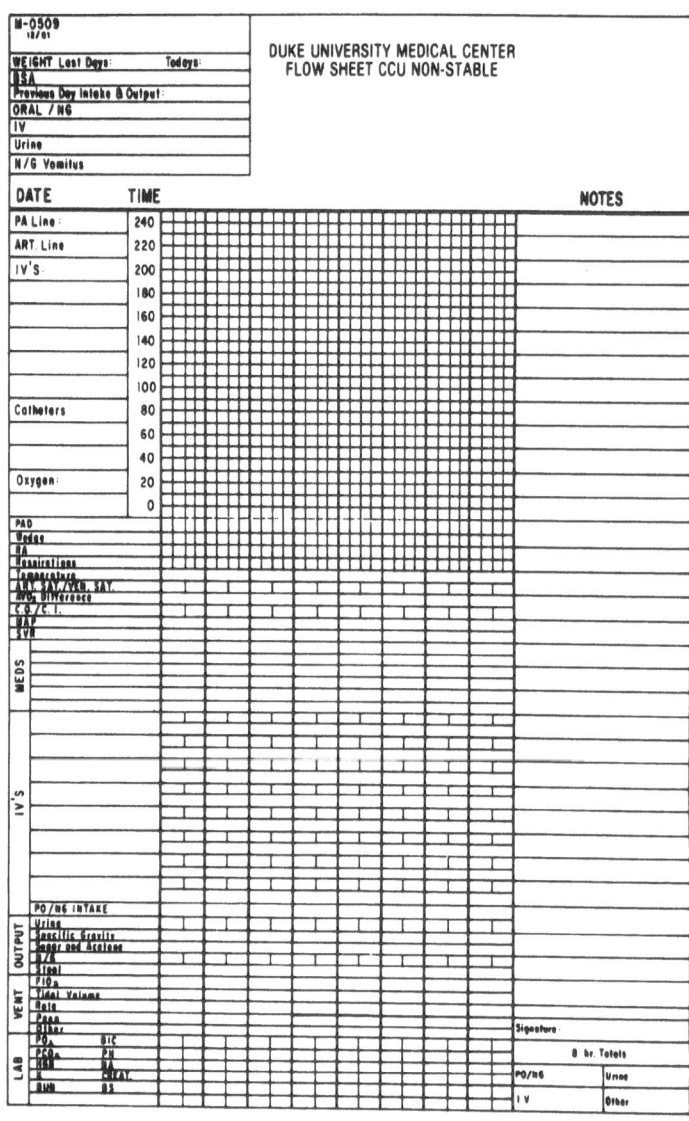

Figure 37-3. Nursing flow sheet for patient requiring hemodynamic monitoring.

tions in a supportive role to the patients and families, nursing staff, and other physicians. In particular, since many different physicians usually admit patients to the CCU, the physician director is responsible for maintaining communication between the admitting physicians and the staff. Criteria for CCU admission and transfer must be established and enforced by the physi-

cian director. Guidelines for acceptable patient care should also be established.

Staff Nurses

Even with an ideal physical layout and excellent leadership, the CCU will not be effective unless competent, motivated staff nurses are present.

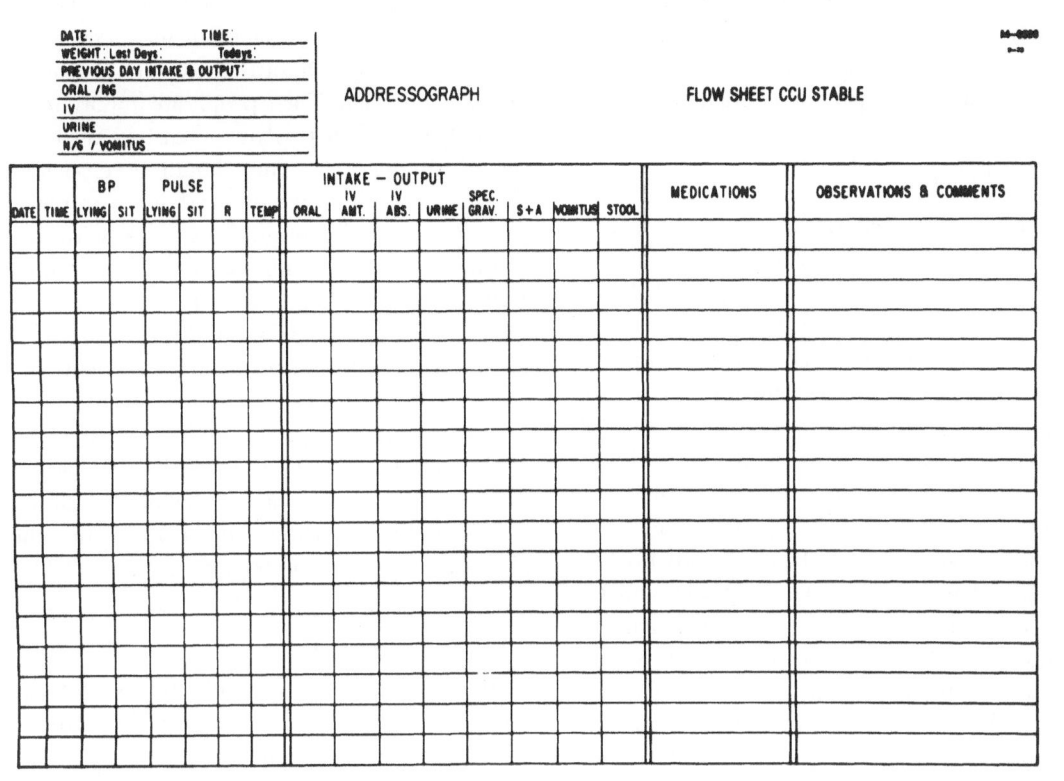

Figure 37-4. Nursing flow sheet for patient not requiring hemodynamic monitoring.

Each CCU nurse should undergo a thorough orientation program prior to assuming patient-care responsibility. Certification in basic life support, basic arrhythmias, venipuncture, and defibrillation should be required. Advanced life-support certification is also recommended and additional training in arrhythmia recognition and management should be considered essential. A thorough working knowledge of all equipment used routinely in the CCU is required, especially the devices used in emergency situations.

Orientation and continuing staff education should be centered around the concept that the nurse should be able to assess the patient, make immediate decisions about the need for emergency care, and evaluate the effectiveness of those decisions. The role of the CCU nurse has expanded to include prevention as well as treatment. Anticipating problems or events can be as crucial as treating problems as they occur. Once a problem is identified, the nurse must be skilled at recording the pertinent information and communicating it to others. A thorough knowledge base and high level of performance can be maintained only with a carefully designed continuing education program and evaluation and feedback about performance on a regular basis.

In addition to competence in the performance of technical procedures, the CCU nurse should be proficient at patient education. The nurse should be able to explain procedures and therapy to the patient and family (see chapter 57). Cardiac rehabilitation efforts should begin in the CCU. Although the rehabilitation program extends into the convalescent post-hospital phase (see chapter 58), the CCU nurse should initiate patient and family orientation to rehabilitation (see chapter 58). The CCU nurse should understand how to prepare the patient and family for imminent death (see chapter 48). The nurse's time can be used most efficiently if a wide variety of educational pamphlets and other teaching materials are readily available in the CCU. A pamphlet containing rules of the unit, names of key people, words or phrases commonly used in the unit, and daily routines of the patient is essential.

Nurse Staffing

Staffing needs are determined by a number of factors. First, the qualifications and training of the nursing personnel must be considered. *Registered nurses* are the best choice to staff a CCU. If this is not possible, *licensed practical nurses* may be used with special training, but only if they are able to give medications. Second, the number of nurses needed depends upon the degree of illness of the patient population. If a great deal of hemodynamic monitoring is done, an increased demand for nurses will exist. If, on the other hand, most of the patients are uncomplicated and require little or no instrumentation, the demand for nurses decreases. Unfortunately, it is very difficult to predict patient needs in a CCU because of the changing status of the patients. The nurse/patient ratio needs to be flexible. Also, flexibility is a mandatory personality trait to consider when accepting a nurse into a CCU position.

Patient Care-Ancillary Services

Often the first contact the patient will have with medical personnel will be the *emergency medical technician* (EMT) or paramedic (see chapter 27). Because the emergency medical service has expanded its role in the health field to include mobile intensive care units, patients are now being treated earlier in the course of their illness. To ensure consistency in patient care, it is important to develop a rapport between the paramedics and CCU personnel. The CCU, if possible, should provide the EMT with both initial and continuing education and clinical experience. The paramedics could offer inservice classes to the CCU staff in their field of expertise. Protocols should be constructed so that they are easily understood by both groups. The patient should be able to observe the trust and rapport between these two groups of people.

Specialized resources should be available to the patient, the family, and the staff during the patient's hospitalization. These include a chaplain (see chapter 48), physical therapist, psychologist, and dietitian. These people are important in the daily care of the patient and are a vital part of the health care team. They should be responsive to patient needs, offer suggestions to improve patient care, and communicate freely with one another, the nurse, and the physician. If possible, a cardiac rehabilitation service should be available during the CCU stay. Personnel trained in cardiac rehabilitation can supplement the CCU nurse's efforts in patient and family education and initiate a program that prepares the patient for both CCU and hospital discharge. These individuals can then work closely with the patient and family throughout the convalescent phase, as described in chapter 58.

Selected References

Sturdavant M: Comparisons of intensive nursing service in a circular and rectangular unit. American Hospital Association.

Hazzard ME: Central care nursing. Garden City NY: Medical Examination, 1978.

Simon N: The psychological aspects of intensive care nursing. Robert J Brady, 1980.

Andreoli K, Fowkes V, Zipes D, Wallace A: Comprehensive cardiac care, 5th edn. St Louis: CV Mosby, 1983.

Turner GO: The cardiovascular care unit: a guide for planning and operation. New York: John Wiley and Sons, 1978.

Blumen HE: CCU design, staffing, and operating policies. Chicago: Rand, 1975.

Clipson C, Wehrer J: Planning for cardiac care: a guide to the planning and design of cardiac care facilities. Health Administration Press, 1973.

Meltzer L, Punning A: Textbook of coronary care. Charles Press, 1972.

Zschoche D: Mosby's comprehensive review of critical care. St Louis: CV Mosby, 1981.

Burrell A, Burrell L: Critical care. St Louis: CV Mosby, 1977.

Grace W, Kayloun V: The coronary care unit. Des Moines IA: Meredith, 1970.

Alpert J, Francis G: Manual of Coronary Care. Boston: Little, Brown and Company, 1980.

38. THE COST-EFFECTIVENESS OF CORONARY CARE UNITS

Lee Goldman

Harvey Fineberg

Since their inception in the early 1960s, coronary care units (CCUs) have undoubtedly saved many lives. However, anecdotal experience cannot substitute for a critical analysis of the impact of coronary care units, or for a comparison of the impact to the costs incurred.

Cost-effectiveness analysis provides a means of comparing the benefits of a new program or innovation with the costs incurred. This type of evaluation typically uses explicit assumptions based on the best available information about the impact of various interventions and their costs. The reliability of the analysis cannot exceed the accuracy of the assumptions on which it is based. In the subsequent discussion, we outline the areas in which data are sufficient to make reasonable judgments. In the subsequent discussion, we outline the areas in which data are sufficient to make reasonable judgments. In these areas, we attempt to compare the cost-effectiveness of coronary care units with that of alternative ways of caring for patients with possible myocardial infarction.

Effectiveness of Coronary Care Units

Early uncontrolled trials of CCUs encouraged their wide adoption. Marshall et al. [1] reported a higher rate of successful resuscitation and a

lower mortality rate in a general hospital with a CCU than among patients treated concurrently by the same physicians in the same city at a Veterans Administration Hospital without a CCU. Two nonrandomized Scandinavian studies [2, 3] similarly showed lower mortalities in CCU patients than in concurrent ward patients, and these differences were especially marked during the first 24 h after admission. Norris et al. [4] found that moderately ill myocardial infarction patients had a lower mortality in a hospital with a CCU than in another hospital without a CCU, though mortality was not significantly lower than it had been in the previous year when a well-organized resuscitation team had been available for the hospital wards. Nevertheless, the Norris group endorsed CCUs because of the logic of centralized monitoring and resuscitation facilities and because the original results of resuscitation on the hospital wards might be hard to sustain.

Subsequent studies have raised questions about the conclusions of these earlier reports. Mather et al. [5] screened 1895 patients with suspected myocardial infarction and randomized 24% of them to home versus hospital care because they were under age 70, had adequate home situations, and did not have any medical conditions that were felt by their physicians to make randomization inappropriate. In these selected patients, survival at 330 days was slightly better among patients randomized to home care. Hill et

This work was supported in part by a grant from the James Hilton Manning and Emma Austin Manning Foundation.

R.M. Califf and G.S. Wagner (eds.), ACUTE CORONARY CARE: Principles and Practice. Copyright © 1985. Martinus Nijhoff Publishing, Boston/Dordrecht/Lancaster.

al. [6] sent a medical team to the homes of 500 patients with suspected myocardial infarction, observed them for 2 h, and then randomized 349 (70%) to home versus hospital care because they had not required resuscitation, had no complications or other diseases requiring hospital admission, and had a suitable social situation for home care. At follow-up six weeks later, the mortality was 13% in the home group and 11% in the hospital group. Although significantly more home-care patients died in the first 24 h, several of the hospital patients who were resuscitated during the first 24 h died subsequently during that hospital stay. Eight patients were resuscitated in their homes by the study team and were never randomized, suggesting that the benefit of medical attention may have been underestimated by the study's requirement that patients remain uncomplicated under observation before randomization was permitted.

Based on the data from the Mather and Hill studies, some critics have suggested that CCUs are not efficacious for patients with suspected myocardial infarction. Nevertheless, the prevailing attitude among many experts in the United States is that CCUs are so clearly valuable that a randomized controlled trial of their efficacy would be unethical. To resolve this striking disagreement about the effectiveness of CCUs, we must examine in greater detail the assumptions about the contribution of CCUs to patient care.

The highest risk of sudden death from acute myocardial infarction is in the first hours after the onset of symptoms; the risk then declines exponentially [7]. Colling et al. [8] found that half of the deaths from acute myocardial infarction occurred nearly immediately and another 21% occurred within the next 2 h. Because the median delay from the onset of symptoms to the arrival of medical care is at least 3 h in nearly all reported studies [6, 8], 70% of the deaths from acute myocardial infarction may occur before patients come to medical attention. Most of these early deaths are from sudden arrhythmias, many of which might be successfully treated if the patient were in a CCU. Thus, we would expect CCUs to be most efficacious in patients who arrive within 2 or, at most, 6 h after onset of symptoms. In patients who arrive within 6 h after the onset of pain, lidocaine in sufficient doses appears to re-duce the risk of ventricular fibrillation [9] (see chapter 40). Such lidocaine doses probably cannot be given as safely in the absence of close nursing supervision and monitoring.

Based on the average delay between onset of symptoms and hospital arrival, about 4%−5% of acute infarction patients can be expected to develop ventricular fibrillation in the absence of severe heart failure after hospital arrival [10]. About 85%−90% of such patients will be successfully resuscitated in the CCU setting and will survive to leave the hospital [10]. These figures are similar to the estimates of Rose [11], who predicted that CCUs probably reduce the mortality from acute myocardial infarction by about 5%.

If the preceding data are accurate, why have the Hill and Mather studies shown no benefit in having CCUs? We believe there are two reasons: patient selection and inadequate sample size. In terms of patient selection, both studies included only patients who were "randomizable," in part because they were seen emergently in their homes and had no problems during the evaluation phase, which in fact is the period of highest risk following infarction. Thus, the randomized patients would be expected to be at low risk, and many of the potential benefits of medical care actually preceded randomization. Second, consider the issue of sample size. If CCUs truly reduced mortality rates from 15% to 10%, a study would need a sample size of 1800 patients to have a 90% chance of demonstrating a statistically significant ($p < 0.05$) reduction in mortality in the CCU group; if such a difference existed, hospital care would be expected to save about 9000 lives per year in the United States. If CCUs have a smaller benefit, such as to reduce mortality from 13% to 11% as in the Hill study [6], a sample size of 11,000 patients might be needed to show statistical significance; nevertheless, CCUs would save about 3500 Americans each year. Thus, the British randomized trials [5, 6] are unlikely to be of sufficient size to show the benefits of CCUs, and the potential risks to the population as a whole are unrecognized if we rely on studies that may be too small to detect clinically important differences.

In contrast to the substantial benefit that the CCU may have for preventing arrhythmic deaths, the efficacy of newer interventions for preventing death from refractory ischemia or heart failure is less clear. Between 1973 and 1978, a period *after* CCUs may have contributed to a decline in sudden arrhythmic deaths, CCU care for patients with acute myocardial infarction did not measurably reduce mortality from ischemic heart disease in 63 hospitals in a defined geographic area near Boston, Massachusetts [12]. Although our data did not represent a randomized controlled trial, our study included almost 5000 patients in each of the two time periods and thus had about a 90% chance of detecting a 2% reduction in mortality if such a reduction had truly occurred. While the monitoring and nursing facilities of CCUs likely reduce sudden deaths, at present no data suggest that the many subsequent innovations in CCU care have substantially contributed to the decline in United States mortality rates despite the occasional example in which an individual is dramatically saved.

If, as in the Hill study [6], a medical team can be in a patient's house during the high-risk early period of an acute myocardial infarction, home care may be almost as safe as hospital care. Nevertheless, we believe that monitoring and resuscitative facilities ideally should be available for 24 h [10]. In the United States, where house calls are uncommon, immediate hospital transfer and admission is much more feasible and probably safer. CCU care need not always extend for three full days, however, because virtually all of the routine benefits of the CCU for uncomplicated patients will be appreciated within the first 24 h.

Costs

The costs of a stay in a CCU depend on the number and type of expensive interventions that are employed on an individual patient. Thus, the cost for routine care of an uncomplicated myocardial infarction will differ dramatically from the cost in a patient who has marked congestive heart failure or unstable angina pectoris that requires hemodynamic monitoring, a prolonged stay, and perhaps emergency catheterization and surgery. Prevention and preparation to deal with the sudden onset of ventricular fibrillation and other complications require only the basic aspects of coronary care. At the present time, it is not possible to perform a reliable analysis of the cost-effectiveness of the many other new innovations that are part of modern coronary care.

Cost-Effectiveness Analysis

When one is measuring the cost-effectiveness of CCUs or of any other medical intervention, one must have a standard for reference. In other words, one must ask how cost-effective are CCUs compared with some alternate management strategy. Although one might perform detailed analyses of a variety of strategies, the limitations of existing data and the political reality of American medical practice indicate that coronary care will remain the preferred management strategy for patients with documented myocardial infarctions.

Three principal strategies might be adopted to improve the efficiency of the care of patients who are currently admitted to CCUs to "rule out" a myocardial infarction. First, one might improve the efficiency of coronary care by truncating the present array of services and by providing only those that are most likely to affect mortality. Second, the present array of services might be provided, though with better criteria for early transfer so that the length of stay could be reduced [13] (see chapter 49). Finally, if it were possible to identify more accurately which patients were truly having myocardial infarctions at the time they were being first evaluated, a portion of the patients admitted to rule out myocardial infarction might not have to be admitted to intensive care (see chapter 30).

We believe the last approach is especially promising because only about 30% of patients who are admitted for suspicion of myocardial infarction actually prove to have infarctions, and over one-half of those with infarctions have obvious electrocardiographic changes on admission [14]. Thus, only about 15% of patients who are admitted to rule out a myocardial infarction actually have an infarction. We believe that these patients, who account for an overwhelming majority of admissions to CCUs, represent the most fertile ground for cost-effectiveness analyses.

We have developed and prospectively validated a computer-derived protocol to aid in the diagnosis of emergency-room patients who have acute chest pain [14]. A prospective trial demonstrated that this protocol could be used to exclude from the CCU about 20 patients without myocardial infarction for each patient with myocardial infarction who would be incorrectly excluded. The dollar savings from adopting the protocol would apply to all excluded patients; the added risks from myocardial infarction would apply only to the patients erroneously excluded. The extent of the risks, as well as savings, depends upon the alternative management strategy selected for patients excluded from the CCU.

In assessing the cost-effectiveness of selective admission, we considered four basic alternatives for patients who have a 5% chance of having an acute myocardial infarction: (a) admit all patients to the CCU (the baseline, current policy), where the full array of services would be available and the patient/nurse ratio would be no higher than 2:1; (b) admit these patients to an intermediate care bed where nursing supervision would permit electrocardiographic monitoring and prophylactic administration of intravenous lidocaine and where resuscitative facilities would be readily available, though the patient/nurse ratio could be higher than 2:1; (c) admit patients to a routine care bed in the hospital; and (d) follow patients on an outpatient basis, with extensive evaluation on each of two days following the initial visit to the emergency room. Under the outpatient strategy, we assume that 25% of patients will require hospital admission because they develop evidence of myocardial infarction, have progressive angina, congestive heart failure, or other reasons for hospitalization.

Our cost estimates include a component for each type of bed-day, (CCU, intermediate care, and routine), for use of ancillary services, and for professional fees. Based on a 5% chance of acute infarction and the 1980 charges at Brigham and Women's Hospital, Boston, the expected savings per MI patient excluded from the CCU are $9980 for the intermediate care strategy, $22,580 for the strategy to admit to a routine care bed, and $54,060 for the outpatient management strategy.

Against the resource savings from nonadmission to the CCU must be weighed the added risk of life lost. As noted above, the principal benefit of CCUs is the ability to prevent sudden arrhythmic death. Let us assume that we are dealing with otherwise uncomplicated patients,

and that our non-CCU strategies provide sufficiently close patient follow-up so that patients can be transferred to a CCU for the management of problems other than sudden arrhythmias. Second, we will consider only primary ventricular fibrillation in the absence of severe heart failure, because it is by far the commonest sudden arrhythmia that occurs in previously uncomplicated patients and that can be prevented or effectively treated in a CCU.

The risk to life in any care setting is the risk of developing the life-threatening event multiplied by the likelihood of death among patients suffering the event. Based on available studies [12, 15 – 18] and unpublished data on the age distribution of patients in Massachusetts with myocardial infarction, we estimate that the risk of primary ventricular fibrillation in patients with acute infarction is 4.5% [10] and that the risk can be reduced by 90% by the use of high-dose prophylactic lidocaine in a CCU [9]. We also estimate the risk of death from primary ventricular fibrillation to be 12% in a CCU [10].

In the intermediate care unit, we might very conservatively assume that prophylactic lidocaine will reduce the prevalence of ventricular fibrillation by half the amount that might be expected in the CCU. Resuscitation of patients with ventricular fibrillation is conservatively assumed to be 66%, no better than survival of patients outside of hospitals when resuscitation begins within 5 min of cardiac arrest [19]. For routine hospital care, we project survival from ventricular fibrillation to be 26%, the same as the average for all out-of-hospital cardiac arrests treated by trained emergency teams [20]. Home care is estimated to produce half the survival from ventricular fibrillation as that obtained outside the hospital in communities with trained emergency teams. This is especially conservative in light of the opportunities for admission to hospital, and the associated reduction of risk, if symptoms or signs suggestive of myocardial infarction are detected in the daily outpatient evaluations. By describing our assumptions as conservative, we mean they tend to favor the current policy of admitting all patients to CCUs.

Table 38-1 summarizes the risks of death due to primary ventricular fibrillation for 1000 myocardial infarction patients under each considered

TABLE 38-1. Consequences of alternative management strategies for 1000 patients with initially uncomplicated myocardial infarctions

	No. of primary ventricular fibrillation deaths/1000 infarctions
Coronary care unit	0.5
Intermediate care unit	7
Routine hospital bed	33
Outpatient	39

TABLE 38-2. Potential savings per life lost from alternate management strategies for patients with a 5% probability of acute myocardial infarction

Intermediate care unit	$1,600,000
Routine hospital bed	$690,000
Outpatient	$1,400,000

strategy. The risks are small in part because fewer than one in 20 patients with myocardial infarction develop primary ventricular fibrillation.

The savings that might be realized from alternative patient management strategies are substantial (table 38-2). The potential savings per life lost ranges from approximately $690,000 for admission to a routine care bed to nearly $1.6 million for admission to an intermediate care bed. The outpatient strategy produces a savings per life lost that is close to that of the intermediate care unit; however, it also has the highest risks (see table 38-1). Despite smaller savings compared with the outpatient strategy, intermediate care saves enough additional lives to make it slightly more cost-effective. Analogous results are obtained when the analysis is made more complex to include risks from complete heart block as well as risks from primary ventricular fibrillation [21].

All strategies produce impressive savings per life lost compared with the current policy of admitting all such patients to the CCU, especially considering the conservatism of our assumptions. The analysis regards patients who are erroneously excluded as typical of all those with uncomplicated myocardial infarctions. Insofar as the excluded patients may have milder infarc-

tions, and hence a lower-than-average risk of complications, our analysis will exaggerate the apparent advantages of CCU admission, and the dollar savings per life lost would be even higher for the alternative strategies than shown in table 38-2. We have also assumed that prophylactic lidocaine can be given only half as effectively in an intermediate care unit as in a CCU. If we ascribe to intermediate care the same ability as a CCU to forestall the development of ventricular fibrillation, then its cost-effectiveness soars above the other alternative strategies.

The intermediate care strategy has the added advantage of being closest to current medical practice. We believe these results support the potential role for algorithms to aid in the screening of emergency-room patients with chest pain [14, 22], followed by admission of those at low risk of myocardial infarction to an intermediate care hospital bed [21]. This strategy is compatible with other efforts, such as more selective use of various components of intensive care services and briefer CCU admissions, to promote the more efficient use of available resources. At the same time, we continue to recommend coronary unit care for patients with definite acute myocardial infarctions or with syndromes that indicate a probability of acute myocardial infarction that is higher than about 5%.

References

1. Marshall RM, Blount SG, Genton E: Acute myocardial infarction: influence of a coronary care unit. Arch Intern Med 122:473−475, 1968.
2. Hofvendahl S: Influence of treatment in a CCU on prognosis in acute myocardial infarction. Acta Med Scand (Suppl) 519:1−78, 1971.
3. Christensen I, Iverson K, Skouby AP: Benefits obtained by the introduction of a coronary-care unit. Acta Med Scand 189:285−291, 1971.
4. Norris RM, Brandt PWT, Lee AJ: Mortality in a coronary-care unit analysed by a new coronary prognostic index. Lancet 1:278−281, 1969.
5. Mather HG, Morgan DC, Pearson NG, et al: Myocardial infarction: a comparison between home and hospital care for patients. Br Med J 1:925−929, 1976.
6. Hill JD, Hampton JR, Mitchell JRA: A randomized trial of home-versus-hospital management for patients with suspected myocardial infarction. Lancet 1:837−841, 1978.

7. Adgey AAJ, Geddes JS, Webb SW, et al: Acute phase of myocardial infarction. Lancet 2:501–504, 1971.

8. Colling A, Dellipiani AW, Donaldson RJ, Mac-Cormack P: Teesside coronary survey: an epidemiological study of acute attacks of myocardial infarction. Br Med J 2:1169–1172, 1976.

9. Lie KI, Wellens HJ, Van Capelle FJ, Durrer D: Lidocaine in the prevention of primary ventricular fibrillation. N Engl J Med 291:1324–1126, 1974.

10. Goldman L, Batsford WP: Risk–benefit stratification as a guide to lidocaine prophylaxis of primary ventricular fibrillation in acute myocardial infarction: an analytic review. Yale J Biol Med 52:455–466, 1979.

11. Rose G: The contribution of intensive coronary care. Br J Prev Soc Med 29:147–150, 1975.

12. Goldman L, Cook F, Hashimoto B, Stone P, Muller J, Loscalzo A: Evidence that hospital care for acute myocardial infarction has not contributed to the decline in coronary mortality between 1973–1974 and 1978–1979. Circulation 65:936–942, 1982.

13. Mulley AG, Thibeault GE, Hughes RA, Barnett GO, Reder VA, Sherman EL: The course of patients with suspected myocardial infarction: the identification of low-risk patients for early transfer from intensive care. N Engl J Med 302:943–948, 1980.

14. Goldman L, Weinberg M, Weisberg M, et al: A computer-derived protocol to aid in the diagnosis of emergency room patients with acute chest pain. N Engl J Med 307:588–596, 1982.

15. Lie KI, Wellens HJ, Durrer D: Characteristics and predictability of primary ventricular fibrillation. Eur J Cardiol 1:379–384, 1974.

16. Lowrie DW, Higgins MR, Goldman MJ: Ventricular fibrillation complicating acute myocardial infarction. Lancet 2:523–528, 1968.

17. Chopra MP, Thadani V, Portal RW, et al: Lignocaine therapy for ventricular ectopic activity with acute myocardial infarction: a double-blind trial. Br Med J 3:668–670, 1972.

18. Bleifield W, Merx W, Heinrich KW, et al: Controlled trial of prophylactic treatment with lidocaine in acute myocardial infarction. Eur J Clin Pharmacol 6:119–127, 1973.

19. Crampton RS, Aldrich RF, Gascho JA, Miles JR, Stillerman R: Reduction of prehospital, ambulance and community coronary death rates by the community wide emergency cardiac care system. Am J Med 58:151–164, 1975.

20. Eisenberg MS, Copass MK, Hallstrom AP, et al: Treatment of out-of-hospital cardiac arrests with rapid defibrillation by emergency medical technicians. N Engl J Med 302:1379–1382, 1980.

21. Fineberg H, Scadden D, Goldman L: Management of patients with a low probability of acute myocardial infarction: cost-effectiveness of alternatives to coronary care unit admission. N Engl J Med (in press), 1984.

22. Pozen MW, D'Agostino RB, Mitchell JB, et al: The usefulness of a predictive instrument to reduce inappropriate admissions to the coronary care unit. Ann Intern Med 92:238–242, 1980.

VIII. CORONARY CARE:
THE CORONARY CARE
UNIT PHASE

39. THE OPTIMAL USE OF TEMPORARY PACING DURING ACUTE MYOCARDIAL INFARCTION

Richard N.W. Hauer

K.I. Lie

Temporary ventricular pacing may be indicated in patients with atrioventricular (AV) nodal or infranodal conduction disturbances complicating acute myocardial infarction. Conduction disturbances in the AV node are usually the consequence of an occlusion proximal to the origin of the AV nodal artery, which in 90% of the cases originates from the right coronary artery [1]. Therefore, conduction disturbances in the AV node are associated with acute inferior wall myocardial infarction [2]. On the other hand, the right bundle branch and the anterior division of the left bundle branch receive their blood supply from the septal perforating branches of the left anterior descending artery [1]. Therefore, right bundle branch block and/or left anterior fascicular block are usually associated with extensive anteroseptal infarction, due to an occlusion proximal to the origin of the septal perforating branches. The posterior division of the left bundle branch has a dual blood supply, from both the posterior descending (a branch of either the right or left circumflex arteries) and the left anterior descending arteries. Therefore, involvement of this division is usually associated with massive myocardial damage, due to two-vessel disease. Several studies using His bundle recordings have established this relationship between the site of block and the site of infarction [3, 4]. Our own observations in 35 patients with ischemic con-duction defects concur with the above. Of the 25 patients with inferior wall myocardial infarction, the block was localized within the AV node in 24 patients and was infranodal in only one patient. In ten cases with an anteroseptal infarction, however, the block was always infranodal.

The different indications for temporary pacing are strongly associated with the different types of conduction disorders, occurring either in inferior or in anteroseptal infarction, as are discussed below.

AV Nodal Conduction Disorders in Inferior Myocardial Infarction and the Indications for Temporary Pacing

In patients with acute inferior myocardial infarction, high-degree AV block is nearly always located in the AV node. A bimodal pattern is found in this clinical setting. Observations from the mobile coronary care units have revealed that, within the first hour after onset of symptoms, short periods of second- and third-degree AV blocks occur in approximately 10% of the patients with inferior myocardial infarction [5] (see chapter 28). The high incidence of both AV nodal conduction disturbances and sinus bradycardia and the immediate response to leg elevation or atropine suggest that vasovagal mecha-

R.M. Califf and G.S. Wagner (eds.), ACUTE CORONARY CARE: Principles and Practice. Copyright © 1985. Martinus Nijhoff Publishing, Boston/Dordrecht/Lancaster.

nisms probably play a very important role in the genesis of these very early conduction disorders. Later appearing (after several hours) second- and third-degree AV nodal blocks are found in approximately 20% of patients hospitalized with inferior myocardial infarction [6]. In our experience, the latest time of onset of AV nodal conduction disturbances was on the fifth day of infarction. Second-degree AV block, in association with acute inferior myocardial infarction, usually manifests as an AV Wenckebach phenomenon. In 91 of our patients with second-degree AV block as a complication of inferior myocardial infarction, approximately half progressed to third degree (complete) AV block. It has been generally believed that, under these circumstances, the escape pacemaker produces an acceptable and dependable heart rate [7, 8]. In our 94 patients with complete AV block, however, 42 (44%) had a ventricular rate of less than 40/min (table 39-1).

Previously it has also been supposed that the escape rhythm, during AV nodal block, usually produces narrow QRS complexes as it originates from a site just below the AV node in the proximal His bundle. However, an escape rhythm with wide QRS complexes (≥ 0.12 s) was seen in 35 (37%) of our 94 patients with AV nodal block. Studies using His bundle recordings have shown that the P waves were not followed by His potentials in almost all patients with inferior myocardial infarction and third-degree AV block with a wide QRS escape rhythm, indicating that the site of block was indeed AV nodal [4]. In some patients the escape complexes showed a right bundle branch block morphology and in others a left bundle branch block pattern. The escape pacemakers with a left bundle branch block pattern had higher ventricular rates compared with those with a right bundle branch block configuration (table 39-2). The underlying mechanism responsible for this remarkable difference was elucidated by electrophysiologic studies [4]. A left bundle branch block morphology originated from a junctional pacemaker with a relatively higher rate and a bradycardia-dependent left bundle branch block, whereas the right bundle branch block morphology originated from a fascicular or ventricular pacemaker with a very slow rate. More than half of our patients with a third-degree AV nodal block and a ventricular

TABLE 39-1. Escape frequency, use of temporary pacing, and mortality in patients with complete or high-degree AV nodal block.

Escape frequency (per min)	No.	PM No.[a]	Mortality no.
≤30	8	7	4
31–40	34	26	6
41–50	32	27	4
51–60	15	9	5
61–70	3	1	1
>70	2	1	0

[a]PM, temporary pacemaker therapy.

TABLE 39-2. Morphology and rate of widened escape complexes during complete AV nodal block and inferior infarction.

Bundle branch block	No.	Rate (per min)
LBBB	10	45–70
RBBB	24	30–35

rate below 40/min had an escape rhythm with right bundle branch block morphology.

The AV nodal conduction disorders in the setting of acute inferior wall myocardial infarction are transient. In our series of 144 patients with second- or third-degree AV block, the duration of block varied from several minutes to 16 days. The conduction defect lasted for more than three days in 33% of the patients. All patients with high-degree AV nodal block who survived resumed 1:1 AV conduction.

In a study of 843 patients with acute inferior infarcts the mean peak SGOT was significantly higher in those with high-degree AV nodal block (140 IU) than in those without AV nodal block (92 IU) (table 39-3). Second- and third-degree AV nodal block was also associated with a higher hospital mortality, since 22% of 144 patients with these blocks died, compared with 9% of 699 patients without AV block. No differences in either estimated infarct size or prognosis were found between patients with second- versus third-degree AV nodal block [9]. In patients with third-degree AV block, the rate of the escape rhythm did not influence the prognosis significantly: ten of 52 with an escape rate higher than

TABLE 39-3. Incidence, age, sex, mean peak serum glutamic—oxaloacetic transaminase (SGOT), and mortality.

	All patients with IMI[a]	Patients without high-degree AV block	Patients with high-degree AV block
No.	843	699	144
Mean age (yr)	63	62	65
Sex			
Male	627	517	110
Female	216	182	34
Mean peak SGOT (IU)	100	92	140
Mortality (%)	12	9	22

[a]IMI, inferior myocardial infarction.

40/min died, compared with ten of 42 patients with an escape rate lower than 40/min (table 39-1). Thus, in patients with inferior myocardial infarction and high-degree AV block, the worse prognosis is independent of the severity of the conduction disorder and its associated severity of bradyarrhythmia. The major factor resulting in a larger infarct size (perhaps including right ventricular involvement) and higher mortality is a more proximal coronary artery occlusion and not the conduction disorder itself (see chapter 21).

The difference in prognosis in patients with and without AV conduction disorders is not a mere reflection of a different natural history associated with lower ventricular rates, as most patients with complete AV block of longer duration or those with a slow escape pacemaker were (lasting more than 24 h) (table 39-1). In our study, 42 of the 144 patients with inferior infarction and conduction disturbances had hemodynamic deterioration coincident with high-degree AV block. Of these 42 patients, 31 had ventricular rates of less than 50/min. Since atropine was rarely effective (response in one of 11), in 29 of these 31 patients treatment with a temporary pacemaker was instituted. Five patients did not respond to pacemaker therapy and died of true cardiogenic shock. The clinical condition improved in the remaining 24 patients and only one died later. If these patients had not been paced, the conduction disturbance itself might have contributed to extension of infarction and a higher mortality.

An additional 11 patients with high-degree

AV block had concurrent hemodynamic deterioration despite ventricular rates of more than 50/min, and had a very poor prognosis. Nine of these 11 patients died from cardiogenic shock and pacing did not influence their courses significantly. Of the remaining 102 patients without hemodynamic deterioration at the time of the onset of high-degree AV block, 17 died. There was no difference in mortality in these 102 patients between those who were paced (16%) and those who did not require temporary pacing (17%) because of an acceptable ventricular rate.

The symptoms of patients with high-degree AV block may either be signs of power failure or Stokes-Adams syncope. These syncopal attacks are mostly due to bradyarrhythmia, but may be the consequence of bradycardia-dependent ventricular tachycardia [10]. Although these tachyarrhythmias are relatively rare, they are very resistant to antiarrhythmic drugs.

From the above discussion, it can be concluded that there are three indications for temporary pacing in patients with high-degree AV block, first appearing between 2 h and several days after the onset of inferior myocardial infarction:

1. A ventricular rate less than 50/min associated with hemodynamic deterioration or Stokes-Adams attacks.
2. Unstable escape mechanisms especially when the escape complexes show a right bundle branch block morphology.

3. Bradycardia-dependent ventricular arrhythmias.

In most patients, 1:1 AV conduction resumes within several days and the duration of pacing can be limited to that period. Occasionally, however, the high-degree AV block may persist during more than one week or even more than two weeks. In these patients the temporary pacing period should be extended. Since all of our surviving patients with high-degree AV block resumed 1:1 AV conduction and since these conduction disorders do not tend to recur, permanent pacing is not necessary.

Patients with inferior myocardial infarction and high-degree AV block appearing within the first hour after onset of symptoms in general respond very well to leg raising or atropine and therefore temporary pacing is not indicated.

AV Infranodal Conduction Disorders in Anteroseptal and Other Myocardial Infarction Sites and the Indications for Temporary Pacing

In 42 of our patients admitted with acute myocardial infarction and preexistent left or right bundle branch block, only one developed complete AV infranodal block (table 39-4). Also in patients with left bundle branch block first appearing after the onset of myocardial infarction, the development of complete AV infranodal block is a rare occurrence [10]. In 25 of the 33 patients with acquired left bundle branch block, this block developed as a consequence of inferior myocardial infarction. In this setting a bradycardia-dependent left bundle branch block usually occurred during second- or third-degree AV nodal block. [4].

In contrast to the low incidence of complete AV infranodal block in patients with preexistent right or left bundle branch block or with acquired left bundle branch block, patients with right bundle branch block complicating acute anteroseptal myocardial infarction are threatened by progression to high-degree AV infranodal conduction disturbances [11]. In 70 of our 73 patients with acquired right bundle branch block collected through 1974, this block occurred as a consequence of anteroseptal infarction (table 39-4). Of these 70 patients, 18 (26%) developed complete AV infranodal block. In all these patients a bifascicular block (right bundle branch block with left anterior fascicular block or with left posterior fascicular block) developed before progression to complete AV block. We have observed both right bundle branch block preceding the fascicular block and the reverse (figure 39-1). Our data indicate that, almost exclusively, patients with acquired right bundle branch block as a consequence of acute anteroseptal infarction are at risk of developing complete AV infranodal block. However, only half of our patients with acquired right bundle branch block actually developed the conduction disorder after admission. In the other half, right bundle branch block was considered a complication of acute anteroseptal infarction if there was (a) absence of right bundle branch block in an electrocardiogram taken within six months before the acute infarction, or (b) a QR pattern in lead V_1 recorded without documented previous infarction. This last criterion is based on a previous study, in which 60 of 70 patients with acquired right bundle branch block and acute anteroseptal infarction had QR complexes in lead V_1, whereas 16 of 18 patients with preexistent right bundle branch block had either a qR pattern or a triphasic QRS complex in lead V_1. The two patients with preexistent right bundle branch block and a QR pattern in V_1 both had a previous anteroseptal infarction [12].

The development of right bundle branch block was registered in ten patients during continuous tape recording. Development of incomplete right bundle branch block occurred in five over a period ranging from several minutes to 2 h. This was followed by the sudden onset of complete right bundle branch block without a change in the preceding RR intervals (figure 39-1). The other five patients abruptly developed complete right bundle branch block without either passing through a phase of incomplete right bundle branch block or a change in the preceding cycle length (figure 39-2). In nine of the ten patients the onset of complete right bundle branch block was associated with a concomitant shift of the frontal QRS axis to the left (figure 39-2). The range of this left-axis shift varied from $10°-30°$. A con-

TABLE 39-4. Incidence of acquired and preexistent bundle branch block and acute myocardial infarction

	Acquired RBBB	Acquired LBBB	Preexistent BBB	No BBB
Total no.	73	33	42	1052
Incidence (%)	6.6	3	3.8	86.6
Mean age (yr)	63.1	64.4	70.4	63.8
Male	54	24	27	765
Female	19	9	15	287
Localization				
Inferior	3	25	14	496
Anteroseptal	70	2	5	195
Anterior	0	6	8	326
Undetermined	0	0	15	35
Mortality (%)	71	21	28	14
Complete infranodal block	18	0	1	0

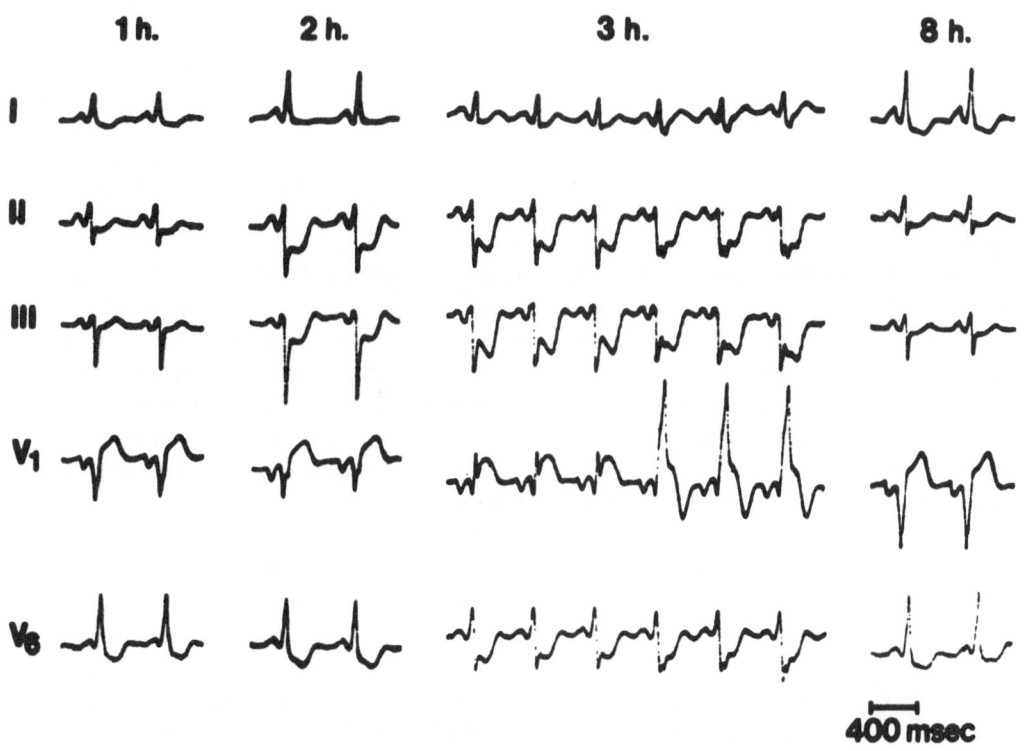

FIGURE 39-1. Development of transient bifascicular block with left anterior fascicular block and incomplete right bundle branch block preceding complete right bundle branch block. From Lie et al. [12], with permission.

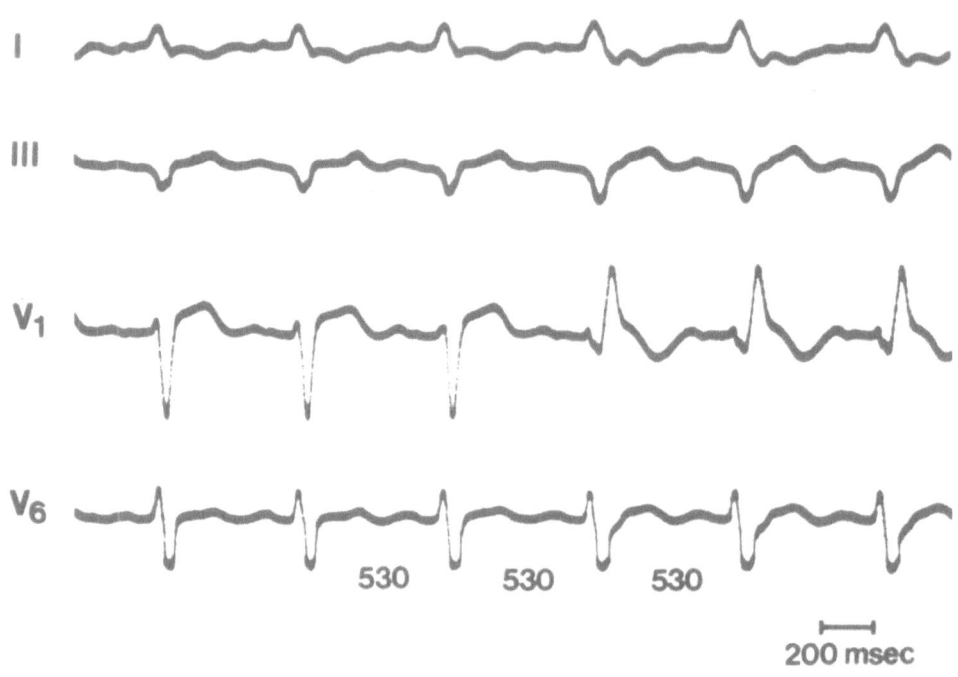

FIGURE 39-2. Sudden onset of complete right bundle branch block without change in the preceding RR intervals. Note the concomitant leftward shift of frontal QRS axis. From Lie et al [12], with permission.

comitant right-axis deviation was observed in only one patient. In the patients with a transient right bundle branch block, the patterns disappeared within one complex. These observations suggest that the conduction disorder is located in the proximal right bundle. Observations by Schuilenburg et al. favor this concept since stimulation with a bipolar catheter 1 cm distal to the His bundle area resulted in normalization of the QRS complex [13]. This suggests that the disappearance of right bundle branch block was caused by overriding of the zone of block in the proximal right bundle.

Continuous tape recording of the electrocardiogram also revealed, as reported above, that complete AV infranodal block was always preceded by a bifascicular block. Diagnosis of left anterior fascicular block or left posterior fascicular block in acute myocardial infarction may be hampered by two factors that influence the frontal QRS axis. First, the frontal QRS axis in transmural myocardial infarction may change to a direction away from the lead showing QS complexes, i.e., away from the site of infarction. Second, in nontransmural myocardial infarction the frontal QRS axis may shift towards the site of infarction as a consequence of intramural conduction block near the site of infarction with delayed activation of this area forming QR complexes.

In an attempt to evaluate the nature of true fascicular block complicating acute myocardial infarction, we observed the pattern and degree of changes in frontal QRS axis in 12 patients with acute anteroseptal infarction who on admission had nonaberrant conduction and subsequently developed complete infranodal block after a phase of bifascicular block. During these observations, the shift in axis occurred gradually over a period of hours, in contrast to the usual sudden development of right bundle branch block. All patients who developed right bundle branch block with left anterior fascicular block achieved a left-axis deviation of at least −60°, and a leftward shift of frontal QRS axis of 60° or more, prior to the development of complete AV infranodal block. Patients who developed right bundle branch block with left posterior fascicular block achieved a right-axis deviation of at least +90°, and a rightward shift of frontal QRS axis of 60° or more, before they progressed to complete AV infranodal block. These data suggest that the classic criteria for diagnosis of fascicular block, regarding deviation of frontal QRS axis, should probably be corrected by a factor of 30° to the left in acute anteroseptal infarction.

We also observed that the classic patterns of fascicular block in the initial aspects of the QRS complex are often not present if the fascicular block complicates acute anteroseptal infarction. The following characteristics may therefore be diagnostically helpful. First, a left or rightward shift of 60° or more in the frontal QRS axis favors the diagnosis of fascicular block as a consequence of acute anteroseptal infarction. Second, if the fascicular block pattern is already present on admission, the diagnosis of acquired fascicular block in acute anteroseptal infarction should be considered when the frontal QRS axis is −60° or less or +90° or more. In 434 of our patients with acute anteroseptal infarction collected through 1978, a right bundle branch block developed in 108 patients (25%). In most of these patients a left fascicular block also developed: a left anterior fascicular block in 47 patients and a left posterior fascicular block in 26 patients. Progression to complete AV infranodal block was observed in 25 (34%) of these patients with bifascicular block. The last percentage is in accordance with that of a large multicenter study reported by Hindman et al. [14], who observed a 35% risk of developing high-degree AV infranodal block in patients with acquired bifascicular block and acute myocardial infarction.

We have previously reported that the HV interval in these patients proved to be a predictor of high risk for development of complete AV infranodal block [11]. Our observations in 34 patients with anteroseptal infarction and bifascicular block reconfirmed the previous conclusions. Progression into complete AV infranodal block occurred in one of 18 patients with bifascicular block and a normal HV interval, whereas this progression occurred in 12 of 16 patients with a prolonged HV interval. The PR interval is of limited value in identifying this high-risk group, as eight of the 22 patients with a normal PR interval had a prolonged HV interval.

Patients with right bundle branch block of short duration (less than 6 h) or of delayed onset (more than 24 h after onset of infarction) tended not to progress to complete infranodal block (tables 39-5 and 39-6). Onset of complete AV infranodal block was usually noted during the first three days after infarction. However, we have observed two patients in which complete AV infranodal block occurred during the second week of infarction. Complete AV infranodal block persisted from several hours to ten days.

In all patients with complete AV infranodal block the escape pacemaker produced a wide QRS complex. In half of these patients the escape pacemaker was unreliable, showing either a very slow ventricular rate or complete ventricular asystole (figure 39-3).

Patients with bundle branch block complicating acute anteroseptal infarction have a poor immediate prognosis [11, 12, 15−17]. Recently, we reported 42 patients with bundle branch block complicating acute anteroseptal infarction with a 57% mortality within six weeks after the onset of infarction [18]. Most of these patients died from cardiogenic shock or cardiac rupture. This poor immediate prognosis is the result of extensive infarction, due to very proximal left anterior descending artery occlusion.

Our data reveal that patients with acute myocardial infarction and acquired left bundle branch block or preexistent right or left bundle branch block seldom progress into complete AV infranodal block. Therefore, prophylactic pacing in these patients is not necessary. One might consider careful electrocardiographic monitoring in those patients with preexistent right bundle branch block and acute inferior myocardial infarction or those with preexistent left bundle branch block and acute anteroseptal infarction, since these subgroups with preexistent bundle branch block are theoretically at higher risk for development of complete AV infranodal block.

The indications for temporary pacing in conduction disturbances following acute anteroseptal infarction are controversial. One report has

TABLE 39-5. Duration of right
bundle branch block in relation to
progression to complete infranodal block

Duration of RBBB	No.	Complete infranodal block
1 – 6 h	16	0
6 – 24 h	9	2
1 – 6	6	3
Persistent until discharge	9	1
Persistent until death	69	19

TABLE 39-6. Onset of right bundle branch block
in relation to progression to complete infranodal
block.

Onset of RBBB	No.	Complete infranodal block
Within 24 h of infarction	78	22
after 24 h of infarction	30	3

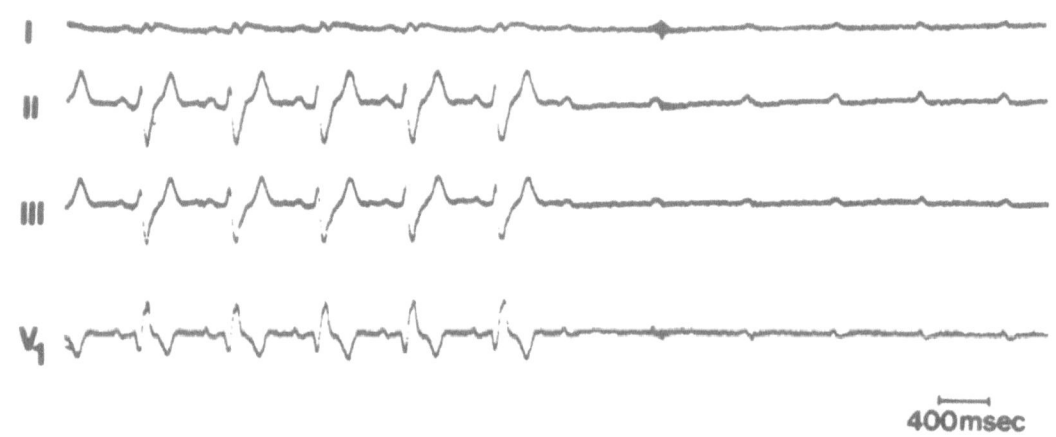

400 msec

FIGURE 39-3. Sudden onset of complete infranodal block in a patient with acute anteroseptal infarction with acquired bifascicular block, resulting in complete ventricular asystole. From Lie and Durrer [10], with permission.

suggested that, in patients with anteroseptal infarction complicated by complete AV infranodal block, temporarily pacing did not affect the immediate prognosis and was associated with a high incidence of catheter-induced ventricular tachycardia or fibrillation [19]. These authors found that, despite temporary pacing, most deaths occurred from complications of the massive myocardial damage. Others have suggested that temporary pacing should be instituted in these patients [11, 15]. We agree with the last opinion since half of our patients with anteroseptal infarction and complete AV infranodal block had a very low ventricular escape rate or ventricular asystole, resulting in hemodynamic deterioration or in Stokes-Adams attacks. Prophylactic temporary pacing should also be instituted in those patients with intact AV conduction at high risk for the subsequent development of complete AV infranodal block, i.e., right bundle branch block with

either left anterior or left posterior fascicular block acquired as a consequence of the anteroseptal infarction. The difficulties in the diagnosis of fascicular block in patients with anteroseptal infarction have been discussed above. His bundle recording may be helpful in identifying those patients at extremely high risk for developing complete AV infranodal block. If facilities for His bundle recording are not available, we recommend institution of temporary pacing in every patient with bifascicular block as a consequence of anteroseptal infarction, since one-third of these will progress to complete AV infranodal block.

We therefore conclude that, in patients with infranodal conduction disorders and acute myocardial infarction, prophylactic temporary pacing is indicated only in those with acquired right bundle branch block with either left anterior or posterior fascicular block as a consequence of the infarction. If the conduction disorder was already present on admission, the following criteria suggest a causal relationship between the anteroseptal infarction and the conduction disorder:

1. Absence of right bundle branch block in an electrocardiogram taken within six months before the acute infarction.
2. QR pattern in lead V_1 without documented previous infarction.
3. Frontal QRS axis $-60°$ or less, or $+90°$ or more.

Patients with anteroseptal infarction and acquired bifascicular block should have the pacemaker in place for five days as the development of complete AV infranodal block usually occurs within this period. If during this time, complete AV infranodal block is documented, some authors suggest subsequent insertion of a permanent pacemaker even if this complete block is only transient [14].

Temporary pacing is probably not necessary in those patients with bifascicular block of delayed onset (later than 24 h) or of short duration (less than 6 h) since the latter subgroups are at low risk for progression to complete infranodal block.

References

1. James TN, Burch GE: Blood supply of the human interventricular septum. Circulation 17:391, 1958.
2. Kostuk WJ, Beanlands DS: Complete heart block associated with acute myocardial infarction. Am J Cardiol 26:380, 1970.
3. Rosen KM, Loeb HS, Chuquimia R, et al: Site of the heart block in acute myocardial infarction. Circulation 42:925, 1970.
4. Lie KI, Wellens HJ, Schuilenburg RM, et al: Mechanism and significance of widened QRS complexes during complete atrioventricular block in acute inferior myocardial infarction. Am J Cardiol 33:833, 1974.
5. Adgey AA, Pantridge JF: Acute phase of myocardial infarction. Lancet 2:501, 1971.
6. Meltzer LE, Cohen HE: The incidence of arrhythmias associated with acute myocardial infarction. Meltzer LE, Dunning AJ (eds) In: Textbook of coronary care, Amsterdam: Excerpta Medica, 1972, p 107.
7. Norris RM: Heart block in posterior and inferior infarction. Br Heart J 31:352, 1969.
8. Rotman M, Wagner GS, Wallace AG: Bradyarrhythmias in acute myocardial infarction. Circulation 45:703, 1972.
9. Tans AC, Lie KI: A-V nodal block in acute myocardial infarction. In: Wellens HJJ, Lie KI, Janse MJ (eds) The conduction system of the heart: structure, function and clinical implications. Leiden: HE Stenfert Kroese, 1976, pp 655−661.
10. Lie KI, Durrer D: Conduction disturbances in acute myocardial infarction. In: Narula OS (ed) Cardiac arrhythmias: electrophysiology, diagnosis and management. Baltimore: Williams and Wilkins,, 1979, pp 140−162.
11. Lie KI, Wellens HJJ, Schuilenburg RM, et al: Factors influencing prognosis of bundle branch block complicating acute anteroseptal infarction. Circulation 50:935, 1974.
12. Lie KI, Wellens HJJ, Schuilenburg RM: Bundle branch block and acute myocardial infarction. In: Wellens HJJ, Lie KI, Janse MJ (eds) The conduction system of the heart: structure, function and clinical implications. Leiden: HE Stenfert Kroese, 1976, pp 662−672.
13. Schuilenburg RM, Lie KI, Durrer D: Localization of the block in patients with acute anteroseptal infarction and complete right bundle branch block. Circulation (Supply 4) 50:245, 1974.
14. Hindman MC, Wagner GS, Jaro M, et al: The clinical significance of bundle branch block complicating acute myocardial infarction. 2. Indications for temporary and permanent pacemaker insertion. Circulation 58:689, 1978.
15. Atkins JM, Leshin SJ, Blomqvist G, et al: Ventricular conduction blocks and sudden death in acute myocardial infarction. N Engl J Med 288:281, 1973.
16. Roos JC, Dunning AJ: Right bundle branch block and left axis deviation in acute myocardial infarction. Br Heart J 32:847, 1970.
17. Ginks WR, Sutton R, Oh W, Leatham A: Long-term prognosis after acute anterior infarction with atrioventricular block. Br Heart J 39:186, 1977.
18. Hauer RNW, Lie KI, Liem KL, Durrer D: Long-term prognosis in patients with bundle branch block complicating acute anteroseptal infarction. AM J Cardiol 49:1581, 1982.
19. Godman MJ, Lassers BW, Julian DG: Complete bundle branch block complicating acute myocardial infarction. N Engl J Med 282:237, 1970.

40. DRUG INTERACTIONS IN CORONARY CARE

W. Wayne Stargel

Drug interactions in patients with acute myocardial ischemia or infarction can be classified by two major types. The first involves interactions that either increase or decrease the plasma concentration of another drug. This is termed *pharmacokinetic drug interaction*. It involves numerous factors, such as changes in absorption, changes in distribution to the site of action, inhibited or enhanced hepatic metabolism, altered protein binding, and increased or decreased renal elimination.

The second major type of drug interaction involves a change in the pharmacologic effect at the receptor, without a change in plasma concentration. This is referred to as *pharmacodynamic drug interaction* and is generally more predictable than the pharmacokinetic drug interactions, provided the pharmacologic actions of both drugs are accurately known.

The clinician should also be aware of the change in dosage requirements as a result of alterations in physiologic parameters associated with acute myocardial infarction, such as congestive heart failure. This chapter discusses the major clinically significant drug—drug interactions involving those drugs commonly used in the treatment of problems associated with acute ischemic heart disease. A brief section also discusses the importance of adjustment in dosage of drugs as a result of the disease process.

Lidocaine

Lidocaine is the most widely used intravenous agent for the acute treatment of arrhythmias associated with acute ischemic heart disease. Pharmacokinetics of lidocaine are important in understanding factors that may be responsible for adverse drug interactions.

Lidocaine is predominately eliminated by hepatic metabolism, with less than 10% excreted as unchanged drug. This hepatic metabolism of lidocaine is primarily dependent upon hepatic blood flow rather than hepatic enzyme activity. Therefore factors known to decrease hepatic blood flow will decrease the clearance of lidocaine, and dosage adjustment may be necessary to avoid toxicity (table 40-1).

Recently both metoprolol and propranolol were reported to affect the elimination of lidocaine [1] by reducing cardiac output and hepatic blood flow. Propranolol appeared to decrease the mean clearance more than metoprolol: 47% vs 31%. The authors also postulated that inhibition of hepatic oxidative enzymes might be partially responsible for the reduction in lidocaine clearance, since neither beta-blocking agent would reduce cardiac output or hepatic blood flow sufficiently to account for the percentage reduction in lidocaine clearance. This observation suggests using caution when administering beta blockers to patients on lidocaine, since toxicity may result from increased lidocaine concentration.

Coadministration of lidocaine and cimetidine is frequently encountered in the coronary care unit, and may result in lidocaine toxicity. Cimetidine has been shown to decrease hepatic clearance of drugs by both inhibition of oxidative metabolism, and reduction of hepatic blood flow. The latter mechanism is presumed the major effect on reducing lidocaine clearance. However, cimetidine has also been reported to reduce the distribution volume of lidocaine, and this may account for higher plasma concentration and toxicity [2]. The magnitude of the decrease in clearance of lidocaine by cimetidine has been reported to be approximately 25%. Recent work with a new H_2-receptor blocker, ranitidine, suggested no interaction with lidocaine [3]. Ranitidine should serve as a substitute for cimetidine to prevent a possible drug interaction. If cimetidine is coadministered with lidocaine, however, the dosage of lidocaine should probably be decreased to avoid toxicity.

A pharacodynamic interaction that may warrant caution is the combination of lidocaine with pentobarbital. It is not uncommon on some coronary care units to use pentobarbital (or other drugs known to suppress respiration) as premedication for cardioversion. Although the combination of lidocaine and pentobarbital is reported to produce apnea in animal studies, very little clinical information is available [4]. This interaction is thought to be caused by an additive depressant effect on the respiratory center. One alternative is to use the combination of lidocaine and diazepam, which has been shown to be well tolerated.

Quinidine

Quinidine has been used in combination with digitalis for over 50 years, but not until the late 1970s did reports appear of a significant drug–drug interaction [5, 6]. The addition of quinidine to patients receiving maintenance regimens of digoxin resulted in a marked increase of digoxin concentration. The mechanism of this interaction is postulated to involve a reduction of both renal and nonrenal clearances of digoxin by quinidine. Digoxin concentration begins to increase within 24 h after quinidine is initiated, and

TABLE 40-1. Factors known to decrease lidocaine clearance

1. Cimetidine
2. Beta blockers (metoprolol, propranolol)
3. Congestive heart failure
4. Liver disease

generally achieves a new steady state within 3–6 days. The magnitude of the increase in digoxin concentration has been reported to range from 25% to 300%. This change in digoxin concentration is dependent upon the dose of quinidine administered. The large individual variability of the quinidine—digoxin interaction makes general dosage recommendations difficult. Most studies have recommended decreasing the digoxin dose by half prior to starting quinidine. This recommendation is based on the clinical studies demonstrating approximately a 100% increase in the digoxin concentration. Close monitoring of the patient and measurement of plasma digoxin concentration may help individualize therapy. Remember that a new steady state of digoxin may be delayed for several days in patients with renal insufficiency.

Quinidine may interact with vitamin-K-dependent anticoagulants. Several cases of quinidine-induced hypoprothrombinemic hemorrhage have been reported in patients concurrently taking other warfarinlike anticoagulants [7, 8]. Quinidine may be capable of inhibiting the synthesis of vitamin-K-dependent clotting factors. This is generally of no clinical significance when quinidine is used alone, but quinidine coadministered with other anticoagulants may be additive in depressing vitamin-K clotting factor synthesis. This interaction does not occur in all patients, but prothrombin times should be monitored when initiating quinidine in patients already receiving anticoagulants.

Quinidine has been reported to potentiate both non-depolarizing and depolarizing muscle relaxants [9, 10]. This interaction increases the intensity and duration of muscle relaxants, and may be an important drug interaction in patients recovering from anesthesia. The mechanism of this drug interaction is not completely understood, but quinidine is postulated to interfere with either acetylcholine release or transport of cations at the neuromuscular junction.

Rifampin is reported to enhance quinidine elimination, presumably through hepatic enzyme induction. A recent study showed a threefold increase in the rate of quinidine elimination by the addition of rifampin [11]. Initiation or discontinuation of rifampin may decrease or increase the pharmacologic effect of quinidine, respectively.

Similar to the quinidine–rifampin interaction is the effect of phenytoin or phenobarbital on quinidine elimination. Concomitant administration of quinidine and the anticonvulsant drugs phenytoin and phenobarbital has been reported to reduce the elimination half-life of quinidine by approximately 50% [12]. This is also believed to be related to the enzyme induction of these drugs resulting in an increased metabolism of quinidine. Administration of either phenytoin or phenobarbital to a patient on quinidine may result in a decrease of the quinidine effect. The opposite is true also: a patient maintained on both quinidine and an anticonvulsant may develop toxicity when the anticonvulsant is stopped.

Cimetidine was recently reported to decrease the elimination of oral quinidine in normal volunteers [13]. The mechanism was postulated to be either hepatic enzyme inhibition, reduced hepatic blood flow, or a combination of these factors. Further studies in patients will determine the clinical significance of this drug–drug interaction.

The amount of quinidine excreted by the kidneys is dependent upon urine pH. Drugs known to increase urine pH (i.e., acetazolamide, or sodium bicarbonate) may result in increased tubular reabsorption of nonionized quinidine [14]. Acidification of the urine has been used in the treatment of quinidine intoxication to enhance elimination. Since the major route of quinidine elimination is hepatic, however, changes in urine pH may be of limited clinical value in altering quinidine concentrations.

Digoxin

In addition to the quinidine–digoxin interaction that has already been discussed, a recent report suggested that calcium antagonists may increase the plasma digoxin concentration [15]. These authors reported an increase in serum digoxin concentration of 45%, 69%, 118% with nifedipine, verapamil, and quinidine, respectively. The increase in plasma digoxin concentration was also related to an increased effect on the heart as measured by both systolic time interval shortening and flattening of the T waves. Careful monitoring of patients treated with digoxin and adjustments in dose may be required with coadministration of these drugs.

The interaction of antacids with absorption of digoxin has most likely been overstated, but single-dose studies have reported approximately 25% reduction in absorption compared with controls [16]. The logical way to avoid this interaction is to stagger the dose, so that at least 2 h separates the digoxin dose from the antacid administration.

Antidiarrheal products that contain kaolin and pectin have been reported to bind digoxin and decrease oral bioavailability [17]. Similar to the antacid interaction, it is best to avoid concomitant administration by allowing for 2 h between doses.

Numerous other drugs may alter the pharmacokinetic properties of digoxin and are summarized in table 40-2.

Hypokalemia increases the risk of cardiac arrhythmias in patients treated with digoxin [18]. Therefore diuretics (i.e., furosemide, thiazides, bumetanide, and ethacrynic acid) that lower serum potassium concentration may increase the potential for digitalis toxicity. This pharmacodynamic drug interaction between digoxin and diuretics is less likely to occur in patients receiving adequate potassium supplementation.

Phenytoin

Phenytoin is primarily eliminated from the body by hepatic metabolism. The hepatic capacity to metabolize phenytoin is limited, and saturation of this enzyme system can lead to accumulation and toxicity. Drug interactions with phenytoin primarily involve either the enhancement or inhibition of enzyme activity, resulting in decreased or increased plasma phenytoin concentrations, respectively (table 40-3).

Phenytoin is also a potent stimulator of he-

TABLE 40-2. Other drug interactions with digoxin

1. Drugs that may decrease digoxin concentration

Drug	Mechanism
Cholestyramine	Decreased absorption
Colestipol	Decreased absorption
Neomycin	Decreased absorption
Sulfasalazine	Decreased absorption

2. Drugs that may increase digoxin concentration

Drug	Mechanism
Spironolactone	Decreased clearance
Amiloride	Decreased clearance
Quinine	Decreased clearance
Amiodarone	Unknown
Antibiotics	Increased absorption
Erythromycin	
Tetracycline	

TABLE 40-3. Drug interactions with phenytoin

Interaction	Drug
May ↑ hepatic metabolism of phenytoin	Barbiturates (low concentration)
	Alcohol
	Carbamazepine
May ↓ hepatic metabolism of phenytoin	Barbiturates (high concentration)
	Cimetidine
	Isoniazid
	Chloramphenicol
	Disulfiram
	Dicumarol
May displace phenytoin from protein-binding sites	Phenylbutazone
	Valproic acid
	Salicylates
	Sulfonylureas

patic enzyme activity, and may be important in increasing the clearance of anticoagulants, glucocorticoids, theophylline, quinidine, disopyramide, and mexiletine [12, 19, 20]. Any drug that induces metabolic enzyme activity may necessitate a higher dose of another drug that is, thereby, cleared more rapidly.

Phenytoin is approximately 90% bound to plasma proteins, with the percentage free being responsible for the pharmacologic effects and the hepatic elimination. As mentioned previously, the amount of phenytoin that is metabolized is limited by the capacity of hepatic enzyme activity. Some drugs have the capability of displacing phenytoin from its albumin-binding sites. This may decrease total phenytoin concentrations by making more free phenytoin available for hepatic metabolism. However, increased free phenytoin may cause saturation of hepatic enzymes responsible for its elimination and thereby lead to toxicity. This protein-binding displacement reaction can be very complex, and like the enzyme activity is very unpredictable. Close monitoring of both free and total phenytoin may help in individualizing therapy.

Administration of intravenous phenytoin to critically ill patients being maintained on dopamine infusion may lead to severe hypotension [21]. Examining this drug interaction in animal studies required that the dogs be made hypovolemic and hypotensive before the interaction could be elicited. Mechanism of this interaction was postulated to be a combination of catecholamine depletion by dopamine and myocardial depression of contractility by phenytoin. Cautious use of intravenous phenytoin should be warranted in patients receiving dopamine.

Beta-adrenergic Blockers

Drug interactions that affect the disposition of beta blockers such as propranolol may be of limited clinical significance because of the wide margin of their safety. More important may be the effect of propranolol on the disposition of other drugs with narrow therapeutic ranges (i.e., lidocaine). Numerous drug interactions have been reported to alter the disposition of propranolol, and these are summarized in table 40-4.

Probably the most classic pharmacodynamic drug interaction is coadministration of an antagonist with an agonist. Propranolol is a competitive antagonist of the effects of catecholamines at the beta-adrenergic receptors. Therefore administration of a beta antagonist (i.e., propranolol) will decrease the response of a beta agonist (i.e., isoproterenol). The antagonism of propranolol at the beta receptor can be overcome by administering higher concentrations of the agonist.

Beta-receptor selectivity may also be important in determining the pharmacologic effect of a given agonist. Propranolol is described as a nonselective beta-adrenergic blocker, because both the beta-1 receptors of the heart and the beta-2 receptors in the lungs and peripheral vessels are equally antagonized. However, metoprolol is a relative selective antagonist of the beta-1 receptor and may elicit different pharmacologic properties in the presence of different catecholamines. An example of the differences between the selective and nonselective antagonism of beta receptors can be illustrated in a

TABLE 40-4. Drug interactions with propranolol

1. Drugs that may decrease propranolol concentrations

Drug	Mechanism
Alcohol	Increased clearance
Aluminum hydroxide gel	Decreased absorption
Phenytoin	Increased clearance
Phenobarbital	Increased clearance
Rifampin	Increased clearance

2. Drugs that may increase propanolol concentrations

Drug	Mechanism
Chlorpromazine	Decreased clearance
Cimetidine	Decreased clearance

patient infused with adrenalin [22]. The infusion of adrenalin in the presence of a nonselective beta antagonist (i.e., propranolol) will result in accentuation of the alpha activity due to beta-2 blockade by propranolol. A marked increase in total peripheral resistance is the result. However, adrenalin infused in the presence of a selective beta-1 blocker (i.e., metoprolol) shows no quantitative change in total peripheral resistance.

Another possible metabolic difference between a selective beta-1 blocker and a nonselective beta blocker involves glycogenolysis, which appears to be controlled by beta-2 stimulation. A recent study showed that the nonselective beta blocker propranolol antagonized the production of glucose during strenuous exercise [23], whereas the beta-1 selective blocker antenolol was reported to be no different from placebo during the same conditions. The authors suggested that the antagonism of glucose production by propranolol may be responsible for decreased exercise tolerance and increased fatigue with strenuous exercise.

Bretylium

Bretylium is limited from chronic administration because of the development of orthostatic hypotension induced by adrenergic neuron blockade. A recent study has reported a drug interaction between bretylium and protriptyline, a tricyclic antidepressant [24]. Bretylium enters postganglionic sympathetic neurons by way of a membrane pump, and thus inhibits neurotransmission by blocking the release of norepinephrine. The authors report that the antiarrhythmic effects of bretylium are not dependent upon adrenergic neuron blockade, and the addition of a tricyclic antidepressant will block the entry of bretylium into the adrenergic neuron. This interaction will prevent the orthostatic drop in blood pressure while maintaining the antiarrhythmic effects of bretylium.

The dosage of catecholamines must be reduced in the presence of bretylium, because of an increase in the pressor response of these agents. The mechanism may be denervation hypersensitivity caused by bretylium. Caution should be exercised when treating the hypotension caused by bretylium with a catecholamine.

Bretylium is known to cause an initial release of norepinephrine from adrenergic neurons after intravenous administration. This increased release of norepinephrine may aggravate digitalis toxicity, and is best avoided unless the etiology of the arrhythmia is clearly not due to digitalis.

Cimetidine

Cimetidine is reported to interact with numerous other drugs through a combination of factors that include: (a) increase in gastric pH, (b) inhibition of hepatic enzymes, and (c) decrease in hepatic blood flow. Drug interactions with cimetidine have been the topic of recent reviews [25–27] and are summarized in table 40-5.

Drug—Disease Interaction

The clinician must not only be aware of drug— drug interactions, but also the affect of the disease process on the dosage requirements of the various drugs. Alterations in both hemodynamic and pharmacokinetic parameters resulting from the disease process may lead to toxicity if appropriate dosage adjustments are not initiated.

Patients experiencing acute myocardial infarction may develop several hemodynamic changes that will affect dosage requirements. One of the most common is the associated reduction of cardiac output. This tends to lower the volume in which the drugs are distributed (volume of distribution). Therefore, loading doses of drugs

TABLE 40-5. Drug interactions with cimetidine

1. Cimetidine may increase the concentration of the following:

Lidocaine	Chlordiazepoxide
Phenytoin	Procainamide
Propranolol	Quinidine
Metoprolol	Morphine
Labetalol	Chlormethiazole
Theophylline	Penicillin
Warfarin	Carbamazepine
Diazepam	

2. Cimetidine may decrease the concentration of the following:
   Ketoconazole

(i.e., lidocaine, procainamide) must be reduced to avoid toxicity.

Low cardiac output states are also responsible for reduction of the glomerular filtration rate, and a reduction of hepatic blood flow. The decrease in glomerular filtration rate will decrease the clearance of drugs known to be eliminated by the kidneys (i.e., bretylium, disopyramide, procainamide). Whereas, a reduction of hepatic blood flow can decrease the elimination of drugs dependent upon the liver for metabolism (i.e., lidocaine, propranolol). Decreases in glomerular filtration rate or hepatic blood flow will require adjustment of maintenance doses to prevent accumulation and toxicity.

Elevation of alpha-1-acid glycoprotein has been reported in patients with acute myocardial infarction [28]. This rise in alpha-1-acid glycoprotein is associated with increased binding of some basic drugs (i.e., lidocaine, propranolol). Because of this increased protein binding, the total plasma concentration will rise, but the free concentration is attenuated. It is a general pharmacologic principle that the therapeutic and toxic effects of a drug are dependent upon free drug concentration (percent unbound). Therefore, some patients may have elevated total plasma concentrations but show no signs of toxicity. Likewise, low concentrations may be ineffective in the setting of increased levels of alpha-1-acid glycoprotein. This increased binding associated with myocardial infarction may also partially explain the accumulation of lidocaine during prolonged infusions [29]. Although more work is needed in this area, monitoring of both total and free concentrations may help in optimizing drug therapy.

References

1. Conrad KA, Byers JM, Finley PR, Burnham L: Lidocaine elimination: effects of metoprolol and of propranolol. Clin Pharmacol Ther 33:133−138, 1983.
2. Feely J, McAllister CB, Wilkinson GR, Wood AJJ: Reduction in lignocaine clearance by cimetidine. Br J Clin Pharmacol 13:591−592P, 1982.
3. Feely J, Buy E: Lack of effect of ranitidine on the disposition of lignocaine. Br J Clin Pharmacol 15:378−379, 1983.
4. LeLorier J: Lidocaine and pentobarbital: a potentially lethal drug−drug interaction. Toxicol Appl Pharmacol 44:657−659, 1978.
5. Leahey EB, Reiffel JA, Drusin RE, Heissenbuttel RH, Lovejoy WP, Rigger JT: Interaction between quinidine and digoxin. JAMA 240:533−534, 1978.
6. Ejvinsson G: Effects of quinidine on plasma concentrations of dignoxin. Br Med J 1:279−280, 1978.
7. Koch-Weser J: Quinidine-induced hypoprothrombinemic hemorrhage in a patient on chronic warfarin therapy. Ann Intern Med 68:511, 1968.
8. Gazzaniga AB, Stewart DR: Possible quinidine-induced hemorrhage in a patient on warfarin sodium. N Engl J Med 280:711, 1969.
9. Schmidt JL, Vick NA, Sadove, MS: The effect of quinidine on the action of muscle relaxants. JAMA 182:143−145, 1963.
10. Way L, Katzung BG, Larson CP: Recurarization with quinidine. JAMA 200:163, 1967.
11. Twum-Barima Y, Carruthers SG: Quinidine−rifampin interaction. N Engl J Med 304:1466−1469.
12. Data JL, Wilkinson GR, Nies AS: Interaction of quinidine with anticonvulsant drugs. N Eng J Med 294:699−702, 1976.
13. Hardy BG, Zador IT, Golden L, Lalka D, Schentag JJ: Effect of cimetidine on the pharmacokinetics and pharmacodynamics of quinidine. Am J Cardiol 52:172−175, 1983.
14. Knouss RF, Gebhardt RE, Thyrum PT, Luchi RJ, Morris JJ: Variation in quinidine excretion with changing urine pH [abstr]. Ann Intern Med 68:1157, 1968.
15. Belz GG, Doering W, Munkes R, Matthews J; Interaction between digoxin and calcium antagonists and antiarrhythmic drugs. Clin Pharmacol Ther 33:410−417, 1983.
16. Brown DD, Juhl RP: Decreased bioavailability of digoxin due to antacids and kaolin−pectin. N Engl J Med 295:1034−1037, 1976.
17. Albert KS, Elliot WJ, Abbot RD, Gilbertson TJ, Data JL: Influence of kaolin−pectin suspension on steady-state plasma digoxin levels. J Clin Pharmacol 21:449−455, 1981.
18. Steiness E, Olesen KH: Cardiac arrhythmias induced by hypokalemia and potassium loss during maintenance digoxin therapy. Br Heart J 38:167−172, 1976.
19. Kessler JM, Keys PW, Stafford RW: Disopyramide and phenytoin interaction. Clin Pharmacokinet 1:263−264, 1982.
20. Begg EJ, Chinwah PM, Webb C. Day RO, Wade DN: Enhanced metabolism of mexiletine after phenytoin administration. Br J Clin Pharacol 14:219−223, 1982.
21. Bevins BA, Rapp RP, Griffen WO, Blouin R, Bustrack J: Dopamine−phenytoin interactions. Arch Surg 113:245−249, 1978.
22. Johnsson G. Regardh CG: Hemodynamic interaction between adrenaline and beta-adrenoceptor antagonists in man and relationship between the effect and plasma levels of beta-adrenoceptor antagonists. Acta Physiol Scand Suppl 440:28, 1976.
23. McLeod AA, Brown JE, Kuhn C, Kitchell BB, Sedor FA, Williams RS, Shand DG: Differentiation of hemodynamic, humoral and metabolic responses to B$_1$- and B$_2$-adrenergic stimulation in man using atenolol and propranolol. Circulation 67:1076−1084, 1983.
24. Woosley RL, Reele SB, Roden DM, Nies AS, Oates JA: Pharmacologic reversal of hypotensive effect complicating antiarrhythmic therapy with bretylium. Clin Pharmacol Ther 32:313−321, 1982.
25. Somogyi A, McLean A, Heinzow B: Cimetidine−procainamide pharmacokinetic interaction in man: evidence of competition for tubular secretion of basic drugs. Eur J Clin Pharmacol 25:339−345, 1983.
26. Somogyi A, Gugler R: Drug interactions with cimetidine. Clin Pharmacokinet 7:23−41, 1982.

27. Sedman AJ: Cimetidine—drug interactions. AM J Med 76:109–114, 1984.

28. Routledge PA, Stargel WW, Wagner GS, Shand DG: Increased alpha-1-acid glycoprotein and lidocaine disposition in myocardial infarction. Ann Intern Med 93:701–704, 1980.

29. Barchowsky A, Shand DG, Stargel WW, Wagner GS, Routledge PA: On the role of alpha-1-acid glycoprotein in lignocaine accumulation following myocardial infarction. Br J Clin Pharmacol 13:411–415, 1982.

41. THE USE OF β-ADRENERGIC AND CALCIUM-BLOCKING DRUGS DURING ACUTE MYOCARDIAL ISCHEMIA AND INFARCTION

Gary L. Stiles

The goal of any therapeutic intervention in acute myocardial ischemia or infarction is to bring the myocardial oxygen supply-and-demand relationship into a favorable balance. Thus, one may attempt to either increase oxygen supply or decrease demand independently or to alter both sides of the relationship simultaneously. This chapter deals exclusively with the use of two classes of drugs: β-adrenergic receptor and calcium-channel-blocking drugs.

A definition of terms seems indicated. An acute myocardial infarction refers to the clinical state in which cardiac muscle dies as a result of an inadequate supply of metabolic substrates. Clinically this can be more precisely defined in terms of a triad: clinical symptoms, electrocardiographic (ECG) changes, and altered serum enzymes. The definition of unstable angina is less well established but usually refers to one of three clinical situations: (a) the recent onset of new angina pectoris usually within the past month to six weeks, (b) the acute exacerbation or progression of angina in terms of severity or frequency of attacks, and (c) the onset of prolonged rest chest pain lasting at least 15−30 min with transient

ECG changes but without enzymatic alterations.

Considering these definitions, one must determine the goal to be achieved with each therapeutic intervention. For unstable angina, a reasonable endpoint would be the elimination of symptoms and the prevention of progression to myocardial infarction. Unfortunately, the natural history of unstable angina is quite variable. Twenty years ago the incidence of developing myocardial infarction within the first few months after the onset of unstable angina ranged from 22% to 80% [1, 2]. Current evidence suggests that myocardial infarction during the acute phase of unstable angina is now probably less than 10% [3]. First-year mortality in unstable angina had been estimated to be as high as 60% [1], but currently the estimates are in the range of 10% [3]. Any comparison between old and new studies on natural history is difficult, however, because definitions of terms as well as practices of medical care have changed significantly (see chapter 55). One wonders whether recently developed therapies such as those considered in this chapter have been responsible for these current relatively favorable outcomes.

For an acute myocardial infarction, the therapeutic endpoint is even more difficult to determine. The ultimate goal of therapy is to decrease the quantity of myocardium undergoing irrevers-

Dr. Stiles is supported by a Clinical Investigator Award from the National Heart, Lung and Blood Institute no. HL 01027.

ible damage and, thereby, to decrease morbidity and mortality. The elimination of clinical symptoms such as pain or ECG changes such as ST-segment elevation are definable, but their relationship to quantitative decreases in myocardial necrosis is not well defined. More sophisticated measures for delineating myocardial salvage are required.

The potential benefits and risks associated with the use of β-adrenergic receptor antagonists and the calcium blockers in ischemic syndromes are shown in tables 41-1 and 41-2, and detailed information is provided in appropriate sections of this chapter.

Unstable Angina

β-ADRENERGIC BLOCKERS
β-Adrenergic blockers are an almost universally accepted therapeutic agent in the treatment of unstable angina pectoris, in spite of the lack of prospective randomized trials versus other therapies. The rationale for β-adrenergic blockers is based on sound physiologic principles. β-blockers have the ability to decrease heart rate, decrease contractility and wall stress, and lower blood pressure, all of which should decrease myocardial

oxygen demand. However, β-blockers have the potential for producing: (a) excessive bradycardia, (b) congestive heart failure with increased diastolic filling pressures and volumes, (c) hypotension, and (d) an increased likelihood of coronary spasm in susceptible individuals. All of these effects would be deleterious by either increasing cardiac demand for oxygen or decreasing supply. The possible occurrence of these effects (particularly the potential for negative inotropy) is important to consider in a rapidly changing clinical situation such as unstable angina.

Early reports were extremely encouraging. Fischl et al. [4] in 1973 reported 20 patients with unstable angina who were treated in a nonrandomized study with propranolol. The patients received an average daily dose of 170 mg, and 17 of the 20 experienced rapid relief of pain, usually within 12 h. There were seven patients who had clinical evidence of mild congestive heart failure prior to initiation of therapy, and the congestive heart failure symptoms improved after propranolol therapy in all. However, three of the seven had digoxin either started concomitantly or increased in dosage. There were no serious side effects associated with propranolol therapy and no acute myocardial infarctions occurred during hospitalization. Although there are no controlled

TABLE 41-1. β-Adrenergic receptor antagonists

Potential benefits	Potential risks
1. Decrease oxygen demand 　a. Decrease heart rate 　b. Decrease contractility 　c. Lower blood pressure 2. Control arrhythmias 　a. Supraventricular 　b. Catecholamine-induced ventricular premature beats	1. Excessive bradycardia 2. Hypotension 3. Congestive heart failure 4. Atrioventricular block 5. Provoke coronary artery spasm

TABLE 41-2. Calcium-channel-blocking drugs

Potential benefits	Potential risks
1. Relieve coronary spasm 2. Decrease MVO$_2$ (demand) 　a. Decrease peripheral vascular resistance (afterload) 　b. Decrease contractility (verapamil) 　c. Decrease heart rate (verapamil) 3. Improve subendocardial/epicardial blood flow	1. Hypotension 2. Heart failure 3. Atrioventricular block 4. Peripheral edema 5. Bradycardia

studies, the preponderance of data strongly suggest that β-adrenergic antagonists are effective in dramatically decreasing the symptoms of unstable angina. Whether β-blockers alter the natural history of unstable angina is much less clear. There are no controlled studies of β-antagonists versus nitrates or other medical therapies, and the rapid emergence of coronary artery bypass surgery has made it virtually impossible to obtain such matched groups of patients. Data from the National Cooperative Study of Unstable Angina [5] suggest that in medically treated patients the inhospital mortality is approximately 3% and the late (30-month) mortality is 7%. The rate of nonfatal myocardial infarction was 8% in the hospital and 11% for the same follow-up period as above. These findings have been interpreted as indicating that β-blockers have altered the natural history of unstable angina. A recent study was reported from Dublin [6] in which patients with unstable angina were treated only with bed rest, reassurance, and sublingual nitroglycerin. They demonstrated that, even without the use of β-blockers, calcium channel blockers or long-acting nitrates, patients had results similar to those reported in the National Cooperative Study. That report [6] does not, however, supply data regarding the presence of stable angina during the follow-up period or the proportion of patients returning to work. Further corroborating studies will be needed to confirm this interesting finding. The study does illustrate that it is possible for a therapeutic intervention to become standard therapy without being proven efficacious.

Currently, β-blockers are an accepted mode of therapy for unstable angina particularly in those patients without evidence of congestive heart failure. In patients with mild congestive heart failure, β-blockers also are a reasonable choice, but dosage should be increased carefully to prevent a precipitous increase in the congestive heart failure with elevated left ventricular filling pressures.

The introduction of β-adrenergic subtype selective antagonists such as atenolol or metoprolol and antagonists with intrinsic sympathomimetic activity (ISA) such as pindolol has raised the question of whether these have advantages compared with nonselective drugs such as propranolol. Subtype selective drugs are selective for β₁-adrenergic receptors (primarily located in the heart) and may, therefore, have fewer side effects such as bronchospasm or exacerbation of peripheral vasoconstriction as seen in Raynaud's phenomenon. There are no data that these subtype selective antagonists produce a more efficacious result regarding ischemic symptoms. Although β-blockers with intrinsic sympathomimetic activity should theoretically have less of a depressive effect on cardiac output and hence be associated with lower left ventricular filling pressures, the possible clinical importance of ISA is still unproven [7].

In a rapidly changing clinical situation such as unstable angina, propranolol or metoprolol, with their relatively short plasma half-lives, would have obvious advantages over longer-acting drugs such as nadolol. Drug levels can be more rapidly increased or decreased as the clinical situation warrants.

In patients with unstable angina who demonstrate ST-segment elevation on ECG during pain, it has been suggested that β-adrenergic receptor blockers might be deleterious rather than beneficial. The rationale is that coronary vasospasm may be the precipitating factor and that β-blockers would remove the dilating effect of catecholamines (a β-adrenergic receptor mediated function) while leaving their constricting effect via α-adrenergic receptors unchecked. This hypothesis remains very tenable and needs to be tested in clinical trials. At the present time the proportion of patients with unstable angina who have coronary vasospasm as an etiologic or contributing factor remains unknown.

CALCIUM CHANNEL BLOCKERS

There are currently three calcium channel blockers available in the United States—nifedipine, diltiazem, and verapamil [8]. Although all of these drugs are calcium channel blockers, each has a unique set of cardiovascular effects. Some of their properties are compared and contrasted in table 41-3 and have been recently reviewed elsewhere [8]. Controlled randomized studies of calcium channel blockers are sparse. Parodi et al. [9] in 1979 reported a controlled study of verapamil versus placebo in 12 patients with angina at rest. They quantified the severity of ischemic attacks by either ECG changes or pain while patients

TABLE 41-3. Cardiovascular effects of the three currently available calcium channel blockers

	Nifedipine	Verapamil	Diltiazam
Decreased heart rate	O	+/−	+
Decreased AV conduction	O	++	+
LV dysfunction	O	+	+
Hypotension	+++	+	+
Coronary dilatation	+++	++	+++

O, absent; +, mild; ++, moderate; +++, marked.

were treated alternately with placebo or 480 mg of verapamil. The treatment periods were characterized by a dramatic reduction in both of the observed aspects of ischemia. Similarly, Previtali et al. [10] assessed the effect of nifedipine in 14 patients with angina at rest who had no evidence of congestive heart failure and who were not on β-blockers or long-acting nitrates. In this acute study, nifedipine, at 60 mg per day, totally relieved symptoms in nine of the 14 patients; and, at 80 mg per day, 11 of 14 patients became pain free. It is of interest to note that five of the 14 patients had documented coronary spasm. These studies suggest that the calcium channel blockers are efficacious in the acute phase of unstable angina. It remains to be determined whether patients with unstable angina who have spasm have different therapeutic requirements than those without spasm.

There are now several excellent studies on the combined use of calcium channel blockers with β-blockers and long-acting nitrates. The Johns Hopkins University group [11] recently reported a randomized study in 138 patients with unstable angina who were given either nifedipine or placebo in addition to a standard nitrate plus propranolol regimen. The two groups were matched regarding risk factors and the dosages of propranolol and nitrates received. After four months the incidence of medical failures (defined by sudden death, myocardial infarction, or urgent coronary bypass) was significantly higher in the placebo-treated group (60%), compared with the nifedipine-treated group (44%). The difference was even more striking when the comparison was made in patients who demonstrated ST-segment elevation with pain (67% vs 33%). Side effects noted upon adding nifedipine to propranolol−

nitrate therapy were minimal and suggest that this is a relatively safe combination.

Moses et al. [12] have studied the short-term efficacy of nifedipine in 19 patients with rest angina refractory to propranolol and nitrates. They found that the addition of nifedipine (30−120 mg daily) abolished the pain in 14 patients, decreased it in two patients, and had no effect in three patients. Of the 19 patients, 16 had coronary arteriography and all had significant coronary artery disease. Ten of the 19 patients had ST-segment elevation with pain, but the incidence of coronary spasm is not known. The side effects noted in this study were also minimal. These studies suggest that calcium channel blockers are an effective therapeutic modality in the short-term management of patients with unstable angina both alone and in combination with nitrates and β-blockers. The long-term efficacy of these drugs in unstable angina remains to be determined.

CURRENT RECOMMENDATIONS IN PATIENTS WITH UNSTABLE ANGINA
Patients who meet the criteria of unstable angina as outlined in the introduction should be hospitalized, given mild sedation, and carefully monitored. Any medical or environmental factors that are contributing to unstable angina should be removed. For the majority of patients, therapy with sublingual, long-acting nitrates or intravenous nitroglycerin in combination with β-adrenergic blockers should be initiated. Dosages should be increased as tolerated until heart rate is slowed to 60 beats/min or less and blood pressure is adequately controlled. This regimen should bring symptoms under control in the vast majority of patients. β-blockers must be discontinued

TABLE 41-4. Compatibility of β-blockers, nitrates, and calcium channel blockers

	Compatible	Avoid
Nifedipine	β-Blockers	Nitrates
Verapamil	Nitrates	β-Blockers
Diltiazem	β-Blockers Nitrates	

if significant congestive heart failure or asthma develops. For patients who remain refractory to this treatment, a calcium channel blocker should be added to help control symptoms. Table 41-4 lists the compatibilities of the various calcium channel blockers with β-blockers and nitrates.

For patients who have primarily rest angina, documented ST-segment elevation with pain, or those who seem to be made worse with β-blockers, calcium channel blockers would seem to be the treatment of choice. This is particularly true for patients known to have a coronary vasospastic component to their angina since the calcium channel blockers are known to be coronary vasodilators. If patients remain symptomatic on calcium channel blockers, then increasing doses of nitrates—sublingual, topical, or IV—should be added. Patients who remain refractory to these medical treatments, and this number should be a very small minority, should undergo coronary arteriography and consideration of coronary artery bypass grafting.

Myocardial Infarction

The quantity of myocardial tissue undergoing necrosis during an acute myocardial infarction appears to be an important determinant of both long- and short-term prognosis [13]. Patients with large myocardial infarctions often exhibit severe symptomatic cardiac dysfunction compared with those with small or moderate-sized infarcts. The rationale for pharmacologic salvage of myocardium during acute myocardial infarction is based on the concept that, if the quantity of infarcted tissue can be limited, then the overall mortality and morbidity should be decreased. There are many reasons why documentation of

the benefits of pharmacologic limitations of infarct size in patients have not been forthcoming. First, for an intervention to have any hope of succeeding it must be given early, probably within the first 4 h during the course of the infarct. After that period of time, most of the irreversible damage has already been completed [14]. A second major problem is that there are currently no methods for directly quantitating infarct size in patients and hence no accurate way to assess whether a treatment is effective. The exact correlation between improvement in ECG or enzymatic parameters and the quantity of tissue infarcted remains to be determined. Thus, only comparisons in morbidity and mortality in the short and long term between large groups of patients with and without a specific therapy can currently be addressed. The rapidity with which necrosis of severely ischemic myocardium occurs suggests that clinical trials aimed at infarct size reduction must begin in either the prehospital or emergency-room phases of patient care.

β-ADRENERGIC BLOCKERS

The use of β-adrenergic blockers during acute myocardial infarction must be considered experimental at the present time and great care must be exercised in their use. Early reports on the effects of β-adrenergic blockers in patients with acute myocardial infarction were encouraging and demonstrated a reduction in early mortality from 29% to 13% when propranolol was administered every 8 h for two weeks [15]. These early results, however, have not been routinely confirmed [16].

In 1978, Peter et al. [17] studied in a randomized fashion a highly select group of patients with acute myocardial infarction. They found that patients treated with propranolol within 4 h of the onset of chest pain and maintained for 24 h exhibited a 27% decrease in creatine kinase levels compared with controls. This change was of borderline statistical significance. Yusuf et al. [18] in 1980 published a preliminary report of a randomized trial of atenolol in 214 patients with suspected myocardial infarction. All patients who were randomized to atenolol received the drug within 12 h of the onset of chest pain. At entry, 135 patients had ECG evidence of infarction; 72 patients received atenolol, which significantly decreased subsequent CPK-MB release compared with controls. In addition, there was enhanced R-wave preservation in the atenolol-treated group. At the time of entry, 79 patients had no ECG evidence of MI and 44 of these did not receive atenolol. Of these 44, 27 (61%) subsequently developed acute MI. In comparison, 35 patients received atenolol of whom only 11 patients (31%) developed acute MI. The data from this study suggest that atenolol is effective in decreasing the release of cardiac enzymes and, by implication, decreasing infarct size. Whether these reports will be corroborated and whether this possible decrease in infarct size will result in decreased mortality and morbidity remain to be determined. The apparent ability of atenolol to decrease the incidence of MI in patients with threatened infarct is exciting and warrants further study.

An important finding in this study [18] is that the overall response was much better when atenolol was given within 4 h of the onset of symptoms rather than later in the clinical course. The incidence of bradycardia and hypotension was higher in the atenolol-treated group, but the authors suggest that these complications were adequately treated by simply stopping the drug.

May reviewed 16 randomized trials of acute-phase β-blocker administration in acute infarction in which mortality results were available: ten studies used oral drug and six studies used intravenous drug [19]. Only the metoprolol trial from Sweden [20] found a dramatic improvement in survival. The interpretation of this study is confounded, however, by the fact that the drug was continued for 90 days so that the independent contribution of early administration is difficult to assess. Importantly, none of the studies intervened routinely within the first 4 h.

CALCIUM CHANNEL BLOCKERS

The use of calcium channel blockers in acute myocardial infarction has a sound physiologic basis and some experimental studies in animals suggest that infarct size may be reduced [21, 22]. At the present time, however, there are only limited human data on the ability of these drugs either to reduce infarct size or to alter morbidity or mortality. Muller et al. [23] have reported a

clinical trial in abstract form in which nifedipine was given at an average of 5.4 h after the onset of chest pain: 110 patients with unstable angina and 81 patients with acute myocardial infarction were randomized to receive either 20 mg each 4 h of nifedipine or placebo. Although pain relief was more rapid in patients treated with nifedipine, no differences in infarct incidence, infarct size as estimated by enzymes, or mortality were observed.

CURRENT RECOMMENDATIONS IN PATIENTS WITH ACUTE INFARCTION

Until large scale studies with early administration of drug during the process of infarction are available, neither calcium channel blockers nor β-blockers can be recommended for treatment of acute infarction. These drugs are not contraindicated, however, if deemed clinically indicated. For example, supraventricular arrhythmias or sinus tachycardia due to a hyperadrenergic state without pump failure might be treated with β-blockers, and postinfarction angina may be treated with calcium channel blockers.

References

1. Beamish RE, Storvie VM: Impending myocardial infarction: recognition and management. Circulation 21:1107–1115, 1960.
2. Wood P: Acute and subacute coronary insufficiency. Br Med J 1:1779–1782, 1961.
3. Russell RO, Rackley CE, Kouchoukos NT: Unstable angina pectoris: management based on available interaction. Circulation (Suppl 2) 65: 72–77, 1982.
4. Fischl SJ, Herman MV, Gorlin R: The intermediate coronary syndrome: clinical, angiographic and therapeutic aspects. N Engl J Med 288: 1193–1198, 1973.
5. Unstable angina pectoris: National Cooperative Study Group to compare medical and surgical therapy. II. In-hospital experience and initial follow-up results in patients with one, two and three vesicle disease. Am J Cardiol 42:839–848, 1978.
6. Mulcahy R, Daly L, Graham Z, Hickey N, O'Donoghue S, Owens A, Ruane P, Tobin B: Unstable angina: natural history and determinants of prognosis. Am J Cardiol 48:525–528, 1981.

7. Aellig WH, Hedges A, Turner P, Waite R: Pindolol: the relevance of intrinsic sympathomimetic activity after 12 years of experience (Symposium). Br J Clin Pharmacol (Suppl 2) 13: 1475−4495, 1982.

8. Braunwald E: Mechanism of action of calcium-channel blocking agents. N Engl J Med 307: 1618−1627, 1982.

9. Parodi O, Maseri A, Simonetti I: Management of unstable angina at rest by verapamil: a double-blind cross-over study in coronary care unit. Br Heart J 41:167−174, 1979.

10. Previtali M, Salerno J, Tavazzi P, Ray M, Medici A, Chimienti M, Specchia G, Bobba P: Treatment of angina at rest with nifedipine: a short-term controlled study. Am J Cardiol 45:825−830, 1980.

11. Gerstenblith G, Ouyang P, Achutt SC, Buckley BH, Becker LC, Mellits ED, Baughman KL, Weiss JL, Flaherty JT, Kallman CH, Llewellyn M, Weisfeldt ML: Nifedipine in unstable angina: a double-blind, randomized trial. N Engl J Med 306:885−889, 1982.

12. Moses JW, Wertheimier JH, Bidenheimer MM, Banks VS, Feldman M, Helfant RH: Efficacy of nifedipine in rest angina refractory to propranolol and nitrates in patients with obstructive coronary artery disease. Ann Intern Med 94:425−429, 1981.

13. Lange LG, Sobel BE: Pharmacological salvage of myocardium. Annu Rev Pharmacol Toxicol 22: 115−143, 1982.

14. Rasmussen MM, Reimer KA, Kloner RA, Jennings RB: Infarct size reduction by propranolol before and after coronary ligation in dogs. Circulation 56:794−798, 1977.

15. Snow PJD: Effect of propranolol in myocardial infarction. Lancet 2:551−553, 1965.

16. Norris RM, Coughey DE, Scott PJ: A trial of propranolol in acute myocardial infarction. Br Med J 2:398−400, 1968.

17. Peter T, Norris RM, Clarke ED, Heng MK, Singh BN, Williams B, Howell DR, Ambler PK: Reduction of enzyme levels by propranolol after acute myocardial infarction. Circulation 57: 1041−1095, 1978.

18. Yusuf S, Peto R, Bennett D, Ramsdale D, Furse L, Bray C, Sleight P: Early intravenous atenolol treatment in suspected myocardial infarction: preliminary report of a randomized trial. Lancet 2:273−276, 1980.

19. May GS: A review of acute-phase beta-blocker trials in patients with myocardial infarction. Circulation 67:I-21−25, 1983.

20. Hjalmarson A, Elmfeldt D, Herlitz J, Holmberg S, Malek I, Nyberg G, Ryden L, Swedberg K, Vedin A, Waagstein F, Waldenstrom A, Waldenstrom J, Wedel H, Wilhelmsen L, Wilhelmsson C: Effect on mortality of metoprolol in acute myocardial infarction. Lancet 2:823, 1981.

21. Reimer KA, Lower JE, Jennings RB: Effect of the calcium antagonist verapamil on necrosis following temporary coronary artery occlusion in dogs. Circulation 55:581−587, 1977.

22. Melin JA, Becker LC, Hutchins GM: Protective effect of early and late treatment with nifedipine during myocardial infarction in the conscious dog. Circulation 69:131−141, 1984.

23. Muller J, Morrison J, Stone P, Rude R, Rosner B, Roberts R, Pearle D, Turi Z, Schneider J, Serfas D, Hennekens C, Braunwald E: Nifedipine therapy for threatened and acute myocardial infarction: a randomized double blind comparison [abstr]. Circulation 68:III-120, 1983.

42. RESPIRATORY CARE FOR PATIENTS WITH ACUTE MYOCARDIAL ISCHEMIA

John D. Hughes

Lewis J. Rubin

The delivery of oxygen to vital organs is dependent on a functional, integrated cardiopulmonary unit. Acute myocardial ischemia may jeopardize tissue oxygen delivery both by compromising the efficiency of the heart as a pump and by limiting the ability of the lungs to exchange gas efficiently. Most interventions in the clinical setting of myocardial ischemia are directed at salvaging ischemic myocardium and preventing the extension of ischemia, but the importance of the respiratory system in maintaining adequate oxygen delivery and acid−base balance in this setting should not be neglected. This chapter focuses on the respiratory complications of acute myocardial ischemia, and provides guidelines for their prevention and management.

Oxygen Transport

The tissues of a normal resting person consume approximately 250 cc of oxygen per minute. By the combination of increasing ventilation, cardiac output, and tissue oxygen extraction, a normal person undergoing strenuous exercise can achieve an oxygen consumption of 2500 cc/min.

Oxygen is carried in the blood in two forms: a small amount (0.003 cc O_2/mmHg O_2/100 cc blood) is dissolved in the water of plasma and red cells; the majority of blood-borne oxygen is reversibly bound to hemoglobin (1.39 cc of O_2 per gram of hemoglobin × hemoglobin content [gm/dl] × percent hemoglobin saturated with oxygen).

The amount of oxygen transported to the tissues, or the systemic oxygen delivery, is the product of the cardiac output and the oxygen content of arterial blood, and is expressed as milliliters of O_2 per minute.

The relationship between the percentage of hemoglobin saturated with oxygen and the partial pressure of oxygen has important implications for systemic oxygen transport (figure 42-1). Increases in PO_2 above 80 mmHg affect negligibly the saturation of hemoglobin and, therefore, the oxygen content of blood. As the PO_2 in blood drops below 55 mmHg, however, hemoglobin saturation and oxygen content fall sharply. Factors shifting the curve to the right such as acidosis, hypercarbia, hyperthermia, and increased 2,3-diphosphoglycerate impair oxygen uptake in the lung, but enhance oxygen unloading at the tissue level. Factors shifting the curve to the left such as alkalosis, hypocarbia, hypothermia, and decreased erythrocyte 2,3-DPG have the opposite effect.

Since myocardial oxygen extraction from blood is nearly maximal under resting conditions, coronary artery disease makes the myocardium exceptionally vulnerable to arterial hypoxemia, anemia, or factors that shift the oxyhemoglobin dissociation curve to the left.

R.M. Califf and G.S. Wagner (eds.), ACUTE CORONARY CARE: Principles and Practice. Copyright © 1985. Martinus Nijhoff Publishing, Boston/Dordrecht/Lancaster.

Gas Exchange Alterations with Myocardial Ischemia

Transient alterations in gas exchange that might adversely affect oxygen transport commonly occur with myocardial ischemia even in the absence of clinical or radiographic evidence of heart failure. Al-Bazzay and Kazemi [1] measured arterial PO_2 in patients recovering from uncomplicated myocardial infarctions and found that the mean PO_2 was 72 mmHg compared with 87 mmHg 2–6 months later. A likely explanation for the observed transient reduction of arterial oxygen tension may be found in the studies by Hales Kazemi [2]: increased closing volumes, an indicator of small airways collapse, may be found in the first two weeks after an uncomplicated myocardial infarction. Closing volumes returned to normal within four weeks of the infarction or could be normalized sooner by diuresis. They concluded that transient left ventricular failure occurs even in "uncomplicated" myocardial infarctions and promotes pulmonary interstitial fluid accumulation, producing premature airway closure. In further support of this concept, Pepine and Weiner [3] used atrial pacing to induce myocardial ischemia and found that, as left ventricular end-diastolic pressure rose, there were increases in airway resistance and decreases in lung compliance.

Pulmonary Effects of Therapy for Myocardial Ischemia

The traditional approach to patients hospitalized for a suspected myocardial infarction or unstable angina has been to place them at bed rest, and administer supplemental oxygen, analgesics, and medication designed to prevent recurrent ischemia. These modalities may have effects on respiratory function that warrant further discussion.

NARCOTICS

Patients with myocardial infarctions usually require narcotic analgesics at the time of their admission to the hospital (see chapter 31). Since lung and cardiac disease frequently coexist, a knowledge of the respiratory effects of narcotics is mandatory.

Morphine and the other narcotic analgesics

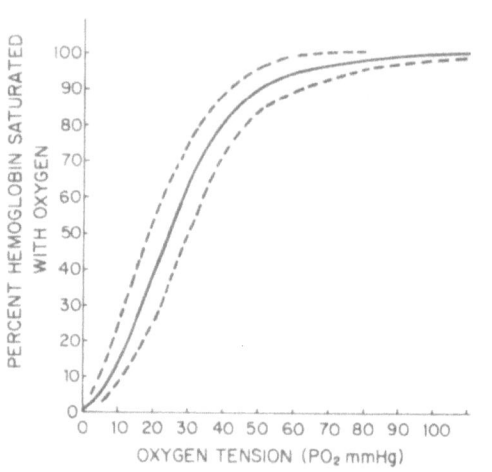

FIGURE 42-1. The oxyhemoglobin dissociation curve. The solid line denotes the relationship between oxygen tension and hemoglobin saturation at normal blood pH, PCO_2, temperature, and erythrocyte 2,3-diphosphoglycerate concentration. Dotted lines represent leftward and rightward shift of PO_2–hemoglobin saturation relationship.

depress respiration even when used in the usual therapeutic doses. Narcotics directly cause a dose-dependent depression of the brain stem respiratory center [4], possibly by blunting sensitivity to increases in blood carbon dioxide tension. The sensitivity to hypoxemia is also somewhat depressed. The combined depressant effects of narcotics on both the hypoxemic and hypercarbic respiratory drives may result in severe depression of ventilation or even apnea in susceptible patients. Narcotics decrease both respiratory rate and tidal volume [5]. They suppress the natural "sigh" reflex, which leads to a decrease in functional residual capacity, resulting in atelectasis and hypoxemia [6]. Narcotics also suppress the cough reflex and may interfere with the normal clearance of secretions. Morphine dilates both peripheral arterioles and venous capacitance vessels. Deaths in cor pulmonale patients have been reported after morphine administration, due perhaps to venodilatation and a profound drop in right ventricular output. This factor could be particularly important in patients with right ventricular infarction (see chapter 21).

Maximal respiratory depression after morphine

administration is seen within 7 min of an intravenous dose, usually within 30 min of an intramuscular dose, and as long as 90 min after subcutaneous injection. Patients with chronic carbon dioxide retention are exceedingly vulnerable to the respiratory depressant effects of narcotics.

Narcotics can be used safely if their actions are understood and anticipated. Patients with lung disease receiving narcotics should be observed carefully. Narcotic antagonists such as nalaxone should be kept readily available.

NITRATES

The nitrates are smooth muscle relaxing agents that have even been used in the treatment of asthma [7, 8]. These agents, however, may have deleterious effects on gas exchange. Kochukosky et al. [9] reported that sublingual nitroglycerin lowered arterial oxygen tension in patients with chronic obstructive pulmonary disease. They postulated that this effect could be due to either a lowering of mixed venous oxygen tension resulting from a decrease in cardiac output and/or an impairment of regional hypoxic pulmonary vasoconstriction producing a diversion of blood to poorly ventilated areas of the lung. Mookherjee et al. [10] reported that sublingual nitroglycerin lowered mean arterial PO_2, increased the alveolar−arterial O_2 gradient, and increased the ratio of dead space to tidal volume in patients undergoing cardiac catheterization to evaluate chest pain. Hales and Westphal [11] measured arterial oxygen tension following sublingual nitroglycerin in four subsets of patients and found there was a significant drop in arterial PO_2 both in normals and in subjects with isolated small airways disease (19 and 14 mmHg, respectively). Curiously, there was an insignificant (4 mmHg) drop in arterial PO_2 in patients with obstructive and restrictive disease. Patients whose arterial oxygen tensions lie at or near the steep part of the hemoglobin dissociation curve should be observed for deterioration in oxygenation after nitrate administration. Supplemental oxygen therapy may be necessary to restore adequate systemic oxygenation.

BETA-ADRENERGIC-BLOCKING AGENTS

Beta-blocking agents have become a mainstay in the therapy of angina (see chapter 41) and are frequently employed for hypertension. Beta-blockers inhibit the actions of several common bronchodilating agents and may precipitate bronchospasm in patients with chronic obstructive lung disease. Patients with bronchospastic obstructive lung disease would be most susceptible to the effect of β-blockers on the airways. A selective $β_1$-blocker such as metoprolol or atenolol may be safer than propranolol in patients with airways disease.

CALCIUM CHANNEL BLOCKERS

As the use of slow channel calcium blocking agents for angina (see chapter 41) and arrhythmias has increased, the effects of these agents on the respiratory system have become better understood. The effects of two of the three agents that have recently been released in the USA, nifedipine and verapamil, have been evaluated in patients with asthma, respiratory failure, and pulmonary hypertension. Both drugs inhibit bronchoconstriction in exercise-induced asthma without modifying basal bronchial tone [12−14]. The calcium antagonists inhibit vascular smooth muscle contraction and lower both pulmonary and systemic vascular resistances [15]. These drugs inhibit hypoxic pulmonary vasoconstriction [15, 16] and have been used to treat pulmonary hypertension [17]. Pulmonary complications were unusual in a series of 3000 patients receiving nifedipine for angina pectoris [18]. Cardiac output is better maintained with the calcium blockers than with the nitrates, perhaps because venous tone is unaffected [19]. The calcium channel blockers may be safer than β-blockers in the angina patient with bronchospastic lung disease because of their minimal effects on basal airway tone.

OXYGEN THERAPY

The administration of oxygen by mask or nasal cannulae has become a standard aspect of care for patients with myocardial infarctions. In the only randomized, double-blinded controlled study on this subject [20], patients with uncomplicated infarctions receiving 6 liters/min of oxygen by mask appeared to derive no significant benefit in terms of mortality, reduction of cardiac enzyme elevation, or reduction in frequency of arrhythmias. Patients whose arterial PO_2 is 75 mmHg or greater are not likely to benefit from supplemental oxygen. In hypoxemic patients hospitalized for ischemic heart disease, however, oxygen therapy is clearly indicated. Supplemental oxygen at low flow rates with careful observation and frequent blood gas monitoring should be instituted initially to patients with chronic hypoxemia and hypercarbia.

THE EFFECT OF BED REST ON PULMONARY FUNCTION

The effects of inactivity on overall cardiovascular health are well chronicled. The supine position is disadvantageous to pulmonary gas exchange, particularly in certain subsets of patients. In the supine position, the abdominal contents push the diaphragm up into the thorax with the effect of reducing the resting lung volume. With a decrease in lung volume, airways supplying dependent lung zones in patients with obstructive lung disease collapse and result in a cessation of ventilation to these areas. The smaller lung volumes in obese patients, coupled with the increased work of breathing, can further compromise respiratory function. In summary, the supine position may result in lower arterial oxygen tensions and increase the work of breathing compared with the sitting position in patients with obstructive lung disease and/or obesity.

EXTERNAL CARDIAC MASSAGE

Thoracic injuries following external cardiac massage are common. Rib fractures are the most common complication, especially in the elderly, and multiple fractures may produce the "flail chest" syndrome [21]. Pneumothorax, hemothorax, mediastinal emphysema, pulmonary lacerations, and bone marrow emboli to the lungs may also occur as a result of resuscitative efforts [22, 23]. When confronted with the problem of a patient with respiratory difficulties following resuscitation, one must consider not only the possible causes of cardiopulmonary arrest, including massive pulmonary embolism and myocardial infarction with pulmonary edema, but the complications stemming from chest trauma during the arrest. Patients with lung lacerations have localized densities radiographically and may have hemoptysis and an accompanying pneumothorax [24]. Patients with intrapulmonary fat emboli

may have tachypnea, hypoxemia, and an overt adult respiratory distress syndrome [25].

When cardiac arrest occurs in a patient with an unprotected airway, aspiration of oropharyngeal or gastric contents commonly occurs. Aspiration must be considered when pulmonary infiltrates are seen on a postarrest chest roentgenogram.

Management of Bronchospasm in the Coronary Care Unit

Patients who simultaneously suffer myocardial ischemia and an exacerbation of obstructive lung disease are a difficult therapeutic challenge because the standard therapeutic modalities for bronchospastic lung disease can increase myocardial oxygen demand and lower the threshhold for arrhythmias.

Theophylline increases heart rate, may increase systemic blood pressure, and increases myocardial contractility [26, 27]. Terbutaline, a sympathomimetic agent, has relatively selective β_2-agonist activity when administered orally, but tachycardia is common. When terbutaline is given subcutaneously its effects are less selective. Metaproterenol and albuterol are selective β_2-agonists that are available in inhaled form. Cardiac effects from these two inhaled agents are minimal when they are used in the suggested dosages.

Theophylline lowers the ventricular fibrillation threshhold in animals [28]. The sympathomimetic agents are thought to have arrhythmogenic potential in proportion to their systemic β_1-agonist activity [29, 30].

Corticosteroids are frequently used in the management of recalcitrant obstructive lung disease. The inhaled forms of beclomethasone are slow acting, but effective, therapy for moderate chronic bronchospasm and produce negligible systemic side effects. High-dose systemic corticosteroids are employed in the therapy of severe bronchospasm, but this mode of therapy has been implicated with an increased incidence of myocardial rupture following transmural myocardial infarction [31] and could, therefore, also result in infarct expansion (see chapter 46).

Although the effects of the bronchodilating agents on the heart may be deleterious, the effects of intense bronchospasm may prove far more harmful to ischemic myocardium. An exacerbation of obstructive lung disease may result in hypoxemia, acid–base disturbances, and a marked increase in the work of breathing.

A rational approach in this setting would be to begin with the therapeutic modality that is least likely to endanger the ischemic heart: oxygen therapy, antibiotics if bronchitis is suspected, and inhaled β_2-adrenergic agonists. The decision regarding theophylline therapy in such a patient must be individualized to the clinical circumstances. If theophylline is begun, serum levels should be checked to assure efficacy without toxicity.

Since left ventricular failure may produce wheezing and since the presence of jugular venous distension is an unreliable indicator of left ventricular filling pressure in patients with lung disease, Swan-Ganz catheterization may be necessary to differentiate congestive heart failure from bronchospasm.

Thromboembolic Disease

Pulmonary embolism is no longer a frequent cause of death in patients with myocardial infarction. Earlier ambulation, aggressive management of deep-vein thrombosis, low-dose heparin, leg exercises, and antiembolism stockings have probably contributed to reducing the frequency of fatal pulmonary embolism in infarct patients to less than 1% [32]. The incidence of deep-vein thrombosis after acute myocardial infarction had been estimated to range from 19% to 37% [33–35]. Warlow et al. [36], in a randomized double-blinded trial, showed that 5000 U of heparin subcutaneously twice daily for ten days, started within 12 h of the onset of myocardial infarction, reduced the incidence of deep-venous thrombosis diagnosed by ^{125}I fibrinogen scanning from 17.2% in the control group to 3.2% in the heparin-treated group. Miller et al. [37] compared the effects of early ambulation on the incidence of deep-vein thrombosis diagnosed by ^{125}I fibrinogen scanning in infarct patients. Of 21 patients who began cautious ambulation within three days of infarction, only two, both of whom had heart failure, developed evidence of thrombosis. In contrast, five of eight infarct patients remaining at complete bed rest for five days

developed evidence of venous thrombosis, of whom four had heart failure. In summary, deep-vein thrombosis appears to be common after myocardial infarction, especially in patients with congestive heart failure. Minidose heparin or early ambulation both appear to reduce the incidence of thrombotic events effectively.

Breathing Disorders during Sleep

Patients with the sleep apnea syndrome or severe chronic obstructive disease can have profound hypoxemia, marked disturbances of cardiac rhythm, and severe aberrations in pulmonary and systemic blood pressure during sleep. Both disorders share epidemiologic characteristics with ischemic heart disease and the coexistence of these breathing disorders with coronary artery disease is not uncommon.

Nocturnal hypoventilation and a small drop in arterial PO_2 are normal physiologic events during sleep. The sleep apnea syndrome occurs when prolonged, frequent episodes of apnea occur during sleep, due either to a lack of respiratory effort or obstruction of the upper airway, or both. Tilkian et al. [38] found six common rhythm disturbances in patients with obstructive sleep apnea: marked sinus arrhythmia, extreme sinus bradycardia (<30 beats/min), asystole ranging from 2.5 to 6.3 s, second-degree AV nodal block, complex premature ventricular beats, and ventricular tachycardia. In an earlier study [39], the same authors noted that nine of 12 sleep apnea patients developed appreciable increases in systemic blood pressure during sleep. Most of these patients had elevations in pulmonary artery pressure, and marked hypoxemia (arterial PO_2 below 50 mmHg) occurred in eight patients.

Patients with severe chronic obstructive pulmonary disease may have significant deteriorations in oxygenation during sleep. In 15 patients with severe stable chronic obstructive pulmonary disease, the mean fall in arterial PO_2 during sleep was 13.5 mmHg [40]. Nocturnal oxygen therapy decreased the frequency and severity of arrhythmias in some hypoxemic patients [41]. Patients in the coronary care unit who manifest arrhythmias and irregular breathing patterns may have some form of nocturnal hypoventilation. During the recovery phase of myocardial ischemia, supplemental oxygen is useful in blunting hypoventilation-mediated hypoxemia. Investigation into the cause of hypoventilation may be warranted at a later date.

Summary

When caring for patients with ischemic heart disease, one should recognize the effect of this disease or its therapy on respiratory function. Hypoxemia may occur as a direct result of myocardial ischemia or indirectly from the therapeutic interventions mentioned above. The management of patients with both heart disease and severe lung disease requires a knowledge of the cardiovascular effects of the bronchodilating agents and the respiratory effects of cardiac drugs. Finally, in patients who develop hemodynamic aberrations or arrhythmias while asleep, nocturnal hypoventilation with hypoxemia must be considered. Arterial blood gases drawn without awakening the patient or noninvasive monitoring of arterial oxygenation with an ear oximeter may elucidate a respiratory etiology for nocturnal cardiac instability.

References

1. Al-Bazzay FJ, Kazemi H: Arterial hypoxemia and distribution of pulmonary perfusion after uncomplicated myocardial infarction. Am Rev Respir Dis 106:721−728, 1972.
2. Hales CA, Kazemi H: Small airways function in myocardial infarction. N Engl J Med 290:761−765, 1979.
3. Pepine CJ, Weiner L: Relationship of anginal symptoms to lung mechanics during myocardial ischemia. Circulation 46:863−869, 1972.
4. Jaffe JH, Martin WR: Opioid analgesics and antagonists. In: Gilman AG, Goodman LS, Gilman A (eds) The pharmacologic basis of therapeutics. New York: MacMillan, 1980, pp 494−534.
5. Nagashima H, Karamanian A, Malovary R, Rodnay P, Ang M, Koerner S, Folder FF: Respiratory and circulatory effects of intravenous butorphanol and morphine. Clin Pharmacol Ther 19:738−745, 1976.
6. Egbert LD, Bendixen HH: Effect of morphine on breathing patterns. JAMA 188:485−488, 1964.
7. Needleman P, Johnson EM: Vasodilators and the treatment of angina. In: Gilman AG, Goodman LS, Gilman A (eds) The pharmacologic basis of therapeutics. New York: MacMillan, 1980, pp 819−833.
8. Hirshleifer I, Arora Y: Nitrates in the treatment of bronchial asthma. Dis Chest 39:275−283, 1961.
9. Kochukosky KN, Chick TW, Jenne JW: The effect of nitroglycerin in gas exchange on chronic obstructive pulmonary disease. Am Rev Respir Dis 111:177−183, 1975.
10. Mookherjee S, Fuleihan D, Warner R, Vardan S, Obeid A: Effects of sublingual nitroglycerin on resting pulmonary gas exchange and hemodynamics in man. Circulation 57:106−110, 1978.
11. Hales C, Westphal D: Hypoxemia following the administration of sublingual nitroglycerin. Am J Med 65:911−918, 1978.
12. Cerrina J, Denjean A, Alexander G, Lockhart A, Duroux P: Inhibition of exercise induced asthma by a calcium antagonist, nifedipine. Am Rev Respir Dis 123:156−160, 1981.
13. Barnes PJ, Wilson NM, Brown MJ: A calcium antagonist, nifedipine, modifies exercise-induced asthma. Thorax 36:726−730, 1981.
14. Patel KR: Calcium antagonists in exercise-induced asthma. Br Med J 282:932−933, 1981.
15. Simonneau G, Escourrou P, Duroux P, Lockhart A: Inhibition of hypoxic pulmonary vasoconstriction by nifedipine. N Engl J Med 304:1582−1585, 1981.
16. Reuben SR, Kuan P: The acute hemodynamic effects of intravenous verapamil in hypoxic lung disease. Bull Eur Physiopathol Respir 302:1269−1273, 1980.
17. McLeod AA, Wise JR, Daly K, Jewitt D: Nifedipine in treatment of primary pulmonary hypertension. Br Heart J 45:619, 1981.
18. Terry RW: Nifedipine therapy in angina pectoris: evaluation of safety and side effects. Am Heart J 104:681−689, 1982.
19. Hagemann K, Lochner W, Niehues B: Studies on the extracardial effects of nifedipine in anesthetized dogs. In: Lochner W, Kroneberg G (eds) The second international adalat symposium. New York: Springer-Verlag, 1975, pp 49−54.
20. Rawles JM, Kenmure ACF: Controlled trial of oxygen in uncomplicated myocardial infarction. Br Med J 1:1121−1123, 1976.
21. Henriksen H: Rib fractures following external cardiac massage. Acta Anaesthesiol Scand 11:57−64, 1967.
22. Guenter CA: Chest trauma. In: Guenter CA, Welch MH (eds) Pulmonary medicine. Philadelphia: Lippincott, 1982, pp 511−554.

23. Grossman JI, Rubin IL: Cardiopulmonary resuscitation. Am Heart J 78:569–572, 1969.
24. Wilson RF, Murray C, Antoneuko DR: Nonpenetrating thoracic injuries. Surg Clin North Am 57:17–36, 1977.
25. Guenter CA, Braun T: Fat embolism: changing prognosis. Chest 79:143–145, 1981.
26. Ogilvie RI, Fernandez PG, Winsberg F: Cardiovascular response to increasing theophylline concentration. Eur J Clin Pharmacol 12:409–414, 1977.
27. Marcus ML, Skelton CL, Grauer LE, Epstein SE: Effects of theophylline on myocardial mechanics. Am J Physiol 222:1361–1365, 1972.
28. Horowitz LN, Spear JF, Moore EN: Effects of aminophylline on the threshhold for initiating ventricular fibrillation during respiratory failure. Am J Cardiol 35:376–379, 1975.
29. Speizer FE, Doll R, Heaf P, Strang LB: Investigation into use of drugs preceding death from asthma. Br Med J 1:339–343, 1968.
30. Kinney EL: Ventricular tachycardia after terbutaline. JAMA 240:2247, 1978.
31. Roberts R, Demello V, Sobel BE: Deleterious effects of methylprednisolone in patients with myocardial infarction. Circulation (Suppl 1) 53: I-204–206, 1976.
32. Hurst JW, King SB, Walter PF, Friesinger GC, Edwards JE: Atherosclerotic coronary heart disease. In: Hurst JW (ed) The heart. New York: McGraw-Hill, 1982, pp 1009–1158.
33. Murray TS, Lorimer AR, Cox FC: Leg vein thrombosis following myocardial infarction. Lancet 2: 792–793, 1970.
34. Nicolaides AN, Kakkar VV, Renney JTG: Myocardial infarction and deep vein thrombosis. Br Med J 1:432–434, 1971.
35. Maurer BJ, Wray R, Shillingford JP: Frequency of venous thrombosis after myocardial infarction. Lancet 2:1385–1387.
36. Warlow C, Terry G, Kenmure ACF, Beattie AG, Ogston D, Douglas AS: A double blind trial of low doses of subcutaneous heparin in the prevention of deep vein thrombosis after myocardial infarction. Lancet 2:934–936, 1973.
37. Miller RR, Lies JE, Caretta RF, Wampold DB, Denardo GL, Kraus JF, Amsterdam EA, Mason DT: Prevention of lower extremity venous thrombosis by early mobilization. Ann Intern Med 84:700–703, 1976.
38. Tilkian AG, Guilleminault C, Schroeder JS, Lehrman KL, Simmons FB, Dement WC: Sleep-induced apnea syndrome: prevalence of cardiac arrhythmias and their reversal after tracheostomy. Am J Med 63:348–358, 1977.
39. Tilkian AG, Guilleminault C, Shroeder JS, Lehrman KL, Simmons FB, Dement WC: Hemodynamics in sleep induced apnea. Ann Intern Med 85:714–719, 1976.
40. Koo KW, Sax DS, Snider GL: Arterial blood gases and pH during sleep in chronic obstructive pulmonary disease. Am J Med 58:663–670, 1975.
41. Tirlapur VG, Mir MA: Nocturnal hypoxemia and associated electrocardiographic changes in patients with chronic obstructive pulmonary disease. N Engl J Med 306:125–130, 1982.

43. OPTIMAL REGULATION OF PRELOAD AND AFTERLOAD DURING ACUTE MYOCARDIAL INFARCTION

Kanu Chatterjee

Alterations in ventricular preload and afterload contribute to the pathogenesis of low-output syndrome—a serious complication of acute myocardial infarction. Likewise, manipulation of preload and afterload is an effective therapeutic principle for the correction of low-output state.

Physiologic Considerations
(see chapter 11)

The terms *preload* and *afterload* stem from the studies of the muscle mechanics with isolated papillary muscles [1]. The load that determines the initial muscle length before contraction is defined as the preload. Afterload is the force that the muscle must develop to match the load against which it shortens after activation.

In the intact heart, the closest approximation of preload is ventricular end-diastolic volume. However, ventricular filling pressure can also be considered as preload. Transmural pressure (i.e., pressure across the ventricular wall at end diastole) is the true ventricular filling pressure. Measurements of transmural pressure require determinations of ventricular end-diastolic pressure and intrapericardial pressure. As, normally, intrapericardial pressure is close to zero, and as it usually does not increase significantly in most pathologic conditions, ventricular end-diastolic pressure can be used to represent filling pressure. It needs to be emphasized that in certain clinical circumstances, such as cardiac tamponade and

acute right ventricular infarction, ventricular end-diastolic pressures cannot be used as their filling pressures because of considerable increase in intrapericardial pressure [2].

Repeated direct determination of left ventricular end-diastolic pressure in critically ill cardiac patients, such as in patients with acute myocardial infarction, is not only impractical but also hazardous. Indirect assessment of left ventricular filling pressure can be accomplished from the measurements of pulmonary capillary wedge or pulmonary artery diastolic pressures, which can be determined relatively safely and repeatedly even in seriously ill cardiac patients with the use of Swan-Ganz catheters [3]. Thus, when manipulation of left ventricular preload is required in patients with acute myocardial infarction, monitoring of pulmonary capillary wedge or pulmonary artery diastolic pressure is frequently employed to determine changes in left ventricular filling pressure.

In the intact heart, afterload is difficult to define. If one extrapolates the conception of afterload as used in the isolated papillary muscle studies, one needs to determine left ventricular wall stress during the isovolumic and the ejection phases of systole. Determination of wall stress requires simultaneous measurements of left ventricular pressure, wall thickness and radius (Laplace relation), which are obviously not feasible during the management of critically ill patients. Thus, other approximations of left ven-

R.M. Califf and G.S. Wagner (eds.), ACUTE CORONARY CARE: Principles and Practice. Copyright © 1985. Martinus Nijhoff Publishing, Boston/Dordrecht/Lancaster.

tricular afterload such as arterial pressure, aortic impedance, and systemic vascular resistance are used in clinical practice.

Systemic arterial pressure is an important determinant of left ventricular afterload as the left ventricle has to generate this pressure to open the aortic valve and maintain ejection. However, arterial pressure is only one of the components that determine left ventricular wall stress. Furthermore, during vasodilator therapy of pump failure, left ventricular stroke volume may increase with reduction of aortic impedances or systemic vascular resistance without any change in arterial pressure. Blood pressure is related to cardiac output and systemic vascular resistance (blood pressure = cardiac output × systemic vascular resistance). During vasodilator therapy of heart failure, when the increase in cardiac output is proportional to the decrease in systemic vascular resistance, blood pressure remains unchanged. In these circumstances, reduction of afterload occurs without any change in arterial pressure. Thus, arterial pressure should be regarded only as a rough approximation of left ventricular afterload.

Some investigators believe that the external force to ventricular ejection (afterload) is better represented by the aortic impedance that can be described by the relation of aortic pulsatile pressure and flow throughout the cardiac cycle [4–12]. In the arterial system, blood pressure and flow exist as pulsatile waveforms superimposed on a mean nonpulsatile component. Thus, total opposition to arterial blood flow encompasses both frequency-dependent pulsatile components and a frequency-independent nonpulsatile steady-state component. Aortic input impedance provides information about both pulsatile and nonpulsatile components of the vascular bed. The influence of each individual component of vascular load on ventricular ejection has been evaluated in experimental animals and human beings. Decreased arterial compliance with constant resistance is associated with reduced stroke volume and mean aortic pressure [10]. Increased resistance alone also decreases stroke volume but increases mean aortic pressure. It has been demonstrated that vasodilators like sodium nitroprusside can decrease impedance and enhance ventricular ejection without changing arterial pressure [13].

Thus, vasodilator-induced increased arterial compliance is a potentially important mechanism for improving left ventricular function during vasodilator therapy. The calculation of aortic input impedance, however, is difficult and cannot be applied in routine clinical practice.

Systemic vascular resistance, which can be determined easily, is related to aortic input impedance. Whereas impedance is the instantaneous relation between pressure and flow, systemic vascular resistance is the average of this relation throughout the cardiac cycle. Systemic vascular resistance is the ratio of the pressure drop across the arterial system (mean arterial pressure/right atrial pressure) and mean flow (cardiac output). The use of systemic vascular resistance to represent afterload not only is helpful in understanding how vasodilators improve cardiac function, but also can be applied in clinical practice. Repeated measurements of cardiac output, and systemic and pulmonary venous pressures, can be performed at the bedside with the use of triple-lumen balloon-tipped flotation catheters [14], with little inconvenience to the patient.

Rationale for the Modification of Preload

In the isolated papillary muscle experiments, initial muscle length (preload) influences the force development; the higher the initial muscle length, the greater is the developed force. In the intact heart, the higher the end-diastolic volume or filling pressure, the larger is the stroke volume. The relation between filling pressure and stroke volume (classic ventricular function curve) is, however, curvilinear (figure 43-1). When the filling pressure is low, the increment in filling pressure is associated with a greater increase in stroke volume (steep portion of the ventricular function curve). In contrast, with a higher initial filling pressure (flat portion of the ventricular function curve), further increments in filling pressure by a similar magnitude as in the previous example will cause very little increase in stroke volume. It is apparent that, if low cardiac output is due to decreased left ventricular preload, increase in preload is associated with increased stroke volume and cardiac output—the rationale for the volume expansion in patients with low output due to hypovolemia.

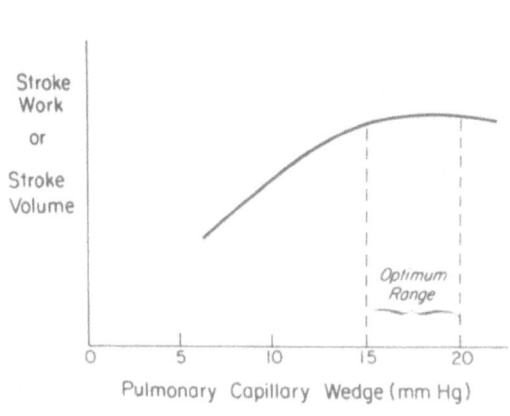

FIGURE 43-1. Representative ventricular function curve. Some measure of ventricular performance, such as stroke work or stroke volume, is plotted as a function of some measure of preload, such as pulmonary capillary wedge (PCW) pressure. In general, there is a greater increase in stroke volume with increasing filling pressure when initial filling pressure is low. The curve flattens out from 15 to 20 mmHg. Any further increase in PCW pressure results in either no change or slight decrease in performance and may result in dyspnea due to pulmonary congestion [29].

Determination of initial filling pressure, however, is essential for the diagnosis of the severity of hypovolemia, particularly in patients with acute myocardial infarction.

The rationale for the reduction of left ventricular preload is primarily to decrease pulmonary venous pressure to avoid symptoms of pulmonary venous congestion. Increased pulmonary capillary wedge pressure is the major hemodynamic determinant of cardiac pulmonary edema. Increase in left ventricular filling pressure is reflected in increased pulmonary venous pressure and reduction in decreased pulmonary venous pressure. Reduction of left ventricular filling pressure is the basis for the use of diuretics and venodilators for the treatment of pulmonary venous hypertension. Reduction of left ventricular preload has relevance in the management of postinfarction angina. Left ventricular wall tension is a major determinant of myocardial oxygen demand. Left ventricular pressure and volume are the two major variables of wall tension; reduction of left ventricular diastolic volume is associated with

decreased myocardial oxygen demand, which is beneficial in restoring the balance between myocardial oxygen demand and supply, and, hence, in preventing myocardial ischemia. The rationale for the use of venodilators such as nitroglycerin, which decreases left ventricular preload in the management of postinfarction angina, is apparent.

Reduction of Afterload

The rationale for the reduction of afterload is to improve left ventricular function in patients with pump failure. In isolated papillary muscle experiments inverse relationships exist between the afterload and both the velocity of muscle shortening and the distance the muscle shortens [1]. With increasing afterload, the velocity of shortening and the distance the muscle shortens progressively decline; conversely, with decreasing afterload, the velocity and the distance of shortening increase (figure 43-2). If one extrapolates this conception to the intact heart, it becomes apparent why increased stroke volume results from decreased afterload or left ventricular ejection impedance. The rationale for the use of vasodilating agents for the treatment of pump failure complicating acute myocardial infarction is to decrease systemic vascular resistance (afterload) and thereby improve left ventricular function.

Clinical Applications of Preload Modification

Maintenance of adequate left ventricular preload is the initial therapy to correct the low-output state due to hypovolemia or predominant right ventricular involvement in patients with acute myocardial infarction.

Preload Increase in Hypovolemic Shock

Relative or absolute hypovolemia is an uncommon complication of acute myocardial infarction. It tends to occur in patients who have been on diuretic therapy prior to the acute infarction or who develop profuse vomiting and diaphoresis at the onset of infarction. The most common cause in clinical practice, however, is the repeated use of potent diuretics and venodilators in attempts to treat "pump failure."

Clinical diagnosis of hypovolemic shock is often difficult in patients with acute myocardial infarction. Pulmonary rales and an S4 gallop, associated with the increased left ventricular end-diastolic pressure that is frequently present at the onset of the acute ischemic process, may persist even after the pulmonary venous pressure returns to normal. The use of diuretics and venodilators in such circumstances precipitates a low-output state due to excessive decrease of left ventricular preload.

Determination of hemodynamics is desirable not only for the diagnosis of hypovolemic shock, but also for the assessment of the response to therapy. The characteristic hemodynamic abnormalities are low right atrial and pulmonary capillary wedge pressures, in the presence of low cardiac output and hypotension. When the low-output state is accompanied by decreased or relatively normal pulmonary capillary wedge pressure, in the absence of decreased right atrial pressure, the decreased left ventricular preload is most likely due to dominant right ventricular infarction rather than to hypovolemia. Thus, monitoring of both right atrial and pulmonary capillary wedge pressures are necessary for the correct diagnosis of hypovolemic shock.

Initial therapy for hypovolemic shock complicating acute myocardial infarction consists of rapid administration of fluids intravenously to increase stroke volume and cardiac output by the Frank-Starling mechanism. The choice of intravenous fluids is less important in these patients as prolonged therapy is usually not necessary. Normal or half-normal saline, dextrose in water, or dextran can be used for volume expansion. Monitoring the changes in hemodynamics during intravenous fluid therapy, however, is essential.

Initially, 100−200 cc of intravenous fluid should be administered rapidly (5−10 min) and the changes in right atrial and pulmonary capillary wedge pressures and cardiac output monitored. If cardiac output increases appreciably with only slight increase in right atrial and pulmonary capillary wedge pressure, fluid administration should be continued and the rate of fluid administration adjusted to maintain pulmonary capil-

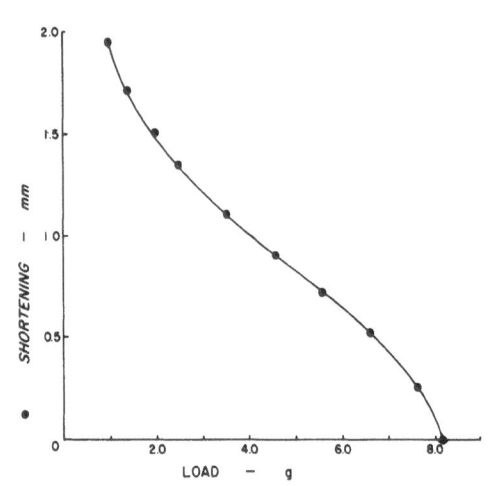

FIGURE 43-2. Relationship between cardiac muscle shortening and imposed afterload in an isolated cat papillary muscle studied in vitro. Initial muscle length is held constant with a preload of 1.0 g. As additional load is added, the distance the muscle can shorten is progressive reduced as the afterload is increased.

lary wedge pressure between 14 and 18 mmHg [15]. If during initial fluid administration, however, pulmonary capillary wedge pressure increases rapidly and exceeds 20−25 mmHg, fluid administration should be discontinued because of the potential risk for precipitating pulmonary edema.

The "optimal filling pressure" to increase stroke volume has been determined in patients with recent myocardial infarction [16]. When one uses mean pulmonary capillary wedge or pulmonary artery diastolic pressure to represent left ventricular filling pressure, the optimal filling pressure is usually between 14 and 18 mmHg in most patients with recent myocardial infarction and without significant cardiomegaly. An increase in wedge pressure to 14−18 mmHg during intravenous fluid therapy is associated with an increase in stroke volume; further increase in wedge pressure beyond 18−20 mmHg usually does not cause any further increase in stroke volume (figure 43-3).

Mean pulmonary capillary wedge pressure is lower than the left ventricular end-diastolic pressure, particularly at higher levels of left ventricular end-diastolic pressures, because of the dif-

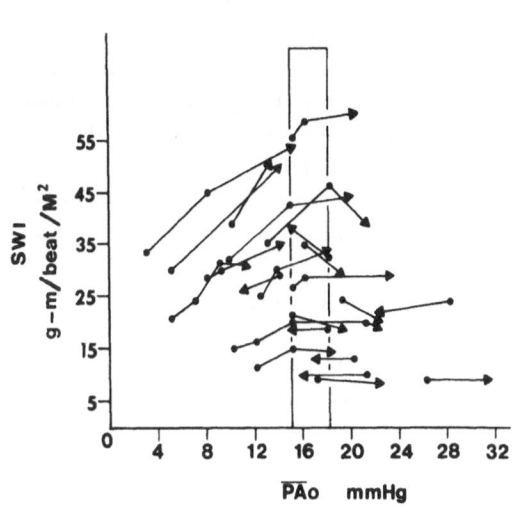

FIGURE 43-3. The highest level of stroke work index appears to lie in the range of 15–18 mmHg of $\overline{P}Ao$ as indicated by the bars. The direction of change in $\overline{P}Ao$ induced by therapy is indicated by the arrows. In all cases, increases in $\overline{P}Ao$ were induced by volume loading, and decreases in $\overline{P}Ao$ by diuresis. From Crexells et al. [16], with permission.

ferences in the compliance of pulmonary veins, left atrium, and left ventricle. If one uses left ventricular end-diastolic pressures instead of pulmonary capillary wedge or pulmonary artery diastolic pressure, optimal filling pressure appears to be between 20 and 25 mmHg [17]. It needs to be emphasized that the pulmonary venous pressure, and not the left ventricular end-diastolic pressure, is the hemodynamic determinant of pulmonary edema. Thus, monitoring pulmonary venous (pulmonary capillary wedge) pressure is preferable during intravenous fluid therapy in these patients.

In some patients, there is an inadequate increase in cardiac output despite maintaining optimal filling pressure with intravenous fluid therapy and the manifestations of low-output state persist (figure 43-3). In such patients, appropriate therapy for pump failure (vasodilators and/or inotropic agents) should be instituted and the optimal filling pressure should be maintained by concomitant administration of intravenous fluids. It is apparent that hemodynamic monitoring is essential and should be performed during

the management of patients with hypovolemic shock complicating acute myocardial infarction.

Preload Increase in Dominant Right Ventricular Infarction (see chapter 21)

Decreased left ventricular preload appears to be an important contributing mechanism in the genesis of low systemic output when right rather than left ventricular infarction is predominant [2]. The mechanism for the decreased left ventricular preload, however, is not entirely clear. In experimental isolated right ventricular infarction, right ventricular diastolic size increases along with an increase in its transmural pressure. Right ventricular stroke volume and stroke work decline due to depressed right ventricular systolic function. Left ventricular diastolic size and its transmural pressure, however, decrease, suggesting that decreased systemic stroke output is related to decreased left ventricular preload. As right ventricular stroke output contributes to the venous return to the left ventricle, depressed right ventricular systolic function appears to be contributory to decreased left ventricular preload [12].

The pericardium also imposes restriction on left ventricular filling in the presence of dominant right ventricular infarction [2]. In experimental right ventricular infarction, intrapericardial pressure increases due to acute and marked right ventricular dilatation within the confinement of the pericardium. Such increase in right ventricular size encroaches upon the intrapericardial space, raises the intrapericardial pressure, and also compresses the left ventricle. Thus, the constraints of pericardium associated with dilatation of the right ventricle cause further decrease in left ventricular preload. Removal of the pericardium in experimental right ventricular infarction is consistently associated with an increase in left ventricular volume. The therapeutic approach to improve systemic output in patients with dominant right ventricular infarction should, therefore, be directed to increase left ventricular preload.

The diagnosis of acute right ventricular infarction needs to be considered whenever the clinical evidence for right ventricular failure is present in the absence of significant left ventricular backward failure with pulmonary arterial hypertension (see chapter 33). Involvement of the free wall of the right ventricle can be further suspected if these clinical abnormalities are present in patients with inferior left ventricular infarction, because dominant right ventricular infarction is a rare accompaniment of acute anterior myocardial infarction. The scalar electrocardiogram aids in the diagnosis of right ventricular infarction; ST-segment elevation or loss of R waves in the precordial lead V_1 or in additional leads V_3R or V_4R is strongly suggestive of dominant right ventricular infarction. Gated blood pool scintigraphy and echocardiography demonstrate depressed right ventricular systolic function, right ventricular dilation, and decreased left ventricular size [2, 18]. A disproportionate elevation of right atrial pressure in relation to pulmonary capillary wedge pressure is the most common hemodynamic abnormality in patients with dominant right ventricular infarction. When low systemic output results from right ventricular infarction, however, "equalization of diastolic pressures," simulating constrictive pericarditis or cardiac tamponade, is frequently observed. Increased intrapericardial pressure consequent upon right ventricular dilatation appears to be the mechanism for the equalization of diastolic pressures [2]. Removal of the pericardium, in experimental right ventricular infarction, abolishes "equalization of diastolic pressures." Tc-99m myocardial scintigraphy provides the definitive diagnosis of right ventricular infarction [18]. However, pyrophosphate imaging is not useful during the management of low-output state complicating right ventricular infarction because low-output state usually develops within a few hours of the onset of infarction and one usually has to wait approximately 24 h to confirm the diagnosis by Tc-99m PyP imaging.

As low systemic output results primarily from decreased left ventricular preload, intravenous fluid therapy improves cardiac output as left ventricular volume increases. The mechanism for increased left ventricular preload during fluid administration is not entirely clear: passive filling of the left ventricle as the primary mechanism for the increased left ventricular preload during intravenous fluid administration has been suggested. In experimental isolated right ventricular

infarction, however, fluid therapy is associated with improved right ventricular systolic function; stroke volume increases along with a further increase in its transmural pressure and diastolic size [19]. Thus, improved right ventricular function appears to be related to utilization of the Frank-Starling mechanism. Increased right ventricular stroke output enhances left ventricular preload. It is necessary to monitor right atrial and pulmonary capillary wedge pressures during intravenous fluid therapy. Excessive fluid administration may precipitate marked dilatation of the right ventricle, which may cause further restriction of left ventricular filling. If right atrial pressure is maintained at 20 mmHg or less, the complications during fluid therapy can be avoided.

If intravenous fluid therapy fails to increase cardiac output adequately, vasodilators can be added to decrease pulmonary vascular resistance. Sodium nitroprusside and nitroglycerin decrease pulmonary vascular resistance (right ventricular afterload), which enhances right ventricular stroke volume and venous return to the left ventricle. However, as these vasodilators may also decrease systemic vascular resistance and systemic venous return, concomitant fluid administration to maintain adequate ventricular preload is essential. The addition of inotropic agents is sometimes necessary in patients with severe low-output state complicating dominant right ventricular infarction. Of the various parenteral inotropic agents available, dobutamine is preferable, as it has the potential to decrease pulmonary vascular resistance in addition to its positive inotropic effect. Dopamine also increases cardiac output, but pulmonary artery pressure and pulmonary vascular resistance may also increase, which may curtail the magnitude of increase in right ventricular stroke output because of increased right ventricular afterload. Pulmonary artery counterpulsation and right ventricular pneumatic pump assists have been used occasionally in patients with severe right ventricular infarct with some success, but the use of such mechanical devices is rarely necessary for the management of low-output state associated with predominant right ventricular infarction.

Temporary transvenous pacing is not infrequently required to maintain adequate heart rate, because of much higher incidence of bradyarrhythmias (approximately 30%) in patients with dominant right ventricular infarction [20]. Ventricular pacing, however, is likely to be associated with further reduction in cardiac output in these patients. Synchronous diastole of the ventricles and atria during ventricular pacing compromises left ventricular filling within the confinement of the pericardium, because of the encroachment on the limited intrapericardial space by the atria during diastole. Atrioventricular sequential pacing provides asynchronous atrial and ventricular diastole, and, therefore, relatively more intrapericardial space is available for the left ventricle to increase its preload. Atrioventricular (AV) sequential pacing in the absence of AV conduction, and atrial pacing in the presence of AV conduction, are preferable to ventricular pacing for the management of bradyarrhythmias complicating dominant right ventricular infarction [21].

Preload Decrease in Postinfarction Angina

Management of postinfarction angina requires reduction of the determinants of myocardial oxygen requirements as well as improved perfusion to the ischemic myocardium. As left ventricular volume contributes to wall stress, reduction of ventricular volume is associated with a significant reduction in myocardial oxygen demand. Nitroglycerin and nitrates are the most effective pharmacologic agents in decreasing left ventricular preload. Nitroglycerin and nitrates are predominantly venodilators, and cause peripheral venous pooling, which decreases systemic venous return and intracardiac volumes. Intravenous nitroglycerin is preferable to nonparenteral nitroglycerin or nitrates for the management of frequent recurrent episodes of rest angina. Hemodynamic monitoring is usually not required in the absence of overt heart failure. In patients with left ventricular failure, however, hemodynamic monitoring helps to determine the magnitude of reduction of pulmonary capillary wedge pressure that will not compromise cardiac output.

Afterload Reduction in Pump Failure

Reduction of left ventricular outflow resistance is associated with increased stroke volume and car-

diac output, and this physiologic principle, therefore, is an effective mode of therapy for pump failure [22]. Vasodilators with the potential to decrease systemic vascular resistance are effective agents for the reduction of left ventricular afterload and, thus, vasodilator therapy has gained widespread acceptance in the management of heart failure. For the treatment of pump failure complicating recent myocardial infarction, intravenous vasodilators with a rapid onset of action and short half-life are preferable: nitroglycerin, sodium nitroprusside, and phentolamine. The hemodynamic effects of nitroglycerin and other nitrates, whether administered sublingually, topically, or intravenously, are qualitatively similar. A reduction of pulmonary capillary wedge and right atrial pressures is the most consistent effect. Pulmonary artery pressure and pulmonary vascular resistance also tend to decrease. There is usually only a modest decrease in arterial pressure, and heart rate remains unchanged. Changes in systemic vascular resistance, stroke volume, and cardiac output are variable. The effects of nitroglycerin on cardiac performance are dependent on the initial level of left ventricular pressure [23] (figure 43-4). In patients with an elevated left ventricular filling pressure that does not decrease to a very low level during treatment, stroke volume and cardiac output either increase slightly or remain unchanged. If the patient has an initally normal filling pressure, further reduction will tend to lower stroke volume as the ventricle moves down the ascending limb of its curve. In such circumstances, hypotension and tachycardia may occur.

Nitroprusside and phentolamine have a relatively balanced effect on both arteriolar and venous beds; they decrease both afterload and preload, in contrast to nitroglycerin's predominant venodilation and thereby reduction of preload. The usual hemodynamic effects of nitroprusside and phentolamine are a reduction of arterial pressure and systemic vascular resistance, and an increase in stroke volume and cardiac output. Pulmonary capillary wedge, right atrial, and pulmonary artery pressures also decrease. Heart rate either decreases or remains unchanged with nitroprusside; with phentolamine, however, some tachycardia may be observed [23].

To determine the relative advantages of the

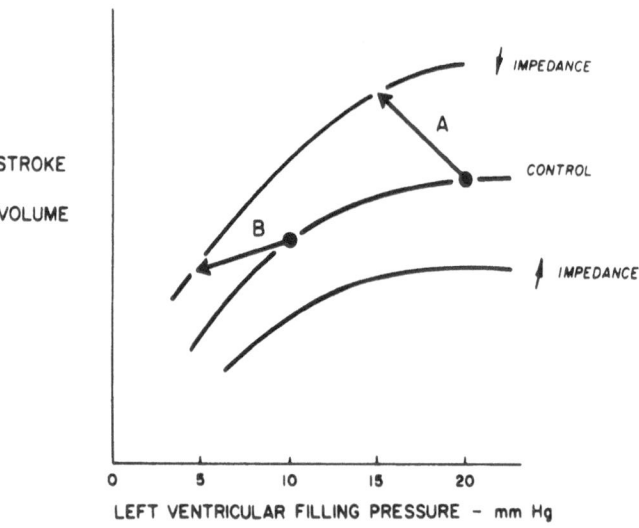

FIGURE 43-4. Left ventricular function curves plotting stroke volume versus left ventricular filling pressure are illustrated under control conditions and after decreased aortic impedance or increased aortic impedance. At a high filling pressure (20 mmHg), with a decrease in impedance, there is a decrease in filling pressure to 15 mmHg (line A) and an increase in stroke volume. Beginning at a low ventricular filling pressure (10 mmHg), there is a similar reduction in the magnitude of filling pressure, but this is accompanied by a reduction in stroke volume (line B). This graph conceptually illustrates the importance of giving vasodilators only to patients with high left ventricular filling pressures. From Chatterjee and Parmley [23], with permission.

various vasodilating agents that are potentially useful for the treatment of heart failure, it is necessary to evaluate their hemodynamic effects in the same patients. The hemodynamic effects of intravenous nitroprusside and nitroglycerin have been compared in the same groups of patients with acute myocardial infarction [24]. A greater increment in the ratio of systemic vascular resistance to pulmonary capillary wedge pressure was noted with nitroglycerin than with nitroprusside at a comparable decrease in arterial pressure. In other studies, however, these differences in the hemodynamic effects of the two agents were less apparent [25]. In most patients, however, nitroglycerin causes only a slight increase in stroke volume and cardiac output, but a marked decrease in left ventricular filling pressure. The changes in stroke volume and left ventricular filling pressure following both the sublingual and intravenous administration of nitroglycerin are shown in figure 43-5. These hemodynamic data have been collected from the published reports [23]. The patients were divided into those with initial pulmonary capillary wedge pressures greater than and less than or equal to 15 mmHg. In patients in whom left ventricular filling pressure was initially low or decreased to a very low level during nitroglycerin therapy, there was a decrease in stroke volume. When left ventricular filling pressure remained above 15 mmHg, there

was no decrease or even a slight increase in stroke volume. In some patients with left ventricular failure and a high left ventricular filling pressure, stroke volume and cardiac output increased significantly. Isosorbide dinitrate has been used sublingually and orally in patients with acute myocardial infarction. The hemodynamic effects of isosorbide dinitrate are very similar to those of nitroglycerin [26].

With sodium nitroprusside, the magnitude of increase in cardiac output and stroke volume appears to be greater in patients with left ventricular failure complicating myocardial infarction. Right atrial and pulmonary capillary wedge pressure decreases significantly along with a

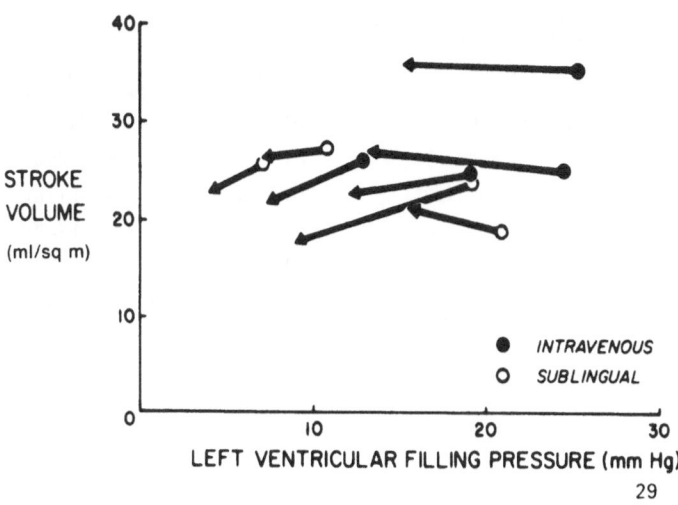

FIGURE 43-5. Effects of intravenous (n = 40) and sublingual (n = 33) nitroglycerin on hemodynamics in patients with acute myocardial infarction. As summarized from the literature, patients were divided as far as possible into those with an initial left ventricular (LV) filling pressure greater than 15 mmHg and those with an initial LV filling pressure less than 15 mmHg. Results of each study in those two categories are indicated by the individual lines. It is apparent that the predominant effect of nitroglycerin is to reduce LV filling pressure, and that a reduction in stroke volume tended to occur in patients whose initial LV filling pressure was low. From Parmley and Chatterjee [29], with permission.

modest decrease in arterial pressure. These beneficial hemodynamic effects can be observed even in patients with severe pump failure with or without clinical features of cardiogenic shock (table 43-1) [27]. The improvement in left ventricular function with nitroprusside, however, is dependent on the level of initial filling pressure. In patients with high initial left ventricular filling pressure, stroke volume increases along with a decrease in filling pressure, indicating improved left ventricular function. In patients with normal filling pressure, on the other hand, stroke volume tends to decrease as filling pressure decreases further, suggesting no change in left ventricular function during nitroprusside therapy (figure 43-6) [23].

The hemodynamic effects of trimethaphan, a ganglion-blocking agent, have been evaluated in a small number of patients with acute myocardial infarction [28]. The majority of these patients were hypertensive despite infarction and, with trimethaphan, there was a significant reduction in arterial pressure without increase in heart rate. Pulmonary capillary wedge pressure decreased but cardiac output did not change. These hemodynamic effects of trimethaphan resembled those of the nitrates, but trimethaphan is rarely used as a primary vasodilator agent because of rapid development of tachyphylaxis, and, at high doses, respiratory depression.

Although the hemodynamic effects of various vasodilator agents used in patients with acute myocardial infarction are qualitatively similar, there are quantitative differences (table 43-2) [29]. The optimal choice of a vasodilator depends on the hemodynamic deficit and the therapeutic objective in each patient. If the major objective is to decrease pulmonary congestion, any vasodilator agent may be useful. However, if there is also a low cardiac output, an agent with greater effect on afterload, such as nitroprusside, is preferred.

Vasodilator Therapy and Myocardial Infarct Size

Controversy exists regarding the effects of vasodilator agents on the extent of myocardial ischemia—

TABLE 43-1. Hemodynamic changes during intravenous vasodilator
therapy in severe pump failure complicating acute myocardial infarction ($n = 43$) [23]

	Control	Vasodilator	P
Heart rate (beats/min)	100 ± 2.4	99 ± 2.7	NS
Arterial pressure (mmHg)	83 ± 1.5	73 ± 1.7	< 0.0005
Pulmonary artery pressure (mmHg)	39 ± 1.2	28 ± 1.1	< 0.0005
Right atrial pressure (mmHg)	13 ± 0.8	9 ± 0.6	< 0.0005
Left ventricular filling pressure (mmHg)	31 ± 1.0	20 ± 0.8	< 0.0005
Cardiac index ($l/min/m^2$)	1.7 ± 0.05	2.2 ± 0.06	< 0.0005
Stroke volume index (ml/m^2)	17.3 ± 0.2	22.8 ± 0.8	< 0.0005
Stroke work index ($g\text{-}m/m^2$)	14 ± 0.7	19 ± 0.9	< 0.05
Systemic vascular resistance ($dyn\ s\ cm^{-5}$)	2023 ± 112	1435 ± 65	< 0.0005

All values are mean ± standard error of the mean.

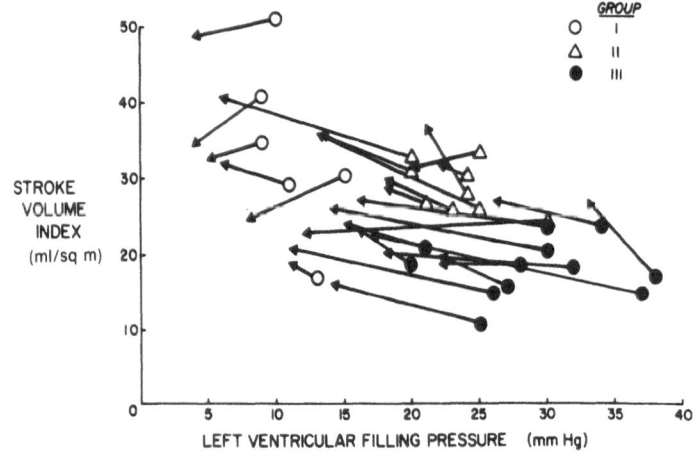

FIGURE 43-6. Effects of nitroprusside on a group of patients with acute myocardial infarction. Group-I patients are those with an initial left ventricular (LV) filling pressure of less than 15 mmHg. Group-II patients had an LV filling pressure greater than 15 mmHg and a stroke work index greater than 20 g-m/m². Group-III patients had an LV filling pressure greater than 15 mmHg and an initial stroke work index less than 20 g-m/m². All patients in group III had severe power failure and many had the classic signs of cardiogenic shock. Note that in group-II and group-III patients, the response to nitroprusside was usually an increase in stroke volume together with a reduction in LV filling pressure. In group-I patients, however, there was a reduction in stroke volume in some patients, which accompanied the reduction in LV filling pressure. From Chatterjee and Parmley [23], with permission.

TABLE 43-2. Summary of hemodynamic effects of various vasodilator drugs used in patients with left ventricular failure complicating recent myocardial infarction [29]

Vasodilator	Heart rate	Blood pressure	Cardiac output	Systemic vascular resistance	Pulmonary capillary wedge pressure
Nitroprusside	No change	Decrease	Increase	Decrease	Decrease
Phentolamine	Increase	Decrease	Increase	Decrease	Decrease
Nitroglycerin	No change	Decrease	Slight or no increase	Decrease or no change	Decrease
Isosorbide dinitrate	No change	Decrease	Slight or no increase	Decrease or no change	Decrease
Trimethaphan	No change	Decrease	Slight or no increase	Decrease or no change	Decrease

injury in patients with acute myocardial infarction. In some studies, nitroglycerin has been shown to decrease the extent of myocardial injury determined by the reduction in the magnitude of ST-segment elevations on electrocardiograms and by decreased creatine-kinase activity [25]. In a prospective randomized study, reduction of infarct size calculated from total creatine kinase (CK) and CK-MB activity curves was observed with intravenous nitroglycerin [30]. In another randomized prospective trial, however, no significant differences were found in peak CK, CK-estimated infarct size, or preservation of precordial R waves between nitroglycerin and placebo-treated patients [31].

In one study, an increase in ST-segment elevation and a higher level of CK with sodium nitroprusside therapy suggested an extension of myocardial injury [25]. In contrast, in a randomized prospective study, reduction of infarct size determined by electrocardiographic or enzymatic methods has been reported [32]. It is apparent that both nitroglycerin and nitroprusside have the potential to decrease myocardial ischemia in appropriate subsets of patients. It should be emphasized, however, that in most patients with acute myocardial infarction, there is a complete interruption of flow by a thrombotic occlusion of a chronically stenosed coronary artery. Increased perfusion to the periinfarction zone, therefore, can occur only if there is an increase in collateral blood flow. The extent to which vasodilators can increase collateral blood flow to infarcting myocardial segments in these patients is unknown. Furthermore, commonly employed enzymatic and electrocardiographic methods for determination of infarct size are imprecise and should not be regarded as conclusive evidence for changes in infarct size during vasodilator therapy.

Vasodilator Therapy and Prognosis in Patients with Acute Myocardial Infarction

The influence of nitroprusside therapy on the mortality of patients with acute myocardial infarction has been evaluated in prospective randomized trials [32–34]. In one study, a significant reduction in mortality at one, two, and four weeks with a decreased incidence of cardiogenic shock and left ventricular failure has been observed in nitroprusside-treated patients [32]. In contrast, in other studies, nitroprusside therapy was not associated with any change in early or late mortality [33,34]. Early intervention with nitroprusside was associated in one study with a worse prognosis [33].

In a few randomized prospective studies, intravenous nitroglycerin was administered to assess its influence on the prognosis of patients with mild or no left ventricular failure [30, 31]. Either no change or only slight reduction in mortality was reported. Thus, no conclusive evidence is available to suggest that the routine use of either nitroprusside or nitroglycerin improves the prognosis of patients with relatively uncomplicated myocardial infarction. It should also be noted that patients with severe pump failure and cardiogenic shock were excluded from these randomized studies.

No controlled study has been performed to assess the effects of vasodilator therapy on the prognosis of patients with severe pump failure or cardiogenic shock. In an uncontrolled study, a lower hospital mortality was reported with vasodilatory therapy compared with the expected mortality with conventional therapy [26]. In patients with an initial stroke work index of 20 g-m/m^2 or less and a left ventricular filling pressure greater than 15 mmHg, the hospital mortality with nitroprusside therapy was 44%, compared with expected mortality of 70% or greater with conventional therapy. However, when the stroke work index was extremely low (less than 10 g-m/m^2) and the left ventricular filling pressure was elevated, the prognosis was extremely poor. The mortality rate in this subset—even with vasodilator therapy—was 82%. In these patients, the use of intraaortic balloon counterpulsation initially and then addition of vasodilator and inotropic agents is occasionally effective.

Guidelines for the Use of Vasodilators in Acute Myocardial Infarction

It is apparent that hemodynamic monitoring is preferable during vasodilator therapy in patients with acute myocardial infarction. Determination of hemodynamics aids in hemodynamic categorization of these patients and in selection of appropriate therapy. In table 43-3, the different hemodynamic subsets and suggested therapeutic intervention in each subset are outlined.

Patients in subset 1 appear clinically stable, have an excellent prognosis, and generally do not require specific therapy. In patients with persistent hypertension or postinfarction angina, vasodilators and beta-adrenergic-blocking agents are used. Although patients in subset 2 may appear to have pump failure, their cardiac performance is generally adequate and their hemodynamic abnormalities are secondary to intravascular hypovolemia. Vasodilators as the initial therapy are

contraindicated in this group as they are likely to produce significant hypotension.

Patients in subsets 3 and 4 have significantly impaired myocardial function and are appropriate candidates for vasodilator therapy. Those in subset 3 with normal perfusion but elevated pulmonary capillary wedge pressure may be treated with diuretics or with intravenous or nonparenteral nitroglycerin or nitrates. Those with moderately depressed stroke work indices (20–40 g-m/m^2), particularly if they are hypertensive, may benefit from a vasodilator such as nitroprusside. Subset-4A patients have both reduced perfusion and elevated left ventricular filling pressure and, therefore, require both preload and afterload reduction. Again, nitroprusside is probably the agent of choice in these patients, but phentolamine has also been employed successfully. In some patients in this subset, hypotension may occur without any significant increase in cardiac output or decrease in pulmonary capillary wedge pressure. In these patients, vasodilator therapy should be discontinued and inotropic therapy and intraaortic balloon counterpulsation therapy should be instituted and then vasodilators added. Patients in subset 4B have more profound hemodynamic impairment and are often hypotensive. Vasodilator therapy frequently produces further hypotension because the increase in cardiac output is inadequate (see chapter 44). Therefore, an initial trial of an inotropic-vasopressor agent to maintain arterial pressure and increase cardiac output is indicated.

The most appropriate therapy in these patients, however, is intraaortic balloon counterpulsation to enhance myocardial perfusion pressure by diastolic augmentation and to decrease left ventricular afterload by systolic unloading (see chapter 44). The favorable hemodynamic and metabolic effects of counterpulsation therapy have been documented in many investigations [35–37]. The augmented diastolic pressure with counterpulsation allows addition of vasodilators that may further decrease left ventricular filling pressure and increase cardiac output, but mortality remains high unless surgically remediable lesions are detected (see chapter 45). In this instance, cardiac catheterization should be performed with a view to corrective surgery.

TABLE 43-3. Hemodynamic subsets and suggested therapeutic intervention

Subset	Clinical presentation	Stroke work index (g-m/m²)	Pulmonary capillary wedge pressure (mmHg)	Suggested therapy
1	Stable	≥40	≤15	Observe
2	Decreased perfusion	<40	≤15	Intravenous fluids
3	Pulmonary congestion	20–40	>15	Diuretics, nitroglycerin, nitro-prusside, phentolamine
4A	Pulmonary congestion, decreased perfusion	10–20	>15	Nitroprusside, phentolamine (inotropes and counterpulsation)
4B	Pulmonary congestion, decreased perfusion	<10	>15	Inotropes–vasopressors, counter-pulsation—then vasodilators, surgery.

Heart Failure Complicating Mechanical Defects

Clinical and hemodynamic improvement is observed during vasodilator therapy in patients whose heart failure is precipitated or exacerbated by mechanical defects such as mitral regurgitation and ventricular septal rupture. The severity of mitral regurgitation is not only related to the degree of anatomic derangement of the mitral valve apparatus, but also to changes in the aortic impedance [38, 39]. An increase in left ventricular ejection impedance is associated with an increased regurgitant volume and decreased forward stroke volume and cardiac output. Vasodilator agents like sodium nitroprusside, hydralazine, and prazosin increase forward stroke volume and cardiac output, and decrease the regurgitant volume as the aortic impedance decreases. Decreased regurgitation is associated with a decreased magnitude of the regurgitant V wave, mean pulmonary capillary wedge, and pulmonary artery pressures (figure 43-7 and table 43-4) [40]. In patients with acute myocardial infarction, sodium nitroprusside is the vasodilator of choice because of its rapid onset of action and short half-life.

The effects of vasodilator agents on the magnitude of left-to-right shunt in patients with ventricular septal rupture are variable. The magnitude of the shunt is not only influenced by the size of the defect, but also by the ratio of the pulmonary and systemic vascular resistance [41]. Increased systemic vascular resistance is associated with an increased shunt volume and a proportional decrease in systemic output. Vasodilators

like sodium nitroprusside, hydralazine, phentolamine, and phenoxybenzamine may reduce the left-to-right shunt and increase the systemic output by decreasing systemic vascular resistance [42, 43], but these vasodilators can potentially also decrease pulmonary vascular resistance and, therefore, should be used with caution.

Although vasodilator agents produce beneficial hemodynamic effects, their clinical application in the management of patients with mechanical defects complicating myocardial infarction has not been clearly defined. In patients with severe mitral regurgitation or ventricular septal rupture, vasodilators can be used for immediate hemodynamic and clinical improvement. However, vasodilator therapy should be regarded as supportive rather than definitive treatment; early surgical correction should be considered (see chapter 45).

Summary

Decreased cardiac output (low-output syndrome) is a serious complication of acute myocardial infarction. Decreased left ventricular preload is the primary mechanism for low systemic output in patients with hypovolemic shock and dominant right ventricular infarction. Intravenous fluid therapy is associated with increased left ventricular preload and increased systemic output.

Increased afterload is associated with further depression of cardiac function in patients with left ventricular failure complicating myocardial infarction. Reduction of afterload with the use of vasodilator agents is associated with improved

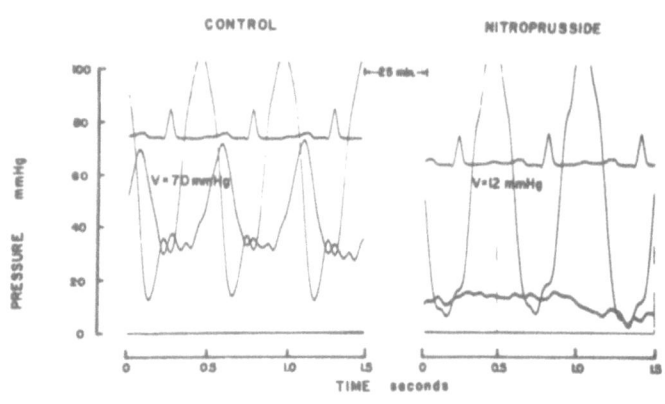

FIGURE 43-7. Hemodynamic effects of sodium nitroprusside in a patient with severe acute mitral regurgitation. Left ventricular pressure and pulmonary capillary wedge pressure are illustrated in each panel. In the left panel, not the large regurgitant V waves (up to 70mmHg) in the pulmonary capillary wedge pressure, and left ventricular end-diastolic pressure returned almost to the normal range and the regurgitant V waves essentially disappeared. This patient illustrates the beneficial effects of vasodilator therapy in patients with mitral regurgitation. From Chatterjee et al. [40], with permission.

TABLE 43-4. Left ventricular volumes both before and during nitroprusside infusion in four patients with mitral regurgitation [40]

	EDV (ml/m²)	ESV (ml/m²)	TSV (ml/m²)	FSV (ml/m²)	RV (%)	EF	EDP (mmHg)
Control	238 ± 51	140 ± 33	96 ± 24	31 ± 7	64 ± 8	0.41 ± 0.07	30 ± 2.5
Nitroprusside	205 ± 46	113 ± 32	93 ± 20	49 ± 9	44 ± 11	0.47 ± 0.08	14 ± 2.3
$P<$	0.01	0.005	NS	0.025	0.05	0.05	0.005

EDV, end-diastolic volume; ESV, end-systolic volume; TSV, total stroke volume; FSV, forward stroke volume; RV, regurgitant volume; EF, ejection fraction; EDP, end-diastolic pressure; NS, not significant

left ventricular function in certain subsets of patients with left ventricular failure. Determination of initial and subsequent hemodynamics, however, is essential during manipulation of preload and afterload to optimize cardiac function in patients with acute myocardial infarction.

References

1. Sonnenblick EH: Force—velocity relations in mammalian heart muscle. Am J Physiol 202: 931—939, 1962.
2. Goldstein JA, Vlahakes GJ, Verrier ED, Schiller NB, Tyberg JV, Ports TA, Parmley WW, Chat-

terjee K: The role of right ventricular systolic dysfunction and elevated intrapericardial pressure in the genesis of low output in experimental right ventricular infarction. Circulation 65: 513−522, 1982.

3. Swan HJC, Ganz W, Forrester JS, et al: Catheterization of the heart in man with the use of a flow-directed balloon-tip catheter. N Engl J Med 283:447−451, 1970.

4. Milnor WR: Arterial impedance as ventricular afterload. Circ Res 36:565−570, 1975.

5. Patel DJ, Defreitas FM, Fry DL: Hydraulic input impedance to aorta and pulmonary artery in dogs. J Appl Physiol 18:134−140, 1963.

6. O'Rourke MF, Taylor MG: Input impedance of the systemic circulation. Circ Res 20:365−385, 1967.

7. Noble MIM, Gabe IT, Renchard D, et al: Blood pressure and flow in the ascending aorta of conscious dogs. Cardiovasc Res 1:9−29, 1967.

8. Nichols WW, Conti CR, Walker WE, et al: Input impedance of the systemic circulation in man. Circ Res 49:451−458, 1977.

9. Murgo JP, Westerhof N, Giolma JP, et al: Aortic input impedance in normal man: relationship to pressure wave forms. Circulation 62:105−116, 1980.

10. Elzinga G, Westerhof N: Pressure and flow generated by the left ventricle against different impedances. Cir Res 32:178−186, 1973.

11. Pepine CJ, Nichols WW: Aortic input impedance in cardiovascular disease. Prog Cardiovasc Dis 24:307−318, 1982.

12. Nichols WW, Pepine CJ: Left ventricular afterload and aortic impedance: implications of pulsatile blood flow. Prog Cardiovasc Dis 24:293−306, 1982.

13. Pepine CJ, Nichols WW, Curry RC, et al: Aortic input impedance during nitroprusside infusion: a reconsideration of afterload reduction and beneficial action. J Clin Invest 64:643−654, 1979.

14. Forrester JS, Ganz W, Diamond G, et al: Thermodilution cardiac output determination with a single flow-directed catheter. Am Heart J 83: 306−311, 1972.

15. Chatterjee K: Pump failure in acute myocardial infarction: fluid and drug therapy. Ann Clin Res 19:124, 1977.

16. Crexells C, Chatterjee K, Forrester J, Dikshit K, Swan HJC: Optimal level of filling pressure in the left side of the heart in acute myocardial infarction. N Engl J Med 289:1263−1266, 1973.

17. Russell RO Jr, Rackley CE, Pombo J, et al:

Effects of increasing left ventricular filling pressure in patients wtih acute myocardial infarction. J Clin Invest 49:1539, 1970.

18. Sharpe DN, Botvinick EH, Shames DM, Schiller NB, Massie BM, Chatterjee K, Parmley WW: The noninvasive diagnosis of right ventricular infarction. Circulation 57:483−490, 1978.

19. Goldstein JA, Vlahakes GJ, Verrier ED, Schiller NB, Botvinick E, Tyberg JV, Parmley WW, Chatterjee K: Volume loading improves low cardiac output in experimental right ventricular infarction. J Am Coll Cardiol 2:270−278, 1983.

20. Chatterjee K: Complications of acute myocardial infarction: medical management. In: Connor WE, Bristow JD (eds) Complications in coronary heart disease. Philadelphia: JB Lippincott, 1984 (in press).

21. Topol EJ, Golschlager N, Ports TA, Di Carlo LA Jr, Schiller NB, Botvinick EH, Chatterjee K: Hemodynamic benefit of atrial pacing in right ventricular myocardial infarction. Ann Intern Med 96:594−597, 1982.

22. Chatterjee K, Parmley WW: Vasodilator therapy for acute myocardial infarction and chronic congestive heart failure. J Am Coll Cardiol 1:133−153, 1983.

23. Chatterjee K, Parmley WW: The role of vasodilator therapy in heart failure. Prog Cardiovasc Dis 19:301−325, 1977.

24. Armstrong PW, Walker DC, Burton Jr, et al: Vasodilator therapy in acute myocardial infarction: a comparison of sodium nitroprusside and nitroglycerin. Circulation 52:1118−1127, 1975.

25. Chiariello M, Gold HK, Leinbach RC, et al: Comparison between the effects of nitroprusside and nitroglycerin on ischemic injury during acute myocardial infarction. Circulation 54:766−773, 1976.

26. Bussman W, Lohner J, Kaltenbach M: Orally administered isosorbide dinitrate in patients with and without left ventricular failure due to acute myocardial infarction. Am J Cardiol 39:91−96, 1977.

27. Chatterjee K, Swan HJC, Kaushik VS, et al: Effects of vasodilator therapy for severe pump failure in acute myocardial infarction on short-term and late prognosis. Circulation 53:797−802, 1976.

28. Shell WE, Sobel BE: Protection of jeopardized ischemic myocardium by reduction of ventricular afterload. N Eng J Med 291:481, 1974.

29. Parmley WW, Chatterjee K: Vasodilator therapy. In: Harvey WP (ed) Current problems in

cardiology. Chicago: Yearbook Medical, 1978.

30. Bussman WD, Passek D, Seidel W, Kaltenbach M: Prospective randomized trial of intravenous nitroglycerin in acute myocardial infarction. [abstr]. Circulation (Suppl 2) 59 and 60:II−164.

31. Flaherty JT, Becker LC, Bulkley BH, et al: A randomized prospective trial of intravenous nitroglycerin in patients with acute myocardial infarction.

32. Durrer JD, Lie KI, Van Capelle FRJ, Durrer D: Effect of sodium nitroprusside on mortality in acute myocardial infarction. N Engl J Med 306: 1121−1128, 1982.

33. Cohn JN, Franciosa JA, Francis CS, et al: Effect of short-term infusion of sodium nitroprusside on mortality rate in acute myocardial infarction complicated by left ventricular failure: results of Veterans Administration Cooperative Study. N Engl J Med 306: 1129−1135, 1982.

34. Hockings BEF, Cope GD, Clarke GM, Taylor RR: Randomized controlled trial of vasodilator therapy after acute myocardial infarction. Am J Cardiol 48:345−352, 1981.

35. Dunkman WB, et al: Clinical and hemodynamic results of intra-aortic balloon pumping and surgery for cardiogenic shock. Circulation 46:465, 1972.

36. McEnany MT, et al: Clinical experience with intra-aortic balloon pump support in 728 patients.

Circulation (Suppl 1) 58:124, 1978.

37. Mueller H, et al: The effects of intra-aortic balloon counterpulsation on cardiac performance and metabolism in shock associated with acute myocardial infarction. J Clin Invest 50:1885, 1971.

38. Wiggers CJ, Feely H: The cardiodynamics of mitral insufficiency. Heart Bull 9:149−183 and 1921−1922.

39. Braunwald E, Welch GH, Sarnoff SJ: Hemodynamic effects of quantitatively varied experimental mitral regurgitation. Circ Res 5:539−545, 1957.

40. Chatterjee K, Parmley WW, Swan HJC, et al: Beneficial effects of vasodilator agents in severe mitral regurgitation due to subvalvular apparatus. Circulation 48:684−690, 1973.

41. Synhorst DP, Laur RM, Doty DB, Brody MJ: Hemodynamic effects of vasodilator agents in dogs with experimental ventricular septal defects. Circulation 54:472−477, 1976.

42. Techlenberg PL, Fitzgerald J, Allaire BI, et al: Afterload reduction in the management of postinfarction ventricular septal defect. Circulation 38: 956−958, 1976.

43. Beckman RH, Rocchini AP, Rosenthal A: Hemodynamic effects of hydralazine in infants with a large ventricular septal defect. Circulation 65: 523−528, 1982.

44. THE MEDICAL MANAGEMENT OF CARDIOGENIC SHOCK DUE TO MYOCARDIAL NECROSIS

R.M. Norris

Definition of Cardiogenic Shock due to Myocardial Necrosis

The term *cardiogenic shock* (as used in this chapter) describes forward failure of the left ventricle due to extensive myocardial necrosis. Forward failure of the left ventricle leads to low cardiac output, low arterial blood pressure, and usually (as a reflex adaptation by the body), high peripheral resistance. The clinical picture in cardiogenic shock—low arterial blood pressure, poorly perfused extremities, oliguria, and frequently mental obtundation—is entirely compatible with these pathophysiologic abnormalities.

Cardiogenic shock due to myocardial infarction is part of a spectrum of hemodynamic disorders, so that any precise definition is artificial. Moreover, forward failure of the left ventricle is always accompanied by backward failure causing high left atrial and pulmonary venous pressures, and leading to the clinical features in less severe cases of gallop rhythm and radiologic pulmonary venous congestion and, in more severe cases, of breathlessness due to pulmonary edema.

Thus defined, cardiogenic shock due to acute myocardial infarction is caused by massive myocardial damage resulting either from the acute infarct or cumulatively from past infarctions. In two autopsy studies [1, 2] the average infarct size of patients dying from cardiogenic shock was 40%−50% of the left ventricle, the range being 25%−72%. By contrast, patients dying after infarction without hemodynamic disturbance preceding death had 15%−40% of the ventricle infarcted [2] (figure 44-1).

Diagnosis of Cardiogenic Shock

There are a number of pitfalls in the diagnosis of cardiogenic shock, all of which have an important bearing on treatment: (a) forward failure of the left ventricle must be distinguished from forward failure of the right ventricle, (b) forward failure must be present in the absence of severe tachyarrhythmia or bradyarrhythmia, (c) the possibility must always be considered that failure may be due to cardiac-depressant drugs such as beta blockers or that hypotension may be caused by vasodilators, and (d) presence of the acute surgical complications of infarction—namely, papillary muscle rupture causing mitral incompetence, rupture of the interventricular septum causing left to right shunt, and subacute rupture of the free wall of the left ventricle—must all be excluded.

Forward failure of the right ventricle (see chapter 33) has been recognized in recent years as an important complication of inferior infarction caused by right coronary artery occlusion and right ventricular infarction [3]. Acute right ventricular failure (possibly made worse by a restrictive action of the pericardium to inhibit ventricular filling [44] leads to underfilling of the left ven-

R.M. Califf and G.S. Wagner (eds.), ACUTE CORONARY CARE: Principles and Practice. Copyright © 1985. Martinus Nijhoff Publishing, Boston/Dordrecht/Lancaster.

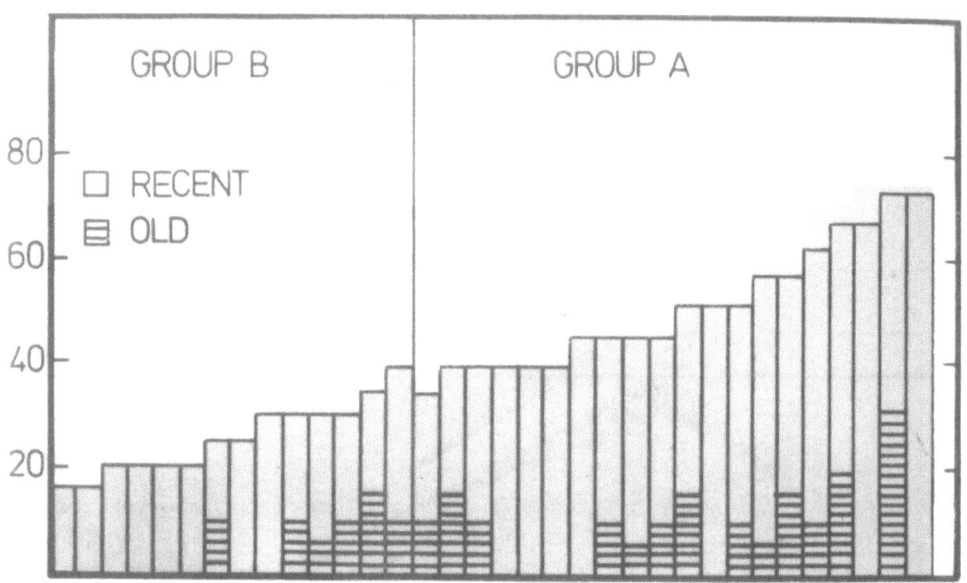

FIGURE 44-1. Cumulative percentage loss of left ventricle from both recent and old infarction: autopsy findings in cardiac patients with (group A) and without (group B) cardiogenic shock. Data of Page and associates [2] adapted by Rude and associates [15] and reproduced with permission.

tricle and, in consequence, forward failure with hypotension and low cardiac output [5]. However, backward failure of the left ventricle is not present—the patient is not breathless, the x-ray shows clear lung fields without pulmonary venous congestion or edema, and the pulmonary capillary wedge pressure is low (<15 mmHg). Acute right ventricular failure occurring in the setting of myocardial infarction has quite different implications from left ventricular failure in that the prognosis is better, the correct treatment is by volume expansion with avoidance of diuretics [6], and sequential atrioventricular pacing can be of added value when high-grade atrioventricular block (common in inferior infarction) is also present [7].

Cardiogenic shock should not be diagnosed in the presence of a correctable tachyarrhythmia such as sustained ventricular tachycardia or uncontrolled atrial fibrillation, or in patients with inferior infarction and bradycardia due to marked vagotonia. Bradycardia and hypotension in this latter group of patients responds to intravenous atropine (0.3−0.6 mg), indicating that the cause is reflex, and not severe left ventricular damage.

With increasing use of intravenous beta blockers and afterload reduction for limitation of infarct size, heart failure and hypotension are pos-

sible complications that must be recognized. Heart failure due to intravenous propranolol is, in our experience, not difficult to treat, provided that the cause is recognized, administration of the beta blocker stopped, and a diuretic administered.

The presence of ruptured papillary muscle or interventricular septum should be suspected when the appearance of a loud systolic murmur coincides with sudden hemodynamic deterioration leading to the development of shock. It is often clinically difficult to distinguish between these two conditions at bedside, although they can be positively differentiated by the appearance of a flail mitral leaflet on echocardiography or a stepup in oxygen saturation in right-sided blood samples obtained through a balloon-tipped catheter. Early ventriculography and coronary arteriography followed by surgical intervention are recommended, as the natural history of both conditions shows a high mortality rate [8]. The condition of subacute left ventricular free-wall rupture [9] is uncommon, but its presence should always be suspected when sudden hemodynamic collapse occurs within a few days of infarction, there is no evidence of reinfarction or arrhythmia, and no systolic murmur is present. Signs of cardiac tamponade are sometimes but not always present. Diagnosis is by demonstration of a pericardial effusion by echocardiography, and treatment is by immediate infarctectomy and patching of the ventricular wall. Subacute cardiac rupture is the only type of left ventricular free-wall rupture that is amenable to treatment. Without surgery, most patients will die from recurrent cardiac rupture, although recovery with development of a left ventricular false aneurysm has been recorded.

Once the presence of forward failure of the left ventricle has been established, and the above causes excluded, an arbitrary cutoff point for hemodynamic abnormality is necessary for precise definition. For a "rule-of-thumb" clinical diagnosis, cardiogenic shock is best defined in terms of systolic blood pressure, because measurement of blood pressure is simple and quick, allowing for immediate treatment, which is usually the only hope for the patient. We consider cardiogenic shock to be present if (in the presence of a recent infarct and signs of left ventricular backward failure) the systolic blood pressure is below 100 mmHg. Left ventricular backward failure is usually readily apparent from the chest x-ray that shows pulmonary venous congestion, interstitial edema, or pulmonary edema. If pulmonary congestion is not obvious radiologically, pulmonary wedge pressure together with right atrial pressure must be measured using a balloon-tipped catheter to exclude the right ventricular infarction syndrome. Some older definitions of shock refer to the patient's condition after relief of pain and anxiety, but there is no evidence that pain and anxiety influence hemodynamic measurements in any consistent way.

The above definition of cardiogenic shock may seem overly simple and arbitrary, in that a cutoff point of 100 mmHg for systolic blood pressure might, on the one hand, include patients who are merely hypotensive and not in shock and, on the other hand, exclude patients in the early phases of shock in whom hypotension had not yet developed. In our experience, however, patients who are merely hypotensive do not have signs of left ventricular backward failure. Those in whom systolic blood pressure is over 100 mmHg in the presence of left ventricular failure, but who are compensating for an obligatory low stroke volume with high peripheral resistance, cool extremities, and sinus tachycardia, may be described as having "preshock." In a study of the effects of intraaortic balloon counterpulsation in one such group of patients [10], we found that most, but not all, progressed to develop cardiogenic shock as described above.

Prognosis in Cardiogenic Shock

All agree that the prognosis in cardiogenic shock is poor, despite optimum treatment. As shock represents a spectrum of hemodynamic disturbance with no natural cutoff point, prognosis for life must be considered as a continuous variable according to the hemodynamic subset. This can be accomplished with reference to arterial blood pressure (figure 44-2) [11] or the relation between cardiac index and left ventricular filling pressure (figure 44-3) [12]. Description of hospital survival in terms of systolic blood pressure on admission to hospital (figure 44-2) gives the more useful information because it can be applied to all unselected cases admitted to general or community hospitals. Description of prognosis in terms of cardiac index and wedge pressure is more accurate, but can be applied only to selected patients. Figure 44-2 shows an increasingly poor prognosis as admission systolic blood pressure fell below 100 mmHg, and figure 44-3 shows a 95% mortality rate for patients in whom cardiac index was less than 2 liters/min/m^2 and left ventricular filling pressure equal to or greater than 15 mmHg.

Occurrence of Cardiogenic Shock

With control of arrhythmias in coronary care units, cardiogenic shock and cardiac failure are now the leading causes of death in patients admitted to hospital (figure 44-4). As shock and failure have a common cause (i.e., massive myocardial damage), the two conditions can be grouped together as "pump failure." Prevention

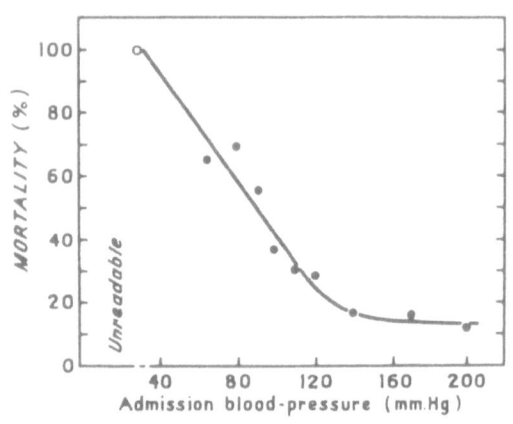

FIGURE 44-2. Relation between systolic blood pressure on admission to hospital and hospital mortality rate in 757 patients with acute myocardial infarction. From Norris et al. [11], with permission.

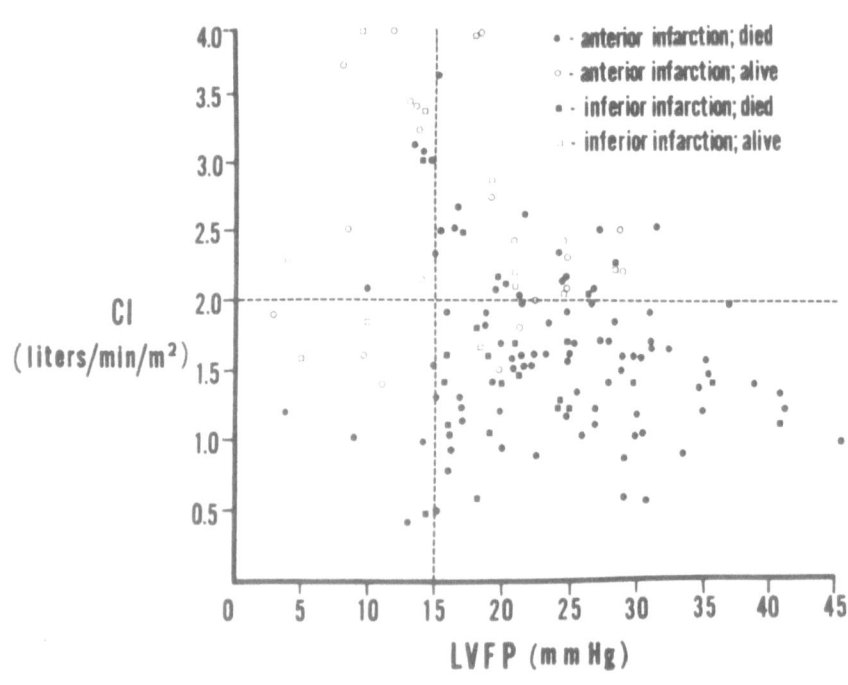

FIGURE 44-3. Hemodynamic data of 152 patients with cardiogenic shock, derived from the Myocardial Infarction Research Units cooperative study data bank [12]. Figures for left ventricular filling pressure (LVFP) are plotted against cardiac index (CI) for each patient. Subsequent death in hospital (closed symbols) was predicted with 95% accuracy from the combination of CI <2.0 liters/min/m^2 and LVFP ≥15 mmHg. Mortality for patients in other hemodynamic subsets ranged from 33% to 58%. From Weber et al. [12], with permission.

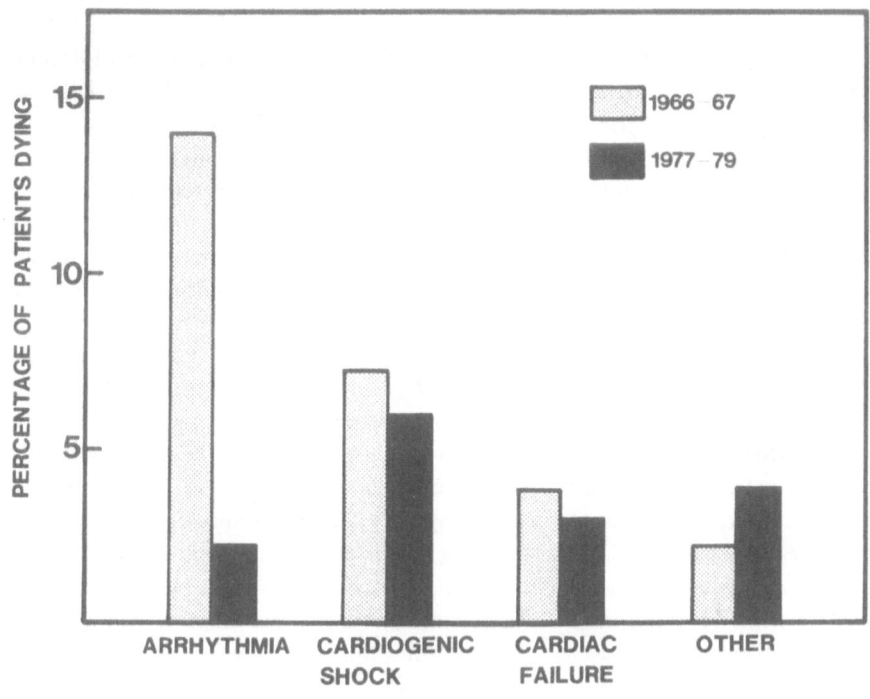

FIGURE 44-4. Contrasting mortality patterns comparing patients treated in hospitals in 1966—67 before the introduction of a coronary care unit with those treated in a coronary care unit during 1977—79. Sudden deaths from arrhythmia have declined markedly in 1977—79, but the proportion of patients dying from shock and cardiac failure has changed but little. From Churchill Livingstone Ltd., with permission.

and control of pump failure is the major therapeutic problem in coronary care units in the 1980s.

Prevention of Cardiogenic Shock

Because cardiogenic shock due to acute myocardial infarction is caused by massive irreversible myocardial damage, the logical therapeutic measure is to prevent the occurrence of myocardial damage or at least to limit its extent; any treatment that is given after damage has become irreversible must be at best palliative. Whether cardiogenic shock can be prevented is presently unknown and is the principal thrust of a large number of studies in progress throughout the world. There is emerging encouraging evidence that shock may prove to be, to some extent at least, a preventable complication of infarction.

It is common experience that patients seldom develop cardiogenic shock at the very onset of an acute infarct, but develop it gradually over a period of 4—12 h after the onset of chest pain. Geddes and colleagues have suggested that early treatment of arrhythmias, autonomic disturbances, and clinically apparent hemodynamic abnormalities can prevent the development of cardiogenic shock; in one series of patients studied by these authors, the incidence of cardiogenic shock was 4% in patients who were treated within 3 h of the onset of myocardial infarction compared with 13% in patients in whom therapy was delayed beyond 3 h [13]. Further evidence for a delayed onset of cardiogenic shock comes from studies showing a prolonged duration of appearance of creatine kinase enzyme in the blood of patients with cardiogenic shock compared with the duration in patients without shock [14]. Our own experience confirms that shock is uncommon at the onset of infarction and is more common in patients whose admission to hospital has been delayed than in those who have been admitted early.

The major thrust of therapies for restriction of infarct size is to prevent deaths from cardiogenic shock and cardiac failure. A large body of literature confirms the efficacy of measures for restriction of infarct size in animals [15], but unfortunately none of these have so far been shown to be effective in patients. One suspects that the reason is that it has proved impossible for logistic reasons to apply these therapies early enough. Ischemic necrosis in experimental infarction advances as a wave front from the center of the ischemic area, being 84% completed within 6 h [16]; it is therefore unlikely that any therapeutic intervention to limit infarct size in patients would be effective more than 4−6 h after the onset of chest pain. One measure for restriction of infarct size that we are currently testing is propranolol (0.1 mg/kg intravenously) within 4 h of the onset of chest pain, and followed by oral therapy over 24 h. We previously showed that this regimen reduced enzyme levels by approximately 30%, provided treatment was started within 4 h of onset of chest pain [17]. Other possible therapies under clinical trial include intravenous hyaluronidase, and reduction of afterload using intravenous infusions of nitroglycerin or sodium nitroprusside.

There is now a real possibility that coronary thrombosis, the cause of transmural myocardial infarction leading to cardiogenic shock, might be reversed by the use of intracoronary streptokinase [18]. Whether clot lysis leads to functional reperfusion of the myocardium, whether reperfusion can limit infarct size, the allowable time limits during which reperfusion could be effective, are all questions that remain to be answered. It seems likely, however, that dissolution of coronary thrombi, or even prevention of thrombosis, is a foreseeable goal during the next decade. Prevention of cardiogenic shock by restriction of infarct size is now a realistic therapeutic strategy.

Treatment of Cardiogenic Shock

INOTROPIC DRUGS AND PRESSOR AMINES
Circulating catecholamine levels are high in patients with cardiogenic shock due to myocardial

infarction so that the heart in shock has its own inotropic stimulation. The infarcting segment of left ventricle (on average 40%−50% of left ventricular mass) cannot respond to this endogenous inotropic stimulation. If it could partially respond, the effect would likely be detrimental by increase in oxygen requirements and consequent increase in infarct size. The remaining 50%−60% of healthy myocardium, however, can respond both to the endogenous and exogenous stimulation; and the use of inotropic and pressor drugs is the cornerstone of treatment for established cardiogenic shock. The aims of treatment with inotropic drugs are to improve tissue perfusion by increasing blood flow, particularly to the brain and kidneys and also to the heart itself. The disadvantage of pressor drugs is that their effects are temporary and symptomatic, and they do nothing for the primary lesion in the heart itself.

Until the mid-1970s, the two most widely used stimulant drugs were isoproterenol and norepinephrine infused intravenously in a dose of 1−4 μg/min for isoproterenol and 1−10 μg/min for norepinephrine. Isoproterenol is a pure beta-adrenergic stimulator, and its infusion in normal subjects causes tachycardia, increased cardiac output, and peripheral vasodilation leading to a slight reduction in arterial pressure. In patients who are in shock, however, the effect of inotropic stimulation may outweigh the vasodilation, so that the blood pressure response is variable. Systolic blood pressure usually rises while diastolic pressure may fall due to vasodilatation, with no resultant change in mean arterial pressure [19]. Norepinephrine is mainly an alpha stimulant with some additional beta-stimulant action, so that its major action in cardiogenic shock is to cause vasoconstriction with little inotropic stimulation. Infusion of norepinephrine in cardiogenic shock causes arterial pressure to rise with little change in cardiac output or heart rate [19].

Thus isoproterenol and norepinephrine cause a pressor effect by different mechanisms—isoproterenol mainly by inotropic stimulation and norepinephrine mainly by peripheral vasoconstriction. The effects on the myocardium are therefore quite different, as is shown by Mueller and her colleagues [19] in an elegant series of experiments in instrumented patients with cardiogenic shock. The experiments showed norepinephrine to be more desirable because it improved oxygenation of the ischemic myocardium. This was indicated by a shift from lactate production to lactate extraction as measured in samples of arterial and coronary sinus blood. Isoproterenol caused oxygenation to deteriorate, as indicated by increased lactate content in the coronary sinus blood. In spite of these effects, mortality remained extremely high with either form of treatment.

Use of both of these drugs has now largely been superseded by the use of dopamine and dobutamine, but there is no documentation that either of the new drugs are more effective than norepinephrine or isoproterenol. The effective infusion rate for both dopamine and dobutamine is 200 μg-1 mg/min (2.5 − 10.0 μg/kg/min). Dopamine [20] is the natural precursor of norepinephrine, and in addition to a positive inotropic action has a selective dilating action in certain vascular beds due to stimulation of specific dopaminergic receptors. Its principle advantages are that it combines (a) inotropic stimulation by beta stimulation with (b) improvement in renal blood flow, and (c) it causes less tachycardia than does isoproterenol. Its inotropic effects, but not its peripheral vascular effects, are blocked by propranolol. Like isoproterenol, however, it tends to exacerbate myocardial ischemia, as evidenced by increased lactate production for the ischemic myocardial segments [21]. Also, dopamine may increase left ventricular filling pressure [22], an undesirable effect in patients with shock due to left ventricular failure.

Dobutamine, a synthetic compound formulated to increase cardiac performance selectively without altering heart rate or blood pressure [23], has the advantage over dopamine that it is less likely to increase filling pressure [22], but has the disadvantage that it increases arterial pressure less than dopamine. Thus dopamine would be preferable to dobutamine for the treatment of shock with marked hypotension, but dobutamine is preferred to dopamine for the treatment of all other instances of cardiogenic shock due to left ventricular failure [22].

The relative hemodynamic effects of norepinephrine, isoproterenol, dopamine, and dobutamine, together with those in intraaortic balloon counterpulsation (IABC) are compared in table 44-1. Although optimally, one would tai-

lor the drug regimen to the hemodynamic subset, it is frequently impossible in practice to obtain full hemodynamic data before treatment is commenced. In such instances, choice of the optimum pressor agent is empirical and it is worthwhile to substitute one agent for another if the first agent does not quickly produce the desired clinical effect. When the systolic blood pressure is below 90 mmHg with signs of peripheral hypoperfusion and/or oliguria with the heart rate 100/min or more, the initial choice might be infusion of dopamine at a dose of 200 μg/min, increasing the dose quickly until the systolic blood pressure reached 95 − 100 mmHg and urine flow was >30 ml/h. If the heart rate was slow with hypotension and hypoperfusion (and atropine did not reverse the abnormality) and the patient was not hypovolemic, isoproterenol 1 − 3 μg/min would be the drug of first choice. When signs of pulmonary congestion were more prominent than those of forward failure, the choice would be dobutamine. The use of norepinephrine should be reserved for refractory cases in which an adequate pressor effect could not be obtained with the other drugs.

Other intropic drugs are not of much value or have not yet become established for use in cardiogenic shock. Digoxin is of no value; its measurable inotropic effects after myocardial infarction are much less than those of dobutamine [24]. Its toxic level may be unpredictably low after myocardial infarction particularly when poor tissue perfusion and consequent acute renal failure are also present. Its use in cardiogenic shock is best avoided.

USE OF OTHER DRUGS IN CARDIOGENIC SHOCK

Whereas inotropic and pressor drugs are used for the treatment of forward failure, powerful diuretics are the drugs of choice for treatment of backward failure. Furosemide is the best diuretic, given intravenously in a dose of 40 − 120 mg once or twice daily. Furosemide reduces left ventricular filling pressure without affecting arterial pressure or cardiac output [25]. It should be used in all patients who have clinical or radiologic signs of pulmonary edema. If furosemide 40 mg intravenously does not cause a diuresis, the outlook is poor, but a larger dose should still be tried.

TABLE 44-1. Comparison of agents for the treatment of cardiogenic shock due to acute myocardial infarction

	Norepinephrine	Isoproterenol	Dopamine	Dobutamine	IABC
Heart rate	↑ ↓	↑ ↑	↑	↑ ↓	↓
Arterial pressure	↑ ↑	↑ ↓	↑	↑ ↓	↑
Cardiac output	↑ ↓	↑	↑	↑	↑
Peripheral resistance	↑	↓	↑ ↓	↓	↑ ↓
LVEDP	(?)	(?)	↑ ↓	↓	↓
Myocardial metabolism	Improves	Deteriorates	Deteriorates	(?)	Improves

IBAC, intraaortic balloon counterpulsation.

Reduction of preload and afterload by vasodilating drugs such as sodium nitroprusside has not been widely used in the treatment of cardiogenic shock because of the risk of aggravation of hypotension and consequent reduction in vital organ perfusion. Of 43 patients with severe pump failure due to myocardial infarction reported by Chatterjee et al. [26], 17 were in cardiogenic shock (systolic blood pressure 90 mmHg or less with signs of diminished organ perfusion and pulmonary edema). These patients did in fact show an improvement in hemodynamic measurements (reduced left ventricular filling pressure and increased cardiac index) during nitroprusside infusion so that aggravation of hypotension was not usually a problem. Hospital mortality, however, for the 17 patients remained high at 53%, increasing to 88% after a mean follow-up time for survivors of two years. This was attributed to the severe and permanent destruction of myocardium that had occurred in all patients. The combination of a pressor drug such as dopamine with a vasodilator such as nitroprusside or glyceryl trinitrate seems a logical measure that is worthy of clinical trial, but whatever drug combination is used, long-term mortality is likely to remain high.

THE USE OF INTRAAORTIC BALLOON COUNTERPULSATION

Intraaortic balloon counterpulsation was first described 30 years ago [27], and it has been used in the treatment of complicated myocardial infarction for 20 years. Its place has still not been adequately defined, however, and the results of its use are disappointing. In theory, it is the most logical way, short of left ventricular bypass, to support the acutely failing left ventricle. A balloon of 30- to 40-ml capacity (figure 44-5) is alternately filled and emptied of helium, the cycles of filling and emptying being triggered by an ECG signal so that filling of the balloon coincides with diastole and emptying with systole. The balloon that is attached to the distal end of a no. 7 catheter is inserted through an arteriotomy in the groin or percutaneously [28], and is positioned in the thoracic aorta, just below the arch. The proximal end of the catheter is attached to a console containing the helium supply, pumping mechanism, pressure transducers, and ECG-triggering mechanism. Filling and emptying of the balloon can be adjusted so that emptying occurs at varying times after the R wave, with filling at about the time of the T wave. Precise timing of inflation and deflation is adjusted to obtain the optimal waveform on a pressure signal recorded with a transducer from a brachial artery catheter. The waveform on alternate beats with and without balloon inflation is shown in figure 44-6. Counterpulsation increases diastolic pressure by impeding distal runoff of blood from the aorta during diastole (balloon inflation) and reduces systolic pressure by providing a potential space of 30−40 ml into which the left ventricle can eject during systole (balloon deflation). Optimal pressure levels during counterpulsation are attained by (a) setting the mechanism to pump during alternate beats, (b) adjusting the timing so that diastolic pressure is maximally augmented during pumped beats, and (c) comparing a nonpumped beat with the preceding pumped beat to maximally reduce systolic pressure.

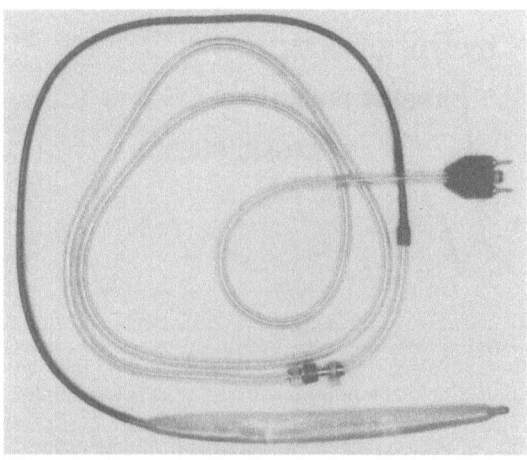

FIGURE 44-5. Intraaortic balloon catheter with connection to helium supply on pumping console. From Churchill Livingstone Ltd., with permission.

Theoretical benefits to the left ventricle of diastolic augmentation by counterpulsation are twofold. First, coronary flow is improved by increasing aortic diastolic pressure; this should improve collateral flow to the infarct and tend to restrict infarct size. Second, left ventricular oxygen requirements should be diminished by reduction of afterload by balloon deflation during left ventricular ejection.

In practice, the hemodynamic effects of balloon counterpulsation during cardiogenic shock are favorable although rather modest. Increase in aortic diastolic pressure is marked, so that diastolic pressure exceeds systolic pressure during pumping (figure 44-6), while mean arterial pressure is increased [29]. After several hours of pumping, cardiac output is increased, while left ventricular filling pressure and heart rate fall [29, 30]. Subjectively, patients usually feel better, although the instrumentation and constant measurements can be uncomfortable and frightening. Complications of counterpulsation can be serious. The most important are ischemia of the leg distal to the femoral arteriotomy and dissection of the aorta, the risks of which can be minimized by careful balloon insertion. Patients having counterpulsation should be heparinized, the leg pulses must be checked frequently, and the balloon removed immediately if necrosis of the leg is threatened.

In general, results of counterpulsation for cardiogenic shock have been disappointing, and few units now advocate its use for the treatment of established shock. The reason is probably that the myocardium has been irreversibly damaged by the time that counterpulsation is started. If counterpulsation could be started during the "preshock" period during which myocardial ischemic injury is progressing but is not yet complete, ischemic myocardium might be salvaged, shock prevented, and mortality reduced. In collaboration with M.F. O'Rourke and colleagues at St. Vincent's Hospital, Sydney, we attempted a randomized trial of counterpulsation in patients seen within 12 h of the onset of infarction, who had left ventricular failure and hypotension but did not yet have fully developed shock [10]. Counterpulsation was started at a mean of 7 h after the onset of chest pain. Seven of 14 treated patients and seven of 16 control patients (standard decongestant and pressor therapy) died. The extent of enzyme rise and clinical disability was similar in treated and control cases. We thought the reason for the absence of any favorable trend toward improvement of prognosis by counterpulsation in "preshock" might have been that intervention at 7 h, although early by many standards, was still too late for salvage of ischemic myocardium to be achieved. For logistic reasons it is very difficult to start counterpulsation much earlier than this. However, percutaneous insertion of balloon catheters [28] might reduce delays and enable counterpulsation to be started immediately after the onset of hemodynamic deterioration in selected cases.

Aortic balloon counterpulsation during infarction is probably best reserved for patients who have a surgically correctable lesion such as ventricular septal rupture or mitral incompetence due to papillary muscle rupture [31]. For patients who do not have these lesions, combination of counterpulsation with emergency revascularization by coronary saphenous vein grafts is a further therapeutic option that is possible only in the largest and best-equipped units. Published results do not justify the widespread use of this combined therapy, although some worthwhile salvage does seem possible with optimum coordination and timing of treatment [32].

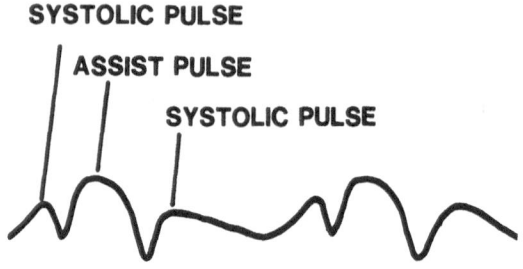

FIGURE 44-6. Form of the arterial pressure wave recorded from the brachial artery when the balloon is set to inflate during alternate cardiac cycles. The first and third systolic pulses, which follow nonassisted beats, show a higher pressure than the second and fourth systolic pulses, which follow assisted beats (systolic unloading). The assist (diastolic) pulses are due to balloon inflation, the brachial artery pressure (reflecting pressure upstream from the balloon) being higher during assisted diastole than during systole. From Churchill Livingstone Ltd., with permission.

References

1. Harnarayan C, Bennett MA, Pentecost BL, Brewer DB: Quantitative study of infarcted myocardium in cardiogenic shock. Br. Heart J 32:728, 1970.
2. Page DL, Caulfield JB, Kastor JA, De Sanctis RW, Sanders CA: Myocardial changes associated with Cardiogenic Shock. N Engl J Med 285:133, 1971.
3. Sharpe DN, Botvinick EG, Shames DM, Schiller MB, Massie BM, Chatterjee K, Parmley WW: The noninvasive diagnosis of right ventricular infarction. Circulation 57:483, 1978.
4. Goldstein JA, Vlakakes GJ, Venier ED, Schiller NB, Tyberg JV, Ports TA, Parmley WW, Chatterjee K: The role of right ventricular systolic dysfunction and elevated intrapericardial pressure in the genesis of low output in experimental right ventricular infarction. Circulation 65:513, 1982.
5. Cohn JN, Guika NH, Broder MI, Limas CJ: Right ventricular infarction: clinical and hemodynamic features. Am J Cardiol 33:209, 1974.
6. Forrester JS, Diamond G, Chatterjee K, Swan HJ: Medical therapy of acute mycardial infarction by application of hemodynamic subsets. N Engl J Med 295:1404, 1976.
7. Topol EJ, Goldschlager N, Posto TA, Dicarlo LA, Schiller NB, Botvinich EH, Chatterjee K: Hemodynamic benefit of atrial pacing in right ventricular myocardial infarction. Ann Intern Med 96:594, 1982.
8. Fox AC, Glassman E, Isom OW: Surgically remediable complications of myocardial infarction. Prog Cardiovasc Dis 21:461, 1979.
9. O'Rourke MF: Subacute heart rupture following myocardial infarction. Lancet 2:124, 1973.
10. O'Rourke MF, Norris RM, Campbell TJ, Chang VP, Sammel NL: Randomized controlled trial of intra-aortic balloon counterpulsation in early myocardial infarction with acute heart failure. Am J Cardiol 47:815, 1981.
11. Norris Rm, Brandt PWT, Caughey DE, Lee AJ, Scott PJ: A new coronary prognostic index. Lancet 1:274, 1969.
12. Weber KT, Janicki JS, Russell RO, Rackley CE: Identification of high risk subsets of acute myocardial infarction: derived from the myocardial infarction research unit cooperative study data bank. Am J Cardiol 41:197, 1978
13. Geddes JS, Adgey AAJ, Pantridge JF: Prevention of cardiogenic shock. Am Heart J 99:243, 1980.
14. Gutovitz AL, Sobel BE, Roberts R: Progressive nature of myocardial injury to selectd patients with cardiogenic shock. Am J Cardiol 41:469, 1978.
15. Rude RE, Muller JE, Braunwald E: Efforts to limit the size of mycardial infarcts. Ann Intern Med 95:736, 1981.
16. Reimer KA, Lowe JE, Rasmussen MM, Jennings RB: The wavefront phenomenon of ischemic cell death. 1. Myocardial infarct size versus duration of coronary occlusion in dogs. Circulation 56:786, 1977.
17. Peter T, Norris RM, Clarke Ed, Heng MK, Singh BN, Williams B, Howell DR, Ambler PK: Reduction of enzyme levels by propranolol after acute myocardial infarction. Circulation 57:1091, 1978.

18. Weinstein J: Treatment of myocardial infarction with intracoronary streptokinase: efficacy and safety data from 209 United States cases in the Hoechst-Roussel registry. Am Heart J 104:894, 1982.

19. Mueller H, Ayres SM, Gregory JJ, Giannelli S, Grace WJ: Hemodynamics, coronary blood flow and myocardial metabolism in coronary shock: response to l-norepinephrine and isoproterenol. J Clin Invest 49:1885, 1970.

20. Goldberg LI: Dopamine: clinical uses of an endogenous catecholamine. N Engl J Med 291: 707, 1974.

21. Mueller HS, Evans R, Ayres SM: Effect of dopamine on hemodynamics and myocardial metabolism in shock following acute myocardial infarction in man. Circulation 57:361, 1978.

22. Francis GS, Sharma B, Hodges M: Comparative hemodynamic effects of dopamine and dobutamine in patients with acute cardiogenic circulatory collapse. Am Heart J 103: 995, 1982.

23. Tuttle RR, Mills J: Dobutamine: development of a new catecholamine to selectively increase cardiac contractility. Circ Res 36:185, 1975.

24. Goldstein RA, Passamani ER, Roberts RA: Comparison of digoxin and dobutamine in patients with acute infarction and cardiac failure. N Engl J Med 303:846, 1980.

25. Dikshit K, Vyden JK, Forrester JS, Chatterjee K, Prakash R, Swan HJ: Renal and extra-renal hemodynamic effects of frusemide in congestive heart failure after acute myocardial infarction. N Engl J Med 288(1)1087, 1973.

26. Chatterjee K, Swan HJC, Kaushik VS, Jobin G, Magnusson P, Forrester JS: Effects of vasodilator therapy for severe pump failure in acute myocardial infarction on short-term and late prognosis. Circulation 53:797, 1976.

27. Kantrawitz A, Kantrawitz A: Experimental augmentation of coronary flow by retardation of the arterial pressure pulse. Surgery 34:678, 1953.

28. Leinbach RC, Goldstein J, Gold HK, Moses JW, Collins MB, Subramanian V: Percutaneous wire-guided balloon pumping. Am J Cardiol 49:1707, 1982.

29. Mueller H. Ayres SM, Giannelli S, Conklin EF, Mazzara JT, Grace WJ: Effect of isoproterenol, l-norepinephrine and intra-aortic counterpulsation on hemodynamics and myocardial metabolism in shock following acute myocardial infarction. Circulation 45:335, 1972.

30. Ehrick DA, Biddle TL, Kronenberg MW, Yu PN: The hemodynamic response to intra-aortic balloon counterpulsation in patients with cardiogenic shock complicating acute myocardial infarction. Am Heart J 93:274, 1977.

31. Gold HK, Leinbach RC, Sanders CA, Buckley MJ, Mundth ED, Austen WG: Intra-aortic balloon pumping for ventricular septal defect or mitral regurgitation complicating acute myocardial infarction. Circulation 47:1191, 1973.

32. Pierri MK, Zema M, Kligfield P, McCabe J, Hoover E, Gay W, Subramanian V: Exercise tolerance in late survivors of balloon pumping and surgery for cardiogenic shock. Circulation (Suppl 1) 62:I-138, 1980.

45. SURGICAL TREATMENT OF CARDIOGENIC SHOCK FOLLOWING ACUTE MYOCARDIAL INFARCTION

Martha J. Radford

Harry R. Phillips

Cardiogenic shock complicates 10%−20% of acute myocardial infarctions, and mortality is high [1]. Attempts to lessen morbidity and mortality following acute myocardial infarction have been focused on patients in shock. Those patients who develop "mechanical" complication of infarction represent a subgroup that clearly benefits from prompt surgical intervention. Surgical intervention in other patients with shock after acute infarction remains controversial [2].

Cardiogenic shock is defined by clinical observations. Arterial hypotension (systolic arterial pressure less than 90 mmHg—higher in hypertensive patients) must be accompanied by evidence of poor tissue perfusion: low urine output, peripheral vasoconstriction, and/or altered mental status. Thus, the diagnosis of cardiogenic shock implies observation of the patient over a period of time, usually at least several hours. Interventions designed to improve the prognosis of cardiogenic shock may be effective only if applied early in the course of hemodynamic deterioration. If successful in reversing the downward hemodynamic trends, such interventions may cloud the definition of cardiogenic shock by preventing it. This chapter, then, may be more properly titled "Surgical treatment of *patients at high risk for* cardiogenic shock following acute myocardial infarction."

R.M. Califf and G.S. Wagner (eds.), ACUTE CORONARY CARE: Principles and Practice. Copyright © 1985. Martinus Nijhoff Publishing, Boston/Dordrecht/Lancaster.

Differential Diagnosis of Shock following Myocardial Infarction

The reasons for cardiogenic shock following myocardial infarction are listed in table 45-1. Prompt identification of the cause of cardiogenic shock is vital to subsequent management. Clues to the presence of a surgically correctable mechanical defect may be gleaned from physical findings, electrocardiogram, and chest radiograph (table 45-2). Shock following first myocardial infarction should heighten the clinician's suspicion of the presence of a mechanical defect. The finding of a new systolic murmur with or without a thrill alerts the clinician to the possible presence of ventricular septal rupture or acute mitral regurgitation, but the presence of shock may render the murmur unimpressive or even absent [3−5]. Although patients with acute mitral regurgitation may demonstrate relatively more pulmonary congestion compared with patients with ventricular septal rupture, there is no physical finding that can clearly differentiate these two mechanical causes of cardiogenic shock.

Precise diagnosis and subsequent management require invasive hemodynamic monitoring using the balloon-tipped pulmonary artery catheter; it is our view that any patient with hemodynamic deterioration suggesting impending cardiogenic shock after myocardial infarction should have

TABLE 45-1. Causes of cardiogenic shock after acute myocardial infarction

Cause	Treatment
Hypovolemia Right ventricular infarction	Volume expansion
Ventricular septal rupture Free-wall rupture Severe mitral regurgitation (papillary muscle rupture or infarction)	Prompt surgical correction of mechanical defect
Multiple myocardial infarction Large myocardial infarction Infarct expansion Infarct extension Postinfarct ischemia	Pharmacologic and counterpulsation support Role of urgent revascularization and/or infarctectomy controversial

such a catheter placed. The most important findings at pulmonary artery catheterization (table 45-3) are low pulmonary capillary wedge pressure (less than $12-16$ mmHg, indicating relative hypovolemia and/or the presence of right ventricular infarction) or the presence of a stepup in the oxygen saturation at the level of the right ventricle (>5 mg%, indicating presence of ventricular septal rupture). The presence of large V waves in the pulmonary capillary wedge tracing suggests the presence of severe mitral regurgitation; this finding may, however, be present in patients without severe mitral regurgitation [6], and may be absent in patients who have significant mitral regurgitation [7]. A rise in pulmonary capillary wedge pressure coincident with chest pain and/or ECG changes in the postinfarct patient strongly suggests the presence of ischemia, infarct extension, or infarct expansion.

Echocardiography may be helpful in elucidating the cause of cardiogenic shock. A large, hypocontractile right ventricle with or without paradoxical septal motion supports the diagnosis of right ventricular infarction, but may also be observed in patients with ventricular septal rupture. Injection of microcavitations may not demonstrate the presence of right-to-left shunt, because, following acute septal rupture, flow is predominantly left to right. Exploration of the interventricular septum using pulsed Doppler echocardiography may demonstrate an area of left-to-right or to-and-fro flow. However, since the defect may consist of multiple small dissections or fenestrations through the septum, it is often difficult to sample adequately all areas of the septum, and a negative study does not rule out septal rupture. In patients with acute mitral regurgitation (MR), left atrial enlargement may not always be present. If a flail mitral leaflet can be visualized, this is a very helpful finding, but its absence does not rule out significant MR. Retrograde systolic flow through the mitral valve can usually be appreciated using Doppler echocardiography, but its degree is difficult to evaluate. A large akinetic or dyskinetic area of myocardium supports the diagnosis of large infarction with or without infarct expansion, but does not exclude the presence of a mechanical defect. The coexistence or well-preserved left ventricular ejection (as estimated by echocardiography or radionuclide angiography) with cardiogenic shock suggests the presence of either right ventricular infarction or a mechanical defect.

The diagnosis of free-wall rupture requires special comment. The usual clinical course is sudden catastrophic decompensation during the first week after myocardial infarction in a patient who has been previously stable. Decompensation has been noted to occur in association with recurrence of chest pain [8, 9], possibly related to infarct expansion [10]. Echocardiography may be helpful [9]; the demonstration of fluid (blood) in the pericardial space suggests free-wall rupture.

Treatment of Shock due to Hypovolemia or Right Ventricular Infarction

The treatment of cardiogenic shock due to relative hypovolemia has been considered in chapter 44. If, however, shock persists after replacement

TABLE 45-2. Clinical findings that may help elucidate the cause of cardiogenic shock

Cause	History	PE	ECG	CXR
Hypovolemia		No JVD No rales No S3		No PVR
Right ventricular infarct		JVD No rales unless ex- tensive LV infarct also present	IMI or PMI ST elevations in right-sided chest leads	Normal unless extensive LV infarct also present May have pleural effusions
Ventricular septal rupture	First infarct Hypertension (25%)	JVD Rales may appear later +/− S3 Murmur +/− Thrill	AMI = IMI Transmural infarct	May be normal, show increased blood flow or pulmonary edema
Free-wall rupture	Pain at time of hemodynamic deterioration	JVD Little pulmonary congestion	Transmural infarct	
Acute mitral regurgitation		JVD CHF prominent Murmur +/− Thrill	IMI > AMI Infarct not necessarily transmural	PVR or pul- monary edema
Multiple infarctions	Previous MI(s)	S3	Old MI(s)	PVR or pul- monary edema
Large single myocardial infarction	First infarct	S3	Usually, AMI with leads involved	PVR or pul- monary edema
Infarct expansion	Occasionally, pain after infarct No rise in CPK	New S3	Transmural MI New or persistent ST elevations	May be normal
Infarct extension	Pain after infarct Rise in CPK	New S3	Transmural or non- transmural MI New ECG evidence of infarction	May be normal
Ischemia	Pain after infarct No rise in CPK	Transient S3 with pain	+/− Ischemic changes with pain, possibly in coronary bed remote from that involved in infarct	May be normal

PE, physical examination; ECG, electrocardiogram; CXR, chest radiograph; JVD, jugular venous distention; PVR, pulmonary vascular redistribution; IMI, inferior myocardial infarction; AMI, anterior myocardial infarction; PMI, posterior myocardial infarction; CPK, creatine phosphokinase.

TABLE 45-3. Findings at pulmonary artery catheterization in patients with shock following myocardial infarction

Relative hypovolemia	PCW < 12 mmHg, RAP < PCW
RV infarction	RAP ≥ PCW, PAS depression May mimic pericardial tamponade
Ventricular septal rupture	Stepup in O_2 saturation at level of right ventricle
Free-wall rupture	May mimic tamponade
Acute mitral regurgitation	PCW > 18 mmHg, large V waves usually present
Multiple infarctions Large single myocardial infarction	PCW > 18 mmHg
Infarct expansion Infarct extension Ischemia after infarct	May have rise in PCW coincident with chest pain and/or ECG changes

of intravascular volume so that pulmonary capillary wedge pressure is 14−18 mmHg, another cause for shock must be investigated. Vigorous volume replacement to maintain left-sided filling pressures is also the treatment for right ventricular (RV) infarction (see chapter 21); occasional patients may require a temporary transvenous pacemaker to correct bradycardia or heart block. Surgical intervention is rarely necessary for shock due to RV infarction; however, one patient has been reported who developed tricuspid regurgitation in association with right ventricular infarction, and required tricuspid valve replacement to be weaned from inotropic and intraaortic counterpulsation support [11].

Ventricular Septal Rupture

Ventricular septal rupture (VSR) following transmural anterior or inferior myocardial infarction leads to cardiogenic shock in at least half of patients with this complication [3]. Shock may occur almost immediately after rupture, or onset may be more gradual. There are virtually no survivors of cardiogenic shock in the setting of postinfarct VSR treated medically [3, 9]. Afterload reduction or intraaortic counterpulsation do not allow more than transient improvement in hemodynamic status [12], probably because both right and left ventricular dysfunction are present [3, 13].

Surgical repair of VSR is recommended for these patients as soon as possible (within hours)

after onset of hemodynamic deterioration. Perioperative mortality for patients in frank cardiogenic shock is high (70%−80%) [3, 4, 9]. This mortality rate is decreased (to 20%−30%) by surgical intervention at the first sign of hemodynamic deterioration, prior to the development of frank shock [3, 14, 15]. Preoperative cardiac catheterization with coronary arteriography (with or without intraaortic counterpulsation as a stabilizing maneuver) is considered optional by some investigators [15], since no hemodynamic parameter predicts survival [3] and results of catheterization cannot be used to choose which patients will benefit from surgical repair of VSR. We recommend preoperative cardiac catheterization to define coronary artery anatomy so that bypass grafting can be performed if deemed necessary.

Several advances in surgical technique have improved survival of patients who suffer myocardial infarction complicated by septal rupture: approach to the septal defect via a left ventriculotomy through the infarct, infarctectomy, and patch replacement of myocardium removed [15]. These techniques were first used for surgical repair of posterior septal rupture [16]. A high incidence of dehiscence or rupture of either the septal repair or the infarcted posterior free wall had been associated with high operative mortality when the defect was repaired using techniques developed for congenital ventricular septal defects [16]. These innovations have been adapted for repair of anterior septal rupture as well [14].

The long-term prognosis of patients surviving repair of septal rupture following myocardial infarction is excellent. In the series with the longest follow-up period (at least four years), only one cardiac death and one nonfatal myocardial infarction have been reported in a group of 17 survivors [3]. No survivors reported disabling cardiac symptoms. The reasons for this favorable long-term prognosis are uncertain. No preoperative hemodynamic parameter, including ejection fraction, pulmonary capillary wedge pressure, or ratio of right-to-left shunt, has been shown to correlate with perioperative survival [3, 14]. The group of patients with VSR has less severe coronary artery disease than do other patients with cardiogenic shock after infarction [3]. Single-vessel coronary disease is found in one-fourth of patients with VSR [3, 14], and survival has not been reported (in the small number of patients studied) to depend on whether coronary artery bypass surgery is performed [3, 14]. Another possible explanation for the favorable functional results in these patients may be that replacement of infarcted myocardium by prosthetic material leads to a more stable ventricular structure, perhaps preventing infarct expansion.

Free-wall Rupture

Sudden shock and death usually quickly follow rupture of the free wall of either ventricle. Occasionally, however, rupture is "subacute," that is, there is time to make the diagnosis. Intraaortic counterpulsation may temporarily stabilize the patient, but prompt surgical intervention is the only successful treatment of shock due to free-wall rupture. Repair involves buttressing the infarcted and ruptured free wall with Dacron felt, with or without infarctectomy. About 50% of patients who undergo repair of free-wall rupture survive, and prognosis in survivors is excellent, perhaps for the same reasons as for ventricular septal rupture [8, 9, 18].

Acute Mitral Regurgitation

From 15% to 20% of patients who develop acute mitral regurgitation (MR) following myocardial infarction will also develop cardiogenic shock [19]. Acute MR follows inferior infarction more frequently than anterior infarction, and is usually, but not always, associated with rupture of the body or head of a papillary muscle. A relatively small nontransmural myocardial infarction may be responsible for the papillary muscle dysfunction or rupture [4, 19], and cardiogenic shock may occur in the presence of a relatively well-preserved ejection fraction. In patients with normal or mildly depressed ventricular function and marked MR, hemodynamic deterioration may be ascribed to disruption of the valve. In patients with markedly depressed ejection fraction and MR, left ventricular dysfunction, changes in ventricular architecture, and disruption of the valvular apparatus may all play a role in hemodynamic deterioration.

In general, cardiac catheterization with coronary angiography is advised for patients with acute MR so that coronary anatomy and left ventricular function may be defined. Intraaortic counterpulsation can be used to stabilize the patients so that catheterization may be carried out more safely.

Long-term survival of medically managed patients with ruptured papillary muscle is extremely rare, and once hemodynamic deterioration to cardiogenic shock has supervened, mortality approaches 100% [5] unless successful surgical intervention can be accomplished. Afterload reduction therapy and intraaortic balloon counterpulsation will stablize some patients [12], but the majority of those in shock will require surgery. Although reported series do not always clearly distinguish patients in shock from those not in shock, the operative mortality for patients in shock is probably 25%−50% [4, 19] versus 2%−30% for those not in shock [4, 20]. The only hemodynamic predictor of long-term survival is the left ventricular ejection fraction [4, 19]. As with ventricular septal rupture, any delay in surgery after onset of cardiogenic shock increases the end-organ damage due to poor tissue perfusion and increases the perioperative morbidity and mortality.

Both mitral valve repair and mitral valve replacement have been advocated for postinfarct mitral regurgitation. Valve replacement in the postinfarct patient is considered a more challenging procedure than valve replacement for rheumatic heart disease [20]. The small left atrium makes exposure of the valve ring more difficult, and the lack of annular thickening, and proximity of the sewing ring to necrotic myocardium, may make the prosthesis less stable. Some surgeons have advocated mitral valve repair for these patients [21], but this practice has not been universally adopted.

The long-term prognosis of patients surviving postinfarct mitral valve replacement has not been as good as that following repaired septal rupture, and depends most critically on the preoperative ejection fraction [19]. Since mortality in patients who have been followed long term is primarily cardiac, coronary artery bypass grafting to jeopardized areas of myocardium at the time of valve replacement has been advocated by most groups. If aneurysmectomy is required at the time of valve replacement, perioperative and long-term survival are less likely [22].

Surgical Treatment of Shock following Myocardial Infarction in Patients without a Mechanical Defect

Although indications for surgical treatment of shock associated with mechanical defects following myocardial infarction are clear, the advisability of and indications for surgery in patients with shock without a mechanical defect are controversial. Surgical intervention in patients with shock and no mechanical defect after infarct has been suggested in two situations. First, some patients who have been stabilized by pharmacologic and counterpulsation support may benefit from coronary angiography and revascularization of all jeopardized areas of myocardium. The assumption inherent in this approach is that at least part of the left ventricular dysfunction leading to shock is due to ischemia, and is therefore reversible by revascularization. Although the recurrence of chest pain and ECG changes may suggest ischemia, it is often difficult to determine the degree to which reversible ischemia plays a role in the generation of cardiogenic shock in any one patient. Infarct extension (further irreversible infarction) and infarct expansion, as well as reversible ischemia, may lead to hemodynamic deterioration associated with chest pain and ECG changes (see chapter 46). Published series have

advocated either surgery for all patients who could not be weaned from counterpulsation support [23], or have applied subjective criteria of "operability," depending on the coronary anatomy [24]. Either approach has been reported to improve survival compared with medical treatment (table 45-4A), but patients who come to operation after a trial of medical therapy represent a selected subgroup of patients with cardiogenic shock, and medical and surgical series may not represent comparable populations. Factors that predict survival have not been firmly established, but may include first myocardial infarction, coronary anatomy favorable for revascularization, short duration of shock, relatively young age, and absence of comorbid condition (diabetes, infection, renal failure, etc.).

The second possible indication for surgical intervention in patients with cardiogenic shock is a large first single infarction that may have undergone expansion either early [24] or late [2] after onset of the infarction. Such patients may benefit from prolonged intraaortic counterpulsation support [24], but a few patients have been reported to require urgent infarctectomy [2, 24].

In recent years, there has been increasing interest in early reperfusion of acutely infarcted myocardium using thrombolytic agents (see chapter 34), percutaneous transluminal coronary angioplasty, or surgical reperfusion (see chapter 35). Such early intervention has been shown to improve left ventricular function [23, 28] and, in a few patients, appears to have reversed the course of cardiogenic shock [23, 30]. In the Western Washington collaborative trial of intracoronary streptokinase, improved survival of those in cardiogenic shock was found in the treated group versus the control group [31].

Emergency surgical revascularization in the early hours of myocardial infarction is an appealing concept, both to reverse shock and possibly to prevent shock. The investigators in Spokane and Des Moines have suggested that complications of infarction including shock may occur less frequently in patients who undergo acute myocardial revascularization [32, 33]. In addition, outcome for patients who are hypotensive at the time of revascularization (there usually is not enough time to establish the diagnosis of shock prior to surgery) may be improved over that of similar

TABLE 45-4. Surgical treatment of shock following myocardial infarction (without mechanical defect present)

	No. of patients	Time to operation	Hospital survival
A. Surgery following trial of medical therapy			
Massachusetts General Hospital [23] (1969–1976)	34	Prob. days	17 (50%)
Loyola [25] (1971–1976)	17	8 h– 18 days	7 (41%)
Cornell [26] (1976–1978)	20	4 h– 7 days	11 (55%)
Stoneybrook [24] (1976–1980)	12	1 day–7 weeks	8 (67%)
B. Immediate surgical revascularization			
Spokane [32] (1971–1980)	22	1.5 h–14 h	20 (91%)
Des Moines [33] (1975–1981)	26	1 h–30 h	20 (77%)

patients treated either medically or by late revascularization (table 45-4B). However, hypotensive patients who undergo early revascularization may represent a different group than those operated on after a trial of medical therapy for cardiogenic shock. Early in the course of myocardial infarction, hypotensive patients may include some whose hemodynamic status might spontaneously improve, as well as some who might die during medical therapy for shock and would not otherwise have become operative candidates.

Summary

An aggressive surgical approach to patients with cardiogenic shock because of a mechanical defect following acute myocardial infarction results in improved survival. A patient with a new systolic murmur, or with hemodynamic deterioration following acute myocardial infarction (particularly first infarction), should have a flow-directed pulmonary artery catheter placed as soon as possible. Urgent echocardiographic study, if available, can also be helpful in diagnosis. Intraaortic counterpulsation may offer temporary stabilization, and allow cardiac catheterization to be performed under more favorable conditions.

If oximetry demonstrates the presence of ventricular septal rupture, surgical repair should be accomplished as soon as possible. Medical management will rarely stabilize these patients, surgical technique is well developed, and long-term postoperative prognosis is excellent. If free-wall rupture is present, urgent surgical repair represents the patient's only hope for survival. Patients with acute mitral regurgitation should also be considered for early operative repair, especially those whose ejection fraction is in the normal range or slightly below. Although patients with left ventricular ejection fractions less than 35% and significant mitral regurgitation have a poorer operative survival, the potential benefits of mitral valve replacement probably outweigh the risks.

Some patients with cardiogenic shock without a mechanical defect may also benefit from surgical intervention, but choosing the appropriate patients is difficult and criteria are controversial. If potentially reversible ischemia is responsible for depression of cardiac function, revascularization may improve prognosis. In a few patients with cardiogenic shock following a first large transmural myocardial infarction, infarctectomy may increase the chance of survival.

References

1. Scheidt S, Ascheim R, Killip T: Shock after acute myocardial infarction: a clinical and hemodynamic profile. Am J Cardiol 26:556–564, 1970.

2. Gunnar RM, Loeb HS: Shock in acute myocardial infarction: evolution of physiologic therapy. J Am Coll Cardiol 1:154–163, 1983.

3. Radford MJ, Johnson RA, Daggett WM, Fallon JT, Buckley MJ, Gold HK, Leinbach RC: Ventricular septal rupture: a review of clinical and physiologic features and an analysis of survival. Circulation 64:545–553, 1981.

4. Killen DA, Reed WA, Wathanacharoen S, Beauchamp G, Rutherford B: Surgical treatment of papillary muscle rupture. Ann Thorac Surg 35:243–248, 1983.

5. Nishimura RA, Schaff HV, Shub C, Gersh BJ, Edwards WD, Tajik AJ: Papillary muscle rupture complicating acute myocardial infarction: analysis of 17 patients. Am J Cardiol 51:373–377, 1983.

6. Bethea CF, Peter RH, Behar VS, Margolis JR, Kisslo JA, Kong Y: The hemodynamic simulation of mitral regurgitation in ventricular septal defect after myocardial infarction. Cathet Cardiovasc Diagn 2:97–104, 1976.

7. Johnson RA, Haber E, Austin WG (eds): The practice of cardiology. Boston: Little, Brown and Company, 1980, p 355.

8. Nunez L, De la Llana R, Sendon JL, Coma I, Aguado MG, Larrea JL: Diagnosis and treatment of subacute free wall ventricular rupture after infarction. Ann Thorac Surg 35:525–529, 1983.

9. Feneley MP, Chang VP, O'Rourke MF: Myocardial rupture after acute myocardial infarction: ten year review. Br Heart J 49:550–556, 1983.

10. Lorell B, Leinbach RC, Pohost GM, Gold HF, Dinsmore RE, Hutter AM, Pastore JO, De Sanctis RW: Right ventricular infarction. Am J Cardiol 43:465–471, 1979.

11. Korr KS, Levenson H, Bough EW, Gheorghiade M, Stone J, McEnany MT, Shulman RS: Tricuspid valve replacement for cardiogenic shock after severe right ventricular infarction. JAMA 244:1958–1960, 1980.

12. Gold HK, Leinbach RC, Sanders CA, Buckley MJ, Mundth ED, Austin WG: Intraaortic balloon pumping for ventricular septal defect or mitral regurgitation complicating acute myocardial infarction. Circulation 47:1191–1196, 1973.

13. Goldman ME, Horowitz SF, Miller J, Mindich B, Teichholz LE: Recovery of right ventricular function following repair of acute ventricular septal defect. Chest 82:59–63, 1982.

14. Kopf S, Meshkor A, Lake HH, Graeme L, Geha AS: Changing patterns in the surgical management of ventricular septal rupture after myocardial infarction. Am J Surg 143:465–472, 1982.

15. Murphy TE, De Buer A: Surgical management of ventricular septal defects following myocardial infarction. In: Moran JM, Michaelis LL (eds) Surgery for the complications of myocardial infarction. New York: Grune and Stratton, 1980, pp 191–210.

16. Daggett WM: Surgical technique for early repair of posterior ventricular septal rupture. J Thorac Cardiovasc Surg 84:306–312, 1982.

17. Hochreiter C, Goldstein J, Corer JS, Tyberg T, Goldberg HL, Subramanian V, Rosenfeld I: Myocardial free-wall rupture after acute infarction: survival aided by percutaneous intraaortic balloon counter-pulsation. Circulation 65:1279–1282, 1982.

18. Windsor HM, Chang VP, Shenahan MX: Postinfarction cardiac rupture. J Thorac Cardiovasc Surg 84:755–761, 1982.

19. Radford MJ, Johnson RA, Buckley MJ, Daggett WM, Leinbach RC, Gold HK: Survival following mitral valve replacement for mitral regurgitation due to coronary artery disease. Circulation (Suppl 1) 60:39–47, 1979.

20. Collins JJ, Cohn LH, Koster JK, Van Devanter SH: Mitral valve replacement for regurgitation following infarction: choice of prosthesis, techniques, results. In: Moran JM, Michaelis LL (eds) Surgery for the complications of myocardial infarction. New York: Grune and Stratton, 1980, pp 177–184.

21. Kay JH, Mendez M, Zubrate P, Yokoyama T, Vanstrom N, Gharavi M: Long term results of operations for mitral insufficiency secondary to coronary artery disease. Cardiovasc Clin 12:75–80, 1982.

22. Planz EJ, Kouchoukos NT: Surgical correction of multiple mechanical defects and revascularization following infarction. In: Moran JM, Michaelis LL (eds) Surgery for the complications of myocardial infarction. New York: Grune and Stratton, 1980, pp 185–190.

23. Mundth ED: Surgical treatment of cardiogenic shock and of acute mechanical complications following myocardial infarction. Cardiovasc Clin 8:241–263, 1977.

24. Hines GL, Mohtashemi M: Delayed operative intervention in cardiogenic shock after myocardial infarction. Ann Thorac Surg 33:132–138, 1982.

25. Johnson SA, Scanlon PJ, Loeb HS, Moran JM, Pifarre R, Gunnar RM: Treatment of cardiogenic shock in myocardial infarction by intraaortic balloon counterpulsation and surgery. Am J Med 62:687−692, 1977.

26. Subramanian VA, Roberts AJ, Zema MJ, Abel RM, McCabe JC, Hoover E, Kligfield P, Gay WA: Cardiogenic shock following acute myocardial infarction: late functional results after emergency cardiac surgery. New York State J Med May: 947−952, 1980.

27. De Wood MA, Heit J, Spores J, Berg R Jr, Selinger SL, Rudy LW, Hensley GR, Shields JP: Anterior transmural myocardial infarction: effects of surgical coronary reperfusion on global and regional left ventricular function. J Am Coll Cardiol 1:1223−1234, 1983.

28. Stack RS, Phillips HR, Grierson DS, Behar VS, Kong Y, Peter RH, Swain JL, Greenfield JC: Functional improvement of jeopardized myocardium following intracoronary streptokinase infusion in acute myocardial infarction. J Clin Invest 72:84−95, 1983.

29. Salvi A, Klugman S, Della Grazia E, Maras P, Camerini F: Myocardial reperfusion after acute occlusion of the left main coronary artery. Am J Cardiol 51:1791, 1983.

30. Mathey D, Kuck KH, Remmecke J, Tilsner V, Bleifeld W: Transluminal recanalization of coronary artery thrombosis: a preliminary report of its application in cardiogenic shock. Eur Heart J 48:4, 1980.

31. Kennedy JW, Ritchie JL, Davis KB, Fritz JK: Western Washington randomized trial of intracoronary streptokinase in acute myocardial infarction. N Engl J Med 309:1477−1481, 1983.

32. Berg R Jr, Selinger SL, Leonard JJ, Grunwald RP, O'Grady WP: Surgical management of acute myocardial infarctions. Cardiovasc Clin 12:61−74, 1982.

33. Phillips SJ, Zeff RH, Kongtahwam C, Skinner JK, Iannone L, Brown TM, Wickemeyer W, Gordon DF: Surgery for evolving myocardial infarction. JAMA 248:1325−1328, 1982.

46. MYOCARDIAL INFARCT EXPANSION AND EXTENSION

Judith S. Hochman

Bernadine Healy Bulkley

Many studies have shown that long-term prognosis after myocardial infarction is related closely to myocardial function, which is determined primarily by the size and location of the infarct. Infarct extension and expansion are two complications occurring early in the postinfarct period that can significantly increase the *functional* infarct size—the former by increasing the mass of necrotic tissue and the latter by thinning and dilating the infarcted zone. Extension and expansion have been associated with increased mortality and morbidity both early and late after myocardial infarction. This chapter examines these complications in terms of incidence, pathogenesis, time course, consequences, and therapeutic implications.

Infarct Expansion

All infarcts, even those of similar size, are not equal. Infarcts involving similar amounts of myocardium may have markedly different effects on the shape of the left ventricle. For example, an infarct involving 20% of the left ventricle may lead to no appreciable distortion of the left ventricular geometry, or may lead to a regional dilatation in the injured region, and consequently altered geometry plus net cavity enlargement. This latter change in left ventricular topography results from infarct expansion, the process by which the infarct zone thins and dilates [1, 2] (figure 46-1). This process is distinct from infarct

extension: in extension there is new necrosis causing increased infarct size; in expansion there is dilatation of the infarcted tissue without new necrosis. Expansion leads to an effective or functional increase in infarct size as measured by percent involvement of left ventricular circumference.

INCIDENCE

The incidence of expansion in one autopsy series examining patients who died within 30 days of an acute myocardial infarction was 59% [1], with one-third of all patients having moderate to severe expansion. Infarct expansion can be identified echocardiographically by observing wall thinning and lengthening of the infarcted segment. A clinical study of sequential two-dimensional echocardiograms in patients with acute Q-wave infarcts identified expansion in 29% [3]. The disparity between the 29% incidence of expansion in the echocardiographic study and the 59% prevalence in the autopsy study may be due in part to the inclusion in the latter of only patients who died within 30 days of infarction. The existence of this disparity suggests that infarct expansion may contribute to or may be a predictor of postinfarction mortality.

The incidence of expansion in experimental models varies greatly among different species. Coronary ligation in the dog, which has rich collaterals, creates infarcts that are extensively nontransmural and have a low incidence of spon-

R.M. Califf and G.S. Wagner (eds.), ACUTE CORONARY CARE: Principles and Practice. Copyright © 1985. Martinus Nijhoff Publishing, Boston/Dordrecht/Lancaster.

taneous expansion [4]. However, large, fully transmural infarcts, created by ligation plus embolic plugs to occlude small vessels and thus block collateral inflow, have an 80% incidence of expansion in this species [4]. Infarcts created in rats by ligation of the left coronary artery are large and fully transmural, and have an incidence of spontaneous expansion of 60%−70%. One-third of these infarcts exhibit severe expansion [2], similar to the human autopsy experience.

PATHOLOGY

Infarct expansion is characterized grossly by reduction of wall thickness in the infarct area, frequently to 50% or less the dimension of uninfarcted walls. Dilatation of the infarct zone produces distortion of the left ventricular topography with alteration of the relative positions of the ventricular landmarks, such as the anterior and posterior papillary muscles. Infarct expansion can result in a discrete bulge of the left ventricular wall; when scar is laid down, this becomes a true left ventricular aneurysm [5].

One can see thin wavy fiber changes by histology early after myocardial infarction, which may represent fiber stretching. Subsequently, polymorphonuclear leukocytes enter the infarct zone, and disintegrate in the areas of necrosis by days 3−4. No removal of necrotic myocardium has occurred by this point, nor have interstitial connective tissue cells proliferated. Therefore the histologic basis of early infarct expansion appears to be stretching and slippage of sheets of necrotic myocardial cells [6]. After one week, macrophages infiltrate the infarct, and subsequently collagen is laid down. In the experimental rat model, one can demonstrate that infarct expansion begins before resorption of tissue, but then progresses in severity as macrophages remove necrotic myocardial cells [2].

TIME COURSE

Paradoxic bulging with systolic lengthening of an ischemic or infarcted zone can occur very rapidly after occlusion of a coronary artery [7−9]. This can be termed "ischemic expansion" and, if the ischemia is reversed, the paradoxic wall motion may be reversed as well. If the ischemia is not reversed, and transmural infarction occurs, infarct expansion can result. The precise time at

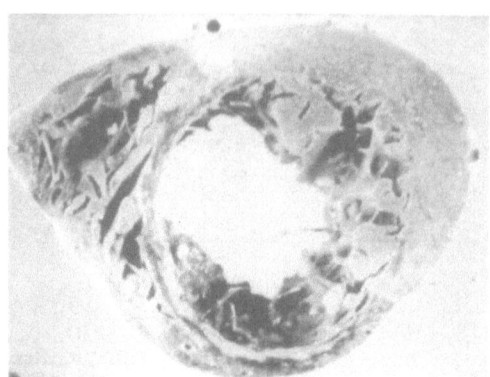

FIGURE 46-1. The heart of an autopsied patient who died of cardiogenic shock. A transmural anteroseptal infarct occurred that involves more than 40% of the left ventricle. Disproportionate dilatation in the region of the transmural infarct is evident, and accounts for overall dilatation of the heart.

which the thinning and dilatation of an infarcted area becomes an irreversible morphologic change is not known.

The autopsy series [1], which identified and measured infarct expansion, showed that the expansion occurred within a few days after the infarction, and was severe by day 5. The echocardiographic studies have shown that expansion can be seen by day 3 after infarction [3, 10] and that it progresses in severity during the first few weeks. After this time period, the infarcted segment continues to expand slightly, but remodeling of the left ventricle is also due to stretching of the uninfarcted segment [11].

Experimental models have confirmed this time course. Rats undergoing left coronary artery ligation develop infarct expansion by 24 h, when only early histologic changes of myocardial necrosis (such as hypereosinophilia) are present [2] (figure 46-2); 80% of animals developing expansion had done so by 24 h. The severity of expansion, however, increases between days 1 and 5 when the inflammatory process is maximum and necrotic myocardial cells are being lysed, but fibrous tissue has not yet been formed. Additionally, early remodeling of uninfarcted left ventricular wall occurs [12]. Both the prevalence and severity of expansion plateau at one week when the reparative process of fibroblast proliferation and collagen formation begins. It should be noted that the histopathologic evolution of infarct heal-

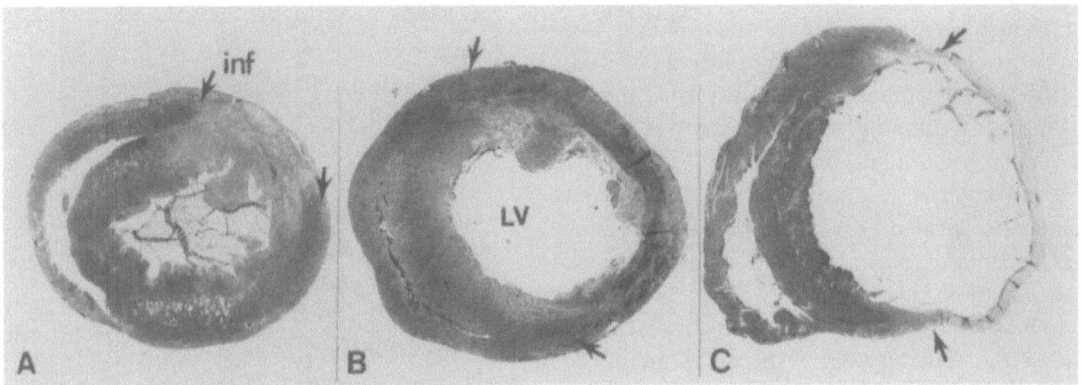

FIGURE 46-2. Infarct expansion in an experimental model of transmural myocardial infarction. (A) A two-day-old transmural infarct (arrows) in which normal cardiac shape is preserved. (B) A large two-day-old infarct with mild to moderate expansion and thinning and regional dilatation of the infarct zone. (C) A large seven-day-old infarct that has undergone marked expansion. From Hochman and Bulkley [2], with permission.

ing is accelerated two- to threefold in rats as compared with humans. Studies in dogs also suggest that infarct expansion occurs early, with immediate diastolic and systolic lengthening of the ischemic zone, and progresses with time.

There are two phases of histopathologic changes: before and after tissue resorption begins. Expansion during the early phase is related to dynamic factors that affect wall stress, such as intracavity volume and pressure and adrenergic tone, and to tensile wall characteristics. The expanded infarct undergoes further changes when edema, inflammation, lysis of fibers, reperfusion, and collagen deposition occur, which may all play important roles in determining the ultimate severity of changes in left ventricular shape. Factors that delay the healing process, such as antiinflammatory drugs, may be detrimental [13, 14].

RISK FACTORS

What causes infarcts to expand? Infarct size has been shown to affect the occurrence and severity of infarct expansion, with larger infarcts being more likely to expand [1, 2, 4]. A critical infarct size of approximately 10% of the left ventricle is

necessary for expansion [4]. This relationship between size and degree of expansion is, however, quite variable, and infarct size alone is of poor predictive value in determining the severity of expansion [2]. Patients with infarct expansion assessed serially by two-dimensional echocardiography had similar serum creatine kinase (CK) peaks as concurrent patients without infarct expansion [3]. Transmurality is a prerequisite for severe expansion, with few nontransmural myocardial infarctions expanding [1, 2, 4]. The extent of transmurality, or the degree to which the epicardium is involved, affects the degree of expansion, with a preserved rim of epicardium tending to inhibit expansion [2, 4].

Infarct location also affects clinical and pathologic sequelae [3, 9, 15−19], including expansion. Anterior infarcts have a tendency to expand, and form aneurysms or rupture more frequently than inferior or posterior myocardial infarctions.

Hemodynamic factors may play a role in determining early infarct expansion before an inflammatory response is begun. Studies in dogs show that increasing intraventricular pressure causes progressive infarct lengthening [20]. A clinical correlate—that hypertension predisposes to postinfarction ventricular aneurysm formation—was recognized years ago [21].

The effect of early exercise on the infarct zone has been of longstanding interest. Both retrospective autopsy series and small experimental studies showed such detrimental effects as left ventricular aneurysm formation and cardiac rupture [21−24]. More recent experimental studies have shown conflicting results regarding the effect of exercise early after myocardial infarction on infarct thinning and dilatation. These differences may be a function of the mode of exercise. In one study in which a small number of rats were subjected to swimming after myocardial infarction, infarct thinning was demonstrated [25]. In several other studies, however, dogs and rats exercised on the treadmill were found to have no increase in incidence of left ventricular aneurysms [26], extent of infarct thinning, or left ventricular dilatation [27].

The second phase of infarct expansion occurs when the inflammatory response is mounted, necrotic myocardial fibers are lysed and resorbed, and the infarct zone undergoes sequential changes in tensile characteristics. At this time, one might expect factors that slow the rate of healing of the myocardial infarction to aggravate expansion. Steroids have been shown to cause delayed healing, infarct thinning, and aneurysm formation [13]. More recently, the nonsteroidal antiinflammatory agent, indomethacin, administered to dogs soon after coronary artery ligation caused marked infarct wall thinning [14]. The mechanism, whether via its effect on the inflammatory reaction or via alterations in coronary blood flow [28], is unclear.

CONSEQUENCES

Infarct expansion has been associated with numerous adverse clinical and pathologic findings (table 46-1). Expansion causes a functional increase in infarct size for a given amount of myocardial necrosis by increasing the percent of left ventricular area and circumference involved by infarction. Early regional left ventricular dilatation can lead to subsequent global dilatation [11]. Patients with early infarct expansion have been found to have increased incidences of worsening Killip class and early mortality [3, 11]. Patients with expansion more frequently had recurrent angina and congestive heart failure [11].

Recurrent ST elevation 3−5 days after myocardial infarction may represent infarct expansion [1] as well as extension. Additionally, infarct expansion may compromise the coronary blood flow to myocardium surrounding the infarct zone with resultant infarct extension [1]. Furthermore, increased left ventricular diameter resulting from expansion [5, 11] would be expected to increase wall stress and therefore myocardial oxy-

TABLE 46-1. Consequences of infarct expansion

1. Functional increase in infarct size
2. Left ventricular dilatation
   A. Regional
   B. Global
3. Congestive heart failure
4. Left ventricular aneurysm
   A. Arrhythmias
   B. Systemic emboli
   C. Congestive heart failure
5. Cardiac rupture
6. Increased mortality
7. Infarct extension (?)
8. Postinfarction angina (?)

gen consumption, predisposing to ischemia in other distributions supplied by critically stenosed coronary arteries. There is a strong association between infarct expansion and cardiac rupture: in one autopsy series of patients who died within three weeks of infarction, 43% with expansion had ruptured compared with 2% of patients without expansion [29]. Lastly, infarct expansion provides the morphologic substrate for the development of left ventricular aneurysm [5], with their associated complications of congestive heart failure, arrhythmias, and systemic emboli.

Infarct Extension

In contrast to infarct expansion, extension results in a larger total mass of infarcted tissue. Extension occurs as a second discrete event following the acute myocardial infarction. It can develop in patients with otherwise uncomplicated infarcts, significantly increasing their morbidity and mortality. Most importantly, there are reasons to believe extension may be preventable.

INCIDENCE

The incidence of infarct extension varies greatly, depending upon the patient population and the definition. An autopsy series [1] studying patients dying within 30 days of infarction showed histologically proven extension in 13 (17%) of 76 cases; 11 (14%) had clinical extensions. There were three additional patients in whom extensions were clinically diagnosed, but who had only infarct expansion at postmortem examination.

Clinical studies report incidences of extension ranging from 9% to 86% [30–37]. The highest estimate [34], based on the inclusion of all patients with reelevation of ST segments, was reduced from 86% to 57% if CK reelevation was required. Infarct expansion may have accounted for some instances of ST reelevation without true extension. The lowest estimate [35], based only on patients in Killip classes I or II with new chest pain, ECG changes, and CK reelevation, increased from 9% to 13% if suspected extension was included. Buda et al. prospectively studied infarct extension by repeated CK determinations and found a 31% incidence of extension at 5.9 ± 0.3 days [36].

PATHOLOGY

Pathologically, infarct extension is diagnosed when the histology shows varying stages of infarct healing with foci of necrosis more recent than the original myocardial infarction [1]. This may take several forms, with extension either at the lateral margins of the infarct or subepicardially [38]. The former generally occurs in transmural infarcts (usually with totally occluded coronary arteries) and the latter in subendocardial infarcts (usually with subtotally occluded arteries). Frequently, contraction band necrosis can be seen at the adjacent lateral or epicardial borders of an older infarct supplied by the same coronary artery, suggesting recent reperfusion injury [1]. This may either result from variation in collateral blood flow or from spontaneous reperfusion of a previously totally occluded coronary artery. Patients who have a stuttering clinical course of infarction, with prolonged pain and CK elevation, have heterogeneous infarcts composed of dead, viable, and variously injured tissue [30]. In patients with a stuttering course, extension accounted for 15% – 24% of the total infarct size [30, 38]. Infarction can also occur in myocardium supplied by a distant diseased coronary artery [30, 39].

The amount of myocardium at risk for "extension" can be theoretically defined. When a coronary artery is occluded by acute thrombosis and blood flow is interrupted, only the myocardium in the distribution of that vessel is the "risk region" in jeopardy (figure 46-3). Using the distribution of the epicardial coronary arteries, an anatomic risk region can be defined. Almost always the myocardial infarction lies within the risk region, but does not involve the entire region at risk. The amount of the region at risk that undergoes infarction varies among patients. This variation is due to both differing myocardial oxygen demands and blood supply of the region at risk. The blood supply includes (a) the antegrade flow through the area of critical stenosis, and (b) retrograde flow via collaterals. Although antegrade flow may be totally interrupted by an acute thrombotic occlusion in the early phase of infarction, in some patients there may be spontaneous thrombolysis or thrombus retraction that reestablishes flow (see chapter 6). Retrograde blood flow via collaterals in the human heart varies greatly from patient to patient with regard to both presence and extent of development, but the extent of collateral development and variation in flow are likely important determinants of the amount of the region at risk for infarcts, and, consequently, the amount at risk for recurrent ischemia and extension. Propagation of thrombus retrograde with occlusion of branch epicardial vessels or antegrade with interruption of collateral inflow are other possible mechanisms for infarct extension.

TIME COURSE

Infarct extension is usually diagnosed as a discrete clinical event after the first 24 h, when a patient has become pain free after the acute myocardial infarction. The time course of this event varies in different series [30–45], with a range of mean times from infarct to extension of 1.25–6.8 days. This type of extension can occur as early as 20 h [30] or as late as 17 days [1]. There is a second type of infarct extension, characterized by a stuttering course of myocardial infarction, where pain and CK elevation continue for several days. Of 40 patients in one series [30], 16 had prolonged CK elevation (peak beyond 30 h) with a slow rise and flat peak of the curve; 11 patients continued to have pain for 2–3 days. Postmortem examination in five of these patients showed heterogeneous healing stages. This syndrome of stuttering and progressive infarction, frequently resulting in death from cardiogenic shock, has been well described [38, 40, 41].

RISK FACTORS

Few studies have attempted to identify which patients are at risk for infarct extension, and could therefore have been identified early. McNeer et al. [33] showed that early extension (within four days after myocardial infarction) could not be predicted, but extension in the late postmyocardial infarction period occurred more often in patients with congestive heart failure, hypertension, and diabetes mellitus. Hutchins and Bulkley's [1] study suggested that patients with infarct expansion were at risk for subsequent infarct extension. Others have suggested that hypotension predisposes to new necrosis at the infarct margins, resulting in a vicious cycle leading to cardiogenic shock [1, 38–42]. Patients with subendocardial infarction are at greater risk for extension than patients with transmural infarctions [37].

Of patients who develop early postinfarction angina, 24% proceed to have subsequent new areas of myocardial necrosis, i.e., infarct extension [43, 44]. Early postinfarction angina developing within the first 7–10 days may occur in as many as 20%–25% of patients who present with acute myocardial infarction. Persistent pain after acute myocardial infarction is a poor prognostic sign, in part because it frequently portends extension. There are two important sources of early postinfarction ischemia. Viable myocardium surrounding the infarct itself and lying within the original risk region of the occluded coronary artery may be the source of persistent ischemic pain (figure 46-3). Such ischemia is particularly important in patients with relatively small nontransmural infarcts, but with a relatively large risk region with severely compromised blood flow. Patients after acute myocardial infarction may be susceptible to a second type of ischemia, namely, ischemia at a distance [43, 44]. In this situation the ischemia and electrocardiographic changes appear to be originating from myocardium outside the region of the acute infarct (figures 46-4 and 46-5), and thus a new vascular territory is in jeopardy.

When ischemia at a distance develops within a few days of acute myocardial infarction, it is likely that it is related to the acute infarct event. There are at least four possible mechanisms that relate the remote ischemia to the initial acute

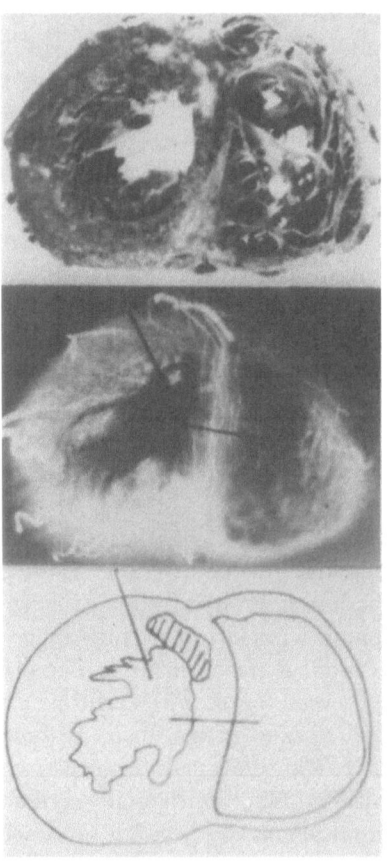

FIGURE 46-3. Infarct size and risk region. (Top) A transverse section of the left ventricle showing an anteroseptal infarct. (Center) Postmortem angiogram demarcates the anatomic risk region defined by the distribution of the left anterior descending coronary artery downstream from the occlusion of the left anterior descending artery. (Bottom) The zone of infarction (hatched area) within the anatomic risk region. The infarct almost always lies within, but involves less than, the anatomic risk region. From Bulkley [46], with permission.

coronary occlusion: (a) The original myocardial injury imposes increased demands on noninfarcted myocardium, causing it to have enhanced oxygen requirements and demand-related ischemia. (b) Multivessel spasm is occurring or resistance alterations in the vascular beds associated with the infarct after net flow. (c) The distant area is supplied by a critically narrowed vessel that is connected by collaterals to the vessel responsible for the infarct; abrupt interruption of blood flow

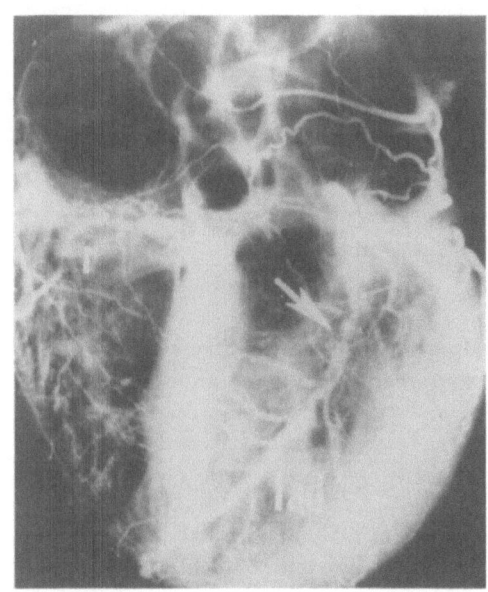

FIGURE 46-4. Ischemia at a distance. Postmortem angiograms from a patient who died with ischemia at a distance, showing the recently occluded left anterior descending coronary artery (arrow) and an "old" totally occluded right coronary artery (R) that is dependent on collaterals. After anteroseptal infarction, ischemia developed in the distribution of the right coronary artery. From Schuster and Bulkley [43], with permission.

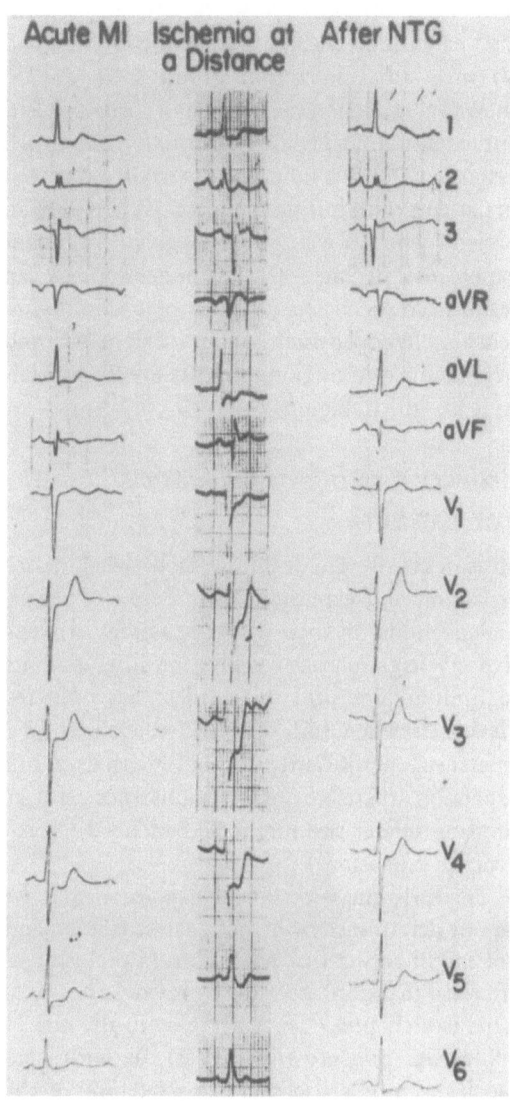

FIGURE 46-5. Ischemia at a distance. After an inferior infarct, postinfarction angina developed and was associated with transient ST-segment depression in a distant vascular territory, the anterior wall. The electrocardiographic changes resolved when the pain was relieved by nitrates and consequently the episode reflected a transient episode of the new ischemia and not "infarct pain." From Schuster and Bulkley [43], with permission.

into the infarct would cause decreased flow into distant myocardium. (d) Given a critical stenosis in the distant bed and vasodilation in the peri-infarct ischemic tissue, a "steal" could occur via collaterals from the distant bed into the myocardium within the original risk region. The latter two explanations would suppose an interdependence of the two vascular beds via well-developed collaterals.

Regardless of the etiology, postinfarction angina represents an early postinfarct complication that is associated with enhanced morbidity and mortality, and it identifies a population at risk for infarct extension.

CONSEQUENCES

Infarct extension results in a larger total infarct size. Numerous studies have shown that large infarct size correlates with poor left ventricular function and increased early and late mortality. Infarct extension correlates temporally with oc-

currence or worsening of congestive heart failure [1], and can cause hypotension, atrioventricular and intraventricular conduction disturbances, and atrial and ventricular arrhythmias [32]. Prognosis is significantly worse in patients with infarct extension. The low-risk (Killip classes I and II) myocardial infarction group studied [35] showed a 91% one-year survival in patients without extension, and a 76% survival for those with extension. A 40% inhospital mortality was seen in patients with infarct extension, versus 20% in patients who had a single CK peak with a monoexponential decline [30]. Cardiogenic shock can result from the vicious cycle of infarction, hypotension, hypoperfusion, infarct extension, and irreversible dysfunction, and has a 90% mortality [39, 40] (table 46-2).

Prevention of Infarct Expansion and Extension

Measures to prevent or inhibit myocardial infarct expansion and extension must be based on an understanding of their pathophysiology. Extensive investigation has centered on interventions to limit infarct size; this subject has been reviewed elsewhere [42, 45, 46] (see chapter 34). Infarct size significantly correlates with degree of expansion; therefore interventions successful at limiting infarct size might be beneficial in preventing expansion.

The early phase of infarct expansion may be largely determined by hemodynamic factors, and one might expect that reductions in preload and afterload that decrease wall stress would be beneficial (see chapter 43). A decrease in the rate of ventricular pressure rise (dP/dt), as with beta blockade, might also decrease stretching of the infarcted zone (see chapter 41). These hypotheses remain to be tested. Measures that preserve an epicardial rim, or increase the tensile strength of the infarct zone, should theoretically limit the degree of expansion as well.

Given their effects on infarct healing, antiinflammatory drugs such as indomethecin and steroids should probably be avoided after myocardial infarction until further knowledge is gained. Interventions that decrease myocardial oxygen consumption or increase blood supply should reduce the incidence of infarct extension. Importantly, subgroups at higher risk, such as patients with postinfarction angina, should be identified and aggressive measures, perhaps in-

TABLE 46-2. Consequences of infarct extension

1. Congestive heart failure
2. Atrioventricular blocks
3. Conduction disturbances
4. Atrial and ventricular arrhythmias
5. Cardiogenic shock
6. Increased mortality

cluding revascularization (see chapter 35), may be warranted in these groups.

References

1. Hutchins GM, Bulkley BH: Infarct expansion versus extension: two different complications of acute myocardial infarction. Am J Cardiol 41: 1127, 1978.
2. Hochman JS, Bulkley BH: Expansion of acute myocardial infarction: an experimental study. Circulation 65:1446, 1982.
3. Eaton LW, Weiss JL, Bulkley BH, Garrison JB, Weisfeldt ML: Regional cardiac dilatation after acute myocardial infarction: recognition by two-dimensional echocardiography. N Engl J Med 300:57, 1979.
4. Eaton LW, Bulkley BH: Expansion of acute myocardial infarction: its relationship to infarct morphology in a canine model. Circ Res 49:80, 1981.
5. Hochman JS, Bulkley BH: The pathogenesis of left ventricular aneurysms: an experimental study in the rat model. Am J Cardiol 50:83, 1982.
6. Weisman H, Bush D, Kallman C, Weisfeldt M, Bulkley B: Cellular mechanism of infarct expansion: stretch vs. slippage [abstr]. Circulation 68: III-253, 1983.
7. Tennant R, Wiggers CJ: The effect of coronary occlusion on myocardial contraction. Am J Physiol 112:351, 1935.
8. Vokonas PS, Pirzada FA, Hood WB: Experimental myocardial infarction. XII. Dynamic changes in segmental mechanical behavior of infarcted and noninfarcted myocardium. Am J Cardiol 37: 853, 1976.
9. Nicklas JM, Becker LC, Bulkley BH: Repeated brief coronary occlusion: effects on regional shape, function and ultrastructure. Clin Res 30:209A, 1982.
10. Asinger RW, Mikell FL, Elsperger J, Hodges M: Evidence of left ventricular thrombosis after acute

transmural myocardial infarction. N Engl J Med 305:297, 1981.

11. Erlebacher JA, Weiss JL, Kallman C, Weisfeldt ML, Bulkley BH: Late effects of acute infarct dilation on heart size. Am J Cardiol 49:1120, 1982.

12. Weisman HF, Bush DE, Bulkley BH: Remote remodeling of normal myocardium due to infarct expansion: distortion at a distance. Clin Res 31:II, 226A, 1983.

13. Bulkley BH, Roberts WC: Steroid therapy during acute myocardial infarction: a cause of delayed healing and of ventricular aneurysm. Am J Med 56:244, 1974.

14. Hammerman H, Schoen FJ, Kloner RA: Early myocardial infarct expansion due to indomethacin administration. Circulation 66:II-83, 1982.

15. Schuster EH, Griffith LSC, Bulkley BH: Preponderance of acute proximal left anterior descending coronary lesions in fatal myocardial infarction: a clinicopathologic study. Am J Cardiol 47:1189, 1981.

16. Strauss HD, Sobel BE, Roberts R: The influence of occult right ventricular infarction on enzymatically estimated infarct size, hemodynamics, and prognosis. Circulation 62:503, 1980.

17. Bulkley BH: Site and sequelae of myocardial infarction. N Engl J Med 305:337, 1981.

18. Lorell B, Leinbach RC, Pohost GM, Gold HK, Dinsmore R, Hutter Am Jr, Pastore JO, De Sanctis RW: Right ventricular infarction. Am J Cardiol 43:465, 1979.

19. Wei JY, Hutchins GM, Bulkley BH: Papillary muscle rupture in fatal acute myocardial infarction: a potentially treatable form of cardiogenic shock. Ann Intern Med 90:149, 1979.

20. Nicklas JM, Maughan WL, Ciuffo A, Sunagawa K, Becker LC, Weisfeldt ML, Bulkley BH: The effect of varied systolic load on acute infarct expansion. Clin Res xx 1983.

21. Schlichter J, Hellerstein HK, Katz LN: Aneurysm of the heart: a correlative study of one hundred and two proved cases. Medicine 33:43, 1954.

22. Sutton DC, Davis MD: Effects of exercise on experimental cardiac infarction. Arch Intern Med 48:1118, 1931.

23. Wessler S, Zoll PM, Schlesinger MJ: The pathogenesis of spontaneous cardiac rupture. Circulation 51:334, 1944.

24. Jetter WW, White PD: Rupture of the heart in patients in mental institutions. Ann Intern Med 21:783, 1944.

25. Kloner RA, Kloner JA: The effect of exercise on healing of myocardial infarction. Circulation 64: IV-99, 1981.

26. Thompson PL, Jenzer HR, Lown B, Lohrbauer LA: Exercise during acute myocardial infarction: an experimental study. Cardiovasc Res 7:642, 1973.

27. Hochman JS, Bulkley BH: The effect of exercise on acute myocardial infarction in rats. Clin Res xx 1983.

28. Friedman PL, Brown EJ, Gunther S, et al: Coronary vasoconstrictor effect of indomethacin in patients with coronary-artery disease. N Engl M Med 305:1171, 1981.

29. Schuster EH, Bulkley BH: Expansion of transmural myocardial infarction: a pathophysiologic factor in cardiac rupture. Circulation 60:1532, 1979.

30. Mathey D, Bleifeld W, Buss H, Hanrath P: Creatine kinase release in acute myocardial infarction: correlation with clinical, electrocardiographic, and pathological findings. Br Heart J 37:1161, 1975.

31. Madias JE, Venkataraman K, Hood WB Jr: Precordial ST-segment mapping. I. Clinical studies in the coronary care unit. Circulation 52:799, 1975.

32. Kronenberg MW, Hodges M, Akiyama T, Roberts DL, Ehrich DA, Biddle TL, Yu PN: ST-segment variations after acute myocardial infarction: relationship to clinical status. Circulation 54:756, 1976.

33. McNeer JF, Wallace AG, Wagner GS, Starmer CF, Rosati RA: The course of acute myocardial infarction: feasibility of early discharge of the uncomplicated patient. Circulation 51:410, 1975.

34. Reid PR, Taylor DR, Kelly DT, Weisfeldt ML, Humphries JO, Ross RS, Pitt B: Myocardial-infarct extension detected by precordial ST-segment mapping. N Engl J Med 290:123, 1974.

35. Fraker TD Jr, Wagner GS, Rosati RA: Extension of myocardial infarction: incidence and prognosis. Circulation 60:1126, 1979.

36. Buda AJ, Macdonald IL, Dubbin JD, Orr SA, Strauss HD: Myocardial infarct extension: prevalence, clinical significance and problems in diagnosis. Am Heart J 105:744, 1983.

37. Marmor A, Sobel BE, Roberts R: Factors presaging early recurrent myocardial infarction ("extension"). Am J Cardiol 48:603, 1981.

38. Alonso DR, Scheidt S, Post M, Killip T: Pathophysiology of cardiogenic shock, quantification

of myocardial necrosis, clinical pathologic and electrocardiographic correlations. Circulation 48: 588, 1973.

39. Blumgart HL, Schlesinger MJ, Zoll PM: Angina pectoris, coronary failure and acute myocardial infarction: the role of coronary occlusion and collateral circulation. JAMA 116:91, 1941.

40. Page DL, Caulfield JB, Kastor JA, De Sanctis RW, Sanders CA: Myocardial changes associated with cardiogenic shock. N Engl J Med 285:133, 1971.

41. Gutovitz AL, Sobel BE, Roberts R: Progressive nature of myocardial injury in selected patients with cardiogenic shock. Am J Cardiol 41:469, 1978.

42. Sobel BE, Braunwald E: The management of acute myocardial infarction. In: Braunwald E (ed)

Heart disease: a textbook of cardiovascular medicine. Philadelphia: WB Saunders, 1980, p 1372.

43. Schuster EH, Bulkley BH: Ischemia at a distance after acute myocardial infarction: a cause of early post-infarction angina. Circulation 62:509, 1980.

44. Schuster EH, Bulkley BH: Early post-infarction angina: ischemia at a distance and ischemia in the infarct zone. N Engl J Med 305:1101, 1981.

45. Maroko PR, Kjekshus JK, Sobel BE, Watanabe T, Covell JW, Ross J Jr, Braunwald E: Factors influencing infarct size following experimental coronary artery occlusions. Circulation 43:67, 1971.

46. Bulkley BH: Pathophysiology of coronary artery disease. Baylor Coll Med Cardiol Ser 6:12, 1983.

47. PERICARDITIS FOLLOWING
MYOCARDIAL INFARCTION

Walter L. Floyd

The occurrence of infarction involving the subepicardial layer of myocardium may be accompanied by a localized inflammation of the overlying pericardium. On occasion, this pericardial reaction will extend beyond the area of infarction to become a more extensive or generalized pericarditis with associated serosanguineous effusion. In patients dying of transmural infarction the incidence of pericarditis observed at autopsy is high [1]. However, since the diagnosis of clinically significant pericarditis is based on observations that may be transient and easily overlooked, the frequency in nonfatal infarction is unknown.

PCIS versus PMIP

Pericarditis may occur either as an early complication of myocardial infarction or remote from the acute event during, or even beyond, the recovery period. The syndrome associated with the delayed form of pericarditis was first described by Dressler and has been considered as a separate entity from the pericardial inflammation associated with acute infarction [2]. The latter syndrome has clinical features identical with the illness occurring after a variety of cardiac injuries including viral pericarditis, all forms of cardiac surgery, blunt and penetrating cardiac trauma, and myocardial perforation at the time of cardiac catheterization or pacemaker implantation. The similarity in the clinical characteristics and timing of pericarditis in patients experiencing these various cardiac injuries suggests a common etiology. Blood in the pericardial space preceding the

onset of symptoms is a common feature and possibly is the agent that incites later pericardial inflammation. Heart-reactive antibodies have been described in the blood of patients after both myocardial infarction and cardiac surgery. A definite autoimmune mechanism has not been established, however, since there is not a strong correlation between the presence of antibodies and the occurrence of pericarditis remote from the injury [3]. The possibility of activation of a virus by the injury, which in turn results in an autoimmune illness, has been suggested by Engle and co-workers [4]. Although pericarditis occurring remote from a myocardial infarction may occur more frequently in patients recognized as having pericarditis at the time of acute infarction [5], it should be considered the same as that which occurs following various forms of cardiac injury. It is best considered under the term *postcardiac injury syndrome* (PCIS) [6]. Such a distinction is likewise important in prognosis and therapy. The occurrence of pericarditis associated with the acute phase of infarction may then be described under the term *postmyocardial infarction pericarditis* (PMIP).

Postmyocardial Infarction Pericarditis

PMIP occurs 2−6 days after the onset of a myocardial infarction and characteristically resolves, or at least becomes clinically inapparent, within several days. The diagnosis is dependent primarily on the observation of a pericardial friction rub. The rub may be transient, lasting only a

R.M. Califf and G.S. Wagner (eds.), ACUTE CORONARY CARE: Principles and Practice. Copyright © 1985. Martinus Nijhoff Publishing, Boston/Dordrecht/Lancaster.

matter of hours, and may be quite localized rather than being heard over the entire precordium. Commonly the extra cardiac sound does not have a typical "three component" character but may have only one or two components during each cardiac cycle. Frequently it is an incidental auscultatory finding that is not associated with symptoms. Such a variability in occurrence, timing, duration, and association with symptoms makes it difficult to estimate the frequency of PMIP. The presence of PMIP probably does not modify prognosis [7], but since it tends to occur in the presence of larger infarcts, higher rates of morbidity and mortality are associated.

The pain of PMIP is characteristically pleuritic, with or without an accompanying friction rub. Thus, close questioning and examining the patient with continuing or recurring pain within the week after infarction is important in making a distinction between pericarditis and myocardial ischemia. Pericarditis is usually a benign, self-limited problem whereas continued myocardial ischemia has grave prognostic implications that have resulted in an increasing frequency of early surgical intervention in the acute phase of the illness (see chapter 46). Accurately distinguishing between these two causes of pain can save the patient unnecessary diagnostic procedures or even inappropriate surgery.

Cardiac tamponade during PMIP is rare except in the presence of anticoagulant therapy. The observation of neck vein distention, positive Kussmaul's sign, or paradoxical pulse is much more commonly the result of right ventricular infarction than of pericarditis (see chapter 21).

Apart from the pattern of pain and the presence of a friction rub, there is little available to the clinician for diagnosing PMIP. Elevation of white blood cell count and erythrocytes edimentation rate is not distinctive from that occurring with the myocardial infarction itself. The persistence of ST-segment or T-wave changes on the electrocardiogram in the early stages of infarction obscures or modifies changes that may result from pericarditis. The degree of pericardial effusion is seldom large and is not distinctive by echocardiography.

In general, the therapy of PMIP is dependent on the severity of pain. Since pain is of relatively short duration, the use of analgesics is sufficient in most patients. Aspirin 600–900 mg q6h or indomethacin 25–50 mg q6h may be used as necessary. In more refractory cases, oral or intravenous steroids will provide prompt and dramatic relief of pain. Indeed, the relief of pericardial pain within hours after the administration of intravenous steroids may be used as a therapeutic trial to distinguish pericarditis from continued myocardial ischemia. If a steroid compound is employed, its use should be brief with nonsteroid drugs being substituted when initial pain relief is achieved.

Postcardiac Injury Syndrome

PCIS usually appears 2–3 weeks after cardiac injury, though, on occasion, it may first appear as late as 60–90 days after infarction. If the syndrome occurs within the first week after injury it must persist beyond that time period to be distinguished from PMIP. The syndrome is relatively rare, occurring in less than 5% of patients with myocardial infarction, but it tends to recur in more than 50% of cases. Multiple recurrences have been observed for more than five years.

PCIS is distinguished by pleuritic pain that occurs in over 90% of patients. Fever, myalgia or a pericardial friction rub occur in two-thirds of patients. A pleural friction rub is less common, being observed in less than 50% of patients. The chest x-ray is abnormal in the majority of patients. The most common finding is mild to moderate pleural effusion. The presence of pericardial effusion is confirmed in roughly one-half of the patients by an enlarged cardiac silhouette and is easily identified by echocardiography. Parenchymal pulmonary infiltrates occur with equal frequency and commonly lead to an erroneous diagnosis of pneumonia.

Leukocytosis, mild anemia, and an elevated sedimentation rate are common laboratory observations. The electrocardiogram may show new ST-segment or T-wave changes, but residual abnormalities of the previous infarction are likely to obscure such observations, and these changes are difficult to distinguish from those occurring with recurrent ischemia. Pericardial and pleural fluid is serosanguineous in appearance and has the laboratory characteristics of an exudate.

Though significant pericardial effusion is present in the majority of patients, cardiac tamponade is uncommon and is more likely to occur in patients on long-term anticoagulant therapy. With tamponade, compromise of cardiac output may occur rapidly and the clinician should be prepared to perform pericardiocentesis promptly. The occurrence of subsequent restrictive pericarditis is likewise rare, but its occurrence should be considered if congestive heart failure occurs beyond the time of recovery from the myocardial infarction. Radionuclide angiography showing relative preservation of myocardial function in the presence of congestive heart failure may be helpful in making the distinction between pericardial restriction and myocardial dysfunction.

Therapy of PCIS is dependent on the severity of symptoms or evidence of hemodynamic compromise. The majority of patients with milder degrees of pain and fever will require only relief of pain and suppression of inflammation with aspirin, indomethacin, or other newer nonsteroidal antiinflammatory drugs. Therapy should be continued for 10–14 days, followed by gradual tapering of doses, the rapidity of which is dependent on the recurrence of symptoms. The patient should be advised of the high probability of recurrence even for extended periods of time, because multiple courses of therapy may be necessary before final spontaneous remission occurs.

The use of oral or parenteral steroid compounds should be avoided, if possible, and reserved for the patients having severe and refractory pain or showing evidence of significant tamponade. When such therapy is necessary an attempt should be made to limit the use of steroids to the initial days of treatment and to depend on the nonsteroidal compounds for the longer-term therapy. Since relapse occurs irrespective of the type of therapy, multiple recurrences should not lead one to consider that treatment with nonsteroidal drugs had failed, and therefore, to institute long-term use of steroid compounds. With time, final spontaneous remission usually will occur and the development of steroid dependence will serve only to compound the patient's illness. Additional simple measures during recurrence such as bed rest or other activity modification and short-term use of nonhabituating analgesic drugs should not be overlooked. The emotional support provided to the patient discouraged by a relapsing and prolonged illness is likely to be the most important therapy that the clinician may provide and avoid iatrogenic factors that may compound and actually prolong the illness.

References

1. Roberts WC, Spray TL: Pericardial heart disease: a study of its causes, consequences and morphologic features. Cardiovasc Clin 7:11–65, 1976.
2. Dressler W: The post myocardial infarction syndrome: a report of forty-four cases. Arch Intern Med 103:28–42, 1959.
3. Kaplan MH, Frengley JD: Autoimmunity to the heart in cardiac disease. Am J Cardiol 24:459–473, 1969.
4. Engle MA, Gay WA Jr, McCabe J, et al: Postpericardiotomy syndrome in adults: incidence, autoimmunity and virology. Circulation (Suppl 2) 64:56–60, 1981.
5. Toole JC, Silverman ME: Pericarditis of acute myocardial infarction. Chest 67:647–653, 1975.
6. Stetzner T, King TE Jr, Antony V, Sahn SA: Postcardiac injury syndrome: help in diagnosis. J Respir Dis 4:27–32, 1983.
7. Niachos AP, McKendrick CS: Prognosis of pericarditis after myocardial infarction. Br Heart J 35:49–54, 1973.

48. PREPARATION OF THE PATIENT, FAMILY AND STAFF FOR IMMINENT DEATH ON A CORONARY CARE UNIT

Ginette Ferszt

Phyllis Taylor

In Ecclesiates 3 it is written, "To everything there is a season and a time to every purpose under the heavens. A time to be born and a time to die. A time to laugh and a time to weep. A time to sew and a time to reap . . . ." This passage beautifully describes the balance of living, a balance drastically disturbed by unexpected death, which is often experienced as a psychological crisis.

As health professionals, we are called to assist the patient and family through this experience. Although death is inevitable, frequently death in the coronary care unit (CCU) is untimely and finds the patient and family unprepared. How can we best help the person who has had a life-threatening myocardial infarct? How can we be helpful to the family? How can we help ourselves? One way that we can be especially helpful is by preparing the patient, family, and staff for the probability of death.

The Patient

It may be quite difficult to prepare the patient for the inevitability of death, especially in a critical care setting. The emotions released by the trauma of the circumstances can block her or his ability to cope.

The word that usually best describes the experience of the patient in the CCU is *fear*: fear of pain, fear of being alone, fear of loss, fear of losing one's control, and fear of the unknown. The patient is additionally burdened by environmental factors that can be frightening. Men in particular may find it difficult or even unacceptable to express their fears.

The use of adequate analgesia to control physical pain is vital in preparing a patient for the probability of death. Emotional pain may also be immobilizing because it produces a high level of anxiety. Statements like "You look frightened," "This must be very frightening for you," or "You look worried" can facilitate a level of communication with the patient that may reduce the emotional pain. As caregivers, we can offer an *acknowledgment* of the patient's experience; we may not be able to prevent death, but we can be present and comforting, and not seem to abandon the patient. In high-stress situations for the patient, the caregiver should be the initiator of communication.

Spiritual pain is another dimension of the patient's suffering. Often this pain is expressed in questions like "How can this be happening to me?" "What did I do to deserve this?" "Is God really a loving and just God?" Offering to pray with the patient can be very helpful in alleviating some of the spiritual pain. Make sure that religious rituals are carried out. The Sacrament of the Sick (Last Rites) for Roman Catholics can

R.M. Califf and G.S. Wagner (eds.), ACUTE CORONARY CARE: Principles and Practice. Copyright © 1985. Martinus Nijhoff Publishing, Boston/Dordrecht/Lancaster.

can provide comfort. One Jewish woman described how members of her family held up her dying father's hands so he could bestow the ritual blessing on the children, since his dying was on a Friday evening, the Sabbath. Being able to sing or chant, have laying on of hands, or whatever is important to that particular patient can be most helpful.

The authors have sometimes described to patients the experiences that others have told them related to dying. These were people who had had cardiac arrests and had been resuscitated successfully. There have been common threads in all of the experiences we have heard, themes of feeling tremendously loved and being without pain, and these have been comforting to our patients who are now facing imminent death.

Another pain that patients have shared with us is that of loneliness and isolation. In response to this, we have tried to work with hospital administration to get permission for a member of the family, a friend, or clergy to be with the patient continually, after they begin the actual dying process. We teach the family how dying might physically appear so that it might not be so mysterious and terrifying. We encourage the family to talk to the patient, to touch, to kiss, to do anything that feels comfortable and appropriate within that family. Children, given good preparation, can be included at this time. It is very important that the staff respect the cultural, national, and religious contexts of the patient and family, and that we do not impose our own contexts on them. Too often the different ways of expressing grief and fear expressed by the patient and family cause the staff to have anxieties. We translate our own anxieties into rules and regulations that might be very alienating to people we want to help.

Through all of this preparation of the patient for imminent death, the caregiver should try to assure that hope is never lost. When asked by a patient if he/she is dying, we have learned that an appropriate response might be that we don't really know, although we do know that they are very ill, but that we hope and pray that they will get better. We also encourage the patient to live each moment to its fullest and to let family and friends know how much they are loved—*now*—

since the "heart attack" has taught how fragile life is.

The Family

Unexpected death can be a catastrophe that has an impact on a patient's family for months or years after the event [1]. Preparation for the probability of death gives the family some time to do important work that may help them in the bereavement period. A family member may need that moment to say "I'm sorry," or "I love you," or "I'll miss you." These brief but valuable moments may be a way to provide some healing in future months. If families are not prepared for the imminent death of the patient, they may feel cheated or robbed of precious time that they will never have again.

It is common for families to feel shock and fear with a sudden change in a patient's status. Some families may feel responsible for the patient's condition, because of something they did or did not do. "If I had only made him see the doctor earlier," "I knew we shouldn't have moved this month, it was just too much stress." Families have their long list of "If only . . ." that can add to their appropriate experience of emotional pain and suffering.

In ambivalent relationships, guilt may accompany anger at the patient for past or present events. Feelings of powerlessness and helplessness may exist because of the reality of being unable to change the situation [2]. The environment of the CCU may add additional stress, with the stimulation of technical equipment, which is frightening and overwhelming. Families are forced to trust professionals whom they do not know or with whom they do not have a comfortable relationship [2].

As a result, it is not surprising to see family members express intense feelings and emotions. These feelings are all-encompassing, often expressed as anger, fear, anxiety, and ambivalence [2]. Families may be demanding, hungering for information, consequently bombarding staff with questions. They may express their feelings through anger directed at all levels of staff. Whatever the family response, the caregiver has the responsibility to intervene with sensitivity. We are frequently handicapped in not having a family history that includes past crises and patterns of coping behavior.

The Initial Family Meeting

The initial meeting with the family can set the stage for the ongoing relationship between family and staff. Therefore, it is important to emphasize this initial contact.

Making time for a *structured* family meeting can result in increased communication and a decrease in the level of anxiety for both the family and staff. Even if the meeting is only 20–30 minutes in length, it is time well spent. Ideally, the physician and nurse together should meet with the family group. This joint effort demonstrates to the family that the team is working together, which can alleviate some of their fears. It also gives the nurse a first-hand opportunity to hear what is told by the physician, thus enabling the nurse to clarify this information in the future. Frequently, families are so anxious during this time that they may not hear all that has been said to them, or may have misunderstandings. This joint meeting is efficient, since the nurse who has been present with the physician will not need to inquire later to find out what the family has been told. It also is a way for health professionals to support each other in a very difficult situation.

It is extremely important that a suitable place be found for this family meeting: a place where the family is not disturbed or distracted, and where the physician and nurse can sit with them comfortably. It is important that the health care team appear *to be present* to the family and not appear hurried. Structure is important during times of stress and anxiety. Presentation of information needs to be clear, direct, and concise.

Begin the family meeting by saying, "We would like to discuss with you what is happening now and what we expect in the next few hours or days. Then we will answer the questions that you have." This opening statement lets the family know that they will have time for their questions, thereby decreasing their anxiety, and facilitating their ability to listen or focus. The physician can then review current symptoms and the meaning of both those symptoms and current treatment. The family is often worried that the patient is in pain. Therefore it is helpful to emphasize this: "We have a special solution in his intravenous line to try to control the extra beats. It is attached to a pump. Often the alarm on the pump sounds even with a slight change in position. The solution does not hurt. Please try not to be too frightened if the alarm sounds while you are visiting." Future plans with expected outcomes should be discussed. "We are going to try . . . , even though we are not certain that it is going to work. This procedure isn't painful. We want to do everything possible without causing unnecessary pain or discomfort." Next it is important to ask the family, "This can be a very frightening experience for people. What concerns or worries do you have?"

This kind of opening statement gives the member of a family a chance to express their worries. Health care professionals may be surprised to learn the concerns expressed by the family. This also gives caregivers an opportunity to gather information as quickly as possible.

At this point in the meeting the family might be asked if they would like to visit the patient. The members of the health care team should accompany the family to the bedside and explain all of the equipment that they see. By touching the patient as well as informing the family, the caregiver can sometimes act as a role model. Family members may feel so overwhelmed or frightened by both the CCU and the critically ill relative that they are immobilized and unable to respond with closeness or touching.

After leaving the patient's room, the nurse and/or physician can then review other issues with the family. An opening statement that can be helpful is: "I hope and pray that your husband will get better, but if he doesn't we feel it is important to review a few things ahead of time. I know this is difficult to talk about, but in my experience, it helps in the long run." Questions we find helpful to ask: "If death becomes imminent, where would you like to be?" "If death becomes imminent, who should be called?" "How do you think you would feel if you were not with your husband when he died?" It is important when exploring these issues that the staff give the family permission to deal with them in their own personal way. Saying something like "People respond differently to situations. Let's talk about how you think you might respond" is helpful. If the family chooses not to be present, assure them that someone will be with the patient to let him know that he is not alone. If they choose to be with the patient, assure them that you will be there to support them.

When the family members are with the patient, offer to include them in aspects of care [3]. People often feel better if they can help. Give them small tasks. Have them put a cold cloth on the patient's head, apply vaseline on lips, speak to the patient even if comatose, touch the patient, and read prayers or scripture according to their religous beliefs. In these ways they can find ways to continue to relate to their loved one and feel useful.

Give the family a set time when you will be able to meet with them to review the patient's situation. This often decreases their anxiety, and puts limits on the number of questions they may have for the staff. If the family is a large one, ask for someone to serve as a spokesperson. Families usually respond well to this, if it is explained to them, "We find it helpful if we can give all the information to one person in the family who can then keep the others informed. It would really be helpful to us if we can communicate in this way."

Religious and cultural traditions need to be considered. Ask if there is a clergyperson whom they would like contacted. Is there a particular family tradition that would be helpful now?

Resuscitation

If there is not going to be resuscitation, the family needs to be included in this decision. Though difficult, it is an important issue, since the family will probably have questions about this in the future. The family also has time to prepare for a situation that could potentially be a crisis.

If there is going to be resuscitation, determine where the family is going to be at that time. Families often would like to be together and near their loved one. Therefore we try to find a private room on the CCU. (It may be the head nurse's office or the resident's sleeping room or a classroom.) During the resuscitation process, a care-

giver should keep the family informed about what is happening. "They are still beating his heart for him." "They are breathing for her." Spend time with the family answering questions, calling people for them or helping them make calls, or perhaps just sitting silently with them. If the resuscitation effort is successful suggest that they may want to visit briefly to reassure themselves that all is "all right for now."

When the Patient Dies

If the resuscitation is not successful, inform the family as soon as possible, since waiting is so terribly difficult. Even when a family has been prepared for the possibility of death, they may still experience shock and profound grief. Loud screams, emotional outbursts, throwing oneself on the body, and crying out, "Oh God, I can't believe this really happened," are not uncommon responses.

There may be more unusual responses by a family member. We have had people ask for a photo. A woman wanted to get in bed with her husband who just died. Another woman wanted to braid and unbraid her deceased daughter's hair. None of these requests were "abnormal," and they needed to be respected.

It is critically important to give the family "permission" to express their feelings, whether those feelings be anger, crying, silence, or numbness. It may be helpful to accompany the family into the room of the deceased. The staff should show reverence for the body by preparing it by putting on clean sheets and a gown before the visit; if the caregiver then touches the deceased, this shows caring and support for the family. We do not recommend even partial shrouding of the body since we have found families sometimes like to hold the hand of the deceased person or stroke the feet.

Have tea or coffee available for the family [3]. If you ask them, they will frequently refuse and say that they do not want to impose [4], but they will welcome this gesture that seems so insignificant, but demonstrates sensitivity and kindness.

Before the family leaves the hospital, it is

important to answer all questions that may remain. It is also important to consider each of the following:

1. Check to assure their transportation for going home.
2. Provide a respectful way to get the patient's belongings home. A paper bag is quite offensive. Address the issue of what to do with a spouse's wedding band.
3. Discuss the issue of autopsy. We try to explain that an autopsy is like an operation except that no anesthesia is used. The face is not mutilated in any way. If families do not want an autopsy, we support them in that decision. Too often we have seen families who have the additional burden of feeling guilty for allowing or not allowing an autopsy.
4. Help the family develop an immediate plan for that day. Let them know how to contact a funeral director. Ask them if they wish their clergyperson be notified.
5. Review with them how they can expect to be feeling and responding during the next few days and weeks. Give them a written guideline that describes the normality of grieving (table 48-1). Some people, during acute grief are frightened by their experience and have stated they "thought they were going crazy." This type of teaching and preparation can prevent additional pain, suffering, and fear.
6. Sending a sympathy card from the staff and from the physician can offer immeasurable support. Families have told us that they felt this gesture gave them the sense that their loved one was really treated as a person and not just another number.
7. Inquire whether there are children in the family and how they think they are going to deal with them. Offer suggestions of ways to help children adjust to the unexpected loss. Giving them written suggestions of points to cover and books to read is also helpful.
8. Finally, if possible, provide for a follow-up visit or phone call in four to six weeks. Families frequently have remaining questions, but do not have a mechanism for having them answered.

TABLE 48-1. Guidelines for the patient's family

The death of a loved one can be so painful that it frightens and overwhelms us. Most people who suffer a loss will experience one or more of the following:

1. Empty feeling in their stomach
2. Tightness in the throat
3. Heaviness in the chest
4. Loss of appetite
5. Difficulty sleeping, feelings of guilt and anger
6. Anger at the loved one for leaving them
7. Preoccupation with the deceased, a sensation of the loved one's presence, like one is expecting her or him to walk through the door, or hearing her or his voice
8. Not wanting to talk about the loss
9. Difficulty concentrating
10. Restlessness
11. Aimlessness
12. Finding it hard to make decisions, hard to complete tasks that are usually routine
13. A sense of denial as though the loss didn't happen
14. Loneliness
15. Mood changes over the slightest thing
16. Crying unexpectedly
17. A need to tell and retell the experience of the loved one's death

These are normal responses. It is important to cry and to talk to others even if this is hard for you.

If you are concerned, worried, or need to talk to someone please call:

_____

_____

The CCU as a Caregiving Environment

The coronary care unit is a tense and highly charged atmosphere for physicians and nurses. These caregivers must be skilled practitioners, and may be able to maintain a large number of relationships under high levels of stress. In critical care units the physician and nurse are bombarded by many external stimuli, including sounds of complex machinery with alarms and flashing lights, all types of tubes and pumps, blood and human excreta, physical and emotional suffering endured by patients and their loved ones [5, 6]. They are also affected by the anxiety and fear of the critically ill patients, the concerned families who are ever-present, the demands of other health care professionals [6], repetitive exposure to dying and death, work overload, lack of gratification, communication problems with administration, and intragroup tensions [5].

The nurse assumes a pivotal position in this complex system and is expected to maintain the balance of objectivity required to make urgent critical decisions, and to provide the warmth and feeling, necessary to comfort patients and families. The compactness of the CCU is advantageous for observation and easy mobility, but it may lead to a lack of objectivity by the nurse in close patient contact [7].

When a patient dies, the CCU staff is confronted with the realities and limitations of medical and nursing science, and with the loss experienced by the family, the patient, and themselves. The busy nature of the CCU makes it difficult for staff to be as available to patients and families as they feel they should be. The life of the CCU continues, with other critical patients demanding time, skill, energy, and concentration. It may also be difficult to build in a mechanism of support for the staff, since they often feel a sense of urgency during the work day and find it unacceptable to focus on themselves. Good physician—nurse communication is essential in this highly stressed area.

Physicians can play a key role in assisting the CCU nurse when a patient is expected to die. It is critically important to keep the nurse informed about changes in and expectations for the patient's progess. If possible, the nurse can join the physician when telling the family that there has been a change in the patient's status. This collaboration is helpful in that it "acknowledges" the nurse as a key member of the team. It is also a way of sharing in a most difficult and stressful situation, which in itself is supportive.

The staff needs to be included as much as possible in the support of the patient and family. This involvement can bring about "healing" for the staff. Feelings of impotence may heighten the staff's grief, and these can be balanced by meaningful interaction prior to the patient's death. It

is very appropriate for staff to cry with the family. Families have expressed that they view this as a measure of how much their loved one was cared about [4] and not as a lack of professionalism by the staff.

Staff may also need someone to provide them with additional support. Peer support with acknowledgment that the staff provided the best possible care is important. Having a skilled professional available to support the staff may also serve to alleviate some of the accumulated stress [5]. This role may be assumed by a psychiatric nurse, clinical specialist, pastoral counselor, psychiatric social worker, mental health professional, or psychiatric consultant. This type of support works best if it is an integral part of the system. The staff may be reluctant to seek out this type of support person. Therefore, the optimum situation is to have such a support person who routinely makes rounds on the CCU and/or who provides episodic support meetings for staff. The ongoing visibility of this support person may make it easier for staff to feel comfortable in seeking help prior to experiencing accumulated stress and "burn out." This support person should become an important part of the system.

If the patient interaction has been particularly difficult for the staff, it may be helpful to have a "wrapup meeting" the week after the death. As many members of the team as possible should be included. It is helpful to have the support person facilitate this meeting.

Holding memorial services during the year is another opportunity for "healing" for the staff. This service provides a time for remembering, grieving, and letting go. It also provides time for the staff to come together as a community, which builds support.

The CCU administration can provide support by allowing and encouraging flexibility of assignments. If a staff member has been particularly affected by the death of a young patient, for example, he or she may need distance from this population for a period of time. This flexibility is a way of acknowledging the humanness of the staff person and providing the type of support needed in these high-stress areas.

We cannot take away the dying and the physical, emotional, or spiritual suffering for the patient, family, and staff, but preparation for imminent death on a coronary care unit can lessen some of the trauma for all involved.

References

1. Holland L, Rogich LE: Dealing with grief in the emergency room. Health Soc Work 5:12−17, 1980.
2. Gardner D, Stewart N: Staff involvement with families of patients in critical care units. Heart Lung 7:105−110, 1978.
3. Rinear E: Helping the survivors of expected death. Nursing 75 5:60−65, 1975.
4. Schultz CA: Sudden death crisis: pre-hospital and in the emergency department. J Emergency Nursing 46−50, June 1980.
5. Hay D, Oken D: The psychological stresses of intensive care nursing. Psychosom Med 34:109−118, 1972.
6. Hoffman R: Stress and the critical care nurse. Supervisor Nurse 20−23, August 1981.
7. Vreeland R, Ellis GL: Stresses on the nurse in an intensive-care unit. JAMA 208:332−334, 1969.

Additional Readings

1. Dubin W, Wolman T: Evaluation and management of the grief reaction. Penn Med 28:19−22, 1979.
2. Hackett TP, Cassem NH, Wishnie HA: The coronary-care unit: an appraisal of its psychological hazards. N Engl J Med 279:1365−1370, 1968.
3. Lindemann E: Symptomatology and management of acute grief. Am J Psychiatry 101:141−148, 1944.
4. Robinson MA: Informing the family of sudden death. Am Fam Physician 23:115−118, 1981.
5. Schnaper N, Cowley RA: Overview: psychiatric sequelae to multiple trauma. Am J Psychiatry 133:883−890, 1976.
6. Sharer PS: Helping survivors cope with the shock of sudden death. Nursing 79 9:20−21, January, 1979.
7. Sourkes BM: The deepening shade: psychological aspects of life threatening illness. Pittsburgh: University of Pittsburgh Press, 1982.

IX. CORONARY CARE: THE PREDISCHARGE PHASE

49. DETERMINATION OF THE OPTIMAL TIME FOR PATIENT MOBILIZATION AND HOSPITAL DISCHARGE FOLLOWING ACUTE MYOCARDIAL INFARCTION

David B. Pryor

Acute myocardial infarction began to be frequently diagnosed in the 1920s and 1930s. Pathology studies at that time demonstrated that myocardial infarctions required $1-2$ months to heal [1]. Consequently, physicians recommended hospitalization for up to two months, including at least two weeks of strict bed rest. By the early 1940s, concern about possible thromboembolic complications and deconditioning effects [2] led to trials of early mobilization. In the 1950s, studies demonstrated no adverse consequences followed mobilization to a chair within the first few days and that the practice might even be beneficial [3, 4]. The duration of hospitalization declined to an average of three weeks over the next two decades [5], and controlled trials attempted to define the optimal duration of hospitalization.

The physician's goal in the management of patients who sustain an acute myocardial infarction is to minimize complications and disability. Unnecessarily prolonged immobilization and hospitalization increase the cost, adversely affect the

This work was supported in part by grant HS-04873 from the National Center of Health Services Research—OASH, training grant LM-07003 from the National Library of Medicine, and a grant from the Andrew W. Mellon Foundation.

patient's sense of well-being, and may lead to complications from thromboembolism and deconditioning. Too brief a hospitalization may also jeopardize the patient's recovery.

The appropriate duration of hospitalization depends upon the patient's course in the coronary care unit and upon the home environment to which the patient will be discharged. Prolonged periods of hospitalization are frequently necessary to manage the complications that may develop from acute infarction. Patients without complications, however, can be discharged after a brief hospitalization, providing their home environments require little activity and continued care is accessible. Since the duration of hospitalization for patients who develop complications is usually dictated by the nature of the complications themselves, this chapter focuses on recognizing uncomplicated patients and determining their appropriate periods of immobilization and hospitalization.

Which Patients Are Uncomplicated?

Determining which patients are uncomplicated is difficult since no universally accepted criteria exist. Furthermore, which day following admission the criteria are applied may significantly affect the likelihood of observing late complications. It is necessary to know both which criteria can be used to identify the uncomplicated patient and when to apply the criteria during the hospitalization to adequately characterize a patient as "uncomplicated."

The most frequently used and validated criteria for characterizing the uncomplicated patient are shown in table 49-1 [6–10]. Ventricular tachycardia and fibrillation, second- or third-degree atrioventricular heart block, pulmonary edema, cardiogenic shock, infarct extension, and persistent hypotension are urgent complications requiring immediate intervention. Sinus tachycardia and sustained supraventricular tachycardia predict likely future complications. These criteria were first reported by McNeer et al. in 1975 [6] in a feasibility study that was designed to determine which patients with acute infarction could be considered uncomplicated and potentially suitable for brief hospitalization. Among 270 patients who met the criteria, mortality at six months was 8%. Using the same criteria, McNeer et al. [7] conducted a prospective trial of 67 patients in 1978. No patients died during the six-month follow-up. The criteria were subsequently validated by Severence et al. [8] in the community hospital setting in 81 patients; mortality was 0% at 30 days and 10% at one year. McNeer's criteria have also been used by two other groups [9, 10] to identify 978 uncomplicated patients for whom the early hospital mortality was only 1%. Using these criteria, about one-half of all patients admitted with acute myocardial infarction are uncomplicated and have a favorable prognosis.

Other investigators have added other criteria to McNeer's seven in order to identify the uncomplicated patient. Some studies [11–13] have suggested that ventricular premature beats are prognostically important. In the early postinfarction period, ventricular premature beats are a common occurrence and by themselves do not appear to have prognostic implications for later in the hospitalization or after discharge [14, 15]. When found in patients with other complications, however, they appear to be a marker of poor ventricular function. Patients with ventricular premature beats and good ventricular function have an excellent prognosis and, barring other complications, can probably be discharged safely after a brief hospitalization.

TABLE 49-1. Characterizing the uncomplicated patient up to day 5 without:

Ventricular tachycardia or fibrillation
Second- or third-degree atrioventricular heart block
Pulmonary edema
Cardiogenic shock
Infarct extension
Persistent hypotension
Sinus tachycardia or sustained supraventricular tachycardia

Right and left bundle branch block complicating acute infarction occurs in patients with extensive myocardial damage. Lie et al. in 1978 [16] noted that 60% of the patients with late inhospital ventricular fibrillation had anterior myocardial infarction complicated by bundle branch block. They prospectively monitored patients with anterior myocardial infarction and bundle branch block for six weeks. A high percentage (36%) developed ventricular fibrillation later during their hospitalization. Almost all of these patients would be considered complicated by other critera; heart failure was noted in 83%.

The importance of other reported criteria is difficult to assess. ST-segment elevation [17], advanced age [18, 19], a previous myocardial infarction within six months [11], and recurrent angina in the postinfarct period particularly when associated with ST-segment changes distant from the site of the infarction [20, 21] have all been used to identify patients at increased risk in the postinfarction period. The independent importance of these criteria beyond those described has not been examined. Discharge time and rehabilitation programs may need to be modified when these criteria occur in otherwise uncomplicated patients.

When to Characterize Patients

It is important to delay characterizing a patient as uncomplicated until five days after admission. Some patients do not develop complications until the third or fourth day. Pozen et al. [22] found that 40% of patients characterized as uncomplicated after only two days subsequently developed complications. This figure fell to 6% when characterization was delayed until day 5. In the feasibility study of McNeer et al. [6], all patients who developed complications did so before the fifth hospital day. It appears prudent, therefore, to delay characterizing a patient as uncomplicated until the fifth day following admission, unless that patient can be accurately placed in a particularly low-risk category. Use of combinations of studies to estimate infarct size may permit those with minimal damage to be so characterized at an earlier time.

Duration of Hospitalization

Determining the appropriate duration of hospitalization for uncomplicated patients is difficult. Studies examining the problem have used different criteria for study entry, different study designs for the timing of mobilization and discharge, and have included relatively small numbers of patients. While most studies conclude that discharge after a brief period of hospitalization is safe, the recommendation is based not on showing decreased morbidity or mortality with earlier discharge, but rather on the lack of finding any difference in the frequency of complications. To conclude that the practice of early discharge is without adverse consequences, the study design should include sufficient numbers of patients to be sure that, if a significant difference in complication rates existed, it would be detected. For example, if a 1% mortality was present for uncomplicated patients discharged after two weeks, to be reasonably (80%) certain that a doubling of this rate would be detected for patients discharged after one week, 4600 patients should be included in the study. No single study incorporates sufficient numbers of patients to provide this certainty. Consequently, recommendations for early discharge are based on combining the information provided by many different studies.

Evidence supporting the safety of early discharge is based on three different types of studies. The natural history studies that identify which patients are uncomplicated illustrate the low morbidity and mortality that accompany uncomplicated infarction. Prospective trials of early discharge have no control groups, but the low rate of complications after discharge for these patients

supports the safety of the practice. Controlled trials, although lacking sufficient numbers of patients in any one study, have all been unable to demonstrate any adverse consequences of early discharge. When the information from all three types of studies is combined, reasonable recommendations for the early discharge of uncomplicated patients can be made.

Table 49-2 lists the ten prospective and controlled trials of early discharge that have included patients discharged within two weeks of admission for acute myocardial infarction [7, 11, 23–30]. Over 1600 patients are included in these studies. The three prospective trials [23–25] demonstrate low complication rates. The 7% mortality rate noted by Gelson et al. [24] would have been 3% if they had used the stricter criteria of McNeer et al. [6–10]. Of the seven controlled trials in table 49-1, six were unable to show any adverse consequences of earlier discharge while one, by Abraham et al. [27], found a significantly lower complication rate for the patients discharged earlier. The study reported by Hill et al. [29] compared home therapy with hospital therapy for patients without complications when first encountered. One-third of the patients initially treated at home required admission to the hospital, raising questions about the advisability of this practice. Together, these studies support the practice of discharging uncomplicated patients after one week of hospitalization.

Mobilization

If uncomplicated patients are to be discharged safely one week after admission, a comprehensive program to prepare them for discharge must begin as soon as possible after they are stabilized in the coronary care unit. Educational programs that include psychological, vocational, and sexual counseling can increase patients' understanding of the risk factors, manifestations, prognosis, and management of coronary artery disease.

Early mobilization with progressive physical activity is necessary to prepare patients for the physical activity required in their home environment. Convalescence in the home environment requires an energy expenditure of 3–4 mets. The patient should be observed at this level of energy expenditure before discharge. Current

TABLE 49-2. Prospective and controlled trials of patients discharged within two weeks of admission

References	No. patients	Discharge time (days)	Study type	Complications or conclusions reached
Chaturvedi et al. [23]	109	68% by day 7	Prospective	2% Mortality at 1 year
Gelson et al. [24]	271	8	Prospective	7% Mortality at 6 weeks (3% with stricter criteria)
Lindvall et al. [25]	46	8	Prospective	2% Mortality at 6 months
Hutter et al. [11]	138	14 vs 21	Controlled	No difference
Hayes et al. [26]	189	9 vs 16	Controlled	No difference
Abraham et al. [27]	129	12 vs 19	Controlled	Fewer complications with early discharge
Oh et al. [28]	190	11 vs 29	Controlled	No difference
McNeer et al. [7]	67	7 vs 11	Controlled	No difference
Hill et al. [29]	266	0 vs 7 or 8	Controlled	No difference overall (mortality in first few days in hospital patients)
Ahlmark et al. [30]	252	8 vs 15	Controlled	No difference

trends [31−33] are to begin with changes in posture, supervised and monitored low-level passive and active isotonic exercises, and self-care activities. Sitting on the side of the bed or in a chair is done as early as the second or third day in the coronary care unit. Activities are gradually increased after the patient leaves the coronary care unit, usually on the fourth or fifth day. During this stage, activities that include longer periods of sitting in a chair, increased self-care, rhythmic exercises of the extremities and trunk, walking in the hall, and even limited stair climbing are performed several times a day. These activities should be monitored for the occurrence of an abnormal heart rate or blood pressure or auscultatory or electrocardiographic changes; a revised regimen must be devised if they occur. Despite the lack of supporting controlled trials, these regimens are practiced widely and no adverse effects have been reported.

A recent trend has been to include limited noninvasive studies, (treadmill) exercise electrocardiography, radionuclide evaluation, or cardiac catheterization either before or soon after discharge to help identify uncomplicated patients who are at increased risk. The safety of the procedures [34−37] has been established, but it is difficult to compare the studies or make recommendations because of the limited sample sizes, different criteria for patient selection, different criteria of an abnormal test response, and the large number of tests. The use of these tests is discussed elsewhere in this text and recommendations for early discharge may need to be modified if significant abnormalities occur.

The patient without early urgent or prognostic complications should not be kept in the hospital beyond one week only for the purpose of a prognostic evaluation. If no spontaneous angina recurs, the electrocardiogram should be observed during the patient's level of exercise achieved by seven days. If there are no signs of ischemia, the patient may be discharged from the hospital. The patient should then return for an outpatient visit in approximately one week for more definitive stress testing and appropriate advancement through a rehabilitation program (see chapter 58).

Summary

In summary, after four days after admission, approximately 50% of all patients with acute myocardial infarction admitted to the coronary care unit are free of the complications outlined in table 49-1. If the home environment is suitable, these uncomplicated patients can be safely discharged after one week, providing an appropriate rehabilitation program was instituted soon after admission. Noninvasive studies during the peri-discharge period may improve identification of high-risk patients. The early discharge of un-complicated patients can reduce the hospital cost, improve the patient's sense of well-being, and decrease the complications from thromboembo-lism and deconditioning.

References

1. Mallory GK, White PW, Salcedo-Salgor J: The speed of healing of myocardial infarction. Am Heart J 18:647−671, 1939.

2. Dock W: The evil sequelae of complete bed rest. JAMA 125:1083−1085, 1944.

3. Levine SA, Lown B: Armchair treatment of acute coronary thrombosis. JAMA 148:1365−1369, 1952.

4. Beckwith JR, Kernodle DT, Le Hew AE, Wood JE Jr: The management of myocardial infarction with particular reference to the chair treatment. Ann Intern Med 41:1189−1195, 1954.

5. Wenger NK, Hellerstein KH, Blackburn HW, Castranova SJ: Uncomplicated myocardial infarc-tion: current physician practice in patient man-agement. JAMA 224:511−514, 1973.

6. McNeer JF, Wallace AG, Wagner GS, Starmer CF, Rosati RA: The course of acute myocardial infarction: feasibility of early discharge of the un-complicated patient. Circulation 51:410−413, 1975.

7. McNeer JF, Wagner GS, Ginsburg PB, et al: Hospital discharge one week after acute myo-cardial infarction. N Engl J Med 298:229−232, 1978.

8. Severence HW, Morris KG, Wagner GS: Cri-teria for early discharge after acute myocardial infarction: validation in a community hospital. Arch Intern Med 142:139−141, 1982.

9. Kennelly BM, Margolis B: Prognostic factors in acute myocardial infarction. S Afr Med J 52:511−514, 1977.

10. Worth RM, Fergusson DJC, Kim JHC, et al: When to discharge a patient surviving acute myo-cardial infarction. Hawaii Med J 38:97−101, 1979.

11. Hutter AM Jr, Sidel VW, Shine KF, De Sanctis RW: Early hospital discharge after myocardial in-farction. N Engl J Med 288:1141−1144, 1973.

12. Moss AJ, De Camilla J, Davis H, Bayer L: The early posthospital phase of myocardial infarction. Circulation 54:58−64, 1976.

13. Moss AJ, De Camilla JJ, Davis HP, Bayer L: Clinical significance of ventricular ectopic beats in the early posthospital phase of myocardial in-farction. Am J Cardiol 39:635−640, 1977.

14. Vismara LA, Vera Z, Foerster JM, Amsterdam EA, Mason DT: Identification of sudden death risk factors in acute and chronic coronary artery disease. Am J Cardiol 39:821−828, 1977.

15. Luria MH, Knoke JD, Margolis RM, Hendricks FH, Kupler JB: Acute myocardial infarction: prognosis after recovery. Ann Intern Med 85:561−565, 1976.

16. Lie KF, Liem KL, Schuilenburg RM, David GK, Durrer D: Early identification of patients devel-oping late in-hospital ventricular fibrillation af-ter discharge from the coronary care unit. Am J Cardiol 41:674−677, 1978.

17. Wilson C, Pantridge JF: ST-segment displace-ment and early hospital discharge in acute myo-cardial infarction. Lancet 1284−1288, 1973.

18. Williams BO, Begg TB, Semple T, McGuinness JB: The elderly in a coronary unit. Br Med J 2:451−453, 1976.

19. Madsen EB, Rasmussen S, Svendsen TL: Short term prognostic index in acute myocardial in-farction: multivariate analysis by Cox model. Eur J Cardiol 10:359−368, 1979.

20. Schuster EH, Bulkley BH: Early post-infarction angina: ischemia at a distance and in the infarct zone. N Engl J Med 305:1101−1115, 1981.

21. Levine FE, Gold HK, Leinbach RC, Daggett WM, Austen WG, Buckley MJ: Safe early revas-cularization for continuing ischemia after acute myocardial infarction. Circulation (Supp 1) I-5−119, 1979.

22. Pozen MW, Stechmiller JK, Voigt GC: Prognos-tic efficacy of early clinical categorization of myo-cardial infarction patients. Circulation 56:816−819, 1977.

23. Chaturvedi NC, Walsh MJ, Evans A, Munro P, Boyle DMC, Barber JM: Selection of patients for early discharge after acute myocardial infarction. Br Heart J 36:533−535, 1974.

24. Gelson ADN, Carson PHM, Tucker HH, Phil-lips R, Clarke M, Oakley GD: Course of patients discharged early after myocardial infarction. Br Med J 1:1555−1558, 1976.

25. Lindvall K, Erhardt LR, Lundman T, Rehnquist W, Sjogren A: Early mobilization and discharge of patients with acute myocardial infarction. Acta Med Scand 206:169−175, 1979.

26. Hayes MJ, Morris GK, Hampton JR: Compari-son of mobilization after two and nine days in uncomplicated myocardial infarction. Br Med J 3:10−13, 1974.

27. Abraham SA, Sever Y, Weinstein M, Dollberg M, Menczel J: Value of early ambulation in patients with and without complications after acute myocardial infarction. N Engl J Med 292:719–722, 1975.

28. Oh W: Early discharge after myocardial infarction: a controlled study. Singapore Med J 17:40–45, 1976.

29. Hill JD, Hampton JR, Mitchell JRA: A randomized trial of home-versus-hospital management for patients with suspected myocardial infarction. Lancet 1:837–841, 1978.

30. Ahlmark G, Ahlberg G, Saetre H, Haglund F, Korsgren M: A controlled study of early discharge after uncomplicated myocardial infarction. Acta Med Scand 206:87–91, 1979.

31. De Busk RF, Spivak AP, Van Kessel A, Graham C, Harrison DC: The coronary care unit activities program: its role in post-infarction rehabilitation. J Chronic Dis 24:373–381, 1971.

32. Wenger NK: Rehabilitation after myocardial infarction. JAMA 242:2879–2881, 1979.

33. Wenger NK, Hellerstein HK, Blackburn H, Castranova SJ: Physician practice in the management of patients with uncomplicated myocardial infarction: changes in the past decade. Circulation 65:421–427, 1982.

34. Ericsson M, Granath A, Ohlsen P, Sodermark T, Volpe V: Arrhythmias and symptoms during treadmill testing three weeks after myocardial infarction in 100 patients. Br Heart J 35:787–790, 1973.

35. Markiewicz W, Houston N, De Busk RF: Exercise testing soon after myocardial infarction. Circulation 56:26–31, 1977.

36. Waters DD, Theroux P, Halphen C, Mizgala HF: Clinical predictors of angina following myocardial infarction. Am J Med 66:991–996, 1979.

37. Theroux P, Waters DD, Halphen C, Debaisieux JC, Mizgala HF: Prognostic value of exercise testing soon after myocardial infarction. N Engl Med 301:341–345, 1979.

50. IDENTIFICATION AND PROPHYLACTIC TREATMENT OF PATIENTS AT HIGH RISK OF LATE POSTINFARCTION SUDDEN DEATH

K.I. Lie

Late inhospital death defined as death after the third day of acute myocardial infarction accounts for at least 45% of all inhospital deaths of patients admitted to the coronary care unit (CCU) [1].

In the majority of patients the mechanism of death is pump failure manifested by severe pulmonary edema or cardiogenic shock (see chapter 44). These patients are usually already in poor hemodynamic condition on admission to the CCU [2] and the subsequent outcome can be predicted on the basis of simple clinical parameters [3, 4]. In a minority of instances, however, late inhospital death may occur suddenly and rather unexpectedly [5].

Earlier studies have indicated that the primary mechanism of late sudden death is ventricular fibrillation [1]. Sudden, nonarrhythmic death has also been reported, at times without a demonstrable cause [6] and also related to cardiac rupture [1, 7]. In this chapter we discuss only the identification and prophylactic management of high-risk candidates for sudden death due to late inhospital ventricular fibrillation.

Late Inhospital Ventricular Fibrillation

IDENTIFICATION OF HIGH-RISK PATIENTS
During the last five years, several studies have

indicated that late inhospital ventricular fibrillation especially occurs in patients with very large infarcts or with cardiac failure in the CCU [8−10]. It is conceivable that prolonged ECG monitoring or antiarrhythmic intervention would probably reduce the hospital mortality of these patients.

In clinical practice, however, indiscriminate prolonged ECG monitoring of all patients with either large infarcts or cardiac failure in the CCU is impractical. In several studies designed to identify high-risk groups, in whom prolonged monitoring would be feasible and justified in cost-effectiveness, bundle branch block complicating acute anteroseptal infarction was the strongest predictive parameter [1, 9, 10]. A minority of these patients progress to complete atrioventricular block (see chapter 39) within the first several days of the acute infarct, and only these will benefit from pacemaker therapy.

In a prospective study [9], approximately one-third of patients with bundle branch block during anteroseptal infarction developed late inhospital ventricular fibrillation within six weeks after discharge from the CCU. This group comprised 75% of all patients who developed unexpected late postinfarction sudden death [9]. These patients usually had right bundle branch block; the presence of concomitant left anterior or posterior hemiblock did not affect the incidence of late

R.M. Califf and G.S. Wagner (eds.), ACUTE CORONARY CARE: Principles and Practice. Copyright © 1985. Martinus Nijhoff Publishing, Boston/Dordrecht/Lancaster.

ventricular fibrillation. In most patients, ventricular fibrillation was initiated by rapid ventricular tachycardia. One-third of patients had runs of ventricular ectopic beats during the 12 h to five days before onset of ventricular tachycardia.

The association between acute right bundle branch block complicating anteroseptal infarction and the subsequent development of late ventricular fibrillation raises the possibility of several pathophysiologic mechanisms. The first relates to the size of the infarction: patients with right bundle branch block and anteroseptal infarction have high serum enzyme levels, a high incidence of pump failure, and hospital mortality rates of 50% or more. Usually these infarcts are a consequence of proximal occlusion of the left anterior descending artery with or without involvement of the other coronary arteries [9−11].

A second mechanism relates to the early development of cardiac aneurysms. More than 90% of patients with anteroseptal infarctions and right bundle branch block, in whom cardiac catheterization was performed, showed cardiac aneurysms [9, 11]. In a subgroup [10] of such patients, this original ventricular tachycardia could be initiated by programmed stimulation. Other types of ventricular tachycardia could also be induced during programmed stimulation, suggesting the possibility of multiple unstable reentrant circuits in these patients. Further elucidation of the mechanism of the ventricular tachycardia using endocardial mapping techniques is now performed [12].

MANAGEMENT AND PROPHYLAXIS

Prolonged ECG monitoring seems justified in patients with acute bundle branch block during anteroseptal infarction since approximately one-third of these will develop late inhospital sudden death due to ventricular fibrillation. Prolonged monitoring should preferably be carried out in intermediate care units. Duration of the monitoring should be extended to 4−6 weeks since during this time these late lethal arrhythmias still may develop. The cause of this bimodal distribution of sudden death is unclear, but may relate to a specific stage of the healing process of large infarcts that facilitates reentrant circuits. During the prolonged monitoring period, two lines of prophylactic antiarrhythmic management can be considered.

Medical Management. In the initial, conservative approach, antiarrhythmic drugs are given, based upon the observation of runs of ventricular ectopic beats or development of ventricular tachycardia. At present, no controlled studies are available on the efficacy of antiarrhythmic drug intervention in these patients. Uncontrolled observations [11] suggest that quinidine and disopyramide are rather ineffective. At present, most patients with these ventricular arrhythmias are treated with either procainamide or amiodarone and reports on long-term efficacy are encouraging [1, 9−11]. The period of electrical instability may be confined to the first six weeks after the onset of the anteroseptal infarction since a rather good prognosis has been shown in these patients who were not on antiarrhythmic therapy after hospital discharge [12].

Surgical Management. Since many patients with late inhospital ventricular fibrillation have recurrences despite rigorous antiarrhythmic intervention and even cardiac pacing, different ways of surgical treatment have been indicated [9, 10]. The outcome of blind aneurysmectomy following medically untractable ventricular tachyarrhythmias is poor. Our data during the last five years showed a mortality rate of more than 50%. Most of the deaths were due to recurrences of the arrhythmia, but it cannot be excluded that further deterioration of cardiac function due to the antiarrhythmic therapy may have influenced the poor prognosis. Therefore we are now inclined to follow a second or alternative line of management.

Recently, surgery for ventricular tachycardia guided by pre- and intraoperative mapping has been advocated. In patients at risk for late postinfarction ventricular fibrillation, endocardial mapping is essential, since multiple minor or major reentrant circuits in the endocardium may be operative. Although the risks of surgical intervention in these patients are very high, a well-designed multicenter trial, comparing various options including a direct surgical approach, should be considered. In such a trial it is important that the medically treated group be well defined with only one or two antiarrhythmic drugs studied according to a comprehensive protocol. At present, such a national cooperative study is in preparation in the Netherlands in collaboration with the Interuniversity Cardiological Institute. We sincerely hope that the results of such a large-scale study will lead to a better management of these patients.

References

1. Norris RM, Sammel NL: Predictors of late hospital death in acute myocardial infarction. Prog Cardiovasc Dis 23:129, 1980.
2. Wackers FJTh, Lie KI, Becker AE, Durrer D, Wellens HJJ: Coronary artery disease in patients dying from cardiogenic shock or congestive heart failure in the setting of acute myocardial infarction. Br Heart J 38:906, 1976.
3. Peel AAF, Semple T, Wang I, Lancaster WM, Dall JLC: A coronary prognostic index for grading the severity of myocardial infarction. Br Heart J 24:745, 1962.
4. Norris RM, Brandt PWT, Caughey DE, Lee AJ, Scott PJ: A new coronary prognostic index. Lancet 1:274, 1969.
5. Thompson P, Sloman G: Sudden death in hospital after discharge from coronary care unit. Br Med J 4:136, 1971.
6. Raizes G, Wagner GS, Hackel DB: Instantaneous nonarrhythmic cardiac death in acute myocardial infarction. Am J Cardiol 39:1, 1977.
7. Van Mantgem JP: Cardiac rupture in acute myocardial infarction. Thesis, 1983.
8. Lawrie DM, Higgins MR, Godman MJ, et al: Ventricular fibrillation complicating acute myocardial infarction. Lancet 2:523, 1968.
9. Lie KI, Liem KL, Schuilenburg RM, David GK, Durrer D: Early identification of patients developing late in-hospital ventricular fibrillation after discharge from the coronary care unit. Am J Cardiol 41:674, 1978.
10. Wellens HJJ, Brugada P, De Zwaan C, Bendermacher P, Bär FW: Clinical characteristics, prognostic significance and treatment of sustained ventricular tachycardia following acute myocardial infarction. In: Wellens HJJ, Kulbertus (eds) The first year after AMI. Mt Kisco NY: Futura, 1983.
11. Lie KI, Liem KL, Durrer D: Management in hospital of ventricular fibrillation complicating acute myocardial infarction. Br Heart J (Suppl) 40:78, 1978.
12. Hauer RNW, Lie KI, Liem KL, Durrer D: Long term prognosis in patients with bundle branch block complicating acute anteroseptal infarction. Am J Cardiol 49:1581, 1982.

51. THE QUANTIFICATION OF RESIDUAL ISCHEMIA IN PATIENTS RECOVERING FROM ACUTE MYOCARDIAL INFARCTION BY EXERCISE THALLIUM-201 SCINTIGRAPHY

Robert S. Gibson

Thallium-201 has emerged as the most clinically applicable radionuclide for assessing capillary-level perfusion in ischemic and nonischemic myocardium [1]. When employed under stress conditions, it offers a unique means of diagnostic evaluation in patients with suspected or known coronary artery disease (CAD). Indeed, no other conventional clinical technique can provide similar information about nutrient blood flow reserve; yet the pathophysiology of ischemic heart disease, its symptomatic manifestations, and its morbidity and mortality are all the direct consequences of inadequate myocardial perfusion. The test is noninvasive, requiring no more than a venipuncture, and is more sensitive and specific for CAD detection than is standardized exercise testing.

Kinetics of Myocardial Uptake and Washout of Thallium-201

It is clear that there are discernible differences in the uptake and washout patterns characteristic of myocardial segments supplied by normal or only mildly nonobstructive coronary arteries and those supplied by arteries with functionally significant stenoses [1, 2]. The correspondence of these gen-

eral patterns to the severity of CAD indicates that quantification of myocardial blood flow reserve is possible with exercise thallium-201 (Tl-201) scintigraphy.

Myocardial kinetics of Tl-201 following a single intravenous injection can be divided into two successive but overlapping phases: initial distribution and redistribution. The initial myocardial concentration of Tl-201 is equal to the product of blood flow delivery of the tracer to the heart (i.e., regional blood flow) and the ability of myocardial cells to extract the tracer from the blood pool. It has been shown that, over a wide range of myocardial blood flows, the uptake of Tl-201 by the heart is proportional to regional perfusion. When the radionuclide is injected at peak exercise, images obtained $8-10$ min thereafter demonstrate the regional blood flow pattern at the time of stress. In normal individuals, distribution of thallium in the myocardium after intravenous injection is relatively homogeneous (figure 51-1). Regions of diminished thallium activity on these initial postexercise images either represent stress-induced ischemia or myocardial scar (figure 51-2). To distinguish these two possibilities, delayed images are obtained $2-3$ h later to ascertain whether the initial postexercise defect remains

R.M. Califf and G.S. Wagner (eds.), ACUTE CORONARY CARE: Principles and Practice. Copyright © 1985. Martinus Nijhoff Publishing, Boston/Dordrecht/Lancaster.

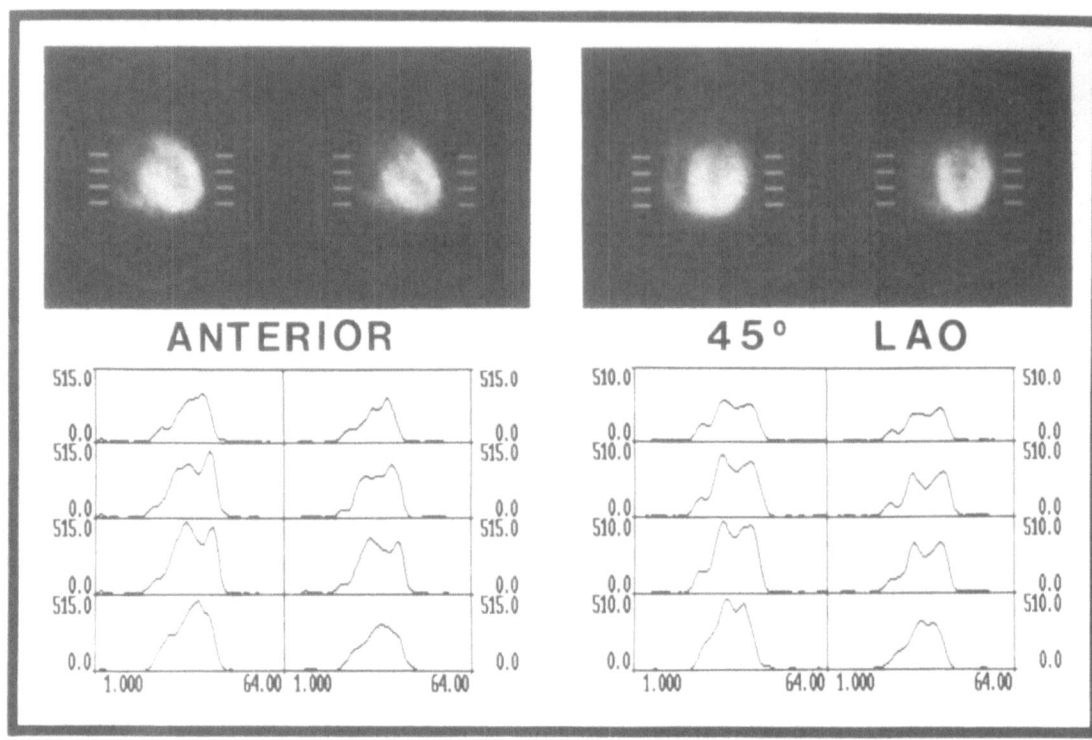

FIGURE 51-1. Anterior and 45° left anterior oblique (LAO) Tl-201 myocardial images obtained 10 min (left-hand image of each pair) and 2½ h after exercise (right-hand image of each pair) in a patient with normal coronary arteries. Uniform thallium uptake is observed throughout the left ventricle on the initial images. Delayed images indicate normal washout. Confirmatory profile plots of Tl-201 activity derived from our quantitative analysis [3] are shown below each image.

FIGURE 51-2. (A) Sequential 45° LAO myocardial images obtained 10 min, 1 h, and 2½ h after exercise in a patient with a prior anterior infarction and multivessel CAD. Time/Activity curves shown below each image confirm normal uptake and washout of Tl-201 in the low posterolateral segment (PDA area), complete redistribution in the high posterolateral segment (circumflex area), and partial redistribution in the anteroseptal segment (LAD area). (B) Sequential 45° LAO myocardial images obtained during low-level exercise in a patient ten days after acute inferior myocardial infarction. The Time/Activity curves confirm normal uptake and washout in the mid-high posterolateral segment, a persistent defect in the inferoapical segment, and an initial defect with delayed redistribution of Tl-201 in the anteroseptal segment. Coronary angiography revealed a normal circumflex artery, total occlusion of the RCA, and a 95% stenosis in the proximal LAD artery.

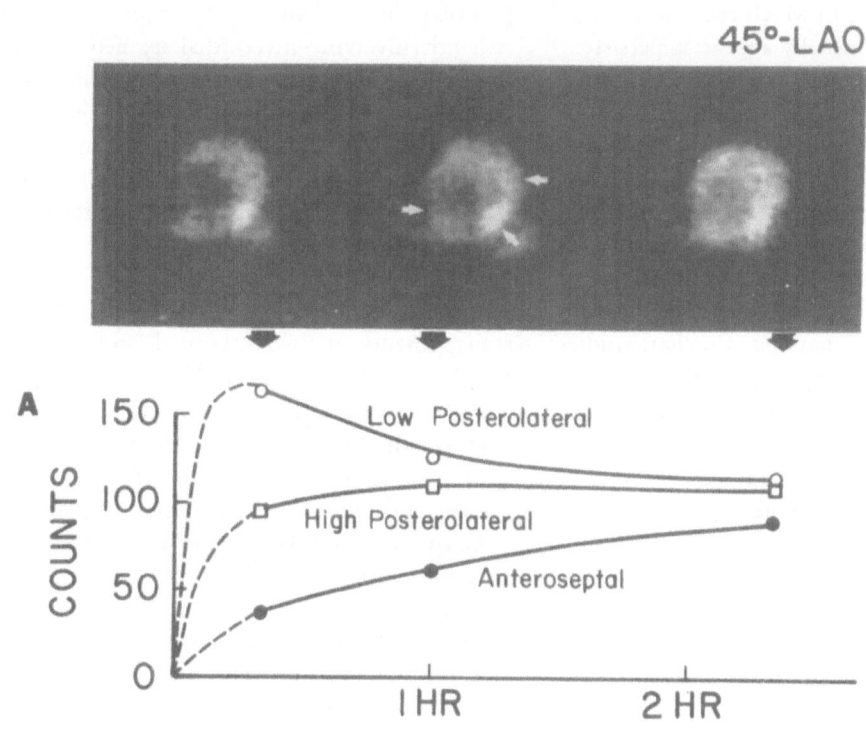

45°-LAO

A

Low Posterolateral

High Posterolateral

Anteroseptal

COUNTS

150

100

50

0

1 HR

2 HR

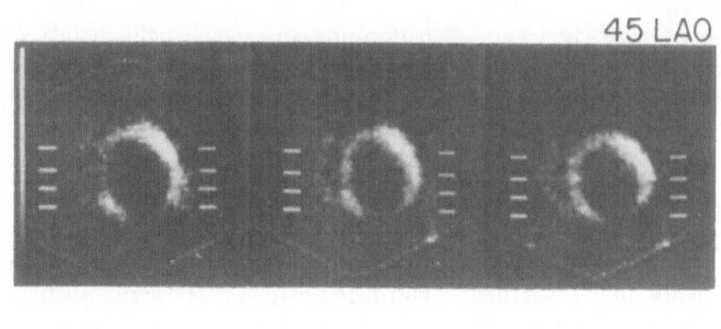

45 LAO

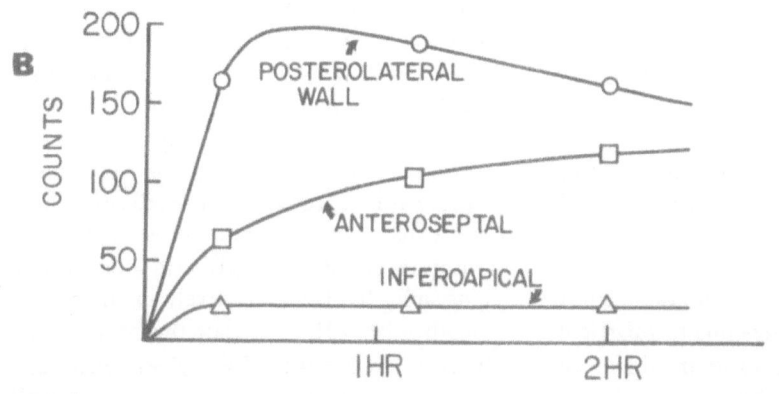

B

200

150

100

50

COUNTS

POSTEROLATERAL
WALL

ANTEROSEPTAL

INFEROAPICAL

1HR

2HR

persistent or demonstrates "redistribution" (delayed normalization), in which the defect disappears. Areas of scar usually appear as persistent defects. In contrast, areas of exercise-induced ischemia will show redistribution with total or partial defect resolution. Partial redistribution can be seen in areas of myocardial infarction, particularly in nontransmural infarcts, and most likely represent a mixture of reversibly and irreversibly damaged myocardium. It can also occur when regional blood flow is markedly reduced in the absence of prior infarction. Previous studies have established that this redistribution phenomenon is the result of more rapid washout of thallium in normal areas in comparison to either less rapid washout or delayed accumulation of thallium in underperfused areas.

Comparison of Thallium-201 Scintigraphy with Other Noninvasive Techniques

A large number of clinical studies have been reported in which the sensitivity, specificity, and predictive accuracy of exercise Tl-201 imaging were compared with stress electrocardiography for CAD detection in patients with chest pain [4]. In the vast majority of these studies, Tl-201 scintigraphy was found to be superior to the stress electrocardiogram. Data from several laboratories indicate that the sensitivity of Tl-201 scintigraphy and stress electrocardiography for disease detection is comparable when patients achieve 85% or more of their maximum predicted heart rate. When patients fail to reach this heart rate endpoint, however, the prevalence of positive ST-segment responses falls off significantly. In these patients with nondiagnostic stress electrocardiograms, the sensitivity of scintigraphy remains quite high, particularly when quantitative methods for image analysis are employed [3, 5]. This capability is especially important following myocardial infarction, since the exercise stress test prior to hospital discharge is, by design, submaximal.

Unlike the stress electrocardiogram, Tl-201 scintigraphy can localize ischemia to a particular area or areas of myocardium subserved by a specific coronary artery (figure 51-3). Because of this

capability, there is the potential to distinguish periinfarction ischemia from more extensive ischemia involving myocardial segments in the distribution of coronary arteries other than those associated with the acute infarction. In our experience, the overall sensitivity for detecting LAD, RCA, and circumflex disease is 91%, 87%, and 63%, respectively [6]. Importantly, this relatively high vessel-by-vessel sensitivity was achieved without loss of specificity. Normal regional Tl-201 uptake and washout were found in 92% of scan segments supplied by normal coronary arteries. Because of this high specificity for individual coronary stenoses, the presence of Tl-201 perfusion abnormalities in multiple different vascular distributions provides strong evidence for the presence of multivessel CAD (figure 51-4).

Currently, only Tl-201 can be used in conjunction with standardized treadmill-exercise testing; the noninvasive measurement of rest and exercise ejection fractions and regional wall motion disorders can be performed easily only in patients performing bicycle ergometry (see chapter 52). This form of exercise is not comparable to upright walking exercise, which in most centers is used to determine the exercise prescription in patients recovering from an acute infarction. Thus, performing an exercise radionuclide angiogram for prognostic purposes may not suffice in the total predischarge evaluation of the patient. Another potential limitation of rest−exercise radionuclide angiography may be in determining the viability status of left ventricular regions with major myocardial asynergy at rest. Since several studies indicate that a low ejection fraction in the postinfarct patient is a powerful predictor of mortality [7, 8], it would appear important to know how much of the observed poor function is due to irreversible myocardial damage and whether there exists a component of severe resting regional myocardial hypoperfusion associated with high-grade coronary artery narrowing in the absence of infarction. In this situation, where poor function and severe asynergy exist at rest, the measurement of exercise ejection fraction often cannot resolve this question. Postnitroglycerin intervention angiography has been effectively utilized to assess viability [9, 10]; of at least theoretical concern, however, is the difficulty in distinguishing artifactual improvement because of passive pulling

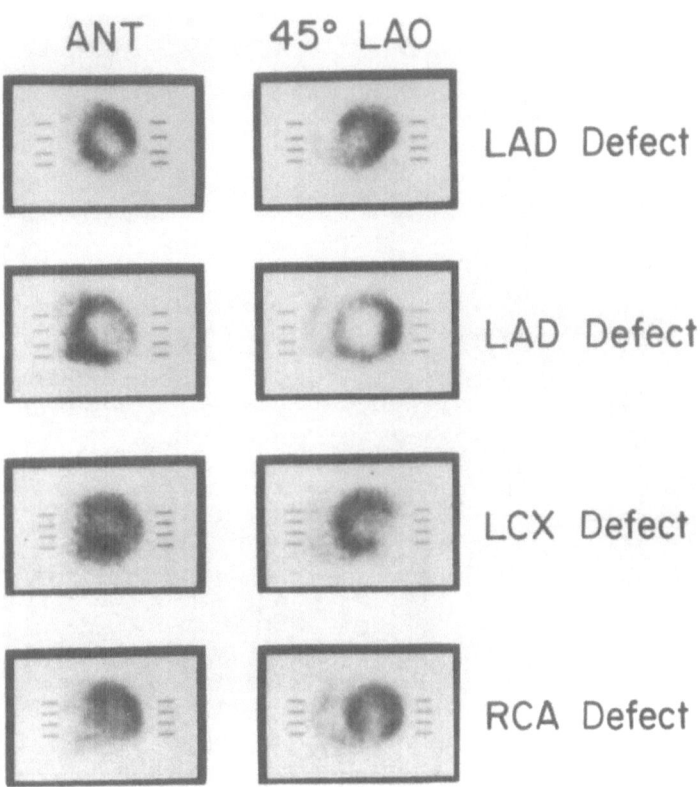

FIGURE 51-3. Anterior (ANT) and 45° LAO post-exercise images from four patients with isolated LAD, circumflex (LCx), and RCA disease. Notice the difference in defect size between the mid-LAD stenosis (top panel) and the more proximal LAD stenosis (second panel).

of a nonviable region by hyperkinetic adjacent segments from true improvement in regional contraction of an akinetic zone. Because Tl-201 uptake and washout depend on nutrient blood flow and cell membrane integrity, this technique has the potential for assessing the presence of viable myocardium. Based on experimental animal studies of transient ischemia and infarction [2, 11–13] and current interpretation of stress-redistribution scintigrams, it may be correctly assumed that myocardial segments showing initial defects after exercise with delayed redistribution represent ischemic but viable muscle. Moreover, it has recently been shown that the presence of redistribution during sequential Tl-201 imaging

can be used to predict accurately the response to surgery of preoperatively asynergic left ventricular segments [14, 15].

Tl-201 stress scintigraphy can also provide the clinician with a clue to the existence of significant, albeit subclinical, left ventricular dysfunction. The presence of abnormally increased lung thallium uptake on the initial postexercise anterior projection image has been investigated in patients with chronic symptomatic CAD and in those recovering from an acute myocardial infarction [16, 17] (figure 51-5). This finding has been described in association with exercise-induced ischemia producing a sudden rise in left ventricular end-diastolic pressure resulting in interstitial

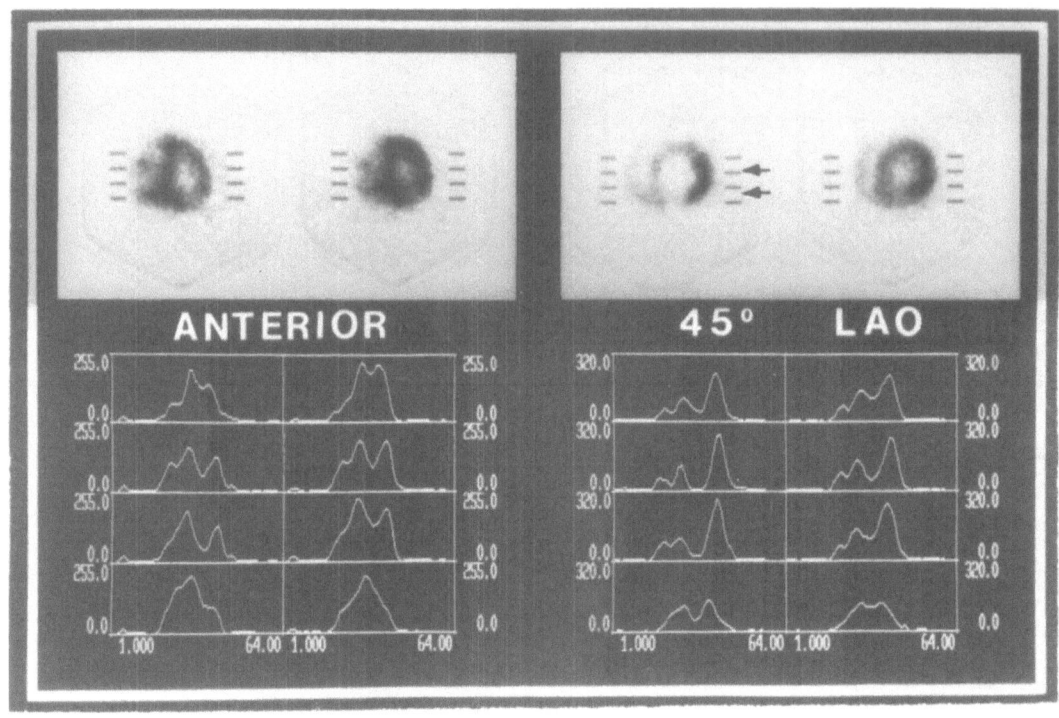

FIGURE 51-4. [25] Anterior and 45° LAO myocardial images obtained 10 min (left-hand image of each pair) and 2½ h (right-hand image of each pair) after low-level exercise in a patient with an acute anterior nontransmural infarction ten days earlier. The posterolateral wall is the only area that shows normal uptake and washout (arrows; 45° LAO image). There is delayed accumulation of Tl-201 indicative of complete redistribution in the anterolateral, apical, and inferior segments and partial redistribution in the anteroseptal segments and infero-apical segments. This scintigraphic study suggested residual ischemia in both the LAD and RCA distributions.

edema during peak exercise. When thallium is injected during peak exercise, it is sequestered temporarily in the lung as it traverses the pulmonary circulation because of the abnormally elevated pulmonary capillary pressure. By 30 min after exercise, with a subsequent decrease in pulmonary venous pressure, the increased lung thallium activity begins to diminish, and it disappears altogether within a time interval consistent with clearance of interstitial lung water [18]. Since lung uptake of Tl-201 during exercise indicates a high likelihood of multivessel CAD even when associated with less extensive perfusion defects, and correlates with greater impairment of exercise tolerance, a higher prevalence of exercise-induced ischemia, and a lower resting ejection

fraction, this finding adds another dimension to conventional stress scintigraphy.

Limitations of Coronary Arteriography for Assessing Prognosis

Since mortality in CAD can be related to the number of vessels with "significant" stenoses, the coronary angiogram has long been used as the standard for evaluating ischemic heart disease. Only recently has it become acceptable among cardiologists to raise the question of whether this invasive assessment of anatomy is always correct in determining whether a patient has functionally significant CAD. We are beginning to see reports hinting that coronary stenotic lesions are

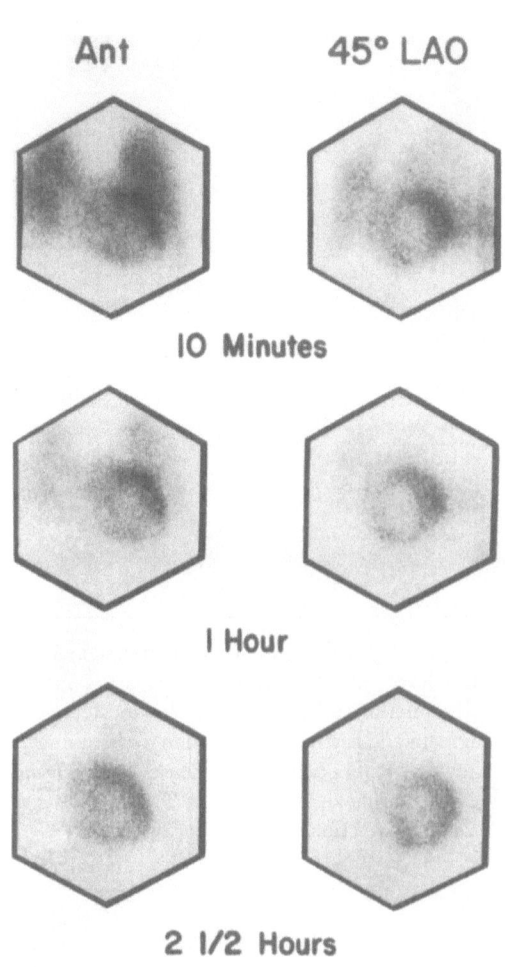

Ant   45° LAO

10 Minutes

1 Hour

2 1/2 Hours

FIGURE 51-5. Conventional unprocessed anterior (left) and 45° LAO (right) scintigrams from a patient with an old inferior nontransmural infarction and multivessel CAD, showing greatly increased lung thallium that diminished over time. The left ventricle is dilated and redistribution of Tl-201 is demonstrated in the inferior, apical, inferoapical, and anteroseptal myocardial segments. The patient developed limiting angina at 5 mets with dyspnea and demonstrated a blunted blood pressure response. The ST-segment motion during exercise was equivocal.

only part of the story; data from these studies indicate that the functional consequences induced by exercise stress of any given anatomic configuration may impinge more upon prognosis than the mere number of vessels with stenosis [19−25]. For example, not all patients with proximal LAD disease, observed in conjunction with an acute inferior infarction and occlusion of the RCA, will behave similarly. In some patients, exercise stress will result in marked ischemia of the apical, anterolateral, and septal regions, indicating a large area of jeopardized myocardium that may be at risk for subsequent infarction (figure 51-6). Other patients with similar anatomy will not demonstrate remote ischemia in the LAD territory and might be expected to do well after recovery from the inferior wall infarction. Several groups have now demonstrated that exercise nuclear imaging can stratify patients with multivessel CAD and also those with single-vessel disease into high- and low-risk groups [20, 22, 23]. In these studies, it has been shown that the amount of myocardial jeopardy appears to be more important for prognostication than mere delineation of the number and location of coronary artery stenoses.

The discrepancy between the anatomic presence of CAD and its functional significance can be seen in a recent study by Marcus et al. [27] in which a newly developed Doppler catheter transducer was used to measure coronary artery flow reserve in patients sent for coronary bypass graft surgery. Coronary artery flow was measured under control conditions and during peak reactive hyperemia after a transient coronary occlusion. Peak reactive hyperemic flow was considered an index of maximum coronary artery flow reserve. In angiographically normal vessels, Marcus and co-workers found a four- to sixfold increase in flow during peak reactive hyperemia. In contrast, patients with severe coronary artery narrowing (i.e., > 90%) had a markedly reduced flow reserve, suggesting that these lesions are hemodynamically significant. In patients with less severe coronary artery narrowing (i.e., 70%−90%), however, flow reserve was at least occasionally normal. Moreover, patients with lesions considered insignificant by angiographic criteria (i.e., < 50%) often had a pronounced reduction in flow reserve, suggesting functional impairment of nutrient blood flow delivery. These studies and others [24, 28] illustrate the hazard of using angiographically determined percent narrowing as the standard for not only judging the utility of noninvasive imaging techniques, but also in evaluating the functional severity of CAD.

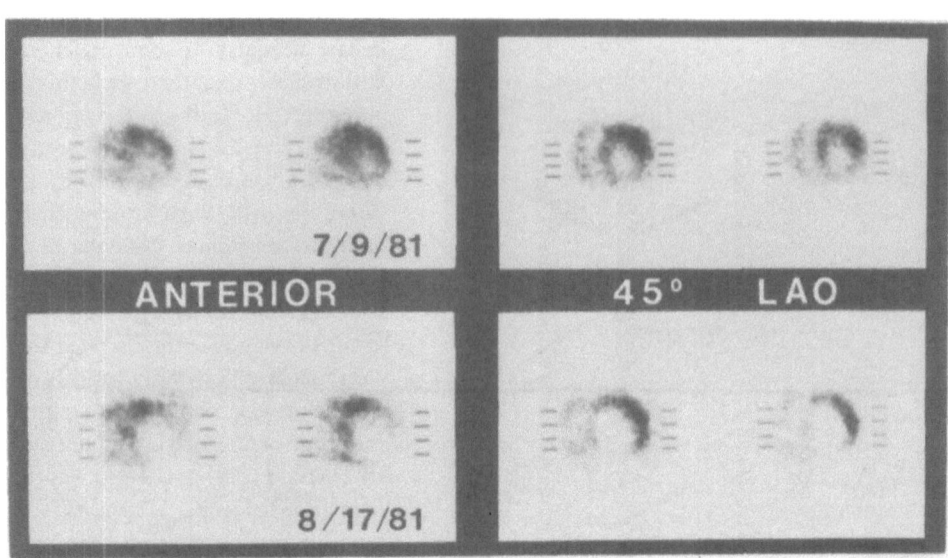

FIGURE 51-6. [25] (Top) Anterior and 45° LAO myocardial images obtained 10 min (left-hand image of each pair) and 2½ h (right-hand image of each pair) following low-level exercise nine days after acute inferior myocardial infarction. Persistent defects are demonstrated in the inferior and inferoapical—low posterolateral segments. Complete redistribution is seen in the anterolateral segment and partial redistribution in the apical and anteroseptal segments. The mid-high posterolateral segment shows normal uptake and washout. (Bottom) Same patient after an extensive anterior infarction. The left ventricle is now dilated and persistent Tl-201 defects are seen in the anterolateral, apical, and anteroseptal segments. The ejection fraction fell from 51% on 9 July 1981 to 34% on 17 August 1981.

Prognostic Value of Thallium-201 Scintigraphy

In clinical practice, before expecting the primary care physician to affirm the usefulness of exercise Tl-201 imaging, it first is necessary to determine the prognostic value of a normal scintigraphic study. This is particularly true since it is an accepted fact that finding normal coronary arteries or only mild nonobstructive disease at cardiac catheterization predicts a very low risk for major cardiac events (table 51-1). To date, only one study has examined the prognostic value of normal exercise scintigraphy in patients presenting for evaluation of chest pain [29]. In this study of 345 patients who had normal scintigrams by quantitative criteria (see figure 51-1), the mean age was 50 years, 60% were male, and in 27% the chest-pain description was considered typical for angina pectoris. During a mean follow-up of

17 months, only three patients died of cardiac causes (0.6% per year) and two patients had nonfatal myocardial infarction (0.4% per year). When these annualized event rates are compared with those in table 51-1, it appears that a normal exercise Tl-201 scintigram offers prognostic information comparable to that obtained with an invasive assessment of coronary anatomy.

Tl-201 scintigraphy soon after acute myocardial infarction is useful in identifying patients with functionally significant multivessel CAD and with jeopardized myocardium who would presumably be at risk of suffering a recurrent cardiac event [6, 25, 26]. By observing the number of vascular regions with diminished perfusion, our group has shown that the extent of underlying coronary obstructive disease can be accurately predicted when low-level exercise Tl-201 scintigraphy is performed within two weeks after myocardial infarction (figure 51-4) [6]. It is important to

TABLE 51-1. Incidence of death and nonfatal infarction in 1146 patients with normal coronary arteries or mild nonobstructive atherosclerosis

| Study[a] | Clinical characteristics | | | | Event rate[c] | |
	Age (yrs)	Sex (% male)	% Pts with typical AP[b]	Follow-up (yrs)	Death (%)	MI (%)
Kemp	47	51	44	3.0	1.0	0
Marchandise	49	56	--	3.0	0	2.4
Pasternak	46	60	34	3.5	0	0.2
Dermaria	--	--	0	2.7	0	0.4
Proudfit	--	62	10	10.0	0.3	0.3[d]
Isner	49	40	--	4.3	0.6	0.7
				Average	0.3	0.7

[a]All studies included ≥ 2000 patient months of follow-up.
[b]Annual event rate.
[c]Includes only Q-wave infarcts.
[d]AP, angina pectoris.

note that we employ quantitative scintigraphy [3] since it permits objective evaluation of both thallium uptake and washout kinetics and is more sensitive than qualitative analysis [5, 30]. This latter point is especially true when information about the degree and extent of physiologic impairment of blood flow is being sought [5].

By examining the full data content of the predischarge exercise Tl-201 scintigraphic study, our group has also shown that this noninvasive imaging technique can stratify postinfarction patients into high- and low-risk groups. To date, we have prospectively followed 140 patients with acute uncomplicated infarction who have undergone predischarge exercise scintigraphy and coronary angiography. In this group, a significantly greater incidence of future cardiac events (death, recurrent infarction, or unstable angina pectoris) was found in patients who demonstrated at least one "high risk" scintigraphic abnormality (figure 51-7). These abnormalities included multiple thallium defects involving different vascular distributions, a redistribution pattern within one or more of these defects and abnormal Tl-201 lung uptake. Importantly, as can be seen in figure 51-7, low-risk patients were best identified by Tl-201 scintigraphy. These patients demonstrated a persistent thallium defect confined to the distribution of their acutely infarcted vessel and showed no evidence of residual ischemia (i.e., no redistribution) or abnormal Tl-201 lung uptake.

In this study, "high risk" scintigraphy identified 47 (94%) of 50 patients who experienced a subsequent cardiac event during a 16 month follow-up period. By comparison, exercise-induced ST-segment depression and/or angina detected only 28 (56%) and the presence of multivessel CAD by angiography identified 37 patients (71%). The reason for this lower sensitivity with angiography compared with scintigraphy was because 13 of the 50 patients who experienced a subsequent cardiac event had a single-vessel CAD. Importantly, 12 of these 13 patients demonstrated redistribution during sequential Tl-201 imaging within the infarct zone. Thus, predischarge scintigraphy was quite useful in identifying a subset of patients with single-vessel CAD and residual periinfarction ischemia who had a future cardiac event. Indeed, the three scintigraphic markers of high risk identified all but three patients who subsequently had a cardiac event and, because of this, the error rate in falsely classifying patients as low risk was less than with exercise testing alone or coronary angiography.

It is not surprising that Tl-201 defects in more than one specific vascular region predict a high likelihood of future cardiac events in postinfarction patients. Several groups have correlated this scintigraphic finding with multivessel CAD [5, 6, 31, 32], a known indicator of prognosis. It has also been shown that thallium imaging may provide objective information concerning the severity of underlying anatomic disease; defects that appear at low levels of exercise stress in postinfarct patients most often denote vessels with 90% or greater obstruction [6]. Also, two independent studies indicate that the number of Tl-201 defects is a powerful predictor of ischemic cardiac events in patients with chronic symptomatic CAD [19, 33].

Our hypothesis that Tl-201 redistribution should be considered a marker of high risk in postinfarction patients appears valid and supported by the results of our study. There is now a substantial amount of experimental and clinical data indicating that redistribution of thallium occurs under conditions of transient ischemia [11−14]. Delayed redistribution also appears to be strongly correlated with an increased risk for major cardiac event in patients with chronic CAD [19]. Moreover, this finding predicts a highly favorable response to coronary revascularization surgery [15]. In studies performed by our group, we have recently shown that 93% of scan segments demonstrating complete redistribution become normal after surgery. As expected, the likelihood of restoring Tl-201 uptake and washout to normal is lower in segments showing partial redistribution; in our study, it was 73%.

Previous observations suggested that increased lung uptake of Tl-201 on the initial postexercise scintigram would correlate with an adverse clinical outcome [16, 17, 19]. In our 140 patients recovering from acute uncomplicated infarction, we found more residual exercise-induced ischemia in patients showing this abnormality. Compared with 97 patients who exhibited normal lung Tl-201 activity, the 43 patients with increased lung uptake had a higher prevalence of ST-segment depression and/or angina (36% vs 53%), Tl-201 redistribution (40% vs 77%), and a greater number of scan segments with redistribution (0.7 vs 1.6 per patient). Thus, these data are in agreement with our hypothesis that acute ischemia during low-level predischarge exercise stress may result in transient myocardial dysfunction, most surely associated with the rise in left ventricular filling and pulmonary capillary pressure. When Tl-201 is injected intravenously during this dysfunctional state, the radionuclide deposits in the pulmonary interstitial space. When ischemia resolves with return of the left ventricu-

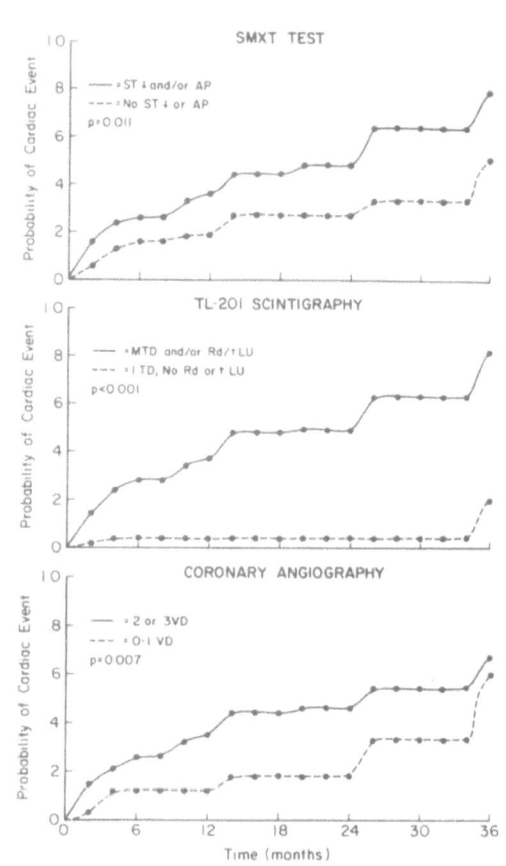

FIGURE 51-7. [25] The cumulative probability of cardiac events as a function of time for different subgroups formed by the exercise test response (top), scintigraphic findings (middle), or angiographic result (bottom) before hospital discharge. The solid and dashed lines indicate the high- and low-risk probabilities, respectively. ST ↓ , 1 mm or more depression; AP, angina pectoris; MTD, multiple thallium defects; Rd, redistribution; ↑ LU, increased lung uptake; 1 TD, thallium defect confined to single vascular region; VD, vessel disease (≥ 50% stenosis).

lar filling pressure to a lower value, the gradient for thallium transport favors movement to the pulmonary capillary blood pool.

Summary and Perspective

Low-level exercise Tl-201 scintigraphy before hospital discharge is quite helpful in assessing risk for subsequent cardiac events in patients recovering from acute infarction. Because of its unique ability to determine nutrient blood flow distribution in a specific myocardial region, it enables us to quantify the extent of residual ischemia and also to distinguish periinfarction ischemia from remote ischemia. Moreover, this noninvasive technique provides important physiologic information in patients with single- or multivessel CAD by angiography. Our studies and others indicate that, in patients with similar coronary pathoanatomy, Tl-201 scintigraphy can be used to further stratify risk based on the presence or absence and extent of inducible myocardial ischemia.

Based on available data, patients who manifest scintigraphic evidence of residual myocardial ischemia at low exercise workloads or heart rates are optimal candidates for intensive or prophylactic medical therapy or for cardiac catheterization and possible coronary bypass surgery or balloon angioplasty. On the other hand, patients with a single-region persistent Tl-201 defect and no increased lung uptake have very little to gain from even a highly effective pharmacologic or surgical intervention since their risk for a future cardiac event is quite low. Such patients, however, are candidates for early rehabilitation and rapid return to productive lifestyles (see chapter 58).

References

1. Gibson RS, Watson DD: Clinical applications of myocardial perfusion scintigraphy with thallium-201. In Beller GA, Yu P, Goodwin JF (eds) Progress in cardiology. Philadelphia: Lea-Febiger, 1983 (in press).

2. Beller GA, Watson DD, Pohost GM: Kinetics of thallium distribution and redistribution: clinical applications in sequential myocardial imaging. In: Strauss HW, Pitt B (eds) Cardiovascular nuclear medicine. St Louis: CV Mosby, 1979, pp 225–242.

3. Watson DD, Campbell NP, Read EK, et al: Spatial and temporal quantitation of planar thallium myocardial images. J Nucl Med 22:577, 1981.

4. Gibson RS, Beller GA: Should exercise electrocardiographic testing be replaced by the radionuclide methods? In: Rahimtoola SH, Brest AN (eds) Controversies in coronary artery disease. Philadelphia: FA Davis, 1982, pp 1–32.

5. Berger BC, Watson DD, Taylor GJ, et al: Quantitative thallium-201 exercise scintigraphy for detection of coronary artery disease. J Nucl Med 22:585, 1981.

6. Gibson RS, Taylor GJ, Watson DD, et al: Predicting the extent and location of coronary artery disease during the early post-infarction period by quantitative thallium-201 scintigraphy. Am J Cardiol 47:1010, 1981.

7. Schulze RA, Strauss HW, Pitt B, et al: Sudden death in the year following myocardial infarction: relation to ventricular premature contractions in the late hospital phase and left ventricular ejection fraction. Am J Med 62:192, 1977.

8. Taylor GJ, Humphries JO, Melletis ED, et al: Predictors of clinical course, coronary anatomy and left ventricular function after recovery from acute myocardial infarction. Circulation 62:960, 1980.

9. Banka VS, Bodenheimer MM, Shahr x, et al: Intervention ventriculography: comparative value of nitroglycerin, postextrasystolic potentiation and nitroglycerin plus extrasystolic potentiation. Circulation 53:632, 1976.

10. Bodenheimer MM, Banka VS, Hermann GA, et al: Reversible asynergy: histopathologic and electrographic correlations in patients with coronary artery disease. Circulation 53:792, 1976.

11. Pohost GM, Zir LM, Moore RH, et al: Differentiation of transiently ischemic from infarcted myocardium by serial imaging after a single dose of thallium-201. Circulation 55:294, 1977.

12. Beller GA, Watson DD, Ackell T, et al: Time course of thallium-201 redistribution after transient myocardial ischemia. Circulation 61:791, 1980.

13. Grunwald AM, Watson DD, Holzgrefe HH, et al: Myocardial thallium-201 kinetics in normal and ischemic myocardium. Circulation 64:610, 1981.

14. Rozanski A, Berman DS, Gray R, et al: Use of thallium-201 redistribution scintigraphy in the pre-operative differentiation of reversible and nonreversible myocardial asynergy. Circulation 64:936, 1981.

15. Gibson RS, Watson DD, Taylor GJ, et al: Prospective assessment of regional myocardial perfusion before and after coronary revascularization surgery by quantitative thallium-201 scintigraphy. J Am Coll Cardiol 1:804, 1983.

16. Boucher CA, Zir LM, Beller GA, et al: Increased lung uptake of thallium-201 during exercise myocardial imaging: clinical, hemodynamic and angiographic implications in patients with coronary artery disease. Am J Cardiol 46:189, 1980.

17. Gibson RS, Watson DD, Carabello BA, et al: Clinical implications of increased lung uptake of thallium-201 during exercise scintigraphy two weeks post-myocardial infarction. Am J Cardiol 49:1586, 1982.

18. Fishman AP: Pulmonary edema: the water-exchanging function of the lung. Circulation 46: 390, 1972.

19. Brown K, Boucher CA, Okada RD, et al: Prognostic value of exercise thallium-201 imaging in patients presenting for evaluation of chest pain: J Am Coll Cardiol 1(4):994, 1983.

20. Nicod P, Corbett JR, Sirth BG, et al: Prognostic assessment after myocardial infarction: comparison between coronary angiography and submaximal exercise testing with radionuclide ventriculography. Am J Cardiol 49:991, 1982.

21. Phillips P, Borer JS, Jacobstein J, et al: Prognostically critical coronary stenosis: identifcation by radionuclide cine angiography. Am J Cardiol 49:991, 1982.

22. Phillips P, Borer JS, Goldstein J, et al: Proximal left anterior descending coronary stenosis: the functional equivalent of triple vessel disease? Am J Cardiol 49:957, 1982.

23. Bonow RO, Kent KM, Rosing DR, et al: Left ventricular function during exercise in mildly symptomatic patients with coronary artery disease: identification of subgroups at risk for left main disease, triple vessel disease, and sudden death. J Am Coll Cardiol 1:654, 1983.

24. Bateman T, Gray R, Rozanski A, et al: Assessment of hemodynamic severity of coronary stenoses using gated wall motion scintigraphy. J Am Coll Cardiol 1:654, 1983.

25. Gibson RS, Watson DD, Craddock GB, et al: Predicting cardiac events after uncomplicated acute myocardial infarction: a prospective study comparing predischarge exercise thallium-201 scintigraphy and coronary angiography. Circulation, 1983 68:321, 1983.

26. Gibson RS, Taylor GJ, Watson DD, et al: Prognostic significance of resting anterior thallium-201 defects in patients with inferior myocardial infarction. J Nucl Med 21:1015, 1980.

27. Marcus M, Wright C, Doty D, et al: Measurement of coronary velocity and reactive hyperemia in the coronary circulation of humans. Circ Res 49:877, 1981.

28. Gould KL, Schelbert HR, Phelps ME: Noninvasive assessment of coronary stenoses by myocardial imaging during pharmacologic coronary vasodilation. Am J Cardiol 43:200, 1979.

29. Pamelia FX, Watson DD, Gibson RS, et al: Prognosis of patients with chest pain and normal thallium-201 exercise scintigrams. J Nucl Med 23:18, 1982.

30. Maddahi J, Garcia ED, Berman DS, et al: Improved noninvasive assessment of coronary artery disease by quantitative analysis of regional stress myocardial distribution and washout of thallium-201. Circulation 64:924, 1981.

31. Massey BM, Botvinick EH, Brundage BH: Correlation of thallium-201 scintigrams with coronary anatomy: factors affected by region sensitivity. Am J Cardiol 44:616, 1979.

32. Dunn RF, Friedman B, Bailey IK, et al: Noninvasive prediction of multivessel disease after myocardial infarction. Circulation 52:726, 1980.

33. Staniloff H, Diamond G, Forester J, et al: Prediction of death, infarction and worsening chest pain with exercise electrocardiography and thallium scintigraphy. Am J Cardiol 49:967, 1982.

52. THE VALUE OF RADIONUCLIDE ANGIOGRAPHY FOR RISK ASSESSMENT OF PATIENTS FOLLOWING ACUTE MYOCARDIAL INFARCTION

Kenneth G. Morris

Mortality in the first year among survivors of acute myocardial infarction is 10% – 15% or approximately three times that of the general population of patients with coronary artery disease. Accurate and reliable methods of risk assessment would be very useful in the clinical management of these patients. High-risk patients could be selected for closer follow-up and more extensive evaluation with angiographic or possibly electrophysiologic testing (see chapter 54), while low-risk patients could be spared the risk and expense of a variety of procedures and interventions, and rehabilitated more rapidly. Also, clinical trials of interventions aimed at altering prognosis following myocardial infarction would be facilitated by stratifying patients by risk prior to randomization, allowing evaluation of the efficacy of the intervention over the spectrum of risk. Sample size requirements might also be reduced by the exclusion of subjects at low risk who are less likely to benefit from an intervention.

Extensive studies have indicated a variety of clinical and laboratory parameters of some prog-

This study was supported in part by a research grant HL 17670 from the National Heart, Lung and Blood Institute, Bethesda, Maryland; HS 03834 from the National Center for Health Services Research—OASH; the Henry J. Kaiser Family Foundation; the Andrew Mellon Foundation; and by the Research Service of the Durham Veterans Administration Medical Center, Durham, North Carolina.

R.M. Califf and G.S. Wagner (eds.), ACUTE CORONARY CARE: Principles and Practice. Copyright © 1985. Martinus Nijhoff Publishing, Boston/Dordrecht/Lancaster.

nostic significance [1–5]. Most of these reflect one of the following pathophysiologic conditions: the severity of left ventricular dysfunction after infarction, the presence of residual potentially ischemic myocardium, and/or electrical instability following recovery from acute infarction. Studies of direct assessment of left ventricular function with contrast angiography have shown that resting ejection fraction is the most important prognostic variable among clinical or angiographic descriptors in survivors [6–8]. The severity of left ventricular dysfunction appears to be linearly related to the extent of the infarction [9]. A second group of prognostic variables, including recurrent angina pectoris or evidence of ischemia during exercise stress testing after infarction [10, 11], and the angiographic severity of coronary artery disease, are indicators of residual potentially ischemic myocardium. Among clinical and angiographic parameters, the number of diseased coronary arteries appears to be the second most prognostically important variable [8]. A third group of variables that may reflect electrical instability of the myocardium would include the late occurrence of ventricular tachycardia or fibrillation or evidence of significant ventricular arrhythmias on Holter monitoring prior to discharge [12] (see chapter 53). In theory, invasive electrophysiologic testing with programmed stimulation of the ventricles may provide more definitive information regarding the electrical stability of the myocardium after infarction (see chapter 54). At present, it is uncertain whether ventricular arrhythmias are prognostically significant independent of those parameters that reflect left ventricular function and, thereby, either ischemic or infarcted myocardium.

Radionuclide angiography (RNA) is an accurate noninvasive method for the evaluation of left ventricular function at rest and exercise. Both the change in ejection fraction from rest to exercise and the exercise ejection fraction correlate with the severity of coronary artery disease [13] and are more sensitive than ST-segment changes for detecting abnormalities due to exercise-induced myocardial ischemia [14]. The amount of left ventricular dysfunction produced acutely by myocardial ischemia appears to vary linearly with the severity of ischemia produced [15]. Thus rest and exercise RNA provide information noninvasively regarding both the severity of left ventricular dysfunction and the amount of potentially ischemic myocardium, two of the three major pathophysiologic mechanisms related to prognosis. It is reasonable to hypothesize that rest and exercise RNA may provide useful prognostic information concerning subsequent mortality and morbidity in survivors of acute myocardial infarction.

Relationship between RNA Measurements and Established Prognostic Variables

Several studies have noted correlations between RNA parameters and other clinical or laboratory parameters that are of known prognostic significance. The results of these studies are summarized in table 52-1. Schulze et al. [12] reported a highly significant correlation between Lown ventricular arrhythmia class III or IV and RNA rest ejection fraction less than 40%. Borer et al. [16] observed that patients with these high-grade ventricular arrhythmias had lower rest and exercise ejection fractions. Battler et al. [17] noted an association between rest ejection fraction and persistent sinus tachycardia. Significant correlations between both Killip and New York Heart Association classes for congestive heart failure with rest ejection fraction have been noted by Shah et al. [18], Battler et al. [17], and Dewhurst and Muir [19]. A significant association between myocardial infarction location and ejection fraction was reported by Shah et al. [18] and Dewhurst and Muir [19], but was not found in the other studies. Dewhurst and Muir observed a significant association between rest ejection fraction as measured by radionuclide angiography and peak creatinine kinase after both anterior and inferior myocardial infarctions.

In studies performed in more than 100 survivors of myocardial infarction at Duke University Medical Center [20], rest ejection fraction was significantly associated with worst Killip class, New York Heart Association class for congestive heart failure, radiographic cardiomegaly, atrial tachyarrhythmias, ventricular arrhythmia score, infarct location, and history of previous myocardial infarction, all variables with established prognostic significance. Exercise ejection fraction was also significantly correlated with most of these variables. The occurrence of ST depression of 0.1 mV or greater during exercise testing was not significantly correlated with rest or exercise ejection fraction, but was significantly associated with the change in ejection fraction from rest to exercise.

The relationship between resting ejection fraction and infarct location in the Duke study as determined by Q waves on the discharge electrocardiogram is demonstrated in figure 52-1: 16 patients had no Q waves resulting from either recent or previous infarct and this group had a mean ejection fraction of 51%. Likewise, patients with inferior and/or posterior infarcts as a group had normal or nearly normal ejection fractions. Patients with precordial Q waves and the single individual with Q waves in leads I and aVL had a mean ejection fraction of only 40%. Patients with both anterior and lateral, or both anterior and inferior Q waves had the most severely depressed ejection fractions with the mean for both groups of less than 30%.

The relationship between functional class for congestive heart failure during recovery after infarction and resting ejection fraction as determined by RNA in the Duke series is shown in figure 52-2. The cumulative distribution function is indicated for each functional class. The median ejection fractions for class-III and class-IV patients were less than 30, and for class-I and

TABLE 52-1. Correlation of RNA parameters with known prognostic variables

Clinical parameter	Rest EF	Exercise EF	Δ EF	Study group
Infarct location	+	+	−	Shaw, Dewhurst, Duke
History previous MI	+	+	−	Duke
Killip class	+	+	−	Duke
MIRU class	+			Battler
NYHA CHF	+	+	−	Dewhurst, Duke
Cardiomegaly	+	+	−	Duke
Atrial tachyarrhythmia	+	+	−	Battler, Duke
Ventricular arrhythmia	+	+	−	Schulze, Borer, Duke
Exercise ST depression	−	−	+	Duke
Peak CPK release	+			Dewhurst

EF, ejection fraction; MI, myocardial infarction.

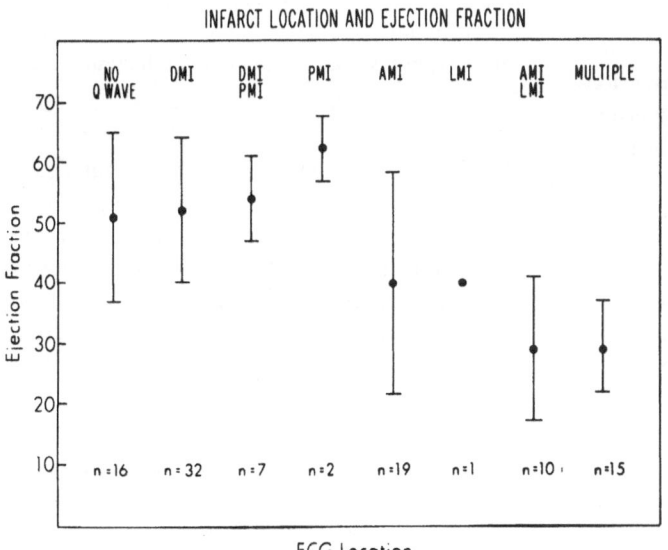

FIGURE 52-1. Relationship between infarct location as determined by location of significant Q waves on discharge electrocardiogram. This includes both recent and old infarcts. DMI, diaphragmatic infarct; PMI, posterior infarct; AMI, anterior infarct; LMI, lateral infarct; and multiple, both diaphragmatic and anterior myocardial infarctions.

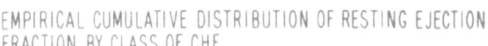
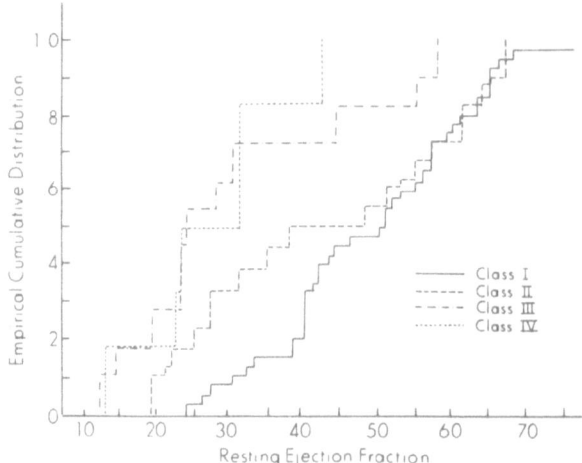

FIGURE 52-2. Relationship between clinical class for congestive heart failure and resting ejection fraction. The cumulative distribution function demonstrates the proportion of patients in each functional class with a given level of ejection fraction. While the significant correlation between clinical class and ejection fraction is seen, significant numbers of patients with low resting ejection fractions are found in each clinical class.

class-II patients were over 45%. It should be noted, however, that 20% of patients classified as New York Heart Association class III for congestive heart failure had normal or nearly normal resting ejection fractions and that 20% of patients with class-I or class-II heart failure had seriously depressed resting ejection fractions. Thus the objective measurement was superior to the clinical class for detecting left ventricular dysfunction.

Prognostic Value of Rest Ejection Fraction

Several small studies have been reported suggesting that resting ejection fraction as measured by RNA treated as a dichotomous variable might provide significant prognostic information regarding subsequent mortality. The results are summarized in table 52-2. Shah et al. [18] reported that the inhospital mortality of patients with acute infarcts with rest ejection fractions of less than 30% was 55%, with six of the seven deaths occurring in that group. Different levels of rest ejection fraction have been considered important by various investigators. Schulze et al. [12] reported a 30% one-year mortality in patients with ejection fractions of less than 40% at the time of discharge, with no mortality in patients with ejection fractions greater than 40%. Similarly,

Borer et al. [16] reported that all four deaths occurring in the first year of follow-up in their group of 45 patients occurred in patients with ejection fractions less than 35%. Subsequently a somewhat larger series by Battler et al. [17] (but with only nine events in the follow-up period) suggested a higher one-year mortality (24%) in patients with ejection fractions less than 52% compared with patients with normal ejection fractions (10%). More recently the Multicenter Postinfarction Research Group [21] has determined, in a series of 799 patients, that a rest ejection fraction of less than 40% was the most important of the variables studied for predicting subsequent mortality.

Califf et al. [22] have observed, however, that the predictive value of rest ejection fraction treated dichotomously and its value viz-à-viz other parameters changes significantly depending on the level of ejection fraction that is assumed to be

TABLE 52-2. Rest ejection fraction (EF) and mortality

Study	Total patients	Total deaths	EF	Mortality		Duration follow-up
Shaw	56	7	≤ 30	6/11	55%	Hospital
Schulze	81	8	< 40	8/45	18%	2−16 months
Borer	45	4	≤ 40	4/17	24%	6−14 months
Battler	87	10	< 52	10/62	16%	2−18 months
MPRG	799	77	< 40	∼ 41/265	15%	1 year

important. They observed in a population with chronic stable coronary artery disease that rest ejection fraction greater or less than 50% was not significantly related to mortality. When the critical level of rest ejection fraction was considered to be 40%, it was the third most important variable. When considered in a continuous fashion, however, rest ejection fraction was the most important predictor of mortality. Our group [23] observed that rest ejection fraction analyzed in a continuous fashion was significantly associated with two-year mortality, and that mortality increased sharply as ejection fraction fell below 40%.

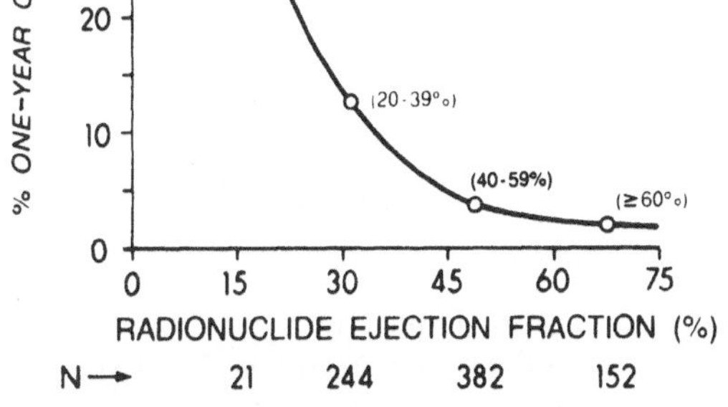

The Multicenter Postinfarction Research Group made a similar observation regarding the univariate association of rest ejection fraction with one-year mortality (figure 52-3) [21]. Patients with ejection fractions greater than 40% had less than 5% one-year cardiac mortality while patients with ejection fractions between 20% and 39% had a one-year mortality above 10% and patients with an ejection fraction less than 20% had a one-year mortality of over 45%. This study also performed multivariate analyses that showed that rest ejection fraction had prognostic significance independent of other clinical and laboratory parameters.

Value of Exercise RNA Parameters

Corbett et al. [24] reported the first study to analyze the prognostic value of exercise as well as resting RNA parameters. Their six-month follow-up study of 61 patients surviving acute myocardial infarction was also the first study that analyzed events other than death in the follow-up period. Discriminant function analysis of multiple RNA parameters treated dichotomously was used to assess their prognostic value with regard to major and minor cardiac events. Major cardiac events (16 patients) included death (four), recurrent myocardial infarction (five), and medically refractory angina (seven). Persistent congestive heart failure (11) and angina pectoris (ten) were considered minor events (21 patients). These investigators found the change in left ventricular ejection fraction with submaximal exercise to be the most important variable distinguishing patients who would subsequently suffer any cardiac event from those who would suffer none. They found rest ejection fraction, left ventricular wall

FIGURE 52-3. Cardiac mortality rate in four categories of radionuclide ejection fraction (EF) determined before discharge. N, the number of patients in the total population in each category. Reproduced by permission of the authors and the NEJM 300:331, 1983.

motion score, and left ventricular end-systolic volume index also to have significant associations with subsequent events. In an extension of this work [25], the authors noted that the peak left ventricular ejection fraction during exercise was the most important variable in distinguishing between these groups if the left ventricular ejection fraction at rest was less than 40%. This variable was also the most significant in those patients with an anterior myocardial infarction. The discriminant function using the change in the left ventricular ejection fraction with exercise was less capable of separating patients who would have major rather than minor cardiac events.

Hung et al. [26] in studies of 117 men recovering from acute myocardial infarcts found the change in ejection fraction from rest to exercise to be the best variable for predicting a combination of cardiac events. "Hard events" (eight) included one sudden cardiac death, one nonfatal episode of ventricular fibrillation, and six recurrent myocardial infarcts (one fatal). Patients with congestive heart failure or chest pain refractory to medical treatment were excluded from evaluation. The left ventricular ejection fraction during exercise was also a significant predictor of "hard medical events" and other events that included hospitalization for unstable angina pectoris (four), congestive heart failure (one), or coronary bypass surgery (nine).

The studies by Corbett and Hung and co-workers clearly demonstrate the ability of exercise RNA variables to predict cardiac events during follow-up. However, it is unclear from the analyses of the events in combination which event or events are actually being predicted and which RNA variable is most closely associated with each specific event.

Initial reports from the Duke series [20] revealed that both rest and exercise ejection fractions were significantly associated with one-year mortality using logistic regression analysis. Other RNA variables such as the occurrence of an exercise-induced wall motion abnormality or the change in ejection fraction with exercise were not significantly associated with mortality at one year. Three other events, all with myocardial ischemia as their underlying pathophysiology, were combined for analysis and included recurrent myocardial infarction, readmission for un-

stable angina pectoris, and coronary artery bypass grafting for disabling medically refractory angina pectoris. RNA variables associated with myocardial ischemia were the best predictors of these nonfatal ischemic events; the change in ejection fraction from rest to exercise was the best predictor of these events at one year. Thus, parameters associated with severe left ventricular dysfunction were the best predictors of mortality while parameters associated with residual myocardial ischemia were associated with the nonfatal ischemic events. Preliminary results of Cox model analysis of the two- and three-year follow-up of these patients has revealed that exercise ejection fraction is a somewhat more potent predictor of subsequent mortality than the resting value [23]. Individual analysis of the nonfatal ischemic events suggests that the change in ejection fraction from rest to exercise is most specifically related to disabling medically refractory angina pectoris requiring coronary artery bypass surgery [23]. Further work is required to establish the relationship between RNA parameters and other nonfatal ischemic events.

Studies by Dewhurst and Muir of the two-year follow-up of 100 survivors of acute myocardial infarction are in agreement with the results of the Duke series. Rest ejection fraction appeared to be significantly related to subsequent mortality while the change in ejection fraction from rest to exercise appeared to be significantly associated with subsequent disabling angina requiring coronary artery bypass grafting. Too few recurrent myocardial infarctions occurred in their study population to allow analysis of that endpoint.

Comparative Prognostic Value of RNA with Other Clinical and Laboratory Parameters

The results of the Duke study and those by Corbett et al. and Dewhurst and Muir all suggest that the RNA variables are more potent predictors of subsequent events than those available through history, physical examination, or ECG. In the discriminant function analyses used by Corbett et al. for their combined event analyses, the RNA variables were ranked higher than clinical variables. In the multivariable Cox models used for the Duke series, a similar result was obtained. Dewhurst and Muir found the RNA variables to be superior to any of the traditional prognostic indices such as those described by Peel, Norris, or Luria.

Exercise electrocardiography has been extensively studied as a prognostic procedure after myocardial infarction. Exercise-induced ST-segment changes were not as potent predictors of subsequent cardiac events as the RNA variables in the Duke series. In the combined event analyses of Corbett and Hung and their co-workers, submaximal exercise test variables such as maximal heart rate, blood pressure, work load, angina, ST changes, and arrhythmias were compared with the RNA variables for prognostic significance; the RNA variables were found to be more significantly related to subsequent events.

Thallium-201 myocardial scintigraphy has also been used prognostically in survivors of acute myocardial infarction. Hung et al. [26] specifically compared thallium-201 myocardial perfusion scintigraphy with rest and exercise radionuclide ventriculography. While they found that the results of thallium scintigraphy were significantly related to subsequent combined events, they determined that the RNA variables were superior to thallium scintigraphy for predicting events in patients recovering from myocardial infarction.

Coronary angiography has been used widely for prognostic purposes. The number of significantly diseased coronary vessels is second only to ejection fraction among clinical and angiographic variables as a predictor of subsequent mortality in patients recovering from myocardial infarction. Little work has been done to compare rest and exercise RNAs with coronary arteriography for predicting subsequent events. Nicod and co-workers [27] have compared these two techniques retrospectively in a relatively small group of patients. They have suggested that submaximal exercise testing with RNA may provide valuable prognostic information regarding subsequent cardiac events, in addition to that available by coronary arteriography. It is a reasonable hypothesis that functional information obtained from rest and exercise RNAs might offer information in addition to that available in an anatomic evalua-

tion. Additional prospective studies, however, are required.

Future Research

The relationships of rest and exercise ejection fractions to subsequent mortality and of the change in ejection fraction from rest to exercise with subsequent medically disabling angina pectoris are likely to be confirmed. Further studies of the relationship of RNA parameters with nonfatal ischemic events, especially myocardial infarction, are required. Much remains to be learned regarding the optimum time of obtaining maximum prognostic information. Our group has reported preliminarily [23] that exercise RNA eight weeks after infarction may provide more information than that available at the time of discharge, especially regarding the occurrence of recurrent nonfatal infarction. Specific predictive models for the relationships between exercise ejection fraction and mortality and other prognostically important endpoints need to be developed and evaluated. These models will need to be validated regarding the accuracy of their predictions and their ability to discriminate between groups with differing prognosis in a variety of patient populations. Studies will be required to examine the influence of the specific exercise protocol and various medications upon the prognostic utility of RNA parameters. These models may then be compared with other parameters such as those presented in chapters 51, 53, and 54 in this volume. Though both RNA and Holter parameters may offer independent prognostic information, it is unclear whether they will be sufficient to render the anatomic information from coronary angiography unnecessary. Finally, if useful models can be developed for stratifying patients by risk, studies can be performed to evaluate the utility of various interventions aimed at reducing morbidity and mortality in survivors of acute myocardial infarction.

References

1. McNeer JF, Wallace AG, Wagner GS, Starmer CF, Rosati RA: The course of acute myocardial infarction: the feasibility of early discharge of

the uncomplicated patient. Circulation 51:410–413, 1975.

2. Luria MH, Knoke JD, Wachs JS, Luria MA: Survival after recovery from acute myocardial infarction: two and five year prognostic indices. Am J Med 67:7–14, 1979.

3. Norris RM, Caughey DE, Deeming LW, Mercer CJ, Scott PJ: Coronary prognostic index for predicting survival after recovery from acute myocardial infarction. Lancet 2:485–488, 1970.

4. Harris PJ, Harrell FE Jr, Lee KL, Behar VS, Rosati RA: Survival in medically treated coronary artery disease. Circulation 60:1259–1269, 1979.

5. Battler A, Karliner JS, Higgins CB, Slutsky R, Gilpin EA, Froelicher VF, Ross J: The initial chest x-ray and acute myocardial infarction prediction of early and late mortality and survival. Circulation 60:1004–1009, 1980.

6. De Feyter PJ, Van Eenige MJ, Dighton DH, Visser FC, De Jong J, Roos JP: Prognostic value of exercise testing, coronary angiography and left ventriculography 6–8 weeks after myocardial infarction. Circulation 66:527–536, 1982.

7. Taylor GJ, Humphries JO, Mellits ED, Pitt B, Schulza RA, Griffith LSC, Ashuff SC: Predictors of clinical course, coronary anatomy and left ventricular function after recovery from acute myocardial infarction. Circulation 62:960–970, 1980.

8. Sanz G, Castaner A, Betriu A, Magrina J, Roig E, Coll S, Pare JC, Mavarro-Lopez F: Determinants of prognosis in survivors of myocardial infarction: a prospective clinical angiographic study. N Engl J Med 306:1065–1070, 1982.

9. Chu A, Morris KG, Cobb FR: Relationship between ventricular function by radionuclide angiography and extent of acute myocardial infarction in conscious dogs. Presented at the 53rd American Heart Association Meeting in Miami, Florida, 16–20 November 1980 [abstr]. Circulation 62:III-77, 1980.

10. Theroux P, Waters DD, Halphen C, Debaisieux J-C, Mizgala HF: Prognostic value of exercise testing soon after myocardial infarction. N Engl J Med 301:341–345, 1979.

11. De Busk RF, Davidson DM, Houston N, Fitzgerald J: Serial ambulatory electrocardiography and treadmill exercise testing after uncomplicated myocardial infarction. Am J Cardiol 45:547–554, 1980.

12. Schulze RA Jr, Strauss HW, Pitt B: Sudden death in the year following myocardial infarction: relation to ventricular premature contractions in the late hospital phase and left ventricular ejection fraction. Am J Med 62:192–199, 1977.

13. Jones RH, McEwan P, Newman GE, Port S, Rerych SK, Scholz PM, Upton MT, Peter CA, Austin EH, Leong K, Gibbons RJ, Cobb FR, Coleman RE, Sabiston DC Jr: Accuracy of diagnosis of coronary artery disease by radionuclide measurement of left ventricular function during rest and exercise. Circulation 64:586–601, 1981.

14. Upton MT, Rerych SK, Newman GE, Port S, Cobb FR, Jones RH: Detecting abnormalities in left ventricular function during exercise before angina and ST segment depression. Circulation 62:341–349, 1980.

15. Schneider RM, Roberts KB, Morris KG, Stanfield JA, Cobb FR: Relation between radionuclide angiographic regional ejection fraction and left ventricular regional ischemia in awake dogs. Am J Cardiol, 1984 (in press).

16. Borer JS, Rosing DR, Miller RH, Stark RM, Kent KM, Bacharach SL, Green MV, Lake CR, Cohen H, Holmes D, Donohue D, Baker W, Epstein SE: Natural history of left ventricular function during 1 year after acute myocardial infarction: comparison with clinical, electrocardiographic and biochemical determinations. Am J Cardiol 46:1–12, 1980.

17. Battler A, Slutsky R, Karliner JS, Froelicher V, Ashburn W, Ross J Jr: Left ventricular ejection fraction and first third ejection fraction early after acute myocardial infarction: value for predicting mortality and morbidity. Am J Cardiol 45:197–202, 1980.

18. Shah PK, Pichler M, Berman DS, Singh BN, Swan HJC: Left ventricular ejection fraction determined by radionuclide ventriculography in early stages of first transmural myocardial infarction: relation to short-term prognosis. Am J Cardiol 45:542–546, 1980.

19. Dewhurst NG, Muir AL: Comparative prognostic value of radionuclide ventriculography at rest and during exercise in 100 patients after first myocardial infarction. Br Heart J 49:111–121, 1983.

20. Morris KG, Califf RM, Palmeri ST, McKinnis RA, Coleman RE, Cobb FR: Prognostic significance of serial rest and exercise radionuclide angiography after acute myocardial infarction. Presented at the 31st Annual Scientific Sessions of the American College of Cardiology, 25–29 April 1982, Atlanta, Georgia. Am J Cardiol 49:901, 1982.

21. The Multicenter Postinfarction Research Group: Risk stratification and survival after myocardial

infarction. N Engl J Med 309:331–336, 1983.

22. Califf RM, Harrell FE, Pryor DB, Lee KL, Rosati RA: Prognostic stratification using ejection fraction. Circulation 68:III-413, 1983.

23. Morris KG, Califf RM, Pameri ST, McKinnis RA, Coleman RE, Cobb FR: Independent prognostic value to rest and exercise radionuclide angiography 3 & 8 weeks after infarction. Presented at the 56th Scientific Sessions of the American Heart Association Meetings, 14–17 November 1983, Anaheim, California. Circulation 68:III-118, 1983.

24. Corbett JR, Dehmer GJ, Lewis SE, Woodward W, Henderson E, Parkey RW, Blomqvist CG, Willerson JT: The prognostic value of submaximal exercise testing with radionuclide ventriculography before hospital discharge in patients with recent myocardial infarction. Circulation 64:535–544, 1981.

25. Corbett JR, Nicod P, Lewis SE, Rude RE, Willerson JT: Prognostic value of submaximal exercise radionuclide ventriculography after myocardial infarction. Am J Cardiol 52:82A, 1983.

26. Hung J, Goris ML, Nash E, Kraemer HC, De Busk R: Comparative value of maximal treadmill testing, exercise thallium myocardial perfusion scintigraphy and exercise radionuclide ventriculography for distinguishing high- and low-risk patients soon after myocardial infarction. Am J Cardiol 53:1221–1227, 1984.

27. Nicod P, Corbett JR, Firth BG, Lewis SE, Rude RE, Huxley R, Willerson JT: Prognostic value of resting and submaximal exercise radionuclide ventriculography after acute myocardial infarction in high-risk patients with single and multivessel disease. Am J Cardiol 52:30–35, 1983.

53. OPTIMAL USE OF AMBULATORY MONITORING PRIOR TO HOSPITAL DISCHARGE FOLLOWING ACUTE MYOCARDIAL INFARCTION

Arthur J. Moss

Ambulatory (Holter) electrocardiographic monitoring was first introduced over 20 years ago [1], and during the past ten years there has been widespread application of this technique to postinfarction patients [2–4]. Advancement in technology and the quality of the Holter recordings has produced an enormous data base that has outstripped our understanding of the clinical significance of the recorded events. Holter monitoring of postinfarction patients prior to hospital discharge is nearly a routine procedure in most institutions, but how can the information generated be utilized to optimize patient care? What are we looking for when we request a Holter recording on a patient after myocardial infarction?

The initial emphasis in Holter monitoring was on the identification of ventricular ectopic beats (VEBs) because these were thought to be harbingers of sudden arrhythmic death. It is now realized that the association between VEBs and ventricular fibrillation is more complex than originally thought. More recently, the usefulness of Holter monitoring in identifying rare events such as transient malignant arrhythmias and in evaluating asymptomatic myocardial ischemia has provided additional reasons for application to postinfarction patients. Furthermore, Holter monitoring is providing increased precision in

the evaluation of postinfarction therapies such as drugs, pacemakers, and "activity prescriptions." It should be emphasized that current recommendations regarding the optimal use of postinfarction Holter monitoring require periodic updating on the basis of accumulating research data and ongoing clinical experience.

Technical Aspects of Ambulatory Electrocardiography

Several types of good-quality 24-h Holter recorders are now available including reel-to-reel and cassette equipment. Desirable features should include the recording of at least two ECG leads, a timing signal, and an event marker that can be activated by the patient at the time of symptoms. Two ECG leads are essential to properly interpret ectopic beats and rhythms (aberration of supraventricular complexes vs ventricular ectopy), to minimize loss of information due to muscle artifact and noise, and to optimize evaluation of ST-segment changes from different regions of the heart. Proper electrode placement with careful cleansing of the skin is an essential requirement for obtaining quality recordings, and technicians should be specially trained in this procedure. Although patient diaries are part of the routine protocol, there is generally a poor correlation

R.M. Califf and G.S. Wagner (eds.), ACUTE CORONARY CARE: Principles and Practice. Copyright © 1985. Martinus Nijhoff Publishing, Boston/Dordrecht/Lancaster.

between recorded events and the diary information.

Commercial analysis units are available with a variety of features including high-speed playback, automated arrhythmia detection, ectopic beat counts according to prespecified criteria, and trend plots of heart rate, ST-segment shifts, and frequency of ectopic beats. The commercial equipment has become progressively more sophisticated, frequently with less than adequate validation of the automated trend data. This problem has been partially rectified by hardcopy printout of the entire 24-h recording in rows of real-time data at slow paper speed. Regardless of the equipment utilized, the key to obtaining quality analyses is the utilization of knowledgeable and experienced personnel who have decision-making capability in their interaction with the system. Quality control procedures must be part of the weekly analysis schedule to establish the validity and the reliability of the rhythm analyses. Without careful attention to quality control, there tends to be a high frequency of false negatives, i.e., failure to identify important events that are present on the recording. Computer techniques are being increasingly utilized in the processing of Holter data [6]. Operator interaction with the computer processing is still required, and it is unlikely that computer analysis will be fully automated at any time in the foreseeable future.

Assessment of Ventricular Arrhythmias

The widespread use of Holter monitoring in postinfarction patients is primarily the result of the interest in ventricular arrhythmias that has been generated from coronary care unit experience. The mechanistic association between VEBs and malignant ventricular arrhythmias in the hyperacute phase of myocardial infarction has been extrapolated to the subacute and chronic phases of ischemic heart disease. The validity of this hypothesis has been questioned since high-risk VEBs during the later phases are often associated with major abnormalities in the mechanical function of the heart. Epidemiologic studies have substantiated an increased risk of cardiac death in postinfarction patients with Holter-recorded frequent or complex VEBs, but these VEBs have an equally strong association with the subsequent occurrence of both sudden and nonsudden cardiac death [7]. The problem is further compounded by a spectrum of VEB classification schemes that have been used and by the absence of any antiarrhythmic drug trials that have substantiated an increased survival with VEB suppression.

Several different approaches have been used for the categorization and grading of Holter-recorded VEBs [8-10]. The six-level Lown grading scheme [8] is the most frequently utilized approach, but it has several shortcomings, as recently reported by Bigger and Weld [10]. The Lown grading scheme has never been validated in a postinfarction population. Close scrutiny of the Lown method indicates that there is insufficient weight given to VEB frequency, and mortality does not increase as a function of the grade. Ruberman et al. [9] have used a three-level (none, simple, and complex) categorization in which the simple category includes noncomplex VEB patterns, i.e., unifocal beats, and the complex category includes multiform, repetitive, early-cycle (R on T), or bigeminal patterns; VEB frequency is not quantitated. We have used the Ruberman scheme in our earlier Holter studies (6-h recordings) and found that VEBs in the complex category identified patients at increased risk of cardiac death. There was no differentiation between patients dying suddenly and nonsuddenly.

Bigger and Weld have recently reported the prognostic significance of 24-h Holter-recorded VEBs in 400 postinfarction patients during a variable 3- to 30-month follow-up period [10]. In this series, the overall cardiac mortality rate was proportional to VEB frequency; repetitive VEBs carried an additional independent risk, and the highest risk was associated with VEBs that were both frequent and repetitive. Early-cycle VEBs, the highest category in the Lown grading system, did not contribute independent risk in the Bigger and Weld analysis.

Recent experience in our Multicenter Postinfarction Risk Stratification Program with 866 enrolled patients revealed that one-year posthospital cardiac mortality progressively increased for increasingly frequent VEBs above a baseline of one per hour on a 24-h Holter recording [11]. Also, VEB frequencies >10/h make significant contributions to cardiac mortality independent of a low radionuclide ejection fraction. Furthermore, both the presence of repetitive VEBs (three or more in a row) and the number of repetitive VEBs in the longest recorded sequence were additional characteristics associated with increased cardiac mortality.

On the basis of these studies and my own clinical experience, I have evolved the grading scheme presented in table 53-1 for evaluating the clinical significance of predischarge VEBs on a 24-h Holter recording following myocardial infarction.

Repetitive VEBs must be at least three in a row. Malignant characteristics of repetitive VEBs are those that relate to rate, duration, or pattern. The definition of "malignant" is still in flux, but coupling intervals <300 ms, durations >10 beats in a row at rates >150/min, or torsades de pointes configurations are generally considered ominous.

This grading scheme permits a rational approach to therapy. Grade-I VEBs do not require consideration of antiarrhythmic therapy since their associated risk is minimal. Even grade-II VEBs probably do not require suppressive therapy. A good argument can be made for the treatment of grade-III VEBs, but satisfactory substantiating studies are not yet available. Both clinical experience and electrophysiologic studies (see chapter 54) indicate the antiarrhythmic and/or

TABLE 53-1. Grading scheme for evaluating clinical significance of predischarge VEBs

Grade I (low risk)	Average VEB frequency <3/h No repetitive VEBs
Grade II (intermediate risk)	Average VEB frequency ≥3/h *or* Repetitive beats without malignant characteristics
Grade III (high risk)	Average VEB frequency ≥3/h *and* Repetitive beats without malignant characteristics
Grade IV (very high risk)	Repetitive beats with malignant characteristics

antiischemic therapy should be administered to suppress grade-IV VEBs.

Detection of Atrioventricular Conduction Disorders

Postinfarction patients are vulnerable to the development of intermittent conduction disorders in the atrioventricular (AV) node and within the intraventricular conducting system (see chapter 39). The clinical significance of these transient conduction disturbances has not been well studied, but special concern is warranted for the individual patient who develops such abnormalities. First-degree AV block and brief periods of second-degree Wenckebach (Mobitz type I) conduction disturbances have minimal significance in the asymptomatic individual, but these arrhythmias may warrant attention in patients receiving cardiac glycosides, beta blockers, antiarrhythmics, or calcium antagonists.

Intermittent higher-grade AV blocks, either Mobitz type-II or complete (third-degree) AV block, are rare Holter events. They almost always appear in patients with established right or left bundle branch block, and always warrant concern because of their pathophysiologic implications. When such findings are observed on a predischarge Holter, hospital discharge should be delayed and further telemetry and/or Holter monitoring instituted. Electrophysiologic studies have rarely provided clinically useful information to guide therapy in this group of patients. Since the need for pacemaker implantation is determined by the presumed risk, it is generally agreed that all postinfarction patients showing Holter-recorded episodes of true Mobitz type-II or complete heart block should receive a prophylactic pacemaker.

Postinfarction patients may manifest transient bundle branch block during Holter monitoring, and it may be difficult to differentiate between left bundle branch block and right bundle branch block (with or without associated fascicular block) from the monitored leads. Regardless of the pattern of the bundle branch block, these transient conduction disturbances have special significance in patients who developed bundle branch block with transient complete AV block during an earlier phase of their acute myocardial infarction (see chapter 39). Permanent pacing is indicated in this subset of patients [12].

Detection of Supraventricular Arrhythmias

Paroxysmal supraventricular arrhythmias have received scant attention in studies of Holter recordings in postinfarction patients. Nevertheless, identification of supraventricular arrhythmias should permit improved care to the individual patient. Short sinus pauses of 1.5 s or less are frequently observed in postinfarction Holter recordings, especially at night and in patients receiving beta-blocking drugs, and such findings carry minimal meaning. Prolonged sinus pauses greater than 2 s or sustained sinus bradycardia less than 40 beats/min indicate either significant sinus node disease or vasovagal episodes (see chapter 12). These bradyarrhythmias may aggravate an already compromised coronary circulation. When these bradyarrhythmias coexist with episodic atrial tachyarrhythmias (brady-tachy syndrome), especially in elderly patients, they are generally poorly tolerated.

Paroxysmal supraventricular tachycardia at rates of 150/min or greater may lead to decompensation in the postinfarction patient and, when documented, appropriate suppressive therapy should be rendered. The Holter recording provides valuable information on the mode of spontaneous onset of the tachycardia, with its important implications for therapy [13].

Paroxysmal atrial flutter or fibrillation often accompanies atrial infarction or atrial overload, and detection of these arrhythmias is important for optimizing individual therapy. These arrhythmias are frequently preceded by progressive sinus bradycardia, occurring at rest or after a meal, and thereby suggesting a vagally induced mechanism. Paroxysmal atrial flutter or fibrillation may cause problems by their ventricular rate, by loss of the atrial kick with its hemodynamic consequences, or by their frequent association with mural thrombi and their potential for systemic embolization. Anticoagulant and antiarrhythmic therapy are often indicated when these arrhythmias are detected.

Evaluation of Ischemic ST-segment Changes

With the technical improvement in Holter recording systems, the frequency response characteristics are sufficient to permit accurate evaluation of ST-segment changes. Thus, some information about the frequency and severity of transient myocardial ischemic episodes during daily activities is available. Myocardial ischemia should be inferred only when there are significant elevations or depressions of the ST segments relative to baseline, often in association with alterations in the T-wave configuration in that lead. Isolated T-wave changes in the absence of associated ST-segment changes must be interpreted with caution since such findings are frequently observed in normals.

The ischemic-type ST-segment changes often occur during asymptomatic periods, and, for the most part, without clear-cut precipitating factors [14]. The frequency of occurrence of ischemic ST-segment changes during sleep in postinfarction patients has not been reported, but almost a quarter of Holter-monitored patients with chronic ischemic disease have such changes [15]. The role of enhanced vasomotor activity in precipitating coronary spasm and myocardial ischemia in postinfarction patients is undergoing active investigation. Holter-recorded episodes of ST-segment elevation are a good marker of vasospastic myocardial ischemia, and such findings may indicate the need for therapy with calcium blockers (see chapter 41).

Stern and Tzivoni have highlighted the potentially dangerous combination of ischemic ST-segment changes and ventricular arrhythmias on Holter recordings [14]. Since myocardial ischemia is a major initiating factor in the genesis of malignant ventricular arrhythmias, and since previous recordings of sudden death have demonstrated ischemic ST-segment depression preceding ventricular fibrillation [16], the coexistence of ischemic and arrhythmic findings should be considered to be ominous.

Heart Rate

A considerable amount of information is contained within the heart rate—the easiest parameter to measure on the Holter recording. The heart rate may be assessed by the average rate over the entire 24-h recording or for specific time intervals during the recording, as zenith and nadir values, and by some measure of variability. In addition, the association between heart rate and specific events such as arrhythmias and myocardial ischemia may provide insight into important pathophysiologic mechanisms.

For patients in sinus rhythm and not receiving cardioactive drugs, the heart rate reflects a complex interplay of intrinsic sinus node function, the balance of vagosympathetic factors, and global cardiac performance. Coumel has pointed out the strong association between either acceleration or deceleration of the sinus rate and the onset of paroxysmal atrial fibrillation [17]. In his selected patients, the episodes of atrial fibrillation did not occur by chance, but were consistently preceded by significant variations of the sinus frequency. He believes that such changes in heart rate reflect catecholamine or vagal activity, i.e., neurophysiologic factors that can alter the threshold for arrhythmia expression. Prior variations in the heart rate may explain, in part, the apparent spontaneity of some serious postinfarction arrhythmias.

The average heart rate over 24 h and its standard deviation, which provides some measure of overall variability, yield important risk-stratifying information. In postinfarction patients not treated with beta-blocking agents, higher average 24-h heart rates are associated with an increased one-year cardiac mortality. It is likely that relative sinus tachycardia in this situation reflects a compensatory mechanism for impaired left ventricular function.

Evaluation of Therapeutic Interventions

Holter recordings are useful for evaluating in the postinfarction patient the efficacy of antiarrhythmic or antiischemic therapy, pacemaker function, and the safety of prescribed or manifest activity. Because of the hour-to-hour and day-to-day variation in Holter-recorded VEB frequency, the physician must be aware of the limitations of a single 24-h recording in the detection of ventricular arrhythmias [18]. When evaluating effi-

cacy of antiarrhythmic therapy, it is difficult to distinguish with single 24-h recordings, one before and one after the intervention, whether the reduction in VEB frequency is due to the therapy or simply the biologic variation. Current evidence indicates that an 80% reduction in VEB frequency between two 24-h monitoring periods (two recordings before and two after therapy) is required to attribute VEB suppression to the antiarrhythmic agent. The practicality and logistics of such recording durations become a problem, and only patients at increased risk, i.e., those with grade-III or grade-IV VEBs on a "routine" predischarge recording, should be considered for additional recordings and antiarrhythmic therapy.

Efficacy of antiischemic therapy is even more difficult to evaluate since no guidelines exist at this time. Nevertheless, flagrant ST-segment alterations on the predischarge Holter recording warrant concern. Presently, I am using such information as an indication for quantitative low-level exercise testing and for possible therapy with antiischemic agents. This is an important area for investigation.

Pacemaker function is easily evaluated by Holter recordings, and it is important to identify any abnormalities in sensing or pacing function of the implanted unit before hospital discharge.

Predischarge Holter monitoring is useful in evaluating rate, rhythm, and ischemic responses to the activities of daily living (see chapter 58). The Holter technique provides complimentary information to low-level exercise testing and gives valuable information about the heart's response to a variety of emotional and exertional stresses as well as the heart's activity during sleep.

Conclusion

Holter monitoring should be routinely performed in posinfarction patients prior to hospital discharge. The recording provides valuable information in the assessment of physiologic risks that may be operative in the individual patient. It provides a means of detecting potentially life-threatening ventricular arrhythmias, important conduction disorders, meaningful supraventricular arrhythmias, ischemic ST-segment changes, and dysfunctional heart rate trends during the activities of daily living. Holter monitoring also provides useful information for evaluating the safety and efficacy of a variety of therapies rendered to postinfarction patients.

References

1. Holter NJ: New method for heart studies. Science 134:1214–1220, 1961.
2. Moss AJ, Schnitzler R, Green R, De Camila J: Ventricular arrhythmias 3 weeks after acute myocardial infarction. Ann Intern Med 75:837–841, 1971.
3. Kotler MN, Tabatznik B, Mower MM, Tominaga S: Prognostic significance of ventricular ectopic beats with respect to sudden death in the late postinfarction period. Circulation 47:959–966, 1973.
4. Schulze RA Jr, Rouleau J, Rigo P, Bower S, Strauss W, Pitt B: Ventricular arrhythmias in the late hospital phase of acute myocardial infarction: relation of left ventricular function detected by gated cardiac blood pool scanning. Circulation 52:1006–1011, 1975.
5. Kleiger RE, Miller JP, Thanavaro S, Province MA, Martin TF, Oliver GC: Relationship between clinical features of acute myocardial infarction and ventricular runs 2 weeks to 1 year after infarction. Circulation 63:64–60, 1981.
6. Lopes MG, Fitzgerald J, Harrison DC, Schroeder JS: Diagnosis and quantification of arrhythmias in ambulatory patients using an improved R-R interval plotting system. Am J Cardiol 35:816–823, 1975.
7. Moss AJ, Davis HT, De Camilla J, Bayer LW: Ventricular ectopic beats and their relation to sudden and nonsudden cardiac death after myocardial infarction. Circulation 60:998–1003, 1979.
8. Lown B, Wolf FM: Approaches to sudden death from coronary heart disease. Circulation 44:130–142, 1971.
9. Ruberman W, Weinblatt E, Goldberg JD, Frank CW, Shapiro S: Ventricular premature beats and

10. Bigger JT, Weld FM: Analysis of prognostic significance of ventricular arrhythmias after myocardial infarction: short-comings of Lown grading system. Br Heart J 45:717–724, 1981.
11. Moss AJ, Bigger JT, Case RB, Gillespie J, Goldstein R, Greenberg H, Krone R, Marcus FI, Odoroff CL, Oliver GC: Risk stratification and prognostication after myocardial infarction. J Am Coll Cardiol 1:716, 1983.
12. Hindman MC, Wagner GS, Jaro M, Aitkins JM, Scheinman MM, De Sanctis RW, Hutter AH, Yeatman L, Rubenfire M, Pujura C, Rubin M, Morris JJ: The clinical significance of bundle branch block complicating acute myocardial infarction. 2. Indication for temporary and permanent pacemaker insertion. Circulation 58:689–699, 1978.
13. Leclercq JF, Slama R: Clinical relevance of supraventricular arrhythmias detected by Holter electrocardiography. In: Roelandt J, Hugenholtz PG (eds) Long-term ambulatory electrocardiography. The Hague: Martinus Nijhoff, 1982, pp 40–50.
14. Stern S, Tzivoni D: Evaluation for ischemic ST-T changes. In: Wenger NK, Mock MB, Ringqvist I (eds) Ambulatory electrocardiographic recording. Chicago: Year Book, 1980, pp 353–360.
15. Stern S, Tzivoni D: Dynamic changes in the ST-T segment during sleep in ischemic heart diseases. Am J Cardiol 32:17, 1973.
16. Hinkle LE, Argyros DC, Robinson T, et al: Pathogenesis of an unexpected sudden death: role of early cycle ventricular premature contractions. Am J Cardiol 39:873–879, 1977.
17. Coumel P: Heart rate trend analysis: patterns and clinical significance. In: Roelandt J, Hugenholtz PG (eds) Long-term ambulatory electrocardiography. The Hague: Martinus Nijhoff, 1982, pp 51–61.
18. Morganroth J, Michelson EL, Horowitz LN, Josephson ME, Pearlman AS, Dunkman WB: Limitations of routine long-term electrocardiographic monitoring to assess ventricular ectopic frequency. Circulation 58:408–414, 1978.

mortality after myocardial infarction. N Engl J Med 297:750–757, 1977.

54. ELECTROPHYSIOLOGIC TESTING TO IDENTIFY HIGH-RISK PATIENTS AFTER ACUTE MYOCARDIAL INFARCTION

Eric N. Prystowsky

Many patients who survive the acute phase of a myocardial infarction are at risk of sudden cardiac death after hospital discharge, often in the first six months after leaving the hospital. Some factors that indicate high frequency of sudden death include substantial ventricular myocardial dysfunction [1] and the occurrence of "complex" premature ventricular depolarizations and nonsustained ventricular tachycardia [2−4]. However, the predictive value of these factors alone for sudden death is not sufficiently accurate for clinical usefulness. In patients who have coronary artery disease but no recent myocardial infarction, electrophysiologic stimulation has a high degree of sensitivity [5] for inducing the patient's clinical arrhythmia, and serial electrophysiologic testing has proven useful for determining the drug therapy that will prevent recurrent arrhythmias [5−8]. Recently, electrophysiologic testing to initiate ventricular tachycardia has been advocated as a technique to identify patients in

Supported in part by the Herman C. Krannert Fund, Indianapolis, Indiana; by grants HL-06308 and HL-07182 from the National Heart, Lung and Blood Institute of the National Institutes of Health, Bethesda, Maryland; and by the Attorney General of Indiana Public Health Trust and by the Roudebush Veterans Administration Medical Center, Indianapolis, Indiana; and by a grant-in-aid from the American Heart Association, Indiana Affiliate, Inc., Indianapolis, Indiana.

R.M. Califf and G.S. Wagner (eds.), ACUTE CORONARY CARE: Principles and Practice. Copyright © 1985. Martinus Nijhoff Publishing, Boston/Dordrecht/Lancaster.

the postmyocardial infarction period most likely to have sudden cardiac death [9, 10]. This chapter discusses the role of programmed ventricular stimulation in patients who have survived an acute myocardial infarction; it evaluates various pacing protocols, the optimum time to perform these studies, and which patients are most likely to benefit from them.

Electrophysiologic Pacing Protocols

In 1978, Greene and associates [11] reported that induction of a repetitive ventricular response (RVR) in man "identifies patients with life-threatening ventricular instability." To test for RVR induction, electrode catheters were inserted into the heart and during atrial pacing the ventricle was stimulated prematurely at various coupling intervals until ventricular refractoriness was reached or until RVRs were induced. Repetitive ventricular responses were defined as two or more premature ventricular complexes in response to a single ventricular stimulus; that is, when the ventricle was stimulated prematurely, the stimulus resulted in a paced ventricular complex followed by at least one nonpaced ventricular complex. Of note, it is important to identify the mechanism of RVRs in each patient because bundle branch reentrant RVRs appear to be physiologic whereas non-bundle-branch reentrant

RVRs occur significantly more often in patients who have ventricular tachycardia [12].

The authors noted that RVRs did not occur in normal patients, but were present in 88% of patients with recurrent ventricular tachycardia. In patients after myocardial infarction, the induction of an RVR presaged a high incidence of symptomatic ventricular tachycardia or sudden death [11]. These results were exciting for they suggested that a relatively simple procedure could predict patients at risk for sudden death. Unfortunately, other laboratories have been unable to duplicate the results [12−14].

We induced non-bundle-branch reentrant RVRs during baseline electrophysiologic studies in one-third of patients with a history of ventricular tachycardia and in an occasional patient with no history of ventricular arrhythmias [12]. In this study, 51 patients with a past history of ventricular tachycardia underwent a repeat electrophysiologic study during drug therapy prior to hospital discharge. The ability to induce a non-bundle-branch reentrant RVR did not predict accurately which patients were at high risk for developing recurrent ventricular tachycardia or sudden death. Thus, data from our laboratory suggest that RVR testing cannot be used to predict patients at risk for developing symptomatic ventricular tachycardia and/or sudden death. Recent data show that results of RVR testing are a poor predictor of sudden death also in patients investigated after an acute myocardial infarction [9, 10].

Two recent manuscripts [9, 10] and one abstract [15] have evaluated the usefulness of electrophysiologic testing with the endpoint of induced ventricular tachycardia to predict sudden death in patients after an acute myocardial infarction. Each group used a different pacing protocol and therefore the studies will be analyzed separately. Hamer et al. [9] investigated 70 patients who had either mechanical (that is, heart failure [$n = 56$] or peripheral circulatory failure [$n = 5$]) or electrical ("disturbances of impulse formation in the atria and ventricles and the development of conduction abnormalities") complications associated with acute myocardial infarction: 41 patients had ventricular electrical disturbances; 13 of these had ventricular fibrillation, nine had ventricular tachycardia, and 19 had frequent

PVCs. All patients were studied prior to hospital discharge, and the study was done a median of 11 days after the last episode of chest pain associated with an increase in cardiac enzymes. The pacing protocol was not the same for all patients in the series, but every patient had one ventricular extrastimulus introduced, both during sinus rhythm and during ventricular pacing with a pulse duration of 2 ms and a current strength of 2 V. A second right ventricular site was tested if no ventricular tachycardia was induced at the first site. The last 33 patients in this series had two ventricular extrastimuli introduced during ventricular pacing with a current of ≤ 10 V. No patient in the study received an antiarrhythmic drug as a consequence of results from electrophysiologic testing. However, some patients who had been taking antiarrhythmic drugs prior to testing continued this therapy after hospital discharge, although the drug therapy was discontinued at the time of programmed ventricular stimulation. A total of 20 patients had ventricular arrhythmias induced during testing: sustained ventricular tachycardia in eight, and self-terminating ventricular arrhythmias were induced in the other 12 (eight with 2−5 complexes and four with more than five complexes). Only 17 of the other 50 patients who had no ventricular tachycardia induced had electrophysiologic testing utilizing a second extrastimulus. Analysis of 24-h continuous electrocardiographic (ECG) recordings demonstrated that spontaneous arrhythmias did not predict the patients who had ventricular tachycardia induced during programmed ventricular stimulation. By the end of 12 months of follow-up, 12 cardiac deaths (nine sudden) occurred, and eight deaths occurred in the first three months after hospital discharge. Analysis of those patients who underwent the more aggressive pacing protocol demonstrated that five deaths (four sudden) occurred in the 20 patients in whom ventricular tachycardia was induced compared with two deaths (one sudden) in those patients in whom ventricular tachycardia was not induced, but this difference was not statistically significant. Significant results did occur, however, when the authors related the occurrence of death to the type of ventricular arrhythmia induced. Thus, all of the deaths among those individuals in whom a positive electrophysiologic study occurred were in patients in whom more than five ventricular complexes were initiated during programmed ventricular stimulation, and only one sudden death occurred in the 25 patients in whom less than five complexes were induced. These authors also stress the need to use more than one ventricular extrastimulus since four patients died suddenly in the group in whom only one extrastimulus was used for testing and in whom no arrhythmias were induced, implying that this technique is insensitive for predictive purposes.

Richards and associates [10] performed programmed ventricular stimulation in 165 patients at a mean of ten days after acute myocardial infarction. Two right ventricular sites were used for pacing, and current strengths of twice diastolic threshold and 20 mA were used. One pacing cycle length, usually 600 ms, and two ventricular extrastimuli were used. Patients were classified as unstable if ventricular fibrillation or ventricular tachycardia lasting longer than 10 s was induced. No patient was included who had spontaneous ventricular tachycardia or fibrillation after the first 48 h of myocardial infarction. Follow-up was up to 12 months: 17 deaths, eight instantaneous, occurred during follow-up; 23% of the patients were designated unstable by programmed ventricular stimulation and the one-year survival in this group was 65%; in the patients designated as stable, the one year survival was 91%. Further, all eight instantaneous deaths occurred in the unstable group of patients. These authors conclude that the predictive accuracy of ventricular electrical stability as a predictor of survival was 94% although the accuracy of instability was only 26% for predicting death. Of note, three patients designated as unstable during programmed ventricular stimulation had their arrhythmias induced only at a pacing current strength of 20 mA.

The third study [15] has been published only in abstract form: 39 patients were included, in whom no ventricular tachycardia or fibrillation occurred after the first 24 h of myocardial infarction. These patients were studied a mean of 22 days after the onset of their infarcts. The pacing protocol included stimulation at the right ventricular apex using twice diastolic threshold and introduction of up to two ventricular extrastimuli. Patients were followed for a mean of 17 months.

Seven patients had ventricular tachycardia induced. Two of the three patients with sustained ventricular tachycardia underwent serial electrophysiologic drug testing and both patients survived during follow-up. Five sudden deaths occurred: one in the inducible group and four in patients in whom ventricular tachycardia was not induced. These differences were not significantly different.

The studies by Hamer et al. [9] and Richards et al. [10] suggest that electrophysiologic testing with initiation of ventricular tachycardia as an endpoint is useful to predict patients in whom sudden death will occur after myocardial infarction, but the study by Marchlinski et al. [15] suggests otherwise. Some of these differences are likely due to methods. For example, two patients who had sustained ventricular tachycardia induced were treated in the study by Marchlinski et al. Further, the group of 39 patients in this study may be too small to determine the predictive value of programmed ventricular stimulation. Additionally, the pacing techniques of Hamer et al. and Richards et al. were "more aggressive" than those used by Marchlinski et al. Although all groups used two ventricular extrastimuli, which appear to be essential for testing patients after acute myocardial infarction, Hamer et al. and Richards et al. used higher current strengths to pace the ventricle. Higher current strengths, in general, allow closer premature coupling intervals to be attained in the ventricle and, most likely, these shorter coupling intervals induced ventricular arrhythmias in at least some of the patients. Further investigations are needed to determine whether higher current strengths or the use of a third ventricular extrastimulus is necessary during programmed ventricular stimulation in these patients, but both pacing techniques will probably increase sensitivity at the expense of loss of specificity. Finally, only pacing at the right ventricular apex was done in the study by Marchlinski et al. In patients with chronic coronary artery disease, especially those with posteromedial wall motion abnormalities, induction of tachycardia with two ventricular extrastimuli occurred in 10% of patients with right ventricular outflow tract pacing in whom tachycardia was not induced with programmed ventricular stimulation at the apex [16].

In summary, if electrophysiologic testing is to be used as a predictor of sudden death in patients after acute myocardial infarction, it appears that at least two and possibly three extrastimuli will be necessary, and that pacing should be done at more than one right ventricular site.

Patients Who Would Benefit from Electrophysiologic Testing

Most communities in the United States have cardiologists who are well trained in the techniques of cardiac catheterization, but relatively few communities have the trained clinical electrophysiologists required to perform programmed ventricular stimulation. Considering the number of patients with acute myocardial infarction, it is inconceivable that all patients could undergo electrophysiologic testing prior to hospital discharge, even if this were an optimal goal for which to strive. Thus, it is imperative to identify the patients who are at highest risk for sudden death after hospital discharge, and to perform programmed ventricular stimulation in these patients as a preliminary study. Patients most likely to benefit from electrophysiologic testing are those with low cardiac ejection fractions as well as those with nonsustained ventricular tachycardia noted during 24-h ECG recording prior to hospital discharge [1, 4].

Recent data suggest that detection of late (delayed) activation potentials by ECG signal averaging techniques from the body's surface appears to be useful to predict patients likely to have ventricular arrhythmias after acute myocardial infarction. Denniss et al. [17] employed this technique to study 110 patients at a mean of 11 days after myocardial infarction to determine whether delayed activation potentials had any predictive value for subsequent ventricular arrhythmias: 79% of patients demonstrated no delayed activation potentials and only one of these had ventricular tachycardia during follow-up. Of 21% of patients who demonstrated delayed activation potentials, four patients developed ventricular tachycardia during follow-up ($p < 0.01$). Thus, use of this technique might allow one to choose those patients in whom electrophysiologic testing would be most beneficial. For example, although 23 patients demonstrated delayed activation potentials, only four developed arrhyth-

mias. Thus, if treatment were given to all patients based on this finding alone, many patients would be treated unecessarily. Results of electrophysiologic testing might determine which patients with delayed activation potentials required therapy, and this therapy could be guided by serial electrophysiologic drug testing. Patients who do not demonstrate delayed activation potentials do not appear to be at high risk for development of ventricular tachycardia, and therefore programmed ventricular stimulation would appear to be less beneficial.

Preliminary data (figure 54-1) from G. Breithardt et al. (personal communication) suggest that this approach may be valid. These authors performed signal averaging and programmed ventricular stimulation [18] on 132 patients a median of 22 days after acute myocardial infarction. No patient had a history of sustained ventricular tachycardia. Follow-up was obtained in 120 patients and was $\geq$ 6 months. During follow-up, nine patients (two of 67 without late potentials and seven of 53 with late potentials) developed sustained symptomatic ventricular tachycardia requiring immediate intervention. These episodes occurred predominantly in patients characterized by (a) the presence of late potentials, (b) at least four consecutive inducible ventricular echo beats, and (c) a rate of induced ventricular arrhythmia of less than 270 bpm (predictive value 35%). Thus, observation of late potentials by signal averaging techniques can be used to select a subgroup of patients with a high risk of subsequent development of sustained ventricular tachycardia and who, therefore, might benefit from further invasive evaluation. Unfortunately, patients who develop bundle branch block with acute myocardial infarction, a group of patients who often are at increased risk for the subsequent development of ventricular arrhythmias [19] (see chapter 50), have not been, and may not be able to be, evaluated with this technique.

In summary, patients who survive acute myocardial infarction should undergo an array of noninvasive tests prior to hospital discharge (see chapters 51-53). These might include radionuclide angiography or two-dimensional echocardiography to determine ventricular function, 24-h continuous ECG recording, and body surface ECG signal average recordings. Patients determined to be at increased risk of sudden death using the

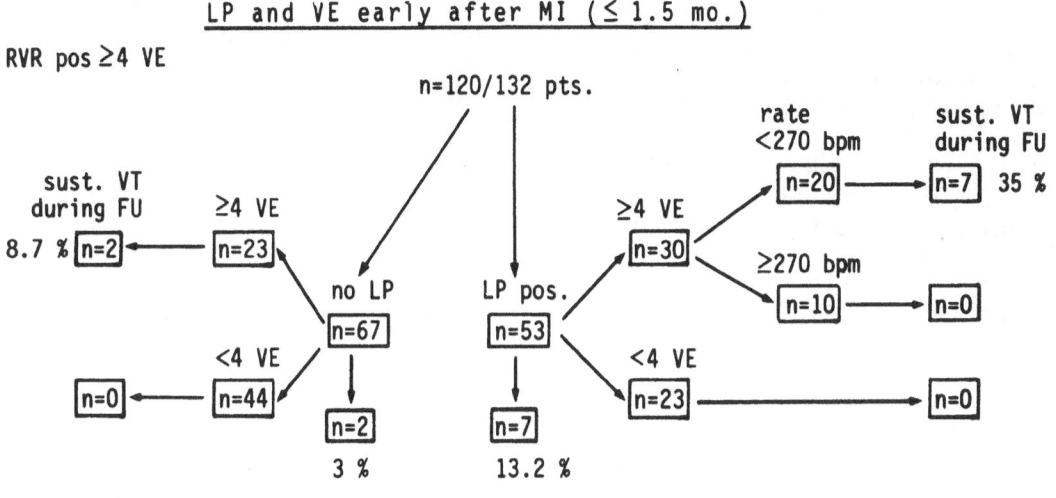

FIGURE 54-1. Prognostic value of signal averaging and programmed ventricular stimulation in patients after recent transmural myocardial infarction. Presence of late potentials (LP pos.) identifies most patients who are at risk of developing subsequent sustained ventricular tachycardia (sust. VT) during follow-up (FU) after acute myocardial infarction (MI): bpm, beats per minute; RVR, repetitive ventricular response: VE, ventricular echo beats.

results of one or more of these noninvasive tests would undergo electrophysiologic testing. Further investigations are needed to determine which arrhythmias induced by programmed ventricular stimulation best predict subsequent occurrences of spontaneous ventricular tachycardia or fibrillation. In patients in whom significant arrhythmias are induced, therapy, either surgery, electrical devices, or antiarrhythmic medications, would be prescribed. In patients in whom no significant arrhythmias are induced, therapy would be withheld. Since the majority of patients will not have a high-risk profile for sudden death determined during noninvasive testing, only a relatively small proportion of patients will undergo invasive electrophysiologic studies.

Appropriate Time for Electrophysiologic Testing

The highest frequency of sudden death after acute myocardial infarction appears to occur within the

first 3–6 months after hospital discharge. Thus, electrophysiologic testing to predict patients at risk for sudden death should be performed prior to hospital discharge. No definitive data are available to suggest that treating patients who are at risk will decrease the occurrence of ventricular arrhythmias or sudden death. However, it appears reasonable to treat these high-risk patients, and to guide their therapy with serial electrophysiologic drug testing. Since the anatomic–physiologic milieu for arrhythmogenesis constantly changes during the months after acute myocardial infarction, antiarrhythmic therapy should be maintained for six months to one year. At this time, the patient could be readmitted to the hospital, antiarrhythmic therapy could be discontinued, and repeat noninvasive and electrophysiologic testing performed. Patients who still appear to be at risk for sudden death should continue therapy, and those patients in whom noninvasive and invasive testing predicts a more benign course could have therapy discontinued.

The changes in results of noninvasive tests with time were demonstrated by Denniss et al. [17], who showed that four of five patients with delayed activation potentials lost the delayed activation potentials spontaneously by six months.

References

1. Schulze RA, Strauss HW, Pitt B: Sudden death in the year following myocardial infarction: relation to ventricular premature contractions in the late hospital phase and left ventricular ejection fraction. Am J Med 62:192, 1977.
2. Ruberman W, Weinblatt E, Goldberg JD, Frank CW, Shapiro S: Ventricular premature beats and mortality after myocardial infarction. N Engl J Med 297:750, 1977.
3. Moss AJ, Davis HT, De Camilla J, Bayer LW: Ventricular ectopic beats and their relation to sudden and nonsudden cardiac death after myocardial infarction. Circulation 60:998, 1979.
4. Bigger JT, Weld FM: Analysis of prognostic significance of ventricular arrhythmias after myocardial infarction: shortcomings of Lown grading system. Br Heart J 45:717, 1981.
5. Naccarelli GV, Prystowsky EN, Jackman WM, Heger JJ, Rahilly GT, Zipes DP: Role of electrophysiologic testing in managing patients who have ventricular tachycardia unrelated to coronary artery disease. Am J Cardiol 50:165, 1982.
6. Mason JW, Winkle RA: Electrode–catheter arrhythmia induction in the selection and assessment of antiarrhythmic drug therapy for recurrent ventricular tachycardia. Circulation 58:971, 1978.
7. Horowitz LN, Josephson ME, Farshidi A, Spielman SR, Michelson EL, Greenspan AM: Recurrent sustained ventricular tachycardia. 3. Role of the electrophysiologic study in selection of antiarrhythmic regimens. Circulation 58:986, 1978.
8. Fisher JD, Cohen HL, Mehra R, Altschuler H, Escher DJW, Furman S: Cardiac pacing and pacemakers. II. Serial electrophysiologic–pharmacologic testing for control of recurrent tachyarrhythmias. Am Heart J 93:658, 1977.
9. Hamer A, Vohra J, Hunt D, Sloman G: Prediction of sudden death by electrophysiologic studies in high risk patients surviving acute myocardial infarction. Am J Cardiol 50:223, 1982.
10. Richards DA, Cody DV, Denniss AR, Russell PA, Young AA, Uther JB: Ventricular electrical instability: a predictor of death after myocardial infarction. Am J Cardiol 51:75, 1983.
11. Greene HL, Reid PR, Schaeffer AH: The repetitive ventricular response in man: a predictor of sudden death. N Engl J Med 299:729, 1978.
12. Naccarelli GV, Prystowsky EN, Jackman WM, Heger JJ, Rinkenberger RL, Zipes DP: The repetitive ventricular response: prevalence and prognostic significance. Br Heart J 46:152, 1981.
13. Ruskin JN, Garan H: Repetitive ventricular responses in patients with life-threatening ventricular arrhythmias. Am J Cardiol 45:406, 1980.
14. Mason JW: Repetitive beating after single ventricular extrastimuli: incidence and prognostic significance in patients with recurrent ventricular tachycardia. Am J Cardiol 45:1126, 1980.
15. Marchlinski FE, Waxman HL, Buxton AE, Josephson ME: Predictive value of programmed stimulation in determining electrical instability after myocardial infarction. J Am Coll Cardiol 1:585, 1983.
16. Prystowsky EN, Naccarelli GV, Rahilly GT, Heger JJ, Zipes DP: Electrophysiologic and anatomic characteristics associated with ventricular tachycardia induced at the right ventricular outflow tract but not at the apex. Am J Cardiol 49:959, 1982.
17. Denniss AR, Cody DV, Fenton SM, Richards DA, Ross DL, Russell PA, Young AA, Uther JB: Significance of delayed activation potentials in survivors of myocardial infarction. J Am Coll Cardiol 1:582, 1983.
18. Breithardt G, Borggrefe M, Quantius B, Karbenn U, Seipel L: Ventricular vulnerability assessed by programmed ventricular stimulation in patients with and without late potentials. Circulation 68:275, 1983.
19. Lie KI, Liem KL, Schuilenburg RM, David GK, Durrer D: Early identification of patients developing late in-hospital ventricular fibrillation after discharge from the coronary care unit: a 5½ year retrospective and prospective study of 1,897 patients. Am J Cardiol 41:674, 1978.

55. STRATEGIES FOR ASSESSING THE RISK STATUS OF PATIENTS FOLLOWING ACUTE MYOCARDIAL INFARCTION OR UNSTABLE ANGINA

Robert M. Califf

Sebastian T. Palmeri

Galen S. Wagner

Admission to a cardiac care unit (CCU) usually signifies a dramatic alteration in the course of a patient's ischemic heart disease. The inhospital predischarge phase, therefore, serves as an important time for the physician and patient to review the past course and plan for the future. Recent information suggesting that risk after hospital discharge may be similar in patients who "rule in" or "rule out" for acute myocardial infarction (MI) highlights the importance of the prognostic evaluation in all post-CCU patients [1, 2]. Patients who are at high risk of subsequent complications should be identified as early as possible so that treatments can be initiated that might prevent recurrent cardiac events. On the other hand, low-risk patients can be enrolled in an accelerated rehabilitation program so that they may more quickly return to productive lives. This chapter discusses the current status of the inhospital evaluation, particularly the roles of a day-3 clinical evaluation and predischarge treadmill exercise testing and cardiac catheterization. Particular emphasis is given to the relationship between estimation of risk and selection of therapy.

Background

A clear understanding of the goals of the prognostic evaluation can improve the efficiency and efficacy of the process. The physician must decide which tests, if any, can help to predict outcome in individual patients. Once the prognosis is estimated, however, the physician must also be prepared to use the information to decide whether any particular therapy might alter the outcome. Finally the patient must be informed about the prognosis and about the specific course of therapy that is recommended. Part of this final step should include specific information about prescribed medications, activity status, and the signs and symptoms that should lead the patient to seek medical attention after hospital discharge [3]. Many aspects of this phase of the predischarge evaluation can be performed most effectively by physician-extenders familiar with the principles of cardiac rehabilitation (see chapter 58).

A source of considerable confusion in the literature is the lack of a clear definition of risk. Prognostic testing in the post-CCU phase can be used to estimate the risk of many different end-

R.M. Califf and G.S. Wagner (eds.), ACUTE CORONARY CARE: Principles and Practice. Copyright © 1985. Martinus Nijhoff Publishing, Boston/Dordrecht/Lancaster.

points: sudden arrhythmic death, recurrent infarction (fatal or nonfatal), recurrent angina, congestive heart failure, and disability (see chapter 58). Different patient characteristics may be important in predicting each of these events since they may be caused by different pathophysiologies and prevented by different therapies.

Patients are usually divided into high- and low-risk groups on the basis of clinical descriptors or test measurements. However, risk can be more accurately defined on the basis of probability; for example, the one-year probability of death in patients in the "high risk" group after MI may range from 15% to 75%. The clinician must remember that a number of factors must be considered when risk is assessed and that these factors most often should be measured on a continuum. Thus, in some studies all patients with an ejection fraction (EF) <40% may be placed in a high-risk group. With this scheme the patient with an EF of 39% will be placed in a different risk group than the patient with an EF of 41%. However, these two patients may have a much more similar risk than the patient with an EF of 39% and other members of the "high risk" group, who may have a markedly depressed EF.

Examination of the shape of the survival curves of patients with acute MI (figure 55-1A) and unstable angina (figure 55-1B) reveals that the risk is highest immediately after the onset of the acute event and then gradually becomes relatively constant. The inhospital mortality averages 10% − 15% for patients with acute MI. Another 5% − 10% of patients die during the first year after discharge, with most deaths occurring in the first three months. Thereafter, mortality averages 3% − 5% per year. The survival curve for patients with unstable angina has a similar shape. Thus, a risk evaluation to select high-risk patients for intervention should be done as soon as possible after the onset of the acute event. Otherwise, many high-risk patients will not be identified before they experience events, some of which may have been preventable.

Characterization of Risk

There are four major factors that must be considered in the risk assessment of an individual patient: the amount of infarcted myocardium, the

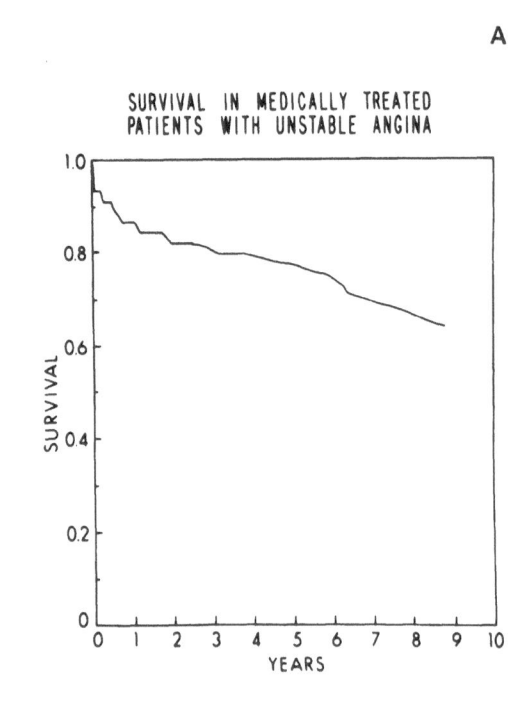

A

SURVIVAL IN MEDICALLY TREATED
PATIENTS WITH UNSTABLE ANGINA

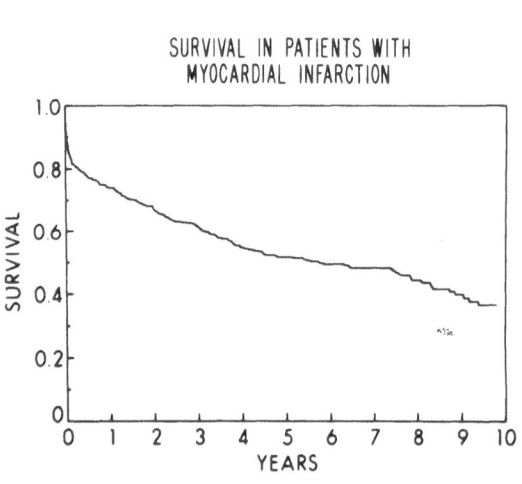

B

SURVIVAL IN PATIENTS WITH
MYOCARDIAL INFARCTION

FIGURE 55-1. (A) Survival of patients admitted to Duke University Medical Center with acute myocardial infarction. Patients transferred from other hospitals because of complications are excluded. (B) Survival of medically treated patients with preinfarction angina after cardiac catheterization at Duke University Medical Center.

amount of remaining viable myocardium "jeop-ardized" by atherosclerotic lesions, the amount of electrical instability, and the propensity for the progression of atherosclerotic process. A variety of historical, physical, and test characteristics can be used to define the risk due to each of these factors (table 55-1). The physician is currently confronted with a bewildering array of potential tests that can be used to define risk, and more tests will become available in the near future. Unfortunately, a consensus has not been reached concerning which tests should be used for which patients.

TABLE 55-1. Characterization of risk

Amount infarcted
    History (CHF, previous MI)
    Exam (S3 gallop, rales, hypotension)
    Hospital course (Killip class, Forrester class, sinus tachycardia, CK-MB)
    ECG (QRS score, infarct location, arrhythmias)
    Chest x-ray (cardiomegaly, pulmonary congestion)
    Echocardiogram (wall motion analysis)
    Radionuclide angiography (wall motion, ejection fraction)
    Thallium (perfusion defect size)
    Technetium pyrophosphate scan
    Cardiac catheterization (ventriculogram)
  * Nuclear magnetic resonance
  * Positron emission tomography
Amount jeopardized
    Hospital course (recurrent angina)
    ECG (recurrent ischemic changes)
    Treadmill exercise test (timing and degree of ST change, angina, hypotension)
    Rest and exercise RNA (exercise EF, wall motion)
    Rest and exercise thallium (new perfusion defect with exercise)
    Cardiac catheterization (coronary anatomy)
Electrical instability
    Hospital course (ventricular arrhythmias)
    Ambulatory monitoring
    Electrophysiologic testing
  * Afterpotential identification
Risk of disease progression
    History (cigarettes, diabetes, hypertension, family history)
    Laboratory (cholesterol—HDL, LDL)
    Exam (blood pressure)
    Psychological testing (type-A behavior)

*Not yet clinically available.

Amount of Infarcted Myocardium

Most complications of acute MI occur more frequently in patients with large infarcts. The clinician can form a general clinical impression of the approximate infarct size by following the clinical course of the patient. Clinical evidence of pulmonary congestion, myocardial dysfunction, and hypoperfusion as estimated by the Killip [4] or Forrester [5] classification systems and cardiomegaly or pulmonary vascular redistribution on chest x-ray [6] are most directly related to infarct size. Many other complications of acute infarction have a less direct, but well-documented, relationship to infarct size. These factors include sinus tachycardia [7], atrial and ventricular tachycardias [8], and bundle branch block [9].

Investigators have also developed more quantitative methods for estimating infarct size with simple clinical data including analysis of CK-MB isozymes (see chapter 18) and of the QRS complex on the 12-lead ECG (see chapter 19). Comparative analysis of the QRS infarct score and peak levels of CK-MB for estimating the extent of the myocardial infarct have indicated that independent prognostic information is contained in these two parameters [10]. The serum isozyme values reflect only the size of the current infarct. The QRS infarct score provides information regarding total infarct size including the acute and prior myocardial infarctions. Currently, however, the QRS score has proven capability only with the initial myocardial infarction. It has not yet been tested in patients with multiple infarcts or in those with confounding factors such as bundle branch block or ventricular hypertrophy on the ECG.

A variety of noninvasive and invasive methods can also be used directly to assess ventricular function as outlined in the previous chapters of this section. The delineation of when each test is indicated and which test is most useful for a particular patient are unresolved issues. A simple clinical guideline is to obtain a direct measure of ventricular function when the other clinical data regarding extent of the infarct are contradictory or unclear. Studies in which multiple testing strategies have been compared for prognostic accuracy in the post-CCU population are not available.

Although the amount of infarcted myocardium is the most important prognostic factor in the post-CCU patient, the appropriate therapy for the patient at high risk due to a large infarct is unclear. Most therapies initiated after the first several hours of the acute event are aimed at the treatment of complications or the reduction of ischemia. No direct method exists for improving left ventricular dysfunction due to infarcted myocardium; however, as more is learned about infarct healing, new methods to reduce infarct size due to "better" healing may be developed (see chapter 46). Currently, initial treatment for the patient with a large infarct should be oriented toward prevention or control of any existing congestive heart failure. No clear evidence exists, however, that chronic treatment with vasodilators, diuretics, or intropic agents lowers mortality [11]. Patients with large amounts of infarcted myocardium appear to be at risk primarily due to sudden, arrhythmic death [12]. The risk in these patients is inversely related to left ventricular ejection fraction in a continuous fashion, although the slope of the curve becomes steeper at lower ejection fractions [13]. Unfortunately, the efficacy of antiarrhythmic drugs in these patients has not been established.

Recent results from the BHAT trial suggest that patients with mechanical problems (pulmonary edema, shock, persistent hypotension, rales, gallop rhythm) during the acute phase of MI, and thus with larger infarcts, have improved survival when placed on beta-blocker therapy prior to discharge [14]. As the authors clearly state, however, this suggestion is based purely on retrospective, subgroup analysis and it therefore does not carry the same degree of confidence as other results of BHAT. In addition, recent results from the Coronary Artery Surgery Study (CASS) suggest that, in patients with large amounts of infarcted myocardium and with angina as the predominant symptom, survival and "quality of life" are improved by coronary artery bypass grafting [15].

Residual Jeopardized Myocardium

In the past, clinicians have relied upon the patient's symptoms and the 12-lead ECG as markers of recurrent ischemia and residual jeopardized myocardium. Schuster and Bulkley demonstrated

that patients with recurrent angina and ECG changes in leads not involved by the initial infarction are at high risk of subsequent mortality [16]. Interestingly, however, the Multicenter Postinfarction Research Group did not find that post-MI angina was a significant independent risk factor [13]. Unstable angina patients with recurrent pain and ECG changes in the hospital have repeatedly been shown to be at high risk [17].

Considerable controversy has arisen over the implications of the occurrence of myocardial infarction without new Q waves (see chapter 10) [18, 19]. Many investigators have concluded that patients with non-Q-wave (subendocardial) infarcts are at high risk of reinfarction due to a large amount of residual myocardium at risk [20,21]. Gibson et al. [22] found that these patients more often have patent infarct-related vessels and high-risk thallium exercise tests compared with patients with Q-wave infarctions (transmural). Some confusion has been caused in other studies by the inclusion of patients with normal and abnormal QRS complexes in the same category. Mahony et al. found an excellent one-year prognosis in patients with a normal QRS complex both before and after infarction, but patients with an abnormal QRS (old MI, bundle branch block, or ventricular hypertrophy) prior to infraction but no *new* Q waves with infarction had a poor one-year prognosis [23]. Until this issue is resolved, a prudent course of action would be to carefully evaluate patients with non-Q-wave infarcts with functional testing, to detect those with large amounts of residual ischemia.

In patients without clinical evidence for recurrent ischemia, a variety of techniques are available to evaluate stress-induced ischemia. Treadmill exercise testing after MI has been performed in large members of patients. The test can detect patients at risk for recurrent events and can be performed with few complications [24]. In addition, the exercise test can be used to formulate an exercise prescription for the patient at the time of discharge. More sophisticated tests such as radionuclide angiography and thallium scintigraphy are described in chapters 51 and 52.

The most commonly used protocols in the post-CCU period are the modified Bruce protocol [25], the modified Balke protocol [26], and the

Naughton protocol [27]. A modified form of the Balke protocol used at Duke Medical Center is outlined in table 55-2. These protocols have the advantage of a gradual increment in work load so that severely deconditioned or unstable patients will not be subjected to a sudden, severe cardio-

vascular stress. Even more gradual protocols can be devised for patients with particular physical limitations. An individualized prescreening process is more important than the particular exercise protocol in avoiding complications. The clinician should use the previously mentioned clinical criteria for detecting large infarcts and residual ischemia to identify high-risk patients who do *not* need further noninvasive prognostic studies. In addition, careful physiologic monitoring by the nursing or physical therapy staff during the patient's inhospital convalescence can detect patients who become unstable at low levels of exercise [28]. A summary of absolute and relative contraindications to exercise testing is listed in table 55-3.

A spectrum of information concerning myocardial dysfunction and residual ischemia can be gained from the routine exercise test. Simply regarding the test as "positive" or "negative", based on the ST-segment response is inadequate. Exercise time and work load provide an imprecise, but inexpensive, estimate of myocardial function. ST-segment response, symptomatic angina, and blood pressure response provide an estimate of residual myocardium at risk. The degree of abnormality in these parameters (i.e., amount, and times of onset, and duration of ST depression and the absolute drop in blood pressure) is also important in estimating prognosis. Ventricular arrhythmias observed before, during, and after testing are related to left ventricular function, but may also provide some information about electrical instability [29]. Each study has found a somewhat different set of characteristics of the test to yield maximal prognostic information, but the general conclusions are: (a) the less the patient's exercise capacity as measured by work load or exercise time, (b) the more the ischemia as judged from symptoms, ST deviation or hypotension, and (c) the more frequent and complex the arrhythmias, the worse the prognosis.

Several important questions remain with regard to the use of early exercise testing during the post-CCU period. Traditionally, exercise testing has been withheld until three weeks after MI. Numerous reports of the safety of exercise at the time of discharge are now available. Few studies have investigated exercise testing in patients who have "cooled off" after an episode of unstable

TABLE 55-2. A modified form of the Balke protocol used at Duke Medical Center

Minute	Speed	% Grade
0−1	2.0	0
1−2	2.5	0
2−3	2.5	2
3−4	2.5	3
4−5	2.5	4
5−6	2.5	5
6−7	2.5	6
7−8	2.5	7
8−9	2.5	8
9−10	2.5	9
10−11	2.5	10
11−12	2.5	11
12−13	2.5	12
13−14	2.5	13
14−15	2.5	14
15−16	2.5	15
16−17	2.5	16
17−18	2.5	17
18−19	2.5	18
19−20	2.5	19
20−21	2.5	20
21−22	2.5	21
22−23	2.5	22
23−24	2.5	23
24−25	2.5	24
25−26	2.5	25
26−27	2.5	26
27−28	2.5	27
28−29	2.5	28
29−30	2.5	29
30−31	2.5	30
31−32	2.5	31
32−33	2.5	32
33−34	2.5	33
34−35	2.5	34

angina. The proper timing of the exercise test is thus in question. Furthermore, in patients taking beta-blocking drugs, the maximal prognostic information can probably be gleaned if the medication is withheld. If this procedure is followed, however, the test cannot be used to formulate an exercise prescription, since the patient's heart rate will be blunted by the beta-blockers prescribed at the time of discharge. The advisability of heart-rate-limited versus symptom-limited tests also has been questioned. Although a heart-rate-limited test intuitively appears to be safer, ample evidence exists that symptom-limited tests can be performed with little risk three weeks after MI. However, no reports of symptom-limited testing at the time of discharge (if this occurs less than three weeks after MI) are available. Some authors have advocated a heart-rate-limited test at the time of discharge, with a symptom-limited test at the time when aerobic activity is resumed (usually six weeks after MI). Finally, the cost/benefit ratio of performing more expensive tests such a radionuclide angiography or thallium scintigraphy compared with simple treadmill exercise testing has not been determined.

Cardiac catheterization provides a direct method for determining the amount of anatomic coronary disease and estimating the extent of jeopardized myocardium. The test is now performed routinely in many centers in patients who have been admitted with unstable angina [30]. A series of studies have recently been published reporting that cardiac catheterization can be performed safely during or after acute MI [31–34] (see chapter 35). In general, the prognostic value of catheterization is similar to that in stable angina: prognosis is directly related to the amount of anatomic disease and to the status of the left ventricle. Although catheterization can be performed with lower risk than previously believed, it is more expensive, more invasive, and more uncomfortable than most other methods of prognostic evaluation. Its performance may lead to surgery simply because of "suitable anatomy" rather than either intractable symptoms or high risk.

Identification of the patient with a large amount of viable myocardium in jeopardy leads to consideration of several therapeutic alternatives aimed

TABLE 55-3. Contraindications to exercise testing prior to hospital discharge

Absolute

Uncontrolled angina, congestive heart failure, hypertension, arrhythmia, metabolic or electrolyte disturbance
Significant aortic stenosis
Severe pulmonary hypertension
Acute infectious diseases (especially myocarditis)
Evidence of significant ischemia, arrhythmia, or heart failure during progressive, supervised, low-level ambulation

Relative

Musculoskeletal or neurologic impairment

at reducing the risk of infarction: intensive medical therapy, percutaneous transluminal coronary angioplasty (PTCA), or coronary artery bypass grafting. Beta-blocking drugs have been shown to reduce the risk of both recurrent MI and death in some selected post-MI patients [35]. No such evidence exists for patients with unstable angina. Calcium-channel-blocking drugs were shown to reduce the risk of "combined medical events" (death, MI, need for surgery) when added to beta-blockers and nitrates [36]. A recent study demonstrated that aspirin therapy reduced the risk of MI in patients with unstable angina [37] (see chapter 16). The best combination of drugs for particular patients remains to be determined.

The use of surgery in the treatment of unstable angina is discussed in chapter 35. Only two randomized studies concerning the use of bypass grafting in asymptomatic post-MI patients are available. Norris et al. studied patients with two previous MIs and found no improvement in survival compared with medically treated patients [38]. More recently, the Coronary Artery Surgery Study (CASS) reported no improvement in either survival or nonfatal infarction rates with surgery in asymptomatic post-MI patients with one-, two-, or three-vessel disease [39]. No information is yet available about the possible benefits of surgery or percutaneous coronary transluminal angioplasty in asymptomatic post-MI patients who have objective signs of ischemia on noninvasive testing.

Electrical Instability

Many post-MI deaths are "sudden," and thus appear to be due to ventricular arrhythmias [40]. Patients are clearly most prone to develop arrhythmias during the acute phase of infarction. The high prevalence of spontaneous ventricular arrhythmias and sudden death in the weeks following acute MI (figure 55-1A) has led to postulate that healing myocardium is "electrically unstable."

Chapters 53 and 54 discuss alternative methods to detect high-risk candidates for sudden death. Ambulatory monitoring can effectively stratify the risk of sudden death, although some authors have questioned the cost-effectiveness of applying this test to all post-CCU patients because of its low predictive accuracy [41]. Preliminary evidence suggests that electrophysiologic testing can also stratify the risk of sudden death and some believe that it can more effectively guide antiarrhythmic therapy. Furthermore, after potentials on the ECG may provide a simple, non invasive marker for patients at highest risk of sudden death. The demonstration that many patients with arrhythmias develop more severe arrhythmias when exposed to antiarrhythmic drugs [42] should encourage clinicians to be cautious about instituting therapy in asymptomatic patients with ventricular arrhythmias. Previous studies on the use of antiarrhythmic drugs in post-MI patients have yielded negative results [43], although these studies all had serious methodologic flaws. Better designed trials are currently planned.

Risk of Disease Progression

The factors that govern the progression of atherosclerosis in patients with previously established disease are poorly understood (see chapter 15). Smoking is the risk factor for which the best evidence exists that modification is effective in secondary prevention [44]. Several recent studies [45, 46], one of which actually directly examined progression of coronary anatomic disease, have found encouraging results when serum cholesterol levels were lowered with cholestyramine. Recent evidence also suggests that control of hypertension [47] and modification of type-A behavior [48] lower event rates in post-MI patients. Although no conclusive trials have been done, the evidence supports the hypothesis that regular exercise in conjunction with risk-factor modification reduces event rates [43]. The cornerstone of all of these therapies is active participation and compliance of the patient. Thus the effective performance of the last phase of the discharge evaluation—transmitting the information to the patient in a manner that will enhance compliance—is crucial [49].

Strategy

Epstein et al. [50] and De Busk et al. [51] have advocated a stepwise approach to the prognostic evaluation. Factors from the history, physical examination, and hospital course should all be considered in the step-1 or clinical evaluation, which should be performed at 48–72 h after admission (figure 55-2). This information adds no cost or risk to the patient's hospitalization. Patients at high risk based on these clinical factors may be spared confirmatory noninvasive testing. If aggressive therapy aimed at myocardial revascularization is considered, the physician can move directly toward cardiac catheterization. Those patients with no urgent complications during the first three days [52] and small infarct size estimated both by CK-MB and the QRS complex [10] are at extremely low risk of experiencing either urgent complications of the initial event or a recurrent ischemic event within the following two weeks. Therefore they can be prepared for early hospital discharge (approximately seven days) if their personal situation permits. Predischarge evaluation can be omitted and a symptom-limited stress test included in the initial outpatient visit at 14–21 days.

The prognosis of patients determined to be at low or intermediate risk based on clinical factors can be further stratified with predischarge noninvasive testing. Support for this approach in which cardiac catheterization is reserved only for patients identified as high risk comes from CASS [39], which demonstrated that coronary artery surgery does not have a dramatic effect on survival in asymptomatic post-MI patients without severely compromised left ventricular function.

A reasonable time to begin planning for discharge in the post-MI patient is 48–72 h after admission, since most of the early complications of MI occur by the third postinfarct day [52]. By prescreening the patient at this time the physician can begin to plan individualized testing and teaching efforts. The prognostic estimate can then be revised if inhospital complications arise. The criteria of McNeer et al. [52] (table 55-4) (see chapter 49) include most characteristics from the hospital course that are known to be important for prognosis [3].

Figure 55-3 is a Venn diagram illustrating the process involved in the early stratification of risk based on simple, clinical parameters. Patients with a significant clinical complication are at high risk. These patients should remain longer in the CCU until stable and their progression throughout the hospital course should be slowed. Even with an uncomplicated initial clinical course, patients with both a CK-MB peak >300 IU and QRS score >6 appear to be at intermediate risk during the hospital course because of their large infarct size. Patients with an uncomplicated clinical course and elevation of only one of the two factors (QRS score and CK-MB) are at lower, but still intermediate, risk, while patients with an uncomplicated clinical course, low CK-MB, and low QRS score are at extremely low risk.

At the time prior to hospital discharge, the entire clinical course of the patients identified to be at intermediate risk via step 1 should be reviewed. Figure 55-2 includes the process of this risk stratification as "Step 2: Specialized testing." These patients enter the predischarge period with a range of risks that can be further stratified only by specialized testing. Considerable further studies are required to delineate which tests should be performed in particular patients. Our recommendation at this time is that a functional test should be the test of first choice. For most practitioners the ECG exercise test (treadmill or bicycle) is the simplest, least expensive, and most readily available. In specialized centers or for patients with conduction disturbances or marked resting ST-T-wave abnormalities, rest and exercise radionuclide, myocardial perfusion (thallium), or blood pool (technetium) studies may be preferable.

The timing and test selection for risk assessment in the unstable angina patient should be somewhat different than for the MI patient. Sta-

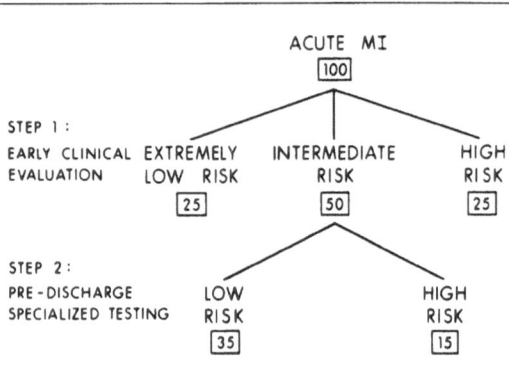

FIGURE 55-2. Stepwise risk stratification in post-MI patients.

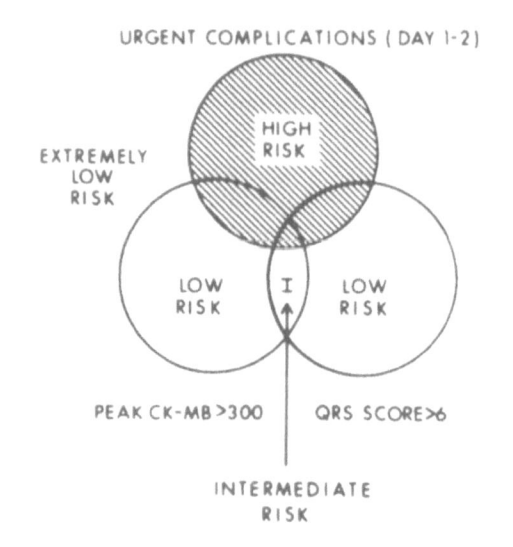

FIGURE 55-3. Risk stratification after MI based on clinical course, CK-MB, and QRS score.

bilization may occur rapidly; by 48 h the patient may be angina free on medical therapy. Based on the findings of the National Cooperative Study of Unstable Angina [53], many experts have recommended cardiac catheterization prior to discharge. This test forms the basis for prognostic stratification with medical therapy and for selection of candidates for surgical therapy. The most prominent reasons for the recommendation for routine catheterization after unstable angina but not after MI are the differences in coronary anatomic findings. Up to 10% of patients with unstable angina will have normal coronary arteries and 10% − 15% will have significant left main stenosis [54]. Both of these findings are unusual in post-MI patients. Unstable angina patients with three-vessel disease often will need to have surgical therapy at a later date [53]. The cost of "crossing-over" may exceed the cost of selecting initial surgical therapy in this three-vessel disease group [55]. The prognostic value of functional testing, after coronary anatomy is known, remains an unresolved issue in the patient who has been stabilized after an episode of unstable angina. We recommend functional testing in all patients who have stabilized although the clinical usefulness of this approach remains to be determined.

Although most of the clinical literature has emphasized the assessment and therapy of the high-risk patient, the identification of the low-risk patient is also very important. An uncomplicated hospital course, low enzyme levels and QRS score, and good functional capacity without evidence for residual ischemia or arrhythmia identify an extremely low-risk patient. The psychological benefits of explicit risk identification may be substantial, especially when integrated into a rehabilitation program [56].

TABLE 55-4. Criteria for uncomplicated infarct

Absense of these "urgent" complications
  Ventricular tachycardia
  Ventricular fibrillation
  2nd- or 3rd-degree atrioventricular block
  Pulmonary edema
  Cardiogenic shock
  Persistent hypotension
  Infarct extension

Absense of any of these "prognostic" complications
  Sinus tachycarida
  Atrial fibrillation/flutter
  Paroxysmal supraventricular tachycardia
  *Recurrent ischemic symptoms

---

*Not in intial McNeer criteria [52].

References

1. Schroeder JS, Lamb IH, Hu AM: Do patients in whom myocardial infarction has been ruled out have a better prognosis after hospitalization than those surviving infarction? N Engl J Med 303: 1−5, 1980.

2. White RD, Grande P, Califf L, Palmeri ST, Califf RM, Wagner GS: Diagnostic and prognostic significance of minimally elevated creatine kinase MB in patients with suspected acute myocardial infarction. Am J Cardiol, 1984 (in press).

3. Pryor DB, Hindman MC, Wagner GS, Califf RM, Rhoads MK, Rosati RA: Early discharge after acute myocardial infarction. Ann Intern Med 99:528−538, 1983.

4. Killip T, Kimball JT: A survey of the coronary care unit: concepts and results. In: Friedberg CK (ed) Acute myocardial infarction in the coronary care unit. New York: Grune and Stratton, 1969, p 281.

5. Forrester JS, Diamond GA, Swan HJC: Correlative classification of clinical and hemodynamic function after acute myocardial infarction. Am J Cardiol 39:137−145, 1977.

6. Battler A, Karliner JS, Higgins CD, Slutsky R, Gilpin EA, Froelicher VF, Ross J Jr: The initial chest x-ray in acute myocardial infarction: predictors of early and late mortality and survival. Circulation 61:1004−1009, 1980.

7. Crimm A, Severance HW, Coffey KS, McKinnis R, Wagner GS, Califf RM: The prognostic significance of isolated sinus tachycardia during the first three days of acute myocardial infarction. Am J Med, 1984 (in press).

8. Harrison DC: Atrial fibrillation in acute myocardial infarction: significance and therapeutic simplifications [editorial]. Chest 70:3, 1976.

9. Hindman MC, Wagner GS, Jaro M, Atkins JM, Scheinman MM, De Sanctis RW, Hutter AM Jr, Yeatman L, Rubenfire M, Pujura C, Rubin M, Morris JJ: The clinical significance of bundle branch block complicating acute myocardial infarction. II. Indications for temporary and permanent pacemaker insertion. Circulation 58: 689−699, 1978.

10. Hindman NB, Anderson TI, Harrison DG, Grande P, Ideker RE, Selvester RH, Wagner GS: Correlation of electrocardiographic and isoenzymatic estimations of myocardial infarct size [abstr]. J Am Coll Cardiol 1:705, 1983.

11. Braunwald E, Colucci WS: Editorial retrospective: vasodilator therapy of heart failure. N Engl J Med 310:459−461, 1984.

12. Califf RM, McKinnis RA, Burks J, Lee KL,

Harrell FE Jr, Behar VS, Pryor DB, Wagner GS, Rosati RA: Prognostic implications of ventricular arrhythmias during 24 hour ambulatory monitoring in patients undergoing cardiac catheterization for coronary artery disease. Am J Cardiol 50:23−31, 1982.

13. The Multicenter Postinfarction Research Group: Risk stratification and survival after myocardial infarction. N Engl J Med 309:331−336, 1983.

14. Furberg CD, Hawkins CM, Lichstein E: Effect of propranolol in postinfarction patients with mechanical or electrical complications. Circulation, 1984 (in press).

15. Alderman EL, Fisher LD, Litwin P, Kaiser GC, Myers WO, Maynard C, Levine F, Schloss M: Results of coronary artery surgery in patients with poor left ventricular function (CASS). Circulation 68:785−795, 1983.

16. Schuster EH, Bulkley BH: Early post-infarction angina: ischemia at à distance and ischemia in the infarct zone. N Engl J Med 305:1101−1105, 1981.

17. Mulcahy R, Daly L, Graham I, Hickey N, O'Donoghue S, Owens A, Ruane P, Tobin G: Unstable angina: natural history and determinants of prognosis. Am J Cardiol 48:525−528, 1981.

18. Phibbs B: "Transmural" versus "subendocardial" myocardial infarction: an electrocardiographic myth. J Am Coll Cardiol 1:561−564, 1983.

19. Spodick DH: Q-wave infarction versus S-T infarction: nonspecificity of electrocardiographic criteria for differentiating transmural and nontransmural lesions. Am J Cardiol 51:913−915, 1983.

20. Hutter AM, De Sanctis RW, Flynn T, Yeatman LA: Nontransmural myocardial infarction: a comparison of hospital and late clinical course of patients with that of matched patients with transmural anterior and transmural inferior myocardial infarction. Am J Cardiol 48:595−602, 1981.

21. Krone RJ, Friedman E, Thanavaro S, Miller JP, Kleiger RE, Oliver GC: Long-term prognosis after first Q-wave (transmural) or non-Q-wave (nontransmural) myocardial infarction: analysis of 593 patients. Am J Cardiol 52:234−239, 1983.

22. Gibson RS, Curling CM, Craddock GB, Watson DD, Beller GA: Prevalence and clinical significance of residual myocardial ischemia two weeks after acute non Q-wave infarction. Circulation (Suppl 3) 68:30, 1983.

23. Mahony C, Hindman MC, Aronin N, Wagner GS: Prognostic differences in subgroups of patients with electrographic evidence of subendo-cardial or transmural myocardial infarction: the favorable outlook for patients with an initially normal QRS complex. Am J Med 69:183−186. 1980.

24. Weiner DA: Prognostic value of exercise testing early after myocardial infarction. J Cardiac Rehab 3:114−122, 1983.

25. Bruce RA, Hornsten TR: Exercise stress testing in evaluation of patients with ischemic heart disease. Prog Cardiovasc Dis 11:371−390, 1969.

26. Wolthuis RA, Froelicher VF, Fischer J, Noguera I, Davis G, Stewart AJ, Triebwasser JH: New practical treadmill protocol for clinical use. Am J Cardiol 39:697−700, 1977.

27. Naughton J, Sevelius G, Balke B: Physiological responses of normal and pathological subjects to a modified work capacity test. J Sports Med 3:201−206, 1963.

28. Sivarajan ES, Bruce RA, Almes MJ, et al: In-hospital exercise after myocardial infarction does not improve treadmill performance. N Engl J Med 305:357−362, 1981.

29. Califf RM, McKinnis RA, McNeer JF, Harrell FE, Lee KL, Pryor DB, Waugh RA, Harris PJ, Rosati RA, Wagner GS: Prognostic value of ventricular arrhythmias associated with treadmill exercise testing in patients studied with cardiac catheterization for suspected ischemic heart disease. J Am Coll Cardiol 2:1060−1067, 1983.

30. Russell RO, Rackley CE, Kouchoukos NT: Unstable angina pectoris: do we know the best management? Am J Cardiol 48:590−591, 1981.

31. Taylor GJ, Humphries JO, Mellits D, Pitt B, Schulze RA, Griffith LSC, Achuff SC: Predictors of clinical course, coronary anatomy and left ventricular function after recovery from acute myocardial infarction. Circulation 62:960−970, 1980.

32. Sanz G, Castaner A, Betriu A, Magrina J, Roig E, Coll S, Pare JC, Navarro-Lopez F: Determinants of prognosis in survivors of myocardial infarction: a prospective clinical angiographic study. N Engl J Med 306:1065−1070, 1982.

33. De Feyter PJ, Van Eenige MJ, Dighton DH, Visser FC, De Jong J, Roos JP: Prognostic value of exercise testing, coronary angiography and left ventriculography 6−8 weeks after myocardial infarction. Circulation 66:527−536, 1982.

34. Roubin GS, Harris PJ, Bernstein L, Kelly DT: Coronary anatomy and prognosis after myocardial infarction in patients 60 years of age and younger. Circulation 67:743−749, 1983.

35. B-Blocker Heart Attack Trial Research Group: A randomized trial of propranolol in patients with

acute myocardial infarction. JAMA 247:1707–1714, 1982.

36. Gerstenblith G, Ouyang P, Achuff SC, Bulkley BH, Becker LC, Mellits ED, Baughman KL, Weiss JL, Flaherty JT, Kallman CH, Llewellyn M, Weisfeldt ML: Nifedipine in unstable angina: a double-blind randomized trail. N Engl J Med 306:885–889, 1982.

37. Lewis HD Jr, Davis JW, Archibald DG, Stenike WE, Smitherman TC, Doherty JE III, Le Winter MM, Linares E, Pouge JM, Sabharwal SC, Chesler E, De Mots H: Protective effects of aspirin against acute MI and death in men with unstable angina: results of a cooperative study. N Engl J Med 309:396–403, 1983.

38. Norris RM, Agnew TM, Brandt PW, Graham KJ, Hill DG, Kerr AR, Lowe JB, Roche AH, Whitlock RM, Barratt-Boyes BG: Coronary surgery after recurrent myocardial infarction: progress of a trial comparing surgical with nonsurgical management for asymptomatic patients with advanced coronary disease. Circulation 63:785–792, 1981.

39. CASS Principal Investigators and their associates: Coronary Artery Surgery Study (CASS): a randomized trial of coronary artery bypass surgery. Circulation 68:939–950, 1983.

40. Moss AJ: Clinical significance of ventricular arrhythmias in patients with and without coronary artery disease. Prog Cardiovasc Dis 23:33–52, 1980.

41. Lesch M, Kehoe RF: Predictability of sudden cardiac death. N Engl J Med 310:255–257, 1984.

42. Velebit V, Podrid P, Lown B, Cohen BH, Graboys TB: Aggravation and provocation of ventricular arrhythmias by antiarrhythmic drugs. Circulation 65:886–894, 1982.

43. May GS, Eberlein KA, Furberg CD, Passamani ER, De Mets DL: Secondary prevention after myocardial infarction: a review of long-term trials. Prog Cardiovasc Dis 24:331–352, 1982.

44. Sparrow D, Dawber TR, Colson T: The influence of cigarette smoking on prognosis after a first myocardial infarction. J Chronic Dis 31:425–432, 1978.

45. The Lipid Research Clinics Coronary Primary Prevention Trial Results: I. Reduction in incidence of coronary heart disease. JAMA 251:351–374, 1984.

46. Brensike JF, Levi RI, Kelsey SF, Passamani ER, Richardson JM, Loh IK, Stone NJ, Aldrich RF, Battaglini JW, Moriarty DJ, Fisher MR, Friedman L, Friedewald W, Detre KM, Epstein SE: Effects of therapy with cholestyramine on progression of coronary arteriosclerosis: results of the NHLBI type II coronary intervention study. Circulation 69:313–324, 1984.

47. Connolly DC, Elveback LR, Oxman HA: Coronary heart disease in residents of Rochester, Minnesota, 1950–1975. III. Effect of hypertension and its treatment on survival of patients with coronary artery disease. Mayo Clin Proc 58:249–254, 1983.

48. Friedman M, Thoresen CE, Gill JJ, Ulmer D, Thompson L, Powell L, Price V, Elek SR, Rabin DD, Breall WS, Piaget G, Dixon T, Bourg E, Levy RA, Tasto DL: Feasibility of altering type A behavior pattern after myocardial infarction. Circulation 66:83–92, 1982.

49. Blumenthal JA, Califf RM, Williams RS, Hindman M: Cardiac rehabilitation: a new frontier for behavioral medicine. J Cardiac Rehab 3:637–656, 1983.

50. Epstein SE, Palmeri ST, Patterson RE: Evaluation of patients after acute myocardial infarction: indications for cardiac catheterization and surgical intervention. N Engl J Med 307:1487–1492, 1982.

51. De Busk RF, Kraemer HC, Nash E, Berger WE, Lew H: Stepwise risk stratification soon after acute myocardial infarction. Am J Cardiol 52:1161–1166, 1983.

52. McNeer JF, Wagner GS, Ginsburg PB, Wallace AG, McCants CB, Conley MJ, Rosati RA: Hospital discharge one week after acute myocardial infarction. N Engl J Med 298:229–232, 1978.

53. Unstable Angina Pectoris Study Group: Unstable angina pectoris national cooperative study group to compare surgical and medical therapy. II. In-hospital experience and initial follow-up results in patients with one, two, and three vessel disease. Am J Cardiol 42:839–848, 1978.

54. Alison HW, Russell RO Jr, Mantle JA, Kouchoukos NT, Moraski RE, Rackley CE: Coronary anatomy and arteriography in patients with unstable angina pectoris. Am J Cardiol 41:204–209, 1978.

55. Charles ED, Kronenfeld JJ, Wayne JB, Kouchoukos NT, Oberman A, Robers WJ, Mantle JA, Rackley CE, Russell RO Jr: Unstable angina pectoris: a comparison of costs of medical and surgical treatment. Am J Cardiol 44:112–117, 1979.

56. Ewart CK, Taylor CB, Reese LB, De Busk RF: Effects of early postmyocardial infarction exercise testing on self-perception and subsequent physical activity. Am J Cardiol 51:1076–1080, 1983.

X. CORONARY CARE:
THE CONVALESCENT PHASE

56. THE ROLE OF OUTPATIENT TRANSTELEPHONIC ECG MONITORING AND SELF-MEDICATION FOLLOWING ACUTE MYOCARDIAL INFARCTION

Daniel David

Elieser Kaplinsky

Malignant ventricular arrhythmias associated with the various consequences of myocardial ischemia constitute the major cause of sudden, out-of-hospital death in the western societies. Among these, a significant subset of patients is the group having sustained a myocardial infarction in the past [1–3]. This chapter considers a potential approach to this problem being investigated in post-myocardial infarction patients by providing medical help to the patient at risk *before* the arrival of emergency medical personnel.

Two technical advances made this study possible: (a) transtelephonic ECG transmission [4] and (b) development of a reliable mode for intramuscular self-injection of drugs. The combination of these two techniques in the management of postmyocardial infarction patients constitutes the subject of our report.

The present study would never have been possible without the devotion, compassion, and enthusiasm of the secretarial, nursing, and medical staff of the Department of Cardiology of our hospital.

R.M. Califf and G.S. Wagner (eds.), ACUTE CORONARY CARE: Principles and Practice. Copyright © 1985. Martinus Nijhoff Publishing, Boston/Dordrecht/Lancaster.

Transtelephonic ECG transmission (TTET)

The two major forms of ambulatory ECG monitoring in out-of-hospital cardiac patients are the Holter monitoring systems (see chapter 53) and transtelephonic ECG transmission (TTET). The latter is based upon the modulation of the ECG signal to audible frequency that can be in turn transmitted via regular telephone lines. On the receiving end the signal is demodulated to reappear as the patient's ECG. The transtelephonic ECG transmitter (the patient unit) is small and easy to carry. The transmitted ECG is interpreted during the telephone contact with the patient, which is maintained for as long as required to solve the presenting problem.

These properties of TTET create a wide range of clinical applications. It is cost effective in patients with symptomatic arrhythmias that last for a sufficiently long period, enabling the patient to contact a surveillance center (advanced TTET devices have, in addition to their transtelephone transmitting capability, a built-in memory). Furthermore, the transmitter can be given to the patient for prolonged periods of time so that even rare episodes of rhythm disturbances could be documented [4]. Thus, the TTET system becomes a valuable approach, complementary to the Holter monitoring devices that cannot be used for extended periods of times. TTET has therefore emerged as an effective additional system for ambulatory therapeutic management of patients with cardiac arrhythmias. Another major advantage of TTET is the direct contact between the patient and the medical team, enabling immediate initiation of management procedures when indicated.

Intramuscular Mode of Drug Administration for Arrhythmias Associated with Myocardial Ischemia

The *intravenous* administration of lidocaine has been long shown to be rapidly effective in the management of ventricular arrhythmias in patients with acute myocardial infarction. Recent studies have shown that the *intramuscular* mode of lidocaine administration is also effective in the control of ventricular arrhythmias in patients with acute myocardial ischemia [6, 7]. The intramuscular injection of 300 mg of lidocaine results in "therapeutic" lidocaine blood levels within 10 min of injection that persist over 60 min [7, 8]. Though Lie et al. failed to establish that a single intramuscular injection of lidocaine (300 mg) could prevent primary ventricular fibrillation in hospitalized patients [9], Valantine et al. [10] and Wennerblom et al. [11] showed (in randomized controlled studies) that an intramuscular injection of lidocaine in the prehospital phase in patients with acute myocardial infarction resulted in reduction of early mortality.

Bradyarrhythmias during acute myocardial ischemia and infarction present yet another problem in the management of patients during the early stages (see chapter 28). While controversy exists regarding the safety of using atropine to reverse slow heart rates in patients in this setting, its controlled use for marked sinus bradycardia and high-degree atrioventricular block probably is beneficial [12, 13]. Atropine is particularly important when the bradyarrhythmia is accompanied by hypotension and, thereby, is associated with hemodynamic instability (see chapter 12).

Combination of TTET and Autoinjection of Medications

The development of automatic syringes for intramuscular self-injections has created a possibility for the lay patient to self-administer medications by the intramuscular route with faster effects than obtained with oral medications and without the attention of professional personnel.

By combining the TTET system with the available automatic intramuscular injections of lidocaine and atropine, a potential for enabling an "on-line" intervention, guided by remote (via the telephone) professional counsel and enacted by the patient, has emerged. The following working hypothesis could then be formulated: Patients at high risk for malignant ventricular arrhythmias, and therefore for sudden death, could be provided the capability of immediate transtelephonic contact to a medical center when symptoms warrant. The subsequent consultation would include transmission of the ECG and, if indicated, the autoinjection of lidocaine and/or atropine. The scope of the program could then be expanded to include preventive measures. Thus, in a high-risk situation, like the appearance of unusual and severe chest pain in a postmyocardial infarction patient, lidocaine might be autoinjected as a possible prevention against the appearance of ventricular arrhythmias, even though no such rhythm disorders were present during transmission.

With this working hypothesis, a multicenter study is currently being conducted in several centers, including ours, and we wish to report our preliminary data. The purpose of the presentation is threefold: to evaluate the feasibility of such an extensive program and its impact on patient management, to investigate the antiarrhythmic potential of the "on-line" interventions, and to determine possible effects the system under investigation might have on prehospital mortality in postmyocardial infarction patients.

Design of the Current Study

Patients hospitalized in the intensive cardiac care unit with a documented acute myocardial infarction were randomly allocated upon discharge from the hospital into one of two groups: (a) The "system" group or (b) the "control" group. The "system" patients were equipped with a transtelephonic ECG transmitter and two automatic syringes, one containing 300 mg of lidocaine and the other 1.5 mg of atropine. Upon leaving the hospital they were trained in handling the transmitter and the automatic autoinjectors. The patients were followed on a regular outpatient basis. They were to call the medical center on a scheduled routine program (routine calls) and whenever unusual symptoms occurred (emergency calls). The medical and nursing staff of the intensive coronary care unit served as the "headquarters" receiving the routine and emergency calls.

Patients were instructed to autoinject lidocaine for unusually severe anginal pain, for significant ventricular arrhythmias (ventricular tachycardia or multiple premature ventricular contractions at a higher than usual level of frequency and severity). A combination of severe bradyarrhythmia and chest pain was the indication for the autoinjection of atropine. In addition, immediately upon the recognition of an emergency situation the mobile coronary care ambulance was sent to bring the patient to the hospital. Whenever lidocaine was autoinjected, a blood sample for the determination of serum lidocaine level was drawn as soon as possible. Telephone contact with the patient or his family was maintained until the mobile unit reached the patient.

Our study has been ongoing for over four years (follow-up time range 1−50 months). In this period a total of 446 patients were randomized into the two study groups. Patients in both groups were similar in age and sex distribution (table 56-1) as well as location of the infarction that resulted in their admission into the study (table 56-2).

Emergency Autoinjection of Drugs

A total of 622 *emergency* calls were recorded, resulting in 127 instructions to autoinject and 112 subsequent admissions to the hospital. Importantly, practically all patients were instructed to autoinject lidocaine. Atropine was injected in only two cases, one due to severe sinus bradycardia, the other in an attempt to accelerate the sinus rate during an episode of accelerated idioventricular rhythm. The remaining 495 emergency calls did not require autoinjection. The most common indication for the autoinjection of lidocaine was severe chest pain in the absence of ventricular arrhythmias (table 56-3). Five patients failed to inject properly due to technical problems and 11 others refused to autoinject, the main reason being fear. In cases in which an arrhythmia was detected in the course of an emergency call *not* associated with chest pain, the decision whether to inject lidocaine or not was based mainly upon the nature and severity of the arrhythmia and the nature of the patient's previous transmissions. Arrhythmias were detected during 102 *routine* calls. However, only eight of these patients were instructed to autoinject (table 56-4), as the presence of ventricular ectopy per se was not regarded as indicative for any intervention.

Antiarrhythmic Effects of Autoinjected Lidocaine

In 39 of 43 patients who injected lidocaine, the rhythm disorder disappeared in less than 25 min (mean 14 min 10 s). In six of the seven patients with ventricular tachycardia, the arrhythmia terminated within less than 15 min. The mean serum lidocaine level for the entire group of patients was 3.05 ± 1.25 ng/ml (well within the therapeutic level). However, the blood sample for the determination of lidocaine serum level was drawn on arrival at hospital and thus at various intervals after the autoinjection of the drug.

Effect of the System on Mortality

Overall mortality was comparable in both the system (30 patients) and control (33 patients) groups (table 56-5). There are, however, some differences that merit special attention.

In evaluating the system, one should be concerned mainly with its potential to prevent prehospital sudden cardiac death. It thus becomes apparent from table 56-5 that there were seven out-of-hospital cardiac deaths in the system patients, three of whom had a very poor left ventricular function (ejection fraction of less than 25%). In contrast there were 17 out-of-hospital cardiac deaths in the control group, 14 of which were sudden in onset (in three it was impossible to ascertain the mode and cause of death). This difference was offset by higher delayed inhospital

TABLE 56-1. Patient population and data

	System	Control	Total
No. of patients	216	230	446
Male	184	191	375
Female	32	39	71
Mean age (years)	59.5	58	
% >55	71	65	

TABLE 56-2. Location of admission myocardial infarction

	Ant/Ext	Ant/Sept	Ant/Lat	Inf	Inf/Lat	Inf post	Post	Rv	Lat	Unknown
System	30.5	10.8	6.2	29	13.9	1.7	4.6	0.7	2.0	0.6
Control	17.5	9.1	8.8	36	11.9	6.7	5.5	0.9	2.3	1.3

Ant = Anterior   Rv = Right Ventricle   Inf = Inferior   Post = Posterior
Lat = Lateral   Ext = Extensive   Sept = Septal

TABLE 56-3. Emergency calls resulting in instruction to inject

Total	127
Severe chest pain	85
Chest pain and premature ventricular contractions	21
Multiple premature ventricular contractions without chest pain	15
Ventricular tachycardia	5
Supraventricular tachycardia	1
Compliance	
Refusals	11
Failures	5

TABLE 56-4. Arrhythmias as detected during routine calls (total 102)

	With injection	No injection
Total	7	95
Premature ventricular contractions	5	86
Ventricular tachycardia	2	0
Atrial tachycardia on fibrillation	0	9

mortality in the system patients. This might have been associated with the higher incidence of prior extensive anterior infarction in the system group.

Left ventricular function data were available on 28 patients who later died, 11 in the system and 17 in the control. It is of importance to note that while only two of 11 of the system patients who died had an ejection fraction of over 25%, in the control 11 of 17 had ejection fraction of over 35%. A possible difference in the cause of death between the two study groups might therefore emerge. In the system group, most of the patients who died had severe myocardial damage. They died mainly in the hospital of terminal

TABLE 56-5. Patient mortality in the system and control groups

	System	Control
Total	30	33
Noncardiac	8 (27%)	8 (24%)
Cardiac	22 (73%)	25 (76%)
Inhospital	15 (68%)	8 (32%)
At home	4 (18%)	7 (28%)
Ambulance	2 (9%)	4 (16%)
Unknown	1 (4%)	6 (24%)

cardiac failure. In the control group, however, most of the mortality was among patients in whom myocardial function was relatively well preserved. A large number of them died suddenly and outside the hospital. With completion of the study, true randomization of baseline variables should be achieved, and it will then be possible to assess the role of this postinfarction coronary care system to reduce mortality.

Perspective for the Future of Posthospital Surveillance Systems

The present report is, of course, a preliminary summary of an ongoing study. While a definitive conclusion cannot be drawn as yet, some directions do emerge.

Transtelephonic ECG monitoring may provide an easy-to-use, relatively inexpensive means for ambulatory management of cardiac patients in whom potentially lethal rhythm disturbances pose the main therapeutic challenge. The system is suitable for prolonged periods of follow-up, such as that necessary in patients after myocardial infarction. We cannot as yet provide a definitive answer as to whether out-of-hospital sudden death can indeed be prevented. Furthermore, even if the favorable difference observed in the out-of-hospital mortality of the control and system groups is proven to be significant, we will not be able to identify the true "antiarrhythmic factor" in the system. The direct and frequent contact with professional personnel whom the patient knows and trusts has an important and most favorable psychological effect upon the patients (see chapter 57). By consulting the service any time, day or night, the patient slowly learns to distinguish between the multitude of symptoms that he encounters upon leaving the hospital after an acute myocardial infarction. He then acquires renewed self-confidence, as evidenced by the gradual reduction in the number of emergency calls with the passing of time and the patient's own feelings of security. Moreover, the TTET provides the treating physician with additional information besides purely ECG data. This may be important in the early detection of heart failure and other complications that, when treated promptly, may stabilize the situation and prevent a potentially harmful deterioration in the patient's condition. The close interaction between the central nervous system and the propensity to lethal arrhythmias only further stresses the potential for arrhythmia reduction via assurance, alleviation of anxiety, and improvement of life quality, all afforded by the total system regardless of the specific effects of its components.

References

1. Ruberman W, Weinblatt E, Goldberg JD, Frank CW, Chaudhary BS, Shapiro S: Ventricular premature complexes and sudden death after myocardial infarction. Circulation 64:297–305, 1981.

2. The Coronary Drug Project Research Group: Prognostic importance of premature beats following myocardial infarction. JAMA 223:1116–1124, 1973.

3. Rappaport E, Remedois P: The high risk patient after recovery from myocardial infarction: Recognition and management. J Am Coll Cardiol 2:391–400, 1983.

4. Hasin Y, David D, Rogel S: Diagnostic and therapeutic assessment by telephone electrocardiographic monitoring of ambulatory patients. Br Med J 2:609–612, 1976.

5. Seidell FR, Markis JE, Groff W, Kaminski A: Enhancement of drug absorption after administration by an automatic injector. J Pharmacokinet Biopharm 2:197, 1974.

6. Bellet S, Roman L, Kostis JB, Fleischmann D: Intramuscular lidocaine in the therapy of ventricular arrhythmias. Am J Cardiol 27:291–293, 1971.

7. Ryden L, Waldenstom A, Ehn L, Holmberg S, Husaini M: Comparison between effectiveness of intramuscular and intravenous lidocaine on ventricular arrhythmias complicating acute myocardial infarction. Br Heart J 35:1124–1131, 1973.

8. Sloman G, Hamer A, Baker G, Hunt D: Use of lignocaine and atropine auto-injection for patients at high risk of sudden death and reinfarction after myocardial infarction. Med J Aust 1 (7) 349–51, 1981.

9. Lie KL, Louridtz WJ, Janse MJ, Willebrands AF, Durrer D: Efficacy of lidocaine in preventing primary ventricular fibrillation within 1 hour after 300 mg intramuscular injection. Am J Cardiol 42:486–488, 1978.

10. Valantine PA, Frew JL, Mashford ML, Sloman JG: Lidocaine in the prevention of sudden death in the prehospital phase of acute myocardial in-

farction. N Engl J Med 291:1327—1331, 1974.

11. Wennerblom B, Holmberg S, Ryden L, Wedel H: Antiarrhythmic efficacy and side effects of lidocaine given in the prehospital phase of acute myocardial infarction. Eur Heart J 3:516—524, 1982.

12. Adgey AAJ, Geddes JS, Mulholland HC, Keegan DAJ, Pantridge JF: Incidence, significance, and management of early bradyarrhythmia complicating acute myocardial infarction. Lancet 2: 1097—1101, 1968.

13. Chadda KD, Lichtstein E, Gupta PK, Choy R: Bradycardia—hypotension syndrome in acute myocardial infarction: reappraisal of the overdrive effects of atropine. Am J Med 59:158—163, 1975.

57. MINIMIZING PSYCHOLOGICAL STRESS FOR PATIENTS AND FAMILY FOLLOWING ACUTE MYOCARDIAL INFARCTION

Michael Rotman

William Harvey, in his book entitled *Exercitatio de Motu Cordis et Sanguinis in Animalibus*, written in 1628, stated that "every affection of the mind that is attendant with either pain or pleasure, hope or fear is the cause of an agitation whose influence extends to the heart" [1]. As crystallized in this statement, a mind—heart interaction occurs in the events of human experience. In the setting of an acute myocardial infarction, psychological "scarring," affecting the patient and his family, can significantly influence the outcome of this event and the rehabilitative potential of the patient [2].

The style of adjustment or adaptation to any life stress, such as sudden illness, is determined by the premorbid personality of the person, and will be influenced by a number of factors centering upon the perception of the stresser and the interpretation of this perception [3—6]. The psychodynamics of the family (specifically the spouse) to the acute illness will be influenced by such factors as the state of the marriage, the communicative abilities of the patient and his family, and the manner in which the family reacts to the acute event [7, 8]. Surrounding the state of "mind" of the patients and their family are the potent influences of the health care team with their own psychological responses and communicative skills. Thus the coping behavior of the patient, the manner in which the family reacts to the acute illness, and the influence of the health care team are all important factors in minimizing psychological stress. In this era of limiting myocardial damage, one may look upon minimizing psychological stress and thus psychological "damage" as improving the immediate and long-term prognosis of the patient.

Insight into the Psychological State of the Acute Event

The mind set of the patient who has had an acute coronary event can be looked at from the perspective of an acute grief reaction [9]. The patient has lost a part of himself, he has a "broken heart," and thus a number of mental mechanisms will develop in response to the acute illness. The psychological response may be one of shock and disbelief, denial, anger, anxiety, depression, and a state of helplessness and hopelessness [10—14]. There may be rebelliousness to the restricted or dependent state with a loss of individuality. As the patient faces the return to the home environment, a number of factors will affect the psychological state; concern over physical capacity, return to work, acceptance by family as a spouse and parent, concern over sexuality, and the need to modify certain risk factors can be an overwhelming and trying task for the patient [7, 15]. An internal monologue of a patient in the setting of the acute event follows:

"This is unreal. I can't tell what day it is. All the hours run together and I feel so helpless lying here. I know it

R.M. Califf and G.S. Wagner (eds.), ACUTE CORONARY CARE: Principles and Practice. Copyright © 1985. Martinus Nijhoff Publishing, Boston/Dordrecht/Lancaster.

is a dream. I'll soon wake up. A heart seizure, is that what I heard? My heart is as solid as ever. Tomorrow I'll be all right. I have to admit that I was frightened, really scared by the pain. It was a confusing feeling, I should never have mentioned it to anyone. I guess I looked sick. It was scary when the ambulance arrived, then I almost blacked out, feeling so heavy on my chest. I feel all right now. It was just a warning. I'll change, I know I have to slow down. I know that my work has me stressed and I feel so pushed by every little thing. I know that I need to stop smoking, but—what if I have had some damage? How much damage? How much of my heart have I lost? Will I be able to work again? I feel so helpless, confused. Will I be all right? Why has this happened to me! I'm scared and I feel alone."

The spouse will herself be going through a number of psychological responses. These include guilt or a feeling of being partially or wholly responsible for the precipitation of her husband's illness, anger and hostility, grief, anxiety, and depression. A fear of losing their spouses and never feeling "safe again" may occur and, as well, a need to protect or nurture their spouses from future acute events. In this setting of "nurturing", a situation of entrapment may develop between being overprotective in this endeavor or being chastened for a noncaring attitude [8, 16–18]. The internal monologue of the spouse in the setting of the acute event follows:

"I feel scared and angry waiting here. Waiting is hell, I feel angry at those officious nurses. I have been through everything with him and now that he might die I am shut out. What harm do they think I will do? I should have driven him instead of waiting for the ambulance. He was so pale, cool and moist when I touched him before we arrived in the Emergency Room. I should have made sure that he took his medication and should have never let him spray those trees this morning. Don't let him die; I promise to do better. What will I do if I am alone, how will I live? How can I stand to lose him? There is so much to say and I feel so alone."

Thus, between the psychodynamics of the patients and their spouses, a situation can occur that can lead to interfamily conflict and a disruption of family equilibrium. The health team

(nurses and physicians) caring for the patient in this setting must understand the mind set of their patients and their families. Only in this way can intervention be appropriately used to help minimize psychological stress.

Minimizing Psychological Stress

Distress is that condition in the human that disrupts the environment and may lead to a loss of adequate coping ability. An acute coronary event such as a myocardial infarction can lead to distress. The successful restoration of this internal balance must occur for a healthy adaptation to the stressful condition [2]. Two important assessments must be made to determine whether the patient is coping properly with this distress: first, what is the patient attempting to cope with, i.e., the stressful situation itself, the stress generated by the situation, or another unrelated situation; and, second, what purpose does the behavior fulfill, i.e., is it helpful or harmful to the patient [19]? Thus, the physician and other health team members must have insight into the patient's coping behavior if they are to minimize psychological stress. The physician must learn to recognize the varying mental mechanisms noted in the previous section. Through open and honest communication, patients and their spouses should be counseled about their feelings, giving them insight into the *"normal"* course of *emotional events*, not *thwarting* these feelings as long as they do not hinder the patient's recovery. In those instances where the behavior patterns are negatively influencing an *adequate* coping state, such as continued grief or denial, channels must be explored to aid the patient and family in handling this disruptive behavior [20, 21].

The physician must communicate through both physical and mental *touching* a feeling of hopefulness and a feeling of concern. It is important to relate to the patient and his family that *dialogue*, at any time and no matter how important or unimportant the subject matter be, is available. The physician must discuss openly those aspects of the recovery process that the patient or spouse may not feel comfortable bringing up, such as sex [22]. Since the patient's future physical and emotional health is significantly influenced by the spouse, her psychological well-being is important. Thus, health care professionals should help promote dialogue between husband and wife as well as other family members. In giving hopeful support to all involved, an emphasis on the non-lethal aspects of coronary disease and a lessening of the "drama" of heart attack need to be made [23].

Giving the patient a feeling of autonomy in the process of recovery is of extreme importance. The patient must understand that he is in "control"; that he is a cause of what happens in his life. This will give the patient the incentive to a satisfying recovery. Progressive physical activity early in the recovery process within the obvious limits of the individual case can make the patient feel an active participant and can potentiate and positively influence the patient's course and lessen the incidence of depression [24].

In the cognitive appraisal of the recovery process, those individuals who feel more competence, less suppressed, and less threatened during the acute phase by enhancing a feeling of *control* and *predictability* will fare better [25]. Thus, procedures that promote choices and encourage participation are important tools in minimizing psychological stress. Patient education in all its forms (video, brochures, and pamphlets), regular didactic programs reviewing the aspects of coronary disease, short-term psychotherapy, behavior modification classes, and biofeedback may all play an important role in giving the patient and his family a feeling of participation and a feeling of control and thus predictability of outcome [19, 20, 21, 25].

In discussions with the patient and his spouse, on the importance of making certain changes in life habits (i.e., stop smoking, lose weight, change dietary habits, regular exercise program), it is important to use a commonsense approach and realize that no one individual can make all changes at once. Reasonable single goals carried out within a reasonable time frame should be emphasized. The patient will feel less distress in the process of making healthy life habit changes when he knows that he has the support of his family and physicians in this endeavor.

The health care team should recognize that heightened psychological distress may be more likely at certain periods of the hospitalization. The transfer or departure from the coronary care unit to a less monitored area may be a time of distress. Studies have shown that, during this time, complications may be more frequent as the output of catecholamines increases [14]. Thus, the uncontrollability and unpredictability of the transfer seem to be factors leading to distress. Communicating to the patient in advance of the transfer, the reasons for the transfer, and the transfer setting will allay anxiety and fear, and help to minimize psychological stress.

Compliance to drug regimens is of utmost importance in the complete care of the patient. The health care team must recognize those factors that have been shown to be important in the setting of behavior compliant to drug regimens. Such factors as the patient's economic status, the manner of instruction of drug use, the number of drugs prescribed, side effects of these drugs, the patient's attitude toward his illness, and the influence of family members are all important factors that can affect compliant behavior. The physician has an obligation to instill upon the patient a feeling of "therapeutic partnership" [26]. The patient should feel that choosing to comply with the medical regimen is to his benefit.

The use of psychotropic agents and beta-blockers should be part of the armamentarium of the physician in helping to minimize stress [27]. Since circulating levels of epinephrine and nor-epinephrine increase in the setting of acute stress and since these "humors" can negatively influence the outcome of the coronary event by inducing serious arrhythmias and increasing cardiac work load, the combination of benzodiazepine psychotropic agents and beta-blockers should be used, unless contraindicated, in the treatment of the patient with an acute myocardial infarction, in order to allay anxiety and other mind sets negatively influencing the patient's course [28, 29].

Minimizing psychological stress after an acute myocardial infarction thus involves a cooperative effort. The patient and his family must be given insight into the psychodynamics of the acute event and the process of coping behavior. The patient must realize that he is truly responsible for the recovery and for maintaining long-term health instead of dis-ease and dis-stress. The patient and his family should feel that the physician and the health care team are available for open and honest dialogue. In his article on "The Physician as Communicator," Norman Cousins speaks about the importance of dialogue when he writes: "Words used by the physician can be gate-openers or gate-slammers. They can open the way to recovery, or they can make a patient dependent, tremulous, fearful, or resistant—the right word can potentiate a patient, mobilize the will to live—the wrong word can produce despair and defeat" [30].

References

1. Harvey W: Exercitatio de Motu Cordis et Sanguinis in Animalibus. 1628.
2. Eliot RS: Stress and the major cardiovascular disorders. Kisco NY: Futura, 1979.
3. Stern MJ, Pascale L, Ackerman A: Life adjustment post-myocardial infarction determining predictive variables. Arch Intern Med 137:1680–1685, 1977.
4. Byrne DG, Whyte HM: Life events and myocardial infarction revisited: the role of measures of individual impact. Psychosom Med 42:1–10, 1980.
5. Totman R: What makes "life events" stressful? A retrospective study of patients who have suffered a first myocardial infarction. Psychosom Res 23:193–200, 1979.
6. Rahe RH: Stress and strains in coronary heart disease. Presented at National Conference on Emotional Stress and Heart Disease, October 1973.
7. Davidson DM: The family and cardiac rehabilitation. J Fam Pract 8:253–261, 1979.
8. Skelton M, Dominion J: Psychological stress in wives of patients with myocardial infarction. Br Med J 2:101–103, 1973.
9. Lindemann E: Symptomatology and management of acute grief. Am J Psychiatry 101:141–148, 1944.
10. Cousins N: Denial: are sharper definitions needed? JAMA 248:210–212, 1982.
11. Schecter N: Psychological aspects of clinical cardiac disease. Psychosomatus 8:166–169, 1967.
12. Spielberger DC: Stress, anxiety and cardiovascular disease. J SC Med Assoc 72:15–22, 1976.
13. Engel GL: A life setting conducive to illness: the giving up–given up complex. Am Int Med 69:293–300, 1968.
14. Scalzi C: Nursing management of behavioral responses following an acute myocardial infarction. Heart Lung 2:62–69, 1973.
15. Bilodeau CB, Hackett TP: Issues raised in a group setting by patients recovering from myocardial infarction. Am J Psychiatry 128:105–110, 1971.
16. Stern MJ, Pascale L: Psychosocial adaptations to post-myocardial infarction: the spouse's dilemma. Psychosom Res 23:83–87, 1979.
17. Mayou R, Foster A, Williamson B: The psychosocial and social effects of myocardial infarctions on wives. Br Med J 1:699–701, 1978.
18. Rahe RH: Group therapy in the outpatient management of post-myocardial infarction patients. Psychosom Med 4:77–82, 1973.
19. Pranulis MF: Coping with an acute myocardial infarction. In: Gentry DW, Williams RB Jr (eds) Psychological aspects of myocardial infarction and coronary care. St Louis: CV Mosby, 1973.
20. Billings CK: Management of psychological responses to myocardial infarction. South Med J 73:1367–1371, 1980.
21. Adsett CA, Bruhn JG: Short term group psychotherapy for post-myocardial infarction patients and their wives. Can Med Assoc J 99:577–589, 1968.
22. Papdopoulos C, Larrimore P, Cardin S, Shelley SI: Sexual concerns and needs of the post-coronary patient's wife. Arch Intern Med 140:38–41, 1980.
23. Bartle SH: Denial of cardiac warnings. Psychosomatus 21:74–77, 1980.
24. Heinzelmann F, Bagley RW: Response to physical activity programs and their effects on health behavior. Public Health Rep 85:905–911, 1970.
25. Krantz DS: Cognitive processes and recovery from heart attack: a review and theoretical analysis. J Hum Stress 6:27–38, 1980.
26. Anderson RJ, Lynn MK: Methods of improving patients compliance in chronic disease states. Arch Intern Med 142:1973–1975, 1982.
27. Frishman WH, Razin A, Swencionis C, Sonnenblick EH: Beta-adrenoceptor blockers in anxiety states: a new approach to therapy? Cardiovasc Rev Rep 2:447–459, 1981.
28. Lown B, Verrier RL, Rabinowitz SH: Neurol and psychologic mechanisms and the problem of sudden cardiac death. Am J Cardiol 39:890–902, 1977.
29. Kones RJ: Emotional stress, plasma catecholamines, cardiac risk factors, and atherosclerosis. Angiology 30:327–336, 1979.
30. Cousins N: The physician as communicator. JAMA 248:587–589, 1982.

58. MINIMIZING DISABILITY AND OPTIMIZING RETURN TO WORK FOLLOWING ACUTE MYOCARDIAL INFARCTION

R. Sanders Williams

Medical management of ambulatory patients with coronary heart disease is a distinctly different task than inhospital care of individuals with acute myocardial infarction. Whereas myocardial infarction is usually an acute, dramatic event, the major problems faced by patients following hospital discharge are more often mundane than dramatic, and are distinctly chronic, not acute. Acute interventions in the coronary care unit are necessary to manage life-threatening complications of myocardial infarction. Successful chronic intervention in the lives of postinfarction patients requires repeated, longitudinal contact with the patient over extended periods of time, with exquisite attention to details of daily living. Recent studies demonstrate the lack of efficacy of brief rehabilitation efforts that are limited to the hospital setting [1], but clinical experience as well as some experimental evidence support the viewpoint that prolonged, longitudinal attention to the postinfarction patient in one of several types of structured programs may offer distinct advantages over less intensive forms of management [2—4].

There are five basic concepts (table 58-1) that summarize a modern approach to minimizing disability and optimizing return to work following acute myocardial infarction.

Continuity of Care

Coordinated efforts to reduce eventual disability from myocardial infarction should begin as soon as life-threatening complications of the infarct have been stabilized (see chapter 49), and should continue without any major hiatus through the remainder of the hospital stay, and into the post-discharge period. For both physiologic and psychological reasons, it is appropriate to delay intensive efforts to limit disability until six weeks after hospital discharge, a common date of entry into many structured cardiac rehabilitation programs. The first few weeks represent a high-risk period for recurrent myocardial infarction or sudden arrhythmic death [5], and efforts to identify patients at higher than average risk for such events should not be delayed.

Likewise, the first few weeks following hospital discharge after myocardial infarction require profound psychological adjustments on the part of patients and their families that can be facilitated by continued contact with health professionals (see chapter 57).

At Duke University Medical Center, during the last half of the hospital stay following a myocardial infarction, patients are introduced to, and seen on a near-daily basis, by members of the rehabilitation staff. Within not more than one week from hospital discharge, most patients undergo functional testing, begin participation in low-intensity group exercise sessions, and are contacted by a rehabilitation nurse or physiologist 3–5 times weekly.

Individualized, Physiologically Rational Rather than Dogmatic Care

It is evident that patients with a myocardial infarction, even when uncomplicated, may differ widely in the degree of their ventricular dysfunction, their subsequent proclivity for serious arrhythmias, and in the extent of myocardial ischemia induced during exercise or emotional stress. Therefore, it should also be evident that fixed schedules for resumption of sexual activity, return to work, or resumption of recreational activities are not rational if these are applied uniformly to a mixed population of infarct survivors. The first step in a program to minimize disability following myocardial infarction should therefore be to quantitate the degree of physiologic disability present as precisely as possible. At the current time this is accomplished best by one or more forms of symptom-limited exercise testing performed near to the time of hospital discharge.

The utility of exercise testing for identifying patients at high risk for subsequent catastrophic events [6, 7] has been discussed in preceding chapters (see chapters 25 and 52). However, the optimal, cost-effective, combination of exercise electrocardiography, hemodynamic monitoring, arrhythmia detection, nuclear scintography, echocardiography, and coronary arteriography that should be applied to selected subsets of patients for the purposes of stratifying risk and for quantitating disability is still the subject of active investigation. At the current time we recommend the routine application of treadmill exercise testing following myocardial infarction, with the addition of radionuclide ventriculography in patients with chest pain, exertional hypotension, asymptomatic ST-segment depression during exercise, multiple infarctions, or ECG evidence for extensive infarction. We usually employ coronary arteriography in postinfarction patients with angina at extremely low exercise work loads or heart rates, or with major reversible impair-

TABLE 58-1. Important concepts for management of ambulatory patients with ischemic heart disease

---

1. Continuity of care
2. Individualized, physiologically rational rather than dogmatic care
3. Coordination of pharmacologic, nonpharmacologic, and operative therapeutic modalities
4. Attention to detail
5. Appreciation of the role of psychological/sociological factors in determining outcomes

---

ments in left ventricular function during exercise scintography.

By stratifying patients into subgroups based on their risk for reinfarction or sudden death, by accurately distinguishing ischemic pain from nonanginal causes of chest pain, and by quantitating the threshold for myocardial ischemia during exertion in terms of heart rate or double-product and in terms of exercise work load, rational, individualized recommendations regarding the patient's return to activities of daily living can be developed.

Coordination of Pharmacologic, Nonpharmacologic, and Operative Therapeutic Modalities

Having quantified the risk status, and the degree of physiologic disability, of the patient who has suffered a myocardial infarction, the modern cardiologist or internist has a formidable and sometimes bewildering diversity of therapeutic modalities from which to choose in the effort to minimize the patient's subsequent degree of disability and risk for cardiac death. It is beyond the scope of this chapter to detail comprehensive management strategies for the diversity of clinical situations presented by patients after myocardial infarction, or to discuss the selection of patients for treatment by specific drug regimens or operative procedures such as transluminal angioplasty, saphenous vein bypass grafting, or ventricular aneurysmectomy.   Rather, this chapter emphasizes the potential value of selected nonpharmacologic, nonoperative therapies. These modalities are often overlooked due to the vastly greater attention directed toward pharmacologic and operative therapies in the medical literature, but can have dramatic effects upon reducing disability following myocardial infarction.

Three nonpharmacologic, nonoperative modalities appear to have merit in increasing the level of activity that patients with coronary heart disease can comfortably and safely perform. These are exercise conditioning, weight loss, and cessation of cigarette smoking.

Detailed descriptions of exercise conditioning programs for coronary patients are available from several sources [8–10] and will not be reviewed here. Suffice it to say that exercise conditioning (defined as the repetitive use of major muscle groups in activities such as walking, jogging, or bicycle ergometry, when performed at least three times weekly for a duration of at least 30 min at an intensity of 60%–85% of the pretraining maximal work capacity) produces profound alterations in a number of cardiovascular and metabolic variables (table 58-2).

Three specific and well-characterized effects of exercise conditioning are most pertinent for reducing disability due to ischemic heart disease: the reduction in heart rate at rest and at any given exercise work load, the reduced peripheral resistance and impedance to left ventricular ejection at any given exercise work load, and the enhanced arteriovenous oxygen extraction in conditional skeletal muscle that permits the performance of any given work load at a lower cardiac output. Reduced heart rate and peripheral resistance (afterload) at standard exercise work loads result in lower myocardial oxygen demand for any given activity, and this relative bradycardia may also increase myocardial oxygen supply by increasing diastolic filling time. In addition, these effects of exercise conditioning occur and extend exercise capacity even in patients already receiving beta-adrenergic antagonists (figure 58-1) [11]. Furthermore, enhancement of functional work capacity by exercise conditioning can occur even in patients with markedly impaired left ventricular function [12] (figure 58-2), and in patients who develop angina pectoris at extremely low levels of exertion [13].

Exercise training often has salutary effects upon risk factors for progression of atherosclerosis such as hypertension, glucose intolerance, and the ratio of HDL to LDL cholesterol, and available data suggest that there may be some survival benefit for postinfarction patients participating in regular exercise conditioning [14]. When compared with the clear evidence for symptomatic

TABLE 58-2. Cardiovascular effects of exercise training

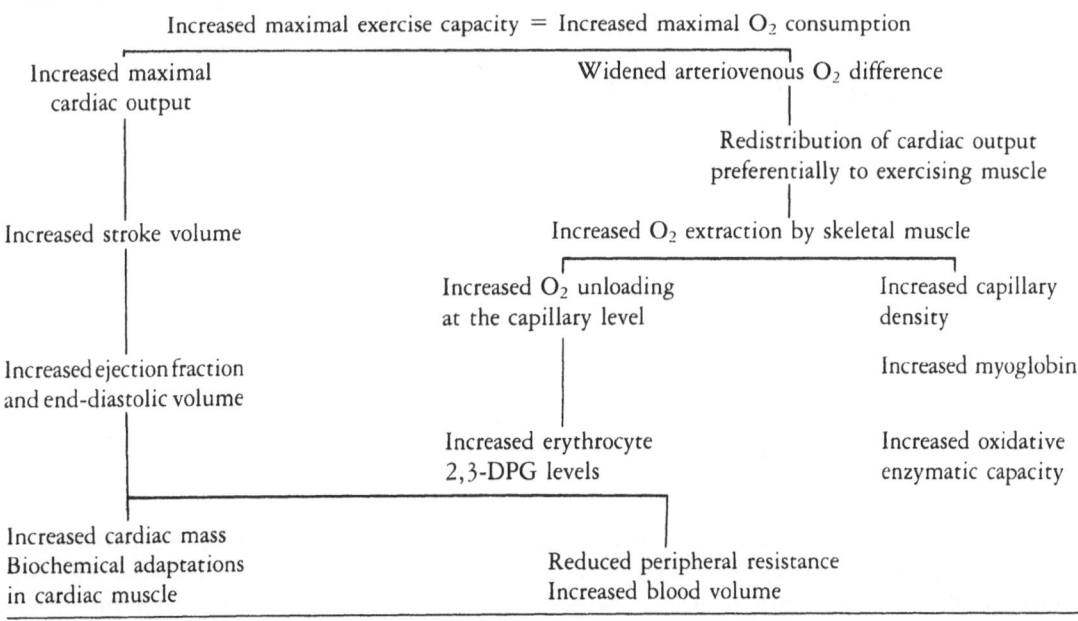

Increased maximal exercise capacity = Increased maximal O_2 consumption

Increased maximal cardiac output

Widened arteriovenous O_2 difference

Redistribution of cardiac output preferentially to exercising muscle

Increased stroke volume

Increased O_2 extraction by skeletal muscle

Increased O_2 unloading at the capillary level

Increased capillary density

Increased ejection fraction and end-diastolic volume

Increased myoglobin

Increased erythrocyte 2,3-DPG levels

Increased oxidative enzymatic capacity

Increased cardiac mass
Biochemical adaptations in cardiac muscle

Reduced peripheral resistance
Increased blood volume

DPG, diphosphoglycerate.

improvement following exercise conditioning, however, this latter effect must continue to be regarded as speculative. Likewise, although animal studies suggest that conditioned hearts maintain more normal mechanical properties than sedentary hearts under ischemic conditions [15], and that exercise conditioning may prevent progression or promote regression of experimental atherosclerosis [16], these merits must also be considered speculative in man.

Weight loss in overweight persons can enhance work capacity due to angina pectoris or

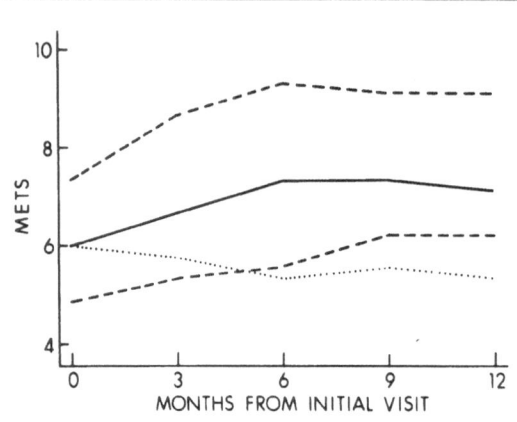

FIGURE 58-1. Response to exercise training in 103 medically treated patients with coronary artery disease and angina pectoris receiving beta adrenergic antagonists. Maximal treadmill work capacity (METS) before the onset of angina in each patient is represented in the baseline measurement and at one or two followup points. The solid line represented the median value and the upper and lower dashed lines indicate the 75th and 25th percentiles respectively. The dotted line is the median baseline work capacity in the population of subjects studied at each followup interval. Median work capacity increased approximately 2 METS or 40% (p < 0.001) over baseline performance in subjects exercising 6 months or more. Patients were receiving similar dosages of beta adrenergic antagonists during baseline and during followup testing sessions.

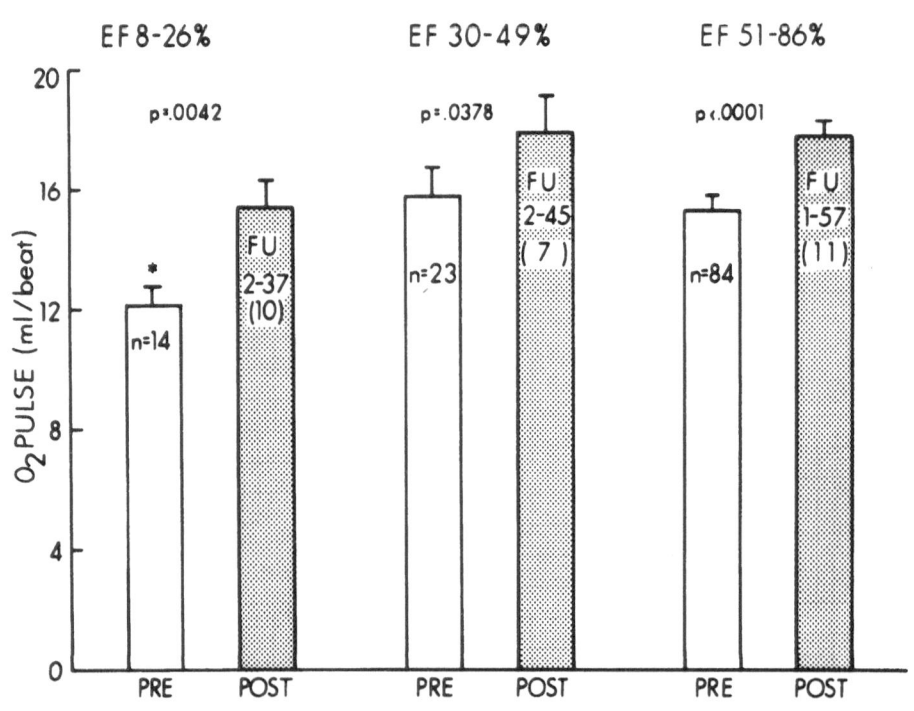

FIGURE 58-2. Effects of exercise training on aerobic fitness of 121 coronary artery disease patients stratified on the basis of resting left ventricular ejection fraction (EF). The range and median (in parentheses) duration of followup in months (FU) are shown. There are no significant differences in posttraining values among the three groups, although the initial level of aerobic fitness was significantly lower (p < 0.04) in the group with the lowest EF than in the other two (n = sample size). (From Williams R.S. *J. Cardiovasc Med* 7:1112, 1982.)

congestive heart failure in persons following myocardial infarction, simply by reducing the requirements for cardiac output and by reducing myocardial oxygen demand during any activities in which the body mass is a determinant of the overall energy costs. Some investigators have theorized that a low-fat diet could shift myocardial substrate utilization from predominantly free fatty acids to predominantly carbohydrates, and thereby reduce myocardial oxygen demand for any given level of activity, by virtue of the reduced requirement for O_2 consumption per mole of ATP produced from the oxidative metabolism of glucose as opposed to fatty acids [17]. However, the clinical utility of this concept remains conjectural.

Continued cigarette smoking after myocardial infarction not only is a risk factor for subsequent cardiac events, but can limit functional work capacity as well. Nicotine increases heart rate and blood pressure and therefore myocardial oxygen demand, and carboxyhemoglobin levels found commonly in cigarette smokers significantly impair oxygen delivery and functional work capacity [18].

Attention to detail

As previously discussed, a variety of factors (table 58-3) that may seem trivial or mundane in the context of managing life-threatening events on the coronary care unit may assume major importance to the patient after discharge following myocardial infarction. Sexual dysfunction, crippling but inappropriate anxiety over performing routine functions of daily living, medication side effects or unrecognized drug interactions, sleep

TABLE 58-3. Therapeutic details often overlooked

1. Proper use of nitroglycerin preparations
2. Drug interactions/side effects, e.g., cimetidine reducing hepatic clearance of nifedipine; nonsteroidal antiinflammatory drugs causing NA^+ retention
3. Criteria for dose titration of beta-blockers
4. Accurate differentiation of anginal versus nonanginal chest pain
5. Inappropriate anxiety over safety of routine activities by patient/spouse
6. Assessment of sexual dysfunction/sleep disorders

disturbances, hypochondriacal symptoms, and depression are widely prevalent after myocardial infarction, but may be overlooked if the physician is preoccupied with the state of the myocardium. Likewise, the patient's lack of understanding of the pathophysiology of coronary disease, and lack of understanding about the rationale for and appropriate use of specific medications, may render the best therapeutic decisions by the physician ineffective. For example, 25% – 50% of patients with angina referred by competent physicians to our rehabilitation program do not use nitroglycerin preparations properly, or are unaware of the potential dangers of sudden cessation of beta-adrenergic antagonists.

In our experience, these details are usually not adequately addressed during brief and infrequent visits to a physician's office. Comprehensive medical care following myocardial infarction requires attention to these, and other, details, and probably necessitates the involvement of trained nonphysician personnel to supplement physician contact and to ensure that these details have not been overlooked.

The Role of Psychological/Sociological Factors in Determining Disability and Return to Work following Myocardial Infarction

In the United States today, it is evident that the personality, occupation, educational background, family environment, and the availability of disability income support are far more important determinants of a patient's return to work following myocardial infarction than are any medical or physiologic factors [19]. White-collar managerial and professional persons often return to work regardless of the severity of the infarct, whereas persons with blue-collar occupations are more likely to remain disabled, regardless of the severity of the infarct, and regardless of the physical demands of the labor. Recent changes in the guidelines determining eligibility for disability income from federal sources may have some impact on this phenomenon, but the major role played by psychological and sociological factors in determining work status is likely to persist.

Nonetheless, potential strategies are available to the practicing physician, even in the absence of a structured rehabilitation program, for maximizing the likelihood that the myocardial infarction patient will return to work. First, early and accurate quantification of the degree of physiologic impairment, and clear communication of these results to the patient, can circumvent an inappropriate expectation of future disability [20]. Patients identified as having low probability for subsequent cardiac events and who have no evidence for myocardial ischemia during exercise should be made aware that they are not candidates for long-term disability income and should return to work within six weeks after their infarction. Currently ongoing or planned studies may demonstrate the safety of even earlier return to work in the future.

In addition to early risk stratification and functional testing, frequent contact with the physician or other knowledgeable health professionals in the first few weeks after the infarct—the continuity of care emphasized previously—can also allay unwarranted anxieties and produce realistic and rational expectations concerning the return to work. Within the constraints of the confidentiality of the doctor–patient relationship, clarification of the patient's medical status to employers and supervisors by the physician can also reduce inappropriate obstacles to the patient's return to work.

Finally, the concepts of individualized care and attention to detail can facilitate return to occupational activities. Monitoring the patient in an actual or simulated work environment can clarify the safety of specific work tasks and provide reassurance to the anxious patient. Accurate differentiation between cardiac and noncardiac causes of chest pain or dyspnea is essential. And, finally, exercise training regimens can, and must, be tailored to increase functional capacity for specific work activities, due to the specificity of many of the cardiovascular adaptations of exercise training to work performed with the trained muscle groups. For example, lowered heart rates (and myocardial oxygen demands) during submaximal exercise produced by exercise conditioning of the legs (jogging, cycling) will be clearly evident during exercise that predominantly uses the leg muscles, but will be less evident during exercise that primarily involves the arms [21].

Comprehensive Treatment Strategies following Myocardial Infarction

In our own center we have developed a comprehensive strategy for minimizing disability following myocardial infarction that builds on the principles outlined above: continuity of care; individualized, rational care; coordination of treatment modalities; and attention to detail. Rehabilitation efforts begin in the hospital, are based on individualized physiologic and psychological assessment of each patient, continue through the immediate postdischarge period, and terminate only when specific goals have been met: elimination of reversible obstacles to the resumption of desired occupational or recreational activities; and elimination of reversible factors producing increased risk for subsequent cardiac events. Our structured program emphasizes the incorporation of effective nonpharmacologic treatment modalities—exercise conditioning, dietary change, and smoking cessation—with appropriate drug therapy and with appropriate selection of patients for revascularization or other operative procedures. We have observed increments in maximum work capacity in approximately 85% of over 800 patients with coronary heart disease participating in our structured program, with an average increase of 40% in treadmill time to angina or fatigue occurring in the first three months, and of over 50% in subjects who remain under follow-up three years from their entry into our program (figure 58-3).

Conclusion

The past 20 years have produced major changes in the management of patients following myocardial infarction. Although a cardiologist from the 1950s suddenly appearing in our midst would be aghast, the safety of markedly shorter hospital stays, greater levels of activity in the hospital and in the early weeks of posthospital management, early symptom-limited exercise testing, and earlier return to work or to recreational activities has been validated experimentally.

Likewise, the efficacy of newer pharmocologic agents, revascularization procedures, and exercise conditioning in limiting disability from coronary heart disease has been established, and

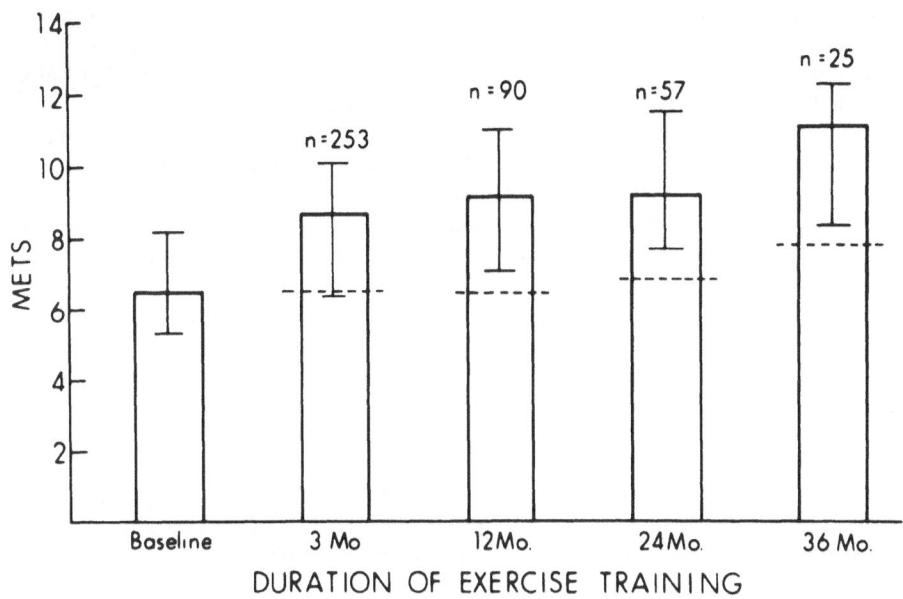

FIGURE 58-3. Functional work capacity in coronary patients undergoing exercise conditioning. The histograms depict the median value of symptom-limited treadmill exercise capacity at the time points indicated, and the vertical lines indicate the interquartile range (25th to 75th percentile). The horizontal dashed lines indicate the median value of baseline work capacity for the individuals tested at each followup period. All followup values are significantly greater than the baseline values (p < .0001).

there is promise that these measures may extend life expectancy following myocardial infarction as well. Coronary heart disease remains a chronic illness that extracts a formidable toll of human suffering. At the current time, however, most patients who have experienced a myocardial infarction can, and should, expect to return to normal or near-normal levels of work and leisure activities. Over the past 50 years, prevailing medical dogma regarding the management of patients following myocardial infarction has probably done as much to impede as to facilitate the well-being of ambulatory postinfarction patients. While many questions remain unanswered, the principles presented in this chapter provide a rational and modern approach that merits serious attention from physicians managing such patients.

References

1. Young DT, Kottke TE, McCall MM, Blume D: A prospective controlled study of in-hospital myocardial infarction rehabilitation. J Cardiac Rehab 2:32, 1982.

2. Williams RS: How beneficial is regular exercise? J Cardiovas Med 7:1112, 1982.

3. Wenger NA: Rehabilitation of the coronary patient: scope of the problem and responsibility of the primary care physician. Cardiovasc Rev Rep 2:1249, 1981.

4. Thomas GS, Lee PR, Franks P, Paffenbarger RS: Exercise and health. Cambridge MA: Oelgeschlager, Gunn, and Hain, 1981.

5. Moss AJ, De Camilla J, Davis H, Bayer L: The early post-hospital phase of myocardial infarction: prognostic stratification. Circulation 54:58, 1976.

6. Davidson D, De Busk R: Prognostic value of a single exercise test 3 weeks after uncomplicated myocardial infarction. Circulation 61:236, 1980.

7. Corbett JR, et al: The prognostic value of submaximal exercise testing with radionuclide ventriculography before hospital discharge in patients with recent myocardial infarction. Circulation 64:535, 1981.

8. Erb BD, Fletcher GF, Sheffield TL: Standards for cardiovascular exercise treatment programs. Circulation 59:1084A, 1979.

9. Pollock ML, Schmidt DH (eds): Heart disease

and rehabilitation. Boston: Houghton Mifflin, 1979.

10. Froelicher VF: Exercise testing and training. New York: Le Jacq, 1983.

11. Pratt CM, Welton DE, Squires WG, et al: Demonstration of training effect during chronic beta adrenergic blockade in patients with coronary artery disease. Circulation 64:1125, 1981.

12. Conn EH, Williams RS, Wallace AG: Exercise responses before and after physical conditioning in patients with severely depressed left ventricular function. Am J Cardiol 49:296, 1982.

13. Cobb FR, Williams RS, McEwen P, et al: Effects of exercise training on ventricular function in patients with recent myocardial infarction. Circulation 66:100, 1982.

14. Froelicher VF, Brown P: Exercise and coronary heart disease. J Cardiac Rehab 4:277, 1981.

15. Bersohn MM, Scheuer J: Effect of ischemia on the performance of hearts from physically trained rats. Am J Physiol 234:H215, 1978.

16. Kramsch DM, et al: Reduction of coronary atherosclerosis by moderate conditioning exercise in monkeys on an atherogenic diet. N Engl J Med 305:1483, 1981.

17. Ornish D: Stress, diet and your heart. New York: Holt, Rinehart and Winston, 1982, p 354.

18. Aronow WS, et al: Effect of cigarette smoking and breathing carbon monoxide on cardiovascular hemodynamics in anginal patients. Circulation 50:340, 1974.

19. Davidson DM: Return to work after cardiac events: a review. J Cardiac Rehab 3:60, 1983.

20. Ewart CK, Taylor CB, Reese LB, De Busk RF: The effects of early postinfarction exercise testing on self perception and subsequent physical activity. Am J Cardiol, 1983 (in press).

21. Clausen JP, et al: Central and peripheral circulatory changes after training of the arms and legs. Am J Physiol 225:675, 1973.

INDEX